THE ILLUSTRATED PRACTICAL BOOK OF
FAMILY HEALTH
AND FIRST

T0097033

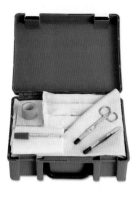

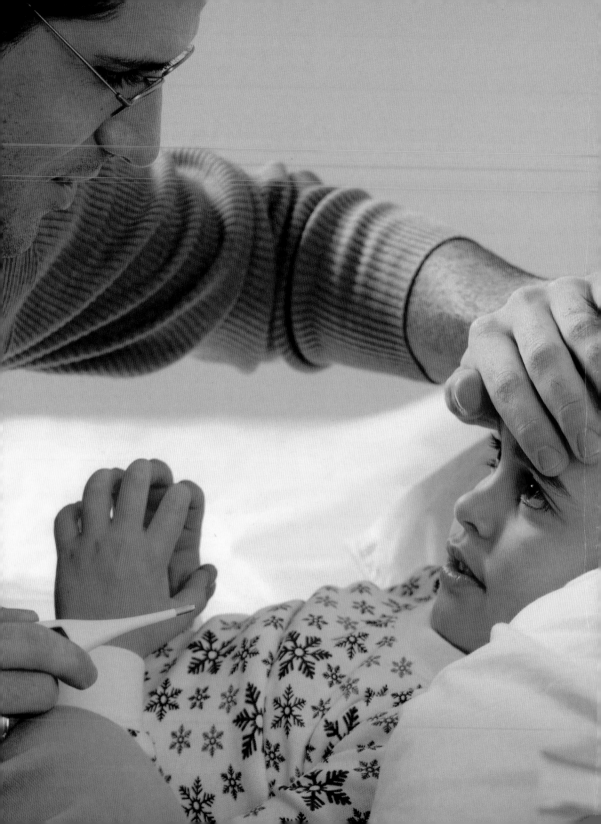

THE ILLUSTRATED PRACTICAL BOOK OF
FAMILY HEALTH AND FIRST AID

From treating cuts, sprains and bandaging in an emergency to making decisions on headaches, fevers and rashes: plus all you need to know about the long-term health and fitness of your family

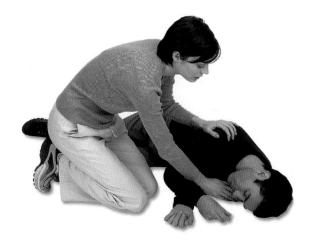

Dr Peter Fermie MA, MB, BS, MRCGP, DCH, DRCOG
Dr Pippa Keech MB, ChB, MRCGP
Dr Stephen Shepherd MB, ChB, MRCGP

southwater

This edition is published by Southwater, an imprint of Anness Publishing Ltd,
Blaby Road, Wigston, Leicestershire LE18 4SE

Email: info@anness.com

Web: www.southwaterbooks.com; www.annesspublishing.com

If you like the images in this book and would like to investigate using them for publishing,
promotions or advertising, please visit our website www.practicalpictures.com for more information.

Publisher: Joanna Lorenz
Editorial Director: Helen Sudell
Project Editors: Melanie Halton, Ann Kay
First aid editorial consultant/additional text: Anne Charlish
Copy-editors: Sue Barraclough, Kim Davies, Tracey Kelly, Mary Lindsay,
Cathy Meeus, Sonya Newland, Nikki Sims, Linda Sonntag
Designers: Nigel Partridge, Lisa Tai
Special first aid photography: Mark Wood
Special effects first aid make-up: Dauphine's of Bristol
Illustrations: Samantha Elmhurst
Production Controllers: Steve Lang, Pedro Nelson

ETHICAL TRADING POLICY
Because of our ongoing ecological investment program, you, as our customer, can have the
pleasure and reassurance of knowing that a tree is being cultivated on your behalf to naturally
replace the materials used to make the book you are holding. For further information about this
scheme, go to www.annesspublishing.com/trees

© Anness Publishing Ltd 2005, 2011

All rights reserved. No part of this publication may be reproduced, stored in a retrieval system, or
transmitted in any way or by any means, electronic, mechanical, photocopying, recording or
otherwise, without the prior written permission of the copyright holder.

A CIP catalogue record for this book is available from the British Library.

Previously published in two separate volumes, *Practical Guide to First Aid*
and *The Complete Family Home Health Encyclopedia*

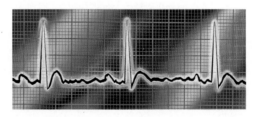

Publisher's Note:
The Illustrated Practical Book of Family Health & First Aid provides information and instructions on
treating a wide range of health matters and tackling life-threatening and emergency situations, but
is not intended as a substitute for professional diagnosis. Anyone with a condition or symptoms
requiring medical attention should consult a fully qualified practitioner as early as possible. While the
advice and information in this book are believed to be accurate at the time of going to press, neither the
authors nor the publisher accept any legal responsibility or liability for any errors, inaccuracies or
omissions, nor for any loss, harm or injury that arises from following instructions or advice in the book.

Foreword

These days, we are constantly bombarded with health advice. It is easy to pick up inaccurate, distorted or partially digested information or to give up altogether and think that only the experts have any chance of knowing what to do in any kind of medical situation – especially in first-aid scenarios.

A skill for life

However, we all need to acquire a certain level of health understanding as a basic life skill – to stay as healthy and fit as we can be and enjoy our lives to the full, to prevent ourselves and others getting into more serious problems and to protect our loved ones. What we need for this is a basic fund of solid, up-to-date information combined with practical, common sense advice. Whether we are soothing a child's headache or giving mouth-to-mouth resuscitation, we often underestimate just how far common sense can literally be a life-saver.

The good news is that this book goes a long way towards providing just such a sensible approach. It has been devised to be your companion through all kinds of day-to-day and emergency situations, as well as offering general advice on a healthy lifestyle and highlighting preventative tips along the way. Remember, however, that nothing replaces a good first-aid course, which gives you the skills needed to tackle emergencies confidently and calmly, and also that you should always consult a medical practitioner when faced with anything other than the most minor of conditions. That said, health is perhaps the most fascinating of subjects, so enjoy reading about your precious body while learning some essential skills.

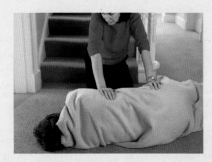
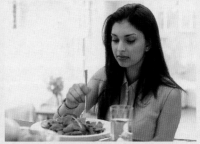

Contents

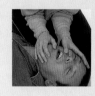

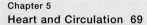

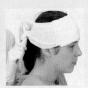

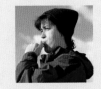
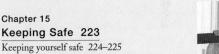
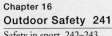

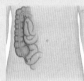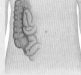

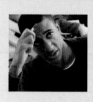
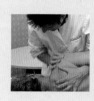
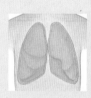

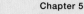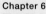

Introduction

TACKLING EMERGENCIES

Understanding the basic techniques of first aid will help you to stay calm and in control in an emergency. This is vital in a crisis, regardless of the level of your specific knowledge. It is also enormously reassuring to the casualty, whatever the eventual outcome, and will often inspire bystanders to offer assistance. Remember, even those with no training can do something really useful, such as phoning for help or comforting the casualty.

WHEN YOU SHOULD DO NOTHING

It is often better to do nothing than to risk doing the wrong thing. In one example, a man dealt with an elderly lady who had collapsed in the street by kneeling beside her and gathering her up so that he was cradling her slumped against his chest. In this position, her head lolled forwards,

making her breathing tortuous. He meant well, but he was actually compromising her breathing – and her chances of survival.

Also, know your limitations. Do not try clambering up a cliff to help someone if you are scared of heights, or attempt a first-aid procedure if you have no idea what you are doing.

BE PREPARED

Another important part of being a potential first-aider, especially when helping people in your circle of family and friends, is thinking through in advance what would need to be done in an emergency. This means, for example, that if a crisis does

◁ Improvisation is a vital health and first-aid skill. Here, a damp facecloth is used to dress an injured hand.

WHAT TO EXPECT AT THE ACCIDENT AND EMERGENCY DEPARTMENT

You may well end up going to hospital with a casualty. If you know what to expect in an accident and emergency (A&E) department, you will cope more calmly when you get there. You will also be able to talk to the casualty about what to expect, which should in turn help to reduce their anxiety.

A nurse should greet you almost as soon as you register at the accident and emergency desk. The nurse's job is to assess what immediate treatment is needed and how urgently the casualty needs to be seen. This is called "triaging". Casualties who need immediate care are often moved to a room called the "resuscitation room". Cases such as

possible heart attacks and asthmatics will be classed as urgent. After this the triage nurse will deal with people who need a bed to lie on, usually classified as a major casualty; the more minor casualties will need to wait a little longer to be treated. Unless the wound or problem is very minor, the nurse will usually ask the casualty to undress and put a hospital gown on. This makes it much easier for medical personnel to examine the patient.

In some hospitals, there may be a separate area for children in A and E, and this spares them the distressing scenes that are often played out in a hospital's emergency department.

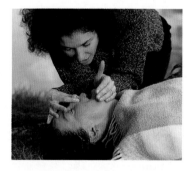

△ Only attempt mouth-to-mouth resuscitation if you really know what you are doing.

arise, you don't end up having to take four children and the family dog to the accident and emergency department.

Advance planning helps you cope with situations more confidently. It might mean thinking about which relatives or friends are close enough to look after the children at short notice, having a list of medication to hand that you or a potential casualty needs, or asking a neighbour if they would feed your animals in a crisis.

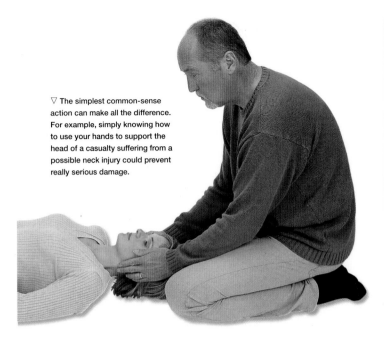

▽ The simplest common-sense action can make all the difference. For example, simply knowing how to use your hands to support the head of a casualty suffering from a possible neck injury could prevent really serious damage.

DON'T DEAL WITH HEALTH PROBLEMS ALONE

➤ If you encounter what you think may be a serious health problem, stay calm and see a doctor immediately. Do not panic or try to push it out of your mind.

➤ Do not be over-confident where self-prescribing is concerned. Ask a professional for advice when buying any medicine, including complementary ones. You may be surprised which ones affect each other adversely.

checks and protecting ourselves and our children from potentially harmful infectious diseases.

SENSIBLE PRECAUTIONS

Whenever you or those around you are ill, always observe a few simple rules. Follow any dosage or other instructions closely and read any accompanying leaflets; they are there for a reason. Don't merrily mix medicines – seek expert advice and always ask a professional if you are worried about anything. Lastly, try to strike a balance between being terrified of every headache and staying well-informed about health – the latter is certainly a much better recipe for long-lasting well-being.

Keeping the following two lists by the phone will help if sudden emergencies arise:
1 A list of the telephone numbers of nearby friends and relatives plus your doctor and the emergency services.
2 A list of all medication taken by any members of your household. Also make sure that you have a record of any intolerances or allergies – this might be invaluable to a doctor or paramedic.

LOOKING AFTER THE FAMILY'S HEALTH

The family health section of this book echoes what we all really know to be true: that maintaining optimum health is something that every single adult has to take personal responsibility for. This emphasis on establishing a healthy lifestyle is reiterated throughout the Family Health Guide's pages and is dealt with in clear, up-to-date detail in the chapter entitled Healthy Living. The main tenets of a healthy and happy life are learning to understand how we can achieve the following as far as we are able:

- Controlling stress levels.
- Following a well-balanced diet.
- Maintaining a healthy personal weight.
- Sticking to a regime of exercise suited to our needs as an individual and to our age and fitness level.
- Avoiding damaging substances.
- Making sure that we have regular health

▽ With children, it can be hard to distinguish mild from serious problems. Learning to recognize tell-tale symptoms is a vital skill.

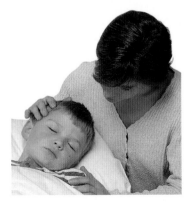

▽ It is important to understand the kinds of substances that may trigger adverse reactions, from certain foods and drinks to dust and pollen.

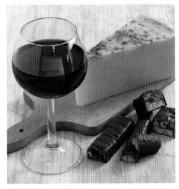

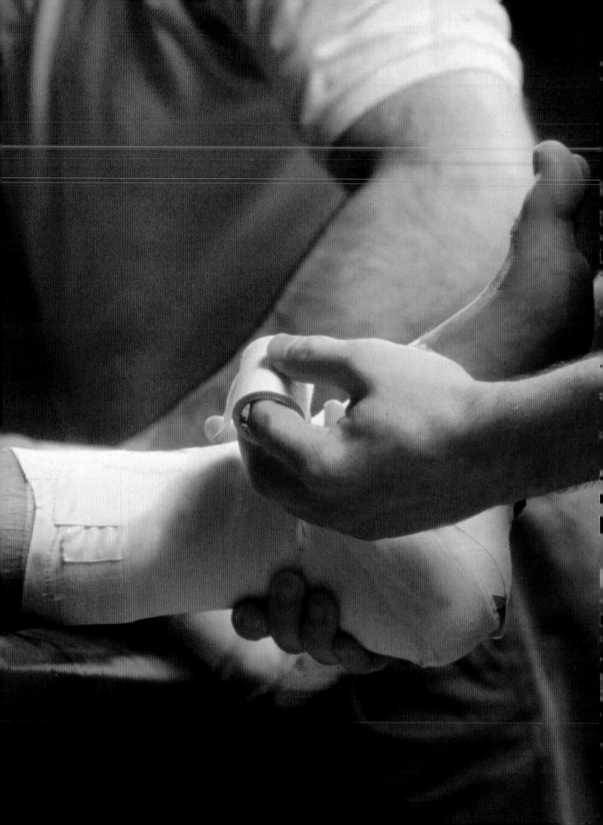

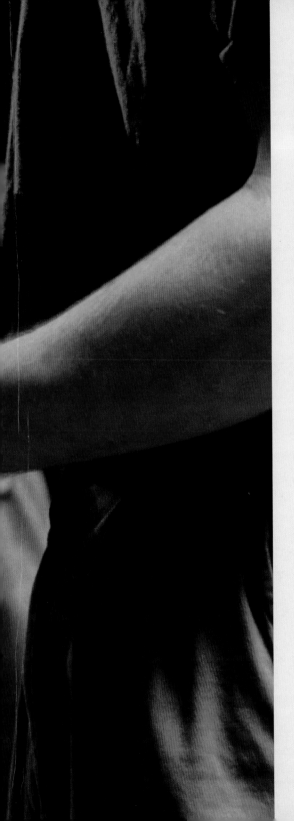

STEP-BY-STEP FIRST AID

This section of the book provides a fully illustrated up-to-date manual of the safest, easiest ways to tackle every kind of first-aid problem. Specially photographed step-by-step sequences deal with everything from bandaging a finger to resuscitation. Information is placed clearly within the context of the body's systems, as with the Family Health Guide section of the book, and special chapters highlight topics such as outdoor safety and first aid for infants. Feature boxes cross-reference and summarize facts throughout and each chapter closes with a checklist of key points covered and major skills learned.

How to use the first-aid chapters

The first-aid manual that follows has been specifically arranged to help readers target the information they need at any one time. Introductory chapters offer special guides on coping with emergencies and devising a life-saving action plan. Other chapters highlight a vast range of vital topics – from children's health to sports injuries – while some deal with a specific body system, placing problems in their proper anatomical context. Each chapter closes with a helpful Skills Checklist – handy summaries that can be ticked off by the reader.

First-aid procedures are presented throughout in a clear step-by-step format, featuring helpful colour photographs and straightforward, jargon-free text, supported wherever necessary by fully annotated colour artworks.

A range of special features, from flow charts to symptoms boxes, has also been used, in order to help readers access vital facts as readily as possible – these are explained below.

See Also boxes
These refer readers to other, related topics in the first-aid section of the book. Cross-references are to whole chapters (in capital letters), or to specific pages.

Flow charts
Lilac-coloured flow charts appear regularly throughout, summarizing the essential steps to follow in all kinds of situations.

Step-by-step sequences
Wherever relevant, procedures are broken down into numbered steps, where techniques can be seen clearly in full-colour photographs.

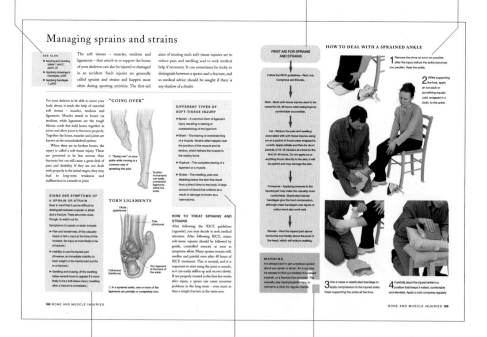

Signs and Symptoms boxes
These blue boxes pick out the major symptoms of each condition, making them easily accessible to first-aiders.

Information boxes
Beige-tinted boxes contain a range of valuable supporting information, from prevention advice and action checklists to useful facts and figures.

Warning boxes
These green-tinted boxes with white crosses alert readers to matters of particular importance. *Always* pay good attention to this advice.

1

ACTION AT AN EMERGENCY

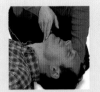

The action that you take at an emergency may have a lasting effect on the casualty. You will need to think quickly and make the correct decisions. Your assessment and examination of the casualty are all-important. This chapter takes you through those initial stages and shows you how to move and handle a casualty who may be badly injured and/or unconscious safely without causing further injury. If you are in any doubt at all about what to do or how to do it, it may be best to do nothing: simply call the emergency services and do what you can to reassure the casualty and keep them warm and safe from further injury.

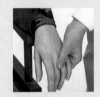

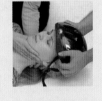

CONTENTS

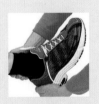

What is first aid?

First aid is literally the very FIRST assistance you give someone who has been injured. All of us should know basic first-aid techniques, in the home, at the office or when out and about. One in three of all accidents takes place in our homes, the majority involving children and the elderly.

Knowing what to do first and recognizing how potentially serious a casualty's condition is may speed recovery and even prove vital to saving a life. Please note that the text on these two pages is a summary and is expanded in detail over subsequent chapters.

First aid help can cover an extremely varied range of scenarios – from simple reassurance after a small accident to dealing with a life-threatening emergency. A speedy response is crucial. Emergency workers refer to the first hour after an accident as the golden hour: the more help given within this hour, the better the outcome for the casualty.

THE GOALS OF FIRST AID

- To keep the casualty alive. The ABC of life support – Airway, Breathing and Circulation – constitutes the absolute top priority of first aid.
- To stop the casualty getting worse.
- To promote their recovery.
- To provide reassurance and comfort to the casualty.

THE DRSABC CODE

Remembering and acting on these can save lives:

D for DANGER
R for RESPONSE
S for SHOUT
A for AIRWAY
B for BREATHING
C for CIRCULATION

WHAT TO DO IN AN EMERGENCY

First, STAY CALM. Secondly, ASSESS THE SITUATION promptly. Now carry out the "DRSABC" sequence, as follows:

1 DANGER

Your assessment should have alerted you to any potential hazards. Now you should:
- Keep yourself out of any danger.
- Keep passers-by out of danger.
- Make safe any hazards, if you can do so without endangering yourself or others. Only move the casualty away from danger in extreme circumstances.

2 RESPONSE

Try to establish the responsiveness level.
- If the casualty appears unconscious or semi-conscious, speak loudly to them – as in "Can you hear me?".
- If this fails to get a response, tap them firmly on the shoulders.

3 SHOUT

If step 2 fails to raise any response:
- Shout out loudly to passers-by for help with the situation.

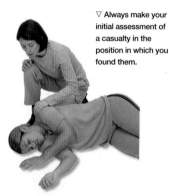

▽ Always make your initial assessment of a casualty in the position in which you found them.

◁ Always try to get help from passers-by. Ideally, ask someone to call the emergency services while you stay with the casualty; keep them warm until trained aid arrives.

4 AIRWAY

Now determine whether the airway (the passage from the mouth to the lungs) is clear enough to allow proper breathing.
- Check the mouth and remove any visible obvious obstructions, such as food, that are at the front of the mouth only.
- Tilt the casualty's head back gently to prevent the tongue from falling back and blocking the airway. Place a hand on the forehead/top of head and two fingers under the jaw. Tilt back gently until a natural stop is reached.

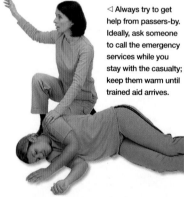

▷ Tilt the head using a hand on the forehead/top of head and two fingers under the jaw. This casualty was found on his back. Avoid moving a casualty on to their back unless you need to start rescue breaths or chest compressions (see steps 5 and 6).

5 BREATHING

Is the casualty breathing?

- LOOK to see if the chest is moving.
- LISTEN for breathing sounds – put your ear against their mouth.
- FEEL for expired air by placing your cheek or ear close to their face.
- CHECK for other signs of life (e.g. body warmth, good colour, ability to swallow).
- If these checks are negative, the casualty is probably not breathing. You must now CALL AN AMBULANCE; ideally, get someone else to go.
- Without delay, start artificial respiration procedures (giving 2 breaths).

6 CIRCULATION

Look for signs of a working circulation.

- Check for breathing, coughing or any movement.
- Never waste time trying to find a pulse unless you are highly experienced in medicine.
- If there are no signs of a circulation, start cardiac massage (chest compressions) – but only if you are trained to do so.

GETTING HELP

Phoning the emergency services is free on all kinds of phone. If the casualty is inside a building and other people are present, ask someone to stand outside the building in order to guide the emergency services. If you are at a house and it's dark outside, switch on any outside lights.

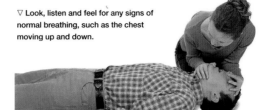

▽ Look, listen and feel for any signs of normal breathing, such as the chest moving up and down.

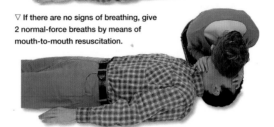

▽ If there are no signs of breathing, give 2 normal-force breaths by means of mouth-to-mouth resuscitation.

INFORMATION FOR THE EMERGENCY SERVICES

- ➤ Whether the casualty is conscious and breathing – information you will have if you have followed DRSABC.
- ➤ Your location (a landmark will do if you know no more) and phone number.
- ➤ Your name.
- ➤ What the problem is and what time it happened.
- ➤ If it is relevant, how many casualties there are, and their sex and age.
- ➤ Report any hazards, such as ice on the road or hazardous substances.
- ➤ Don't hang up the telephone until the authorities tell you to do so.

◁ Tell the emergency services useful information such as the presence of a medical alert/ID tag.

▷ If someone falls from a height, keep them warm and do not move them – unless it is necessary for resuscitation.

VITAL NUMBERS

Some national emergency services numbers:

➤ UK: 999

➤ US: 911

➤ Australia: 000

On mobile phones, use these numbers or 112 (but check with your network).

DON'T MOVE THEM!

There are good reasons for leaving a casualty in place until more skilled personnel arrive. Injuries to the spine, especially to the neck, are possible after accidents and falls, and further movement can cause serious damage to the spinal cord. You may have to use some movement to deal with an injury, but the golden rule after an accident is not to move an injured person unless they are in danger, need to be resuscitated, or are unconscious and should be put into the recovery position. If moving a casualty is unavoidable, you should be very careful with their neck.

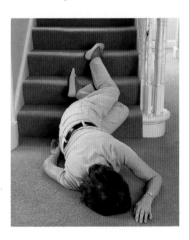

Making your assessment

SEE ALSO

➤ What is first aid?, p16

➤ Examining the casualty, p20

➤ Moving and handling safely 1 and 2, pp24, 26

Your initial assessment may be of major importance to the outcome of an accident. Remember DRS (Danger, Response, Shout) and ABC (Airway, Breathing, Circulation). Together these form DRSABC, which you can also remember as "the doctors' ABC". Once you know a casualty is conscious and breathing, you can start to identify the nature of the problem. Ask if they can remember what happened. Look around for clues to the accident. Appearing as calm as possible will help to give vital reassurance to the casualty.

Once you have checked DRSABC and established that breathing and circulation are functioning, you have more time to address the casualty's specific problems. They may be simple and the remedy straightforward. If the situation is less clear, however, the "Signs and Symptoms" box indicates what you should look out for.

In general, after completing DRSABC, a first-aider should gather basic initial information (what has happened, plus vital medical facts such as whether the casualty is diabetic), call for any emergency aid, and locate and treat – as far as possible – any obvious physical injury. They may then go on to gather further information from the casualty about the incident and their medical history, and carry out a more thorough examination – by looking, feeling, and questioning the casualty.

TAKING A HISTORY

This involves gathering information by asking questions and listening. Remember that it is very reassuring for everyone concerned to see that something is being done for a friend or relative, and this information may be vital for the ambulance and medical staff later on. Begin by questioning the casualty; if their answers are vague or unhelpful, ask anyone else who may know something useful.

1 Ask their name. It is very comforting to be called by name, and useful to use if the casualty starts to lose consciousness.

2 Ask children their age and, if they are old enough to have the information, ask them how you can contact a parent or carer.

3 What is the problem? Let the casualty talk for a while. They may end up telling you not only what their current problem is, but also useful details about previous similar episodes and what their causes were. If they are still vague, you may find it useful to ask about possible symptoms relating to different systems of the body such as the:

- **Nervous system** – Headache, dizziness, weakness of arms or legs, tingling, pins and needles, loss of movement or sensation.
- **Chest** – Cough, shortness of breath, wheeze, pains in the chest – especially on taking a deep breath.
- **Heart** – Chest pains, swollen ankles.
- **Gut** – Vomiting, diarrhoea, stomach or pelvic pain.

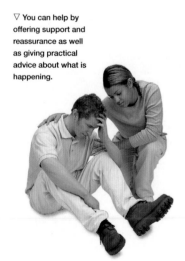

▽ You can help by offering support and reassurance as well as giving practical advice about what is happening.

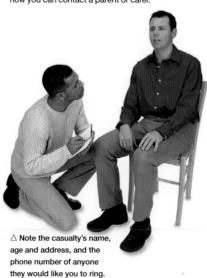

△ Note the casualty's name, age and address, and the phone number of anyone they would like you to ring.

▽ If the child is old enough to know, try to find out how to contact one of their parents or carers.

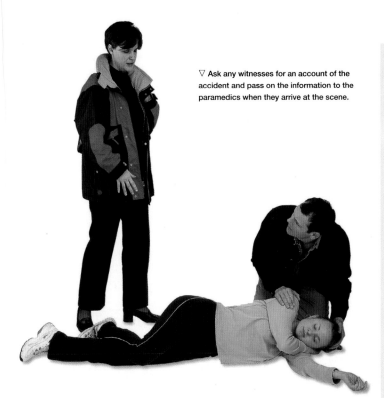

▽ Ask any witnesses for an account of the accident and pass on the information to the paramedics when they arrive at the scene.

SIGNS AND SYMPTOMS

➤ **Symptoms** – What can the casualty tell you about their injury or illness? Are they in pain or stiff, feeling anxious, hot, cold, dizzy, nauseous, faint or thirsty? Is there a sensation of tingling, weakness or memory loss?

➤ **Visual signs** – What can you see in relation to the casualty's condition? Anxious or painful expression, unusual chest movement, burns, sweating, bleeding, bruising, abnormal skin colour, swelling, deformity, vomiting or incontinence? Look for foreign bodies and objects related to substance abuse, such as aerosol cans and small plastic bags. Check for a medical ID tag.

➤ **Other signs** – What can you feel, hear or smell in relation to the casualty? Dampness, abnormal temperature, groaning, sucking sound, alcohol, acetone, solvents or glue, gas or fumes, vomit, urine or faeces?

➤ **Vital signs** – In what state are the casualty's pulse, respiration, colour and temperature? Sum up their general condition.

4 Ask about known medical problems such as diabetes, heart attacks or strokes, which may give you a clue as to what has happened this time.

5 Ask for information about any medication they are currently taking and whether they have any known allergies.

6 Ask when they last ate. If they are going to need emergency surgery, this is a very important question, and it may also be vital if they have diabetes.

GATHERING INFORMATION

Never underestimate how useful bystanders' information can be. People often become ill when they are out by themselves, and passers-by may see what has happened but don't accompany the casualty to hospital; the information is then lost. Exact sequences of events are vitally useful to the medical staff, because they often give big clues about the cause of a collapse or illness.

Sick or injured people may be very vague about what has happened to them, and will not know if, for example, they had a convulsion while they were unconscious. They may not know that one side of their face drooped for a short time, or that they lost their speech. These events will determine what investigations are carried out at the hospital. Ultimately, long-term outcomes – such as whether they will be allowed to drive home or not – depend very much on what actually happened. Any information you can gather and relay to the emergency services is very useful.

IDENTIFICATION DEVICES

If a casualty is alone and collapses, medical ID tags, which are worn as a necklace or bracelet, can be life-saving. One side often features a staff-and-snake emblem (an international medical symbol), and the other will have useful information about the casualty, for example if they suffer from diabetes or epilepsy. Tell the emergency services about the information on the tag.

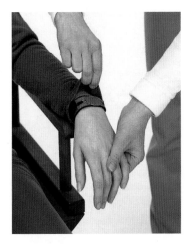

△ Always check a casualty's neck, wrists and ankles for a medical ID tag and pass on the information it carries to the paramedics.

Examining the casualty

SEE ALSO

▶ What is first aid?, p16

▶ Removing clothing and helmets, p22

▶ Responsiveness and the airway, p32

▶ The recovery position, p40

Once you are happy that a casualty is conscious and breathing, try to identify the problem by carrying out an examination. One of the first steps is to look at their face – are they very pale, for example? Don't move them at this stage, especially the neck or back. Now check the body for injury. Start with the head and finish with the arms and legs. Always try to gain a casualty's consent before starting an examination ("I just need to examine you to check for injuries; is that OK?") and keep the casualty and any friends or relatives informed as you go along.

You can tell a lot from looking at people, even before you touch them. Are they grey and anxious? Are they breathing easily, or is breathing laboured, painful or noisy, with wheezing or choking sounds? Remember that ensuring that a casualty's airway is clear is a top priority before any physical check. The feel and colour of skin is another hint. People in shock have pale, cold, clammy skin; a fever makes skin hot, dry and often flushed. Blue skin and lips suggest a heart that is not pumping well, or breathing problems that are preventing enough oxygen from reaching the blood.

Examine people in a systematic, gentle but businesslike way. Place unconscious but breathing casualties in the recovery position (on one side; explained elsewhere) before examining them. If you suspect any injuries that may worsen with movement, especially spinal injuries, examine them first. Always ensure that you protect the casualty's spine.

WHAT TO CHECK FOR

▶ Bruising, swelling, puncture wounds, burns and tender or painful areas.

▶ Changes in the casualty's appearance, breathing or state of consciousness.

▶ The presence of a medical ID tag.

▶ Any medication carried by the casualty, such as an inhaler.

VITAL NOTE: Anyone with a suspected spinal injury (see Step 5) must be kept as still as possible (especially the head) as you check. Ideally, hold them still while a helper checks areas other than the back.

HEAD-TO-TOE EXAMINATION

1 HEAD
Check the scalp for injury – swelling, depressions, cuts and bleeding. Also look out for blood or clear fluids in the nose or ears. Check the mouth for any objects or fluids (such as vomit) that could obstruct breathing and remove if very easy to do (only remove dentures that are loose or broken and easy to extract). Smell the casualty's breath for alcohol, but do not be too eager to dismiss people simply as "drunks" – medical matters are often not that simple. Experienced first-aiders might also check the eyes for pupil size. If they are different sizes and the casualty has been in an accident, there may be bleeding into their brain. If their pupils are like tiny pinpoints, they may have taken drugs or medication (but again, don't jump too quickly to conclusions).

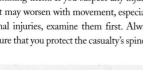

2 NECK
Make sure clothing is not tight, and check for a medical ID tag. Working very gently, feel along the back of the neck, without moving the head, for swelling or tenderness. Some people who have undergone a tracheotomy have a surgical opening called a stoma at the front of the neck that acts as an airway, so make sure that nothing obvious is blocking it.

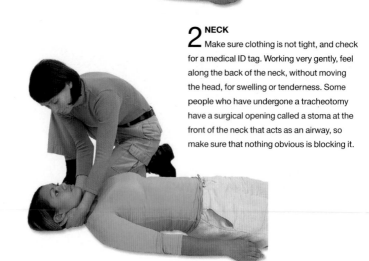

3 CHEST

Is the chest moving normally? Are there very tender places over the ribs (these may be rib fractures)? If there is an object stuck in the chest, leave it there. Feel the collarbones for swelling and tenderness. In some cases, it may be necessary to remove clothing to look at the chest, to check for obvious lacerations or bruises, for example. Typically, you might do this if the emergency services are delayed, but always proceed with sensitivity.

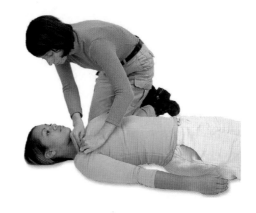

4 ABDOMEN

Feel the stomach gently for any large swellings or tender places. If the casualty is conscious, they will flinch, moan or cry out if you touch an area that is painful.

5 LOWER BACK

If you suspect a spinal injury, from the circumstances of the accident or from what the casualty says, do not try examining the back – even the tiniest amount of movement could risk further damage (see also What to Check For box). If you do not suspect spinal injury, gently feel the back for any tender areas.

6 PELVIS

Note any tender places over the hips. Maintain a very light touch because a pelvic injury can be excruciatingly painful.

7 ARMS AND LEGS

Look for injuries. Now test the limbs' function by asking whether the casualty can feel you touching their arms and legs. Ask them to grip your hand with theirs and to try tensing their leg muscles.

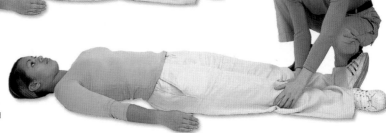

Removing clothing and helmets

SEE ALSO
➤ Examining the casualty, p20
➤ Moving and handling safely 1 and 2, pp24, 26

Removing a casualty's clothing should not be an automatic reaction. It is often unnecessary, especially if the casualty will soon be seen at a hospital, and can make people feel anxious and vulnerable, as well as exposing them to the elements. The movement required may also cause further injury. Only remove clothing if the emergency services are delayed and you feel it is absolutely essential in order to treat the casualty effectively. Do not attempt it if you are unpractised, as you may cause harm, and always seek consent and respect people's privacy.

You may need to look at a wounded site that is hidden by clothing in order to assess and deal with the injury. It may be possible to undress the casualty by unfastening and sliding off clothing but often it is necessary to cut the garments before removing them.

POINTS TO CONSIDER

➤ People can get upset at having their clothes removed by a stranger. Unless it is absolutely necessary, it is usually best to wait until they reach hospital. Remember, you can often feel injuries adequately through clothing.

➤ If you are in any doubt about removing an item of clothing or footwear, or if you are causing the casualty increased pain, it is best to wait for the paramedics.

➤ Try to seek the casualty's consent for your actions and explain what you are doing, so that they are not alarmed.

➤ Remove clothes and shoes with the minimum of movement, to avoid further injury and pain – never pull at clothing.

➤ The injured area will be very sensitive, so try to keep clothing away from it.

➤ Cutting clothes may injure the skin, especially if you are not using scissors designed for this job.

➤ The easiest route for cutting is along the seams.

➤ With leg and foot injuries, try to take off shoes or boots before the leg and ankle become so swollen that it is more painful to remove the footwear.

SWEATERS AND T–SHIRTS

If the injury is in the upper part of the body, then you may need to remove the casualty's top garment. Make sure that you do not attempt to do this if there is any chance that the casualty may have sustained a spinal injury.

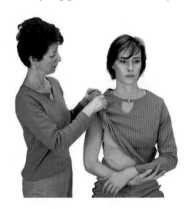

1 Release the uninjured arm carefully, before trying to undress the injured arm. Roll the garment up to the shoulder.

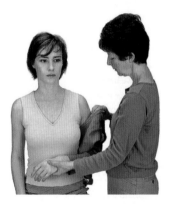

2 Pull the garment over the head, then slowly and very gently pull it down over the injured arm and smoothly off the hand.

SHOES

Removing shoes can be tricky because the foot or ankle may have become swollen. Undo the shoe entirely and support the foot under the ankle with one hand, while gently sliding the shoe off the heel and then over the toes with the other hand.

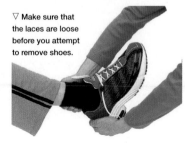

▽ Make sure that the laces are loose before you attempt to remove shoes.

SOCKS

The tight fit of socks causes problems for removal. If there is no swelling or pain you can try rolling the sock down over the foot. If the ankle or foot is very swollen, it is easier to cut off the sock. Pull the material away from the skin as you cut.

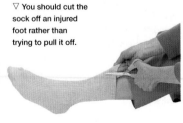

▽ You should cut the sock off an injured foot rather than trying to pull it off.

TROUSERS

If trousers are too tight to pull up from the ankle to reach a leg wound, you may need to cut them along the seam.

▽ Hold the trousers clear of a leg injury while pulling them up.

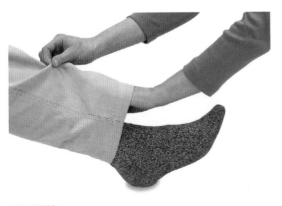

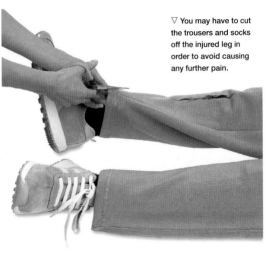

▽ You may have to cut the trousers and socks off the injured leg in order to avoid causing any further pain.

HELMETS

Only remove helmets as a last resort – as a rule of thumb, do so only if they are impeding a casualty's breathing. If the casualty is breathing and has an unrestricted airway, leave removal to the experts. If you have to proceed urgently, try to get someone to assist you so that the neck is supported, in a straight line with the head and spine if possible, while the helmet is taken off.

Full-face helmets

Ideally, two people are needed to remove a full-face helmet. One person is in charge of supporting the casualty's neck and holding on to the lower jaw; the second person undoes (or cuts) the straps and places their fingers under the helmet's rim. Sitting behind the casualty's head, the second person starts to ease off the helmet. The first person must keep the head still. The helmet may have to be tilted back to get it over the chin, and then forwards in order to lift it over the back of the head.

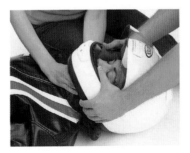

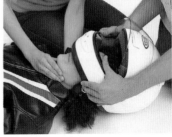

1 One helper firmly supports the casualty's neck and jaw while the other carefully undoes the straps and eases the helmet up.

2 The first helper maintains neck and jaw support while the other helper slowly lifts the helmet over the chin and over the head.

Open-face helmets

These helmets should also be removed by two people, if possible. One person supports the neck and jaw while the second person undoes (or cuts) the chin strap. The second person then grips the sides of the helmet from the inside and pulls the straps apart. The helmet can then be lifted off without causing pain or further injury.

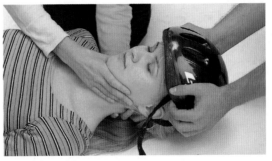

◁ To remove this type of open-face helmet, often used by cyclists, one helper supports the jaw and neck and the other releases or cuts the strap and then gently lifts the helmet away from the head.

Moving and handling safely 1

Never move a casualty if there is any chance that they could have a spinal injury, especially in the neck area. Sometimes, however, you will have no choice in the matter – the injured person may not be breathing and the airway must always take first priority, although there are ways of protecting the neck during resuscitation. Very rarely, it may be vital to move the casualty away from danger into a safer environment, perhaps because of fire or danger of explosion, or because there is a risk of hypothermia or sunstroke.

There are various reasons for having to move a casualty, such as needing to get to water if someone has serious chemical burns, or to reach other injured people. You must know how to move people without causing further injury or endangering yourself. And never forget: if someone is a stretcher case, they need an ambulance.

Causing further injury is always a risk with moving people, so doing nothing may be wise – it is a question of weighing up the relative perils. Always observe the rules of safe lifting, listed below. Also, think laterally and don't automatically rush to drag people all over the place. It may be easier to remove the danger from the casualty than the other way around. So, if a casualty is lying in a busy road, you might be able to park your car so that others will drive around the incident area.

SAFE MOVING

If moving another adult, you must be certain that this is necessary and that you are strong enough to do so. It is vital to protect your own back, so always remember to:

- Lift or move someone only if you are trained or if it is a dire emergency.
- Get the casualty to move himself or herself if possible.
- Keep your feet slightly apart.
- Use your legs to lift, not your back.
- Do not twist or turn as you lift.
- Keep your back straight and locked.
- Keep the weight that is being lifted close to your body.

MOVING A CASUALTY SINGLE-HANDEDLY

The moving techniques shown below and on the opposite page are for when there is just one rescuer at the accident scene. Here the options for moving a casualty are more limited than if there are two or more rescuers. Careful thought must be given to the technique you choose: consider your strength and fitness, the weight of the casualty, whether they are conscious and whether there could be a spinal injury.

Unconscious casualty

An unconscious person is unable to protect their airway so you must ensure there is no danger of their head flopping forwards and blocking their airway when you move them. Dragging is the best way to move the casualty in this instance.

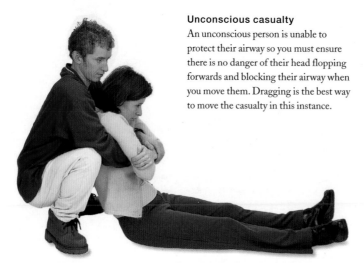

Dragging can also be used when the casualty is too heavy to lift.

Mobile casualty

If the casualty can still walk in a limited way you can try the human crutch. This helps to stabilize their walking.

Immobile casualty

If the casualty cannot move, they may have a spinal injury. If there is any risk of this, never move a casualty – call the emergency services immediately.

DRAGGING

You may have to drag a casualty away from the risk of further injury, such as in a fire. Bend down at the knees, lock your arms around the casualty's chest and keep them as close to you as possible as you move back. Do not drag the casualty sideways.

THE HUMAN CRUTCH

If the casualty is still at all mobile, this highly useful "assisted walk" technique allows the casualty to use your body as a crutch, to give them greater stability. Place a supporting arm firmly around their waist and grasp their nearest hand in your other hand. Make sure that you tell them about any obstacles in their path or changes in floor level, and take only small steps.

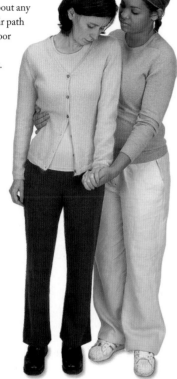

CRADLE CARRY

This method works particularly well with children and helps them to feel reassured and safe. Never attempt this lift on someone unless they are a great deal lighter than you, as you may damage your back; there is also the danger of dropping the casualty and causing further injury.

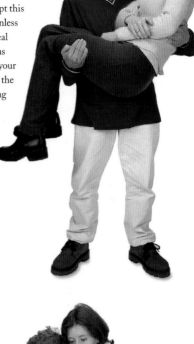

PIGGYBACK

Use this only in a severe emergency and if confident of your strength. Your approach will vary depending on how tall, heavy and strong you are in relation to the casualty. With your back to the casualty, bend forward and get the casualty to put both arms over your shoulders. Pull them on to your back and grasp their thighs. If you can, take hold of their hands. Try to keep your knees slightly bent. If lifting a small, light casualty, you may choose to crouch down in front of them and grasp their thighs before coming up gradually with your back kept straight.

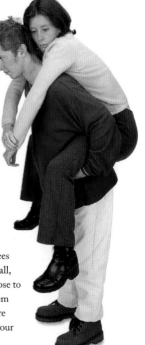

WHICH SINGLE-HANDED CARRY TO USE

➤ Try to use the human crutch wherever possible, especially if you are small and light. This excellent technique poses minimum risk to the rescuer, and little risk of damaging the casualty's internal organs. Ideally, the cradle and piggyback carries are usually best left for lifting someone about half your weight or less, making them particularly suitable for children.

➤ Avoid the "fireman's lift" (where the casualty is carried over the rescuer's shoulder), as this is tricky to do well and safely and could potentially cause severe damage to the casualty.

Moving and handling safely 2

MOVING A CASUALTY WITH TWO OR MORE HELPERS

It is much easier and less likely to cause further injury if you can move or lift a casualty with two or more people helping. This is because you have more control over the move, and your combined strength means you are sharing the burden of weight. At the scene of an accident, always try to enlist help from any bystanders before attempting to move the casualty single-handedly. Explain step-by-step exactly what you intend to do and ensure they understand the importance of coordinating every move.

Unconscious casualty
If the casualty is unconscious or is immobilized as a result of their injuries, you can attempt a fore and aft carry. This can also be used if the person is conscious, but it should be avoided if the arms, shoulders or ribs are injured. If four helpers are available and you have a blanket or piece of cloth handy, a blanket lift provides a safe, supportive method of transporting an injured person – except when spinal injury is suspected, in which case, avoid it. If there is an immediate risk to life, such as

fire or water, that outweighs the danger of movement, very carefully roll the victim away from the danger with as many helpers as possible supporting and controlling the body to minimize damage. All helpers must act in sync when rolling the casualty.

Conscious casualty
The two-hand seat carry can be used if the casualty is conscious and able to move into a sitting position. If the casualty is extremely heavy, then do not try to lift them – leave this to the experts.

FORE AND AFT CARRY
With an unconscious or immobile casualty and two helpers, the stronger should take the upper body and the other the legs. Make sure you synchronize your actions and move in the same direction. Move slowly and carefully and watch out for any obstacles such as steps or stairs.

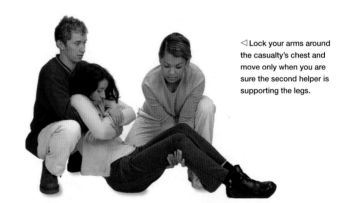

◁ Lock your arms around the casualty's chest and move only when you are sure the second helper is supporting the legs.

TWO-HAND SEAT
This move should be used when the casualty is conscious. Squat one on each side of the casualty and cross arms across their back. Hold on to the casualty's clothes, then pass your other hands under the casualty's knees and grip each other's wrists. Keep close to the casualty and lift together, keeping knees bent.

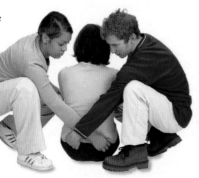

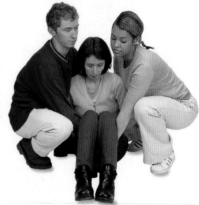

1 Get as close to the casualty as you possibly can in order to reduce strain on your own back. Bend at the knees and take hold of the casualty's clothes, on or just above the buttocks, with your hands crossed.

△ Detail of hand grip.

2 With your other hands, support the casualty's legs. Lock wrists with the other helper and lift, keeping your back straight.

BLANKET LIFT

This rudimentary "stretcher" is the safest, easiest way of moving an unconscious or immobile casualty if there are at least four helpers – doing it with fewer risks further injury. You need a blanket, sheet, rug or any large piece of fabric such as a coat, opened out. Use this to carry the casualty a short way or to transfer them to a proper stretcher. All helpers must move the casualty in a synchronized action. Note that you should never attempt to improvise any kind of stretcher if you are uncertain what to do.

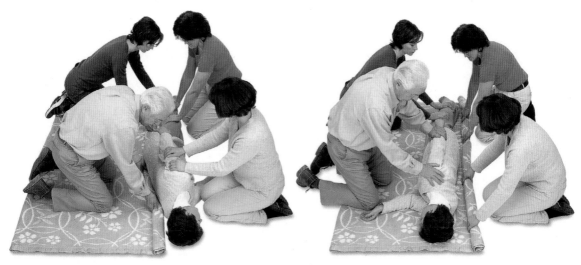

1 With the casualty placed on their side, and the blanket edge rolled up lengthways, position the roll against the casualty's back.

2 Move the casualty over the rolled edge, on to their other side. Make sure the casualty's head isn't close to the edge.

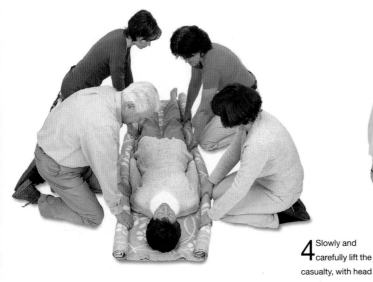

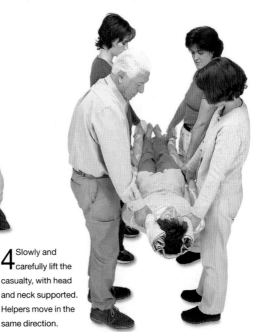

3 Roll up the other long edge of the blanket. The two helpers on either side of the casualty grasp the roll firmly with both hands.

4 Slowly and carefully lift the casualty, with head and neck supported. Helpers move in the same direction.

SKILLS CHECKLIST FOR
ACTION AT AN EMERGENCY

KEY POINTS

- Always do the DRSABC ☐

- Assess the situation promptly but with thought – do not rush in impulsively ☐

- Do not move the casualty before the paramedics arrive unless it is absolutely necessary ☐

- Always treat casualties with respect; seek permission for actions of a personal nature where possible, and keep them well informed of what you are doing ☐

SKILLS LEARNED

- The principal rules of approaching and dealing with emergencies safely and effectively ☐

- The basics of life-saving: what the DRSABC of Danger, Response, Shout, Airway, Breathing, Circulation is all about ☐

- Assessing the nature of the problem ☐

- When and how to remove clothing and helmets, without causing further injury ☐

- Handling and moving a casualty safely ☐

2

LIFE-SAVING PRIORITIES

For the best possible outcome, it is essential that life-saving techniques are carried out in the correct order. Once you have assessed DRSABC (see the previous chapter), you need to concentrate on issues such as continuing resuscitation, possibly moving the casualty into the recovery position, or deciding which technique is best to use for choking, depending on whether the casualty is conscious or unconscious. You must also consider the impact of shock on any casualty and do your best to calm and reassure them at every stage of the emergency.

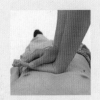

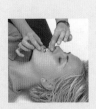

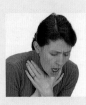

Understanding resuscitation

You could save someone's life by applying basic resuscitation skills. Equipped with these, you should be able to maintain a person's breathing and circulation, and this greatly increases their chances of survival once the emergency services arrive. The key elements of resuscitation are ensuring that oxygen gets into the lungs and that oxygenated blood gets to the brain. Resuscitation should only be attempted by those who have received proper training and practice in these techniques, which are explained in full detail in this chapter.

WHAT IS CARDIOPULMONARY RESUSCITATION (CPR)?

CPR is the technique of providing basic life support using chest compressions and artificial ventilation. The latter is also called "the kiss of life", mouth-to-mouth resuscitation, or rescue breathing. Although the technique has been used for over 50 years, it was not until the 1970s that the idea of training the public in these skills began.

CPR is needed after a cardiac arrest, that is, when the heart suddenly stops beating and circulation of the blood around the body ceases. A person who has had a cardiac arrest is unresponsive to voice or touch, is not breathing and has no pulse. Since two-thirds of cardiac arrests occur unexpectedly and not in hospitals, it makes sense for members of the public to be able to carry out resuscitation.

After only 3–4 minutes without oxygen, the brain can suffer irreversible damage, and this can be fatal, so you should act swiftly.

(There have been some instances of successful resuscitation up to 40 minutes after cardiac arrest when it occurred in cold water, but this is the exception as most incidents occur on dry land.) In most cases, a little knowledge and training can definitely save lives. If CPR is started within seconds of the cardiac arrest, the victim has a significantly improved chance of surviving.

NORMAL CIRCULATION

Blood flows through the blood vessels in one direction at a fairly constant rate. The heart is at the centre of the circulatory system, pumping blood around the body. The heart pumps blood to the lungs where it absorbs oxygen and gives up the carbon dioxide collected as it travels around the body. The blood then returns to the heart, and the oxygenated blood is sent to all parts of the body including the brain. The brain controls all body functions, including those of the heart and lungs, and the working of these three organs is closely linked. If any one fails, it does not take long for the other two organs to fail too.

◁ Unless unconsciousness in an adult is the result of injury or choking, summon the emergency services first and then carry out resuscitation.

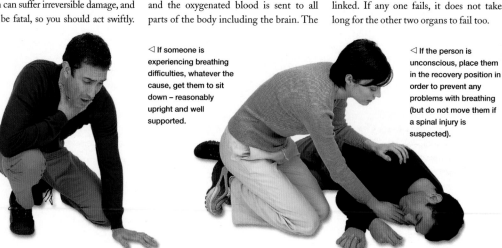

◁ If someone is experiencing breathing difficulties, whatever the cause, get them to sit down – reasonably upright and well supported.

◁ If the person is unconscious, place them in the recovery position in order to prevent any problems with breathing (but do not move them if a spinal injury is suspected).

THE "CHAIN OF SURVIVAL"

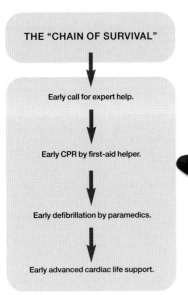

↓

Early call for expert help.

↓

Early CPR by first-aid helper.

↓

Early defibrillation by paramedics.

↓

Early advanced cardiac life support.

BASIC LIFE SUPPORT PRINCIPLES FOR AN UNRESPONSIVE CASUALTY

1 Follow the "ABC" of DRSABC by ensuring that the casualty's AIRWAY is clear: check their mouth for obvious obstructions such as vomit and remove them if you can. Tilt the head back and look, listen and feel for BREATHING for up to 10 seconds. If they are not breathing, call an ambulance and give 2 rescue breaths.

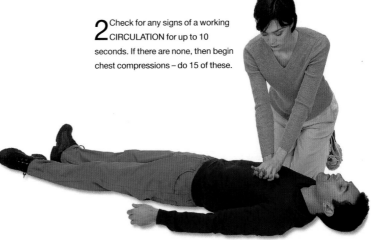

2 Check for any signs of a working CIRCULATION for up to 10 seconds. If there are none, then begin chest compressions – do 15 of these.

3 Now give 2 rescue breaths and then continue a cycle of 2 rescue breaths and 15 chest compressions until the paramedics arrive.

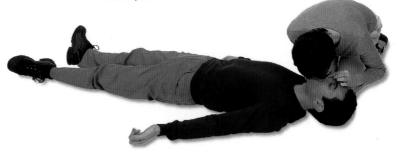

HOW CPR WORKS

Keeping the casualty's airway open, breathing for them and doing chest compressions means that an oxygenated blood supply continues to reach their brain. This "buys" really valuable time for the casualty by keeping their brain alive until more specialized help is available.

ARTIFICIAL VENTILATION

If someone has stopped breathing, their brain will soon be deprived of oxygen, and there will be a build-up of toxic carbon dioxide in the blood. You can breathe for them by artificial ventilation, but if the heart has stopped as well, you must give chest compressions to help move the oxygenated blood around the body.

CHEST COMPRESSIONS

The blood is kept circulating by the use of external chest compressions. By pressing down on the breastbone, blood is forced out of the heart and forced into the rest of the casualty's body. When pressure is released, the heart fills up with more blood, ready for the next compression, and so on. This is done at a rate of 100 compressions per minute.

Responsiveness and the airway

SEE ALSO

➤ What is first aid?, p16
➤ Moving and handling safely 1 and 2, pp24, 26
➤ Coping with neck injuries, p160 (for "log roll" technique)

You must assess a casualty's responsiveness before acting. In the first instance, obtain basic responsiveness information that will tell you whether or not a casualty is conscious – look for signs of life and try for a verbal response – before dealing with any urgent breathing issues and assessing injuries. After performing these essential steps, you might consider a casualty's precise level of consciousness, as explained below. Other issues you need to understand are whether you should move an unresponsive casualty and how to keep their airway open.

If a casualty has any level of response, then they don't need to be resuscitated, but it is very important that the first-aider maintains a vigilant watch on their ABC (Airway, Breathing, Circulation). Offer reassurance while you wait for the paramedics to arrive.

People who have collapsed have different levels of consciousness, from fully alert to a deep coma. Once you have dealt with the immediate dangers (DRSABC and assessing the extent of any injuries), you might try to determine this level (experienced first-aiders only may be able to run through this checklist very rapidly at an early stage) – such additional responsiveness information may be useful, and you can pass it on to the paramedics when they arrive. Professionals use the letters AVPU for the levels of consciousness – Alert, Verbal, Painful and Unresponsive.

RESPONSIVENESS ASSESSMENT IN DETAIL – THE AVPU CODE

ALERT

An alert casualty is awake and will be able to talk to you spontaneously. Reassure them that help is on the way and that you will do all you can to make them comfortable. Then try and find out exactly what happened.

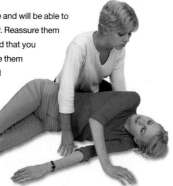

VERBAL

The casualty may seem to be unconscious but will respond to a verbal prompt. Shout "Are you OK?" close to their ear, and they will respond as if being roused from sleep. You could also try tapping them on the shoulder, or even giving them a gentle shake (but not if there is any possibility of a spinal injury).

PAINFUL

If shouting and gentle tapping or shaking does not wake the casualty, they might respond to a painful stimulus such as rubbing hard on their breastbone with your knuckles or giving a gentle pinch. Do not do anything that could draw blood, such as pricking them with a pin or sharp object.

UNRESPONSIVE

This is when the casualty does not respond at all, in any way – you may well have decided this when going through DRSABC initially. If you run through A, V and P, and none of these techniques works, then the casualty is considered unresponsive.

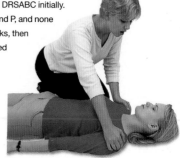

SHOULD YOU MOVE AN UNRESPONSIVE CASUALTY?

If, while following the DRSABC procedure, your initial conclusion is that a casualty is unresponsive, then you must assess their breathing and circulation. Always make your first assessment of a casualty in the position in which you find them. Only move them if absolutely necessary – if this is the only way you can check their vital signs and keep their airway unobstructed, or if you have to get them into a position where you are able to perform resuscitation.

If there is any likelihood at all of injury, take great care to protect the injured person's spine if you move them. Ideally, move them by using the log-roll technique – although at least three helpers are needed to do this safely.

1 If it is essential to move an unresponsive casualty on to their back (most notably, to perform resuscitation), first straighten the casualty's legs and put their arms as close to their sides as possible. Make sure their airway is always kept clear by ensuring the head does not drop down towards their chest.

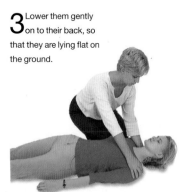

2 Cradle the head and neck with one hand, while holding the lower shoulder with your other hand.

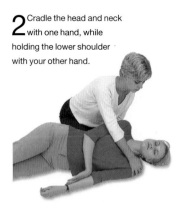

3 Lower them gently on to their back, so that they are lying flat on the ground.

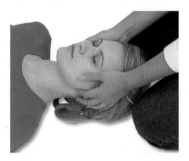

KEEPING THE AIRWAY CLEAR

The airway is just that – a passage through which air passes. This passage stretches from the nose and mouth, through the throat (pharynx), then into the windpipe (trachea), and down to the lungs. Food also passes through the upper part of this tube – the mouth and throat. The airway must be clear for the casualty to be able to breathe, either alone or by means of rescue breaths.

The most common things that block a casualty's airway are the tongue, blood and vomit. When checking an airway, look in the mouth. Do not sweep your finger around blindly, don't risk getting your fingers bitten, and avoid the throat area altogether; never risk pushing something further in. Scoop out objects such as sweets and food with two fingers. If an obstruction is likely to slip further down, or if there is liquid in the mouth, turn the person on their side in order to remove it.

Opening the airway

In an unconscious casualty, the tongue flops to the back of the throat and blocks the airway. To prevent this, put your hand on their forehead and tilt the head back; with two fingers under the chin and thumb on top, lift the jaw. If the casualty is upright, you can support their neck and tilt their head back to open the airway.

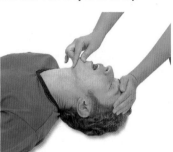

△ Carrying out the simple move of opening the airway can be enough to save someone's life.

If there is a possibility of spinal injury, you must adapt your manoeuvre. Your priority is to get a person breathing, so if they cannot breathe and have a possible neck injury, it is important to open the airway without further injury. Instead of tilting the head back, lift the jaw forwards by pushing upwards at the angle of the jaw.

△ In a suspected neck injury, push up at the sides of the jaw, as shown, to open the airway.

Rescue breathing

Rescue breathing (also called "kiss of life", mouth-to-mouth respiration and artificial ventilation) is a technique that supplies oxygen to the lungs of a person who is not breathing. Usually performed mouth to mouth, it may be done mouth to nose (if the mouth is damaged), mouth to mouth and nose (for babies) or mouth to stoma (a hole in the neck seen in people who have had a tracheotomy). Never let hygiene fears hold you back – infection is unlikely. There are special masks available, but these should be used only by those who are trained in their use.

MOUTH-TO-MOUTH RESCUE BREATHING

1 Following the DRSABC procedure, assess the casualty's airway and breathing. Kneeling beside the casualty, ensure that obstructions are removed from the mouth, and tilt the head back. Keeping the airway open, look, listen and feel for breathing for up to 10 seconds. If you decide that breathing is absent, call an ambulance and prepare to give rescue breaths as follows.

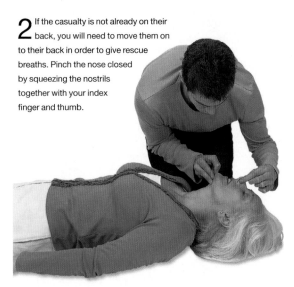

2 If the casualty is not already on their back, you will need to move them on to their back in order to give rescue breaths. Pinch the nose closed by squeezing the nostrils together with your index finger and thumb.

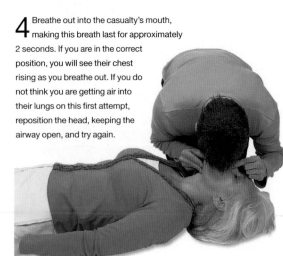

3 Maintaining the head tilt and pinching the nose, open your mouth wide and take a deep breath. Put your mouth against the casualty's mouth and make a tight seal with your lips around their mouth, so that when you breathe out no air escapes around the sides.

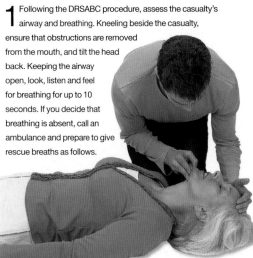

4 Breathe out into the casualty's mouth, making this breath last for approximately 2 seconds. If you are in the correct position, you will see their chest rising as you breathe out. If you do not think you are getting air into their lungs on this first attempt, reposition the head, keeping the airway open, and try again.

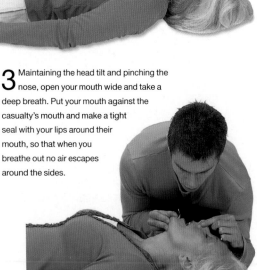

5 Continuing to keep the airway open, remove your mouth and look down towards the casualty's chest. Watch the chest falling as the air comes out. Take a deep breath in again and give another rescue breath. Make no more than 5 attempts to give 2 effective breaths before moving on to step 6.

6 Check for circulation signs: breathing, coughing or movement. If there are signs of circulation, continue rescue breaths until the paramedics arrive. Every 10 breaths (about once a minute), spend a few seconds checking for signs of a circulation. If there are no circulation signs, start cardiac compressions – as explained elsewhere.

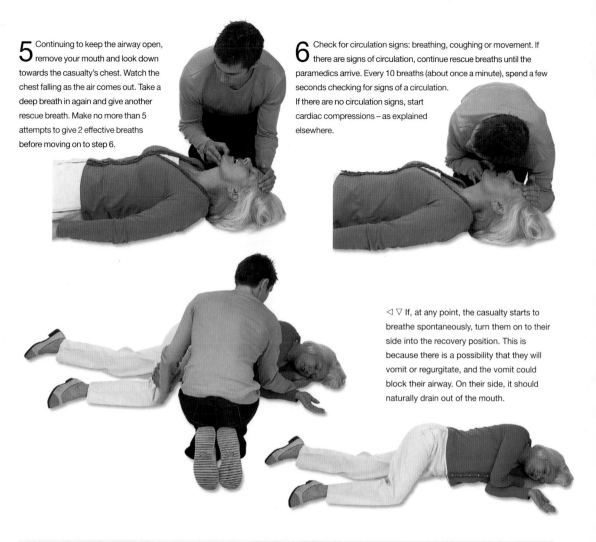

◁ ▽ If, at any point, the casualty starts to breathe spontaneously, turn them on to their side into the recovery position. This is because there is a possibility that they will vomit or regurgitate, and the vomit could block their airway. On their side, it should naturally drain out of the mouth.

MOUTH-TO-MOUTH PROBLEM-SOLVING

If the chest is not rising after each rescue breath:

➤ Check the position of the casualty's head and neck – is the airway open? Often people do not tilt the head back far enough.

➤ Check their mouth for any obvious obstructions.

➤ Check that there is a good mouth-to-mouth seal and the nostrils are completely closed.

If air is filling the stomach:

➤ You may be blowing in too much air, or blowing it in too fast. Stop breathing into their chest when it stops rising. Do not press on their distended abdomen – they might vomit and there is a danger that they might inhale the vomit.

If the mouth is bruised or battered:

➤ Use the mouth-to-nose resuscitation technique if the casualty's mouth is so badly injured that you cannot form an effective seal.

1 Open the airway by tilting the casualty's head back and lifting their chin.

2 Keeping the casualty's mouth closed, take a deep breath and form a seal around their nose with your lips – the seal should be good but do not squeeze the nose shut.

3 Let the air come out of the casualty's mouth by allowing the mouth to open as the chest deflates.

Cardiac compressions

SEE ALSO

➤ What is first aid?, p16
➤ Understanding resuscitation, p30
➤ Full resuscitation sequence, p38

Cardiac compressions are also known as chest compressions, or as cardiac/chest/heart massage. These compressions form part of the CIRCULATION stage of DRSABC. If you are faced with a casualty who is not breathing and who appears to have no obvious signs of a circulation, then you must start to give compressions along with rescue breaths – a combination known as cardiopulmonary resuscitation (CPR). However, you should never carry out cardiac compressions if you have not been trained to do so.

For cardiac compressions to be effective, the casualty should be lying flat on their back on a firm surface such as the floor – or the ground if they are outside. If your hands are in the wrong place, or if you use the wrong technique, the heart massage may not work, and you might also cause some unnecessary damage to surrounding structures, such as the ribs or the liver. Although it is a good idea to practise finding the CPR compression site, never carry out practice compressions on conscious volunteers, as you may cause harm. Always use a first aid dummy.

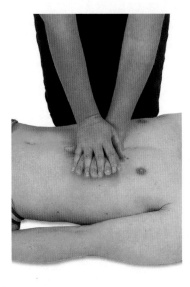

▷ When carrying out cardiac compressions, the heel of only one of your hands should come into contact with the compression site.

WARNING

In general, do not check for a pulse when assessing a person unless you are highly trained and can check it rapidly, without wasting vital seconds. It is not easy to find a pulse, even for trained people, especially in the recommended 10 seconds. The UK and US resuscitation councils have agreed that it is safer if the average first-aider does not check for a pulse before beginning CPR. People die when first-aiders mistakenly feel a non-existent pulse, and fail to resuscitate. Instead of checking for a pulse, look for signs of circulation such as movement, coughing or breathing. Do this for no more than 10 seconds before taking appropriate action.

HOW TO FIND THE COMPRESSION SITE

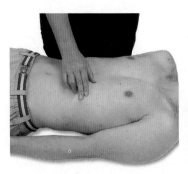

1 Kneel beside the casualty and run the fingers of your hand nearest the waist along the lower ribs until they meet the breastbone at the centre of the ribcage.

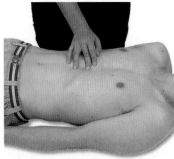

2 Keeping your middle finger at this notch, place the index finger of the same hand over the lower end of the breastbone.

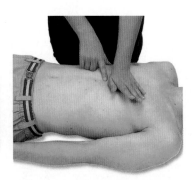

3 Place the heel of the other hand on the breastbone, and slide it down to lie beside the index finger already there. The heel of your hand is now on the compression site.

HOW TO GIVE CARDIAC MASSAGE

1 Kneel down at right angles to the casualty, so that you are positioned roughly halfway between their shoulders and waist.

2 Locate the compression site, and place the heel of one hand over this area. Place the heel of the other hand on top with both sets of fingers interlaced. Do not let the fingers touch the chest. Keep your elbows locked and arms straight all the time.

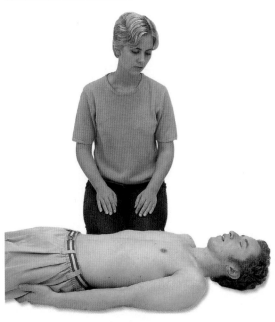

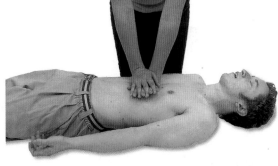

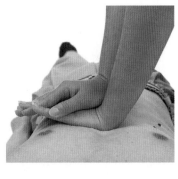

3 Place your shoulders directly over your hands so you are leaning over the casualty. This will concentrate pressure at the compression site. Compress the chest wall down by about 4–5cm (1½–2in). Release the pressure without taking your hands off the chest or bending your elbows.

4 Compress the chest at a rate of 100 compressions per minute. After 15 compressions, you must give 2 rescue breaths. Continue the cycle of compressions and rescue breaths until help arrives. Try to keep going until someone else, or the paramedics, can take over.

Full resuscitation sequence

Here, all of the component skills of cardiopulmonary resuscitation are shown in action together, to give the complete CPR sequence. Remember that CPR can buy valuable time for a casualty before paramedics arrive. You are keeping the casualty's brain alive by breathing for them (the "kiss of life") and performing chest compressions to keep the blood circulating. Perform 2 breaths for every 15 chest compressions at a rate of 100 compressions per minute. Practice on a dummy will help you remember the correct sequence.

HOW TO RESUSCITATE

The DRSABC resuscitation sequence should be followed exactly, with no short cuts or changes of order. Each step has been described in detail separately, but this sequence shows how all the individual elements fit together.

Breathing check
To check for breathing:
• Look for chest movement.
• Listen at the mouth for breath sounds.
• Feel for breath on your cheek.

When to get emergency help
In general:
• If you have a helper: get them to go for help as you start rescue breaths. Continue resuscitation until paramedics arrive.
• If you are alone, and the casualty is adult: call an ambulance, then begin resuscitation. However, if you are treating a victim of injury, drowning, choking, drug or alcohol intoxication, or an infant or child, then give CPR for about 1 minute before you go for help.

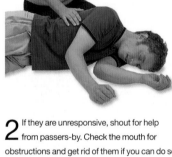

1 Check for responsiveness. If the casualty is responsive and breathing, they do not need to be resuscitated, and should be left in the position they were found in. Tap them firmly on the shoulder, and ask if they are alright.

2 If they are unresponsive, shout for help from passers-by. Check the mouth for obstructions and get rid of them if you can do so easily. Tilt the head back gently, to keep the airway open. Look, listen and feel for breathing.

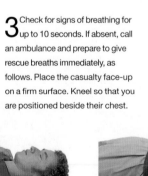

3 Check for signs of breathing for up to 10 seconds. If absent, call an ambulance and prepare to give rescue breaths immediately, as follows. Place the casualty face-up on a firm surface. Kneel so that you are positioned beside their chest.

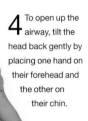

4 To open up the airway, tilt the head back gently by placing one hand on their forehead and the other on their chin.

5 Now give your 2 effective rescue breaths via mouth-to-mouth: pinching the casualty's nose, keeping their airway open and sealing your lips around their mouth. Breathe with normal force – do not blow air forcefully. You should see their chest rise. Make up to 5 attempts to give 2 effective rescue breaths.

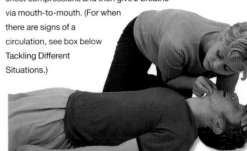

6 Check for a circulation by looking for breathing, coughing or movement. If there are no signs of circulation, perform 15 chest compressions and then give 2 breaths via mouth-to-mouth. (For when there are signs of a circulation, see box below Tackling Different Situations.)

7 Continue, in cycles of 2 breaths to 15 chest compressions, until the emergency services arrive.

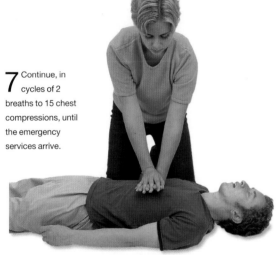

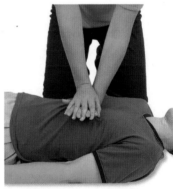

8 You must continue until aid arrives because the casualty's circulation is very unlikely to resume functioning without advanced techniques such as defibrillation – you are just keeping things going until help arrives with specialized equipment.

TACKLING DIFFERENT SITUATIONS

If the casualty is unconscious but breathing:

➤ Turn the casualty into the recovery position.

You should be able to see the chest rising visibly as you give rescue breaths. If it is not rising:

➤ Recheck the mouth for obvious obstructions – sweep with your fingers, and sweep/hook objects out, but try not to put your fingers past their teeth and don't risk pushing objects down the throat.

➤ Recheck that the head is tilted backwards and the chin lifted up so that the airway is clear.

➤ Check that there is a good mouth-to-mouth seal, and pinch the nostrils together.

If the casualty has signs of a circulation:

➤ If you notice movement suggesting that they have a circulation but they are not breathing, continue with rescue breathing until they start breathing again or the emergency services arrive.

➤ Check for signs of a circulation every 10 breaths. If the casualty resumes breathing spontaneously, turn them into the recovery position and continue to watch their breathing.

The recovery position

SEE ALSO

➤ What is first aid?, p16
➤ Understanding resuscitation, p30
➤ Responsiveness and the airway, p32

This is for casualties who are unconscious but breathing. An unconscious casualty is not in control of their airway and, because of this, it can easily become blocked. If the airway remains blocked for more than a few minutes, the lack of oxygen will quickly lead to a cardiac arrest. To ensure that this does not happen, it is best to place the casualty on their side, so that their tongue falls forwards and any fluids, such as vomit or blood, drain out of their mouth instead of down their airway. This is known in first aid as the recovery position.

PLACING A CASUALTY IN THE RECOVERY POSITION

Placing a casualty in the recovery position means that they are in a secure pose that ensures an open airway for easier breathing, and also allows any fluid to drain out of their mouth. Plan the direction in which you will roll the casualty in such a way that they remain accessible to help and are not exposed to potential further injury.

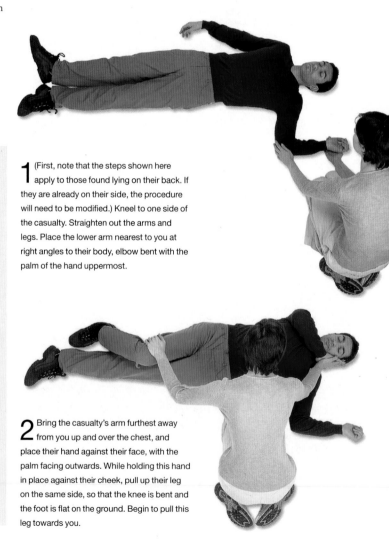

MODIFIED RECOVERY POSITION

In the following situations, you may have to alter the recovery position:

➤ If you feel that there is any possibility at all that the casualty has sustained a spinal injury, then keep them in the position in which you found them, if they are breathing. However, if you think they are in danger of inhaling vomit, then you must roll them on to their side, making sure that their head is kept in alignment with the rest of their body and not twisted or bent at the neck.

➤ If the limbs have been injured and cannot be bent, use rolled-up blankets or similar rolls of material, or even paper, in order to support them in a secure position.

➤ If the casualty's condition suggests multiple injuries and you have extra helpers available, use them to support the casualty and prevent them from toppling over.

1 (First, note that the steps shown here apply to those found lying on their back. If they are already on their side, the procedure will need to be modified.) Kneel to one side of the casualty. Straighten out the arms and legs. Place the lower arm nearest to you at right angles to their body, elbow bent with the palm of the hand uppermost.

2 Bring the casualty's arm furthest away from you up and over the chest, and place their hand against their face, with the palm facing outwards. While holding this hand in place against their cheek, pull up their leg on the same side, so that the knee is bent and the foot is flat on the ground. Begin to pull this leg towards you.

3 Continuing to support their hand against their face, pull them by the leg towards you, until their bent knee touches the ground. You can use your knees to stop them rolling all the way over on to their front.

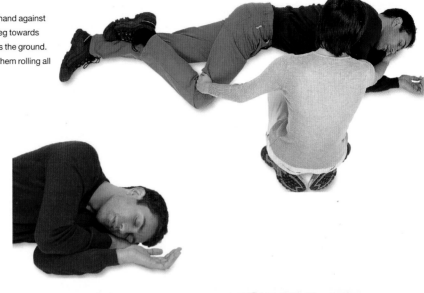

4 Check the airway, tilting their head back to keep the airway open. You may need to adjust the hand under their cheek, so that it is in the correct position to keep their airway open.

5 Adjust the leg so that the thigh is at right angles to the hip, as shown, and the casualty is completely stable. The knee acts as a prop and prevents them rolling forwards.

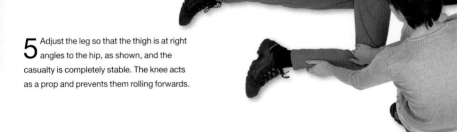

6 This is the recovery position. Note that you may need to separate out the arms if you feel that they are in a position where the circulation might be impeded. You should, ideally, have called the emergency services by now, if you have followed DRSABC. However, if you are alone and do need to leave the casualty for any reason, then the recovery position is a safe and secure one in which to leave them. On your return, continue to check their airway, breathing and circulation every few minutes until expert help arrives.

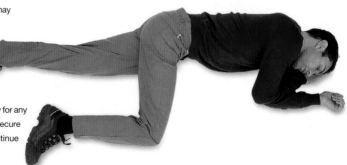

Coping with choking 1

This common hazard can cause death if prompt action is not taken. The brain can suffer irreversible damage if it is deprived of oxygen for as little as 3–4 minutes. Choking is most likely when people are eating, particularly if they are talking or laughing at the same time. In the elderly, poor teeth or dentures may make proper chewing difficult, or a stroke might have affected their swallowing abilities. Choking victims of all ages are best checked out at a hospital even if the object has been successfully expelled, as it may have harmed the airway lining.

Although food is most often the culprit, any foreign body may partially or completely block the airway if it is stuck at the back of the throat. The airway may also be obstructed by the tongue dropping back, especially in people who are unconscious.

COMPLETE OBSTRUCTION

Someone with a completely blocked airway will be unable to speak or cough. They may clutch their neck, or point frantically at their throat, and open their mouth wide. Initially the victim will be red-faced as they struggle for air; then they will become pale and their lips will turn blue as oxygen fails to reach their lungs. Eventually they will lose consciousness, and all chest movements will stop as they cease breathing. An effective circulation will quickly stop unless the airway is cleared and air starts getting through to the lungs once again.

INCOMPLETE OBSTRUCTION

A person may be choking but still be able to get air past the obstruction and into their lungs – this is an incomplete or partial obstruction. Do not interfere with their breathing efforts in any way, apart from encouraging them to cough. If they can cough, there must be enough room around the foreign body for air to pass, and a sharp cough might dislodge and expel it. You may decide to keep the victim seated, in order to reduce the body's demand on an imperfect supply of oxygen.

Other signs of partial blockage include:
• Snoring, gurgling and wheezing.
• Blue or grey lips, earlobes and tongue, even though the person is breathing.
• Breathing that alternates between normal and difficult/laboured.

CLEARING THE AIRWAY

There are three principal ways in which the first-aider should deal with a blocked airway, depending in the first instance on whether the person who is choking is conscious or unconscious:

FOR CONSCIOUS CASUALTIES:
• Back slaps, if coughing alone will not shift the obstruction.
• Abdominal thrusts.

FOR UNCONSCIOUS CASUALTIES:
• Chest thrusts.

These techniques can be used singly or in combination, depending on the circumstances, and on how well a method seems to be working.

Whichever technique you need to use, keep reassuring the person who is choking and stay as calm as possible yourself, as people who are choking tend to panic, quite understandably, and this makes breathing difficulties much worse. If the casualty loses consciousness, open the airway and check for breathing: as the muscles relax this may start spontaneously. If not, you will need to attempt rescue breaths and begin chest compressions.

CLEARING THE AIRWAY OF A CONSCIOUS CASUALTY

1. BACK SLAPS

This simple method is the first technique you should try on a conscious casualty, and is an instinctive reaction when you see someone choking. First encourage them to lean forwards and cough sharply and deeply in order to help move the foreign body. If this proves ineffective, stand to the side and slightly behind the casualty. Keeping them leaning forwards, support their chest with one hand and with your other hand flat, give up to 5 hard slaps between the shoulder blades. If this fails, move on to abdominal thrusts.

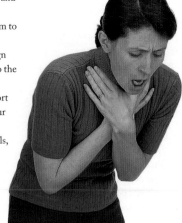

▷ People who think they are choking can panic very easily. Try to keep them calm.

2. ABDOMINAL THRUSTS

This is the other technique used with conscious casualties, but it should never be used on a pregnant casualty. It relies on pressing forcefully into the abdomen to cause an artificial cough, which may force enough air against the blockage to shift it. This method can be used whether the casualty is standing up or sitting down.

If someone is too large for you to get your arms around them, perform the thrusts with the casualty standing up with their back against a wall. Kneel in front of the casualty and, with one of your hands over the other, push upwards and inwards over the abdomen.

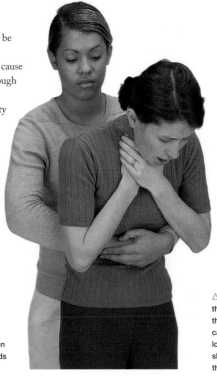

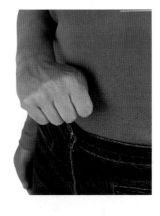

▷ Stand behind the person who is choking. Now slide your arms around the victim and wrap them around their trunk just below the bottom of the ribcage. Use the grip shown on the right. With your elbows out, press inwards and upwards in quick, sharp thrusts.

△ When holding someone for an abdominal thrust, one of your hands should form a fist. The thumb side of the fist is placed against the casualty's abdomen, between their navel and lower ribs, as shown above. Your other hand should be placed over the fist, grasping it, as in the picture on the left.

CLEARING THE AIRWAY OF AN UNCONSCIOUS CASUALTY

CHEST THRUSTS

These are used on unconscious casualties. They are similar to the chest compressions in cardiopulmonary resuscitation (CPR), but are sharper and slower, with each thrust attempting to relieve the obstruction.

Chest thrusts are sometimes used on conscious victims. For example, with a pregnant woman, it would be unsafe to perform abdominal thrusts. Also, where the casualty is too large for you to fit your arms around them, you could use chest thrusts instead of doing abdominal thrusts from the front (see above). To perform chest thrusts on a conscious casualty, get them to stand or sit with their back firmly against a wall, and push against their chest with your hands from the front.

▷ To perform chest thrusts on an unconscious person, they should be lying on their back. Kneel to one side of them and make sharp cardiac compressions, but at a slower rate than for cardiac victim resuscitation. This should be done as part of a full emergency routine where the person's state of consciousness and breathing has been assessed, help has been called for and rescue breaths carried out (see Coping with Choking 2).

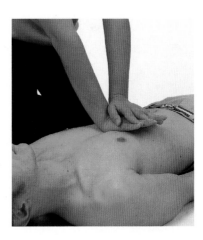

▷

Coping with choking 2

PUTTING IT ALL TOGETHER

The individual techniques detailed in Coping with Choking 1 can now be slotted into full sequences. Time is vital when someone is choking – assess the situation and act as swiftly as possible. To recap: with conscious victims, try to calm them down – this will make your job much easier. Encourage them to dislodge the obstruction with a few deep coughs. If this fails, you will need to proceed to abdominal thrusts, if necessary. If a casualty is unconscious, or loses consciousness as you are helping them, call the emergency service and start resuscitation swiftly, as shown, using chest thrusts to shift the obstruction.

HELPING A CONSCIOUS CASUALTY

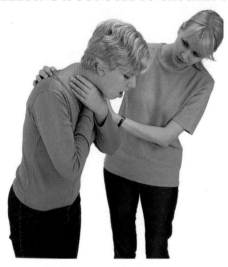

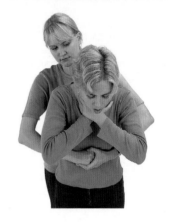

1 If the person who is choking is still managing to breathe, but feels that something is lodged in their airway, they will probably panic. Ask them to cough to try to dislodge the foreign body, but do not do anything else. Attempt to calm them, and summon emergency help.

2 If the situation worsens, or if the casualty cannot cough, speak or breathe and is beginning to look pale, give them 5 sharp back blows.

3 If coughing does not expel the object, give them abdominal thrusts. Continue until the foreign body has moved, or until the emergency services arrive.

HELPING AN UNCONSCIOUS CASUALTY

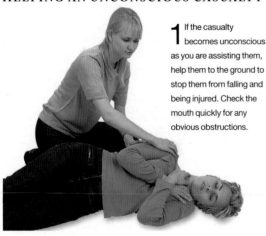

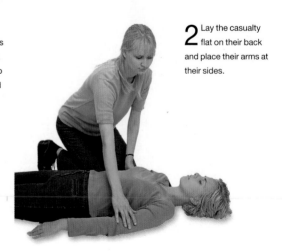

1 If the casualty becomes unconscious as you are assisting them, help them to the ground to stop them from falling and being injured. Check the mouth quickly for any obvious obstructions.

2 Lay the casualty flat on their back and place their arms at their sides.

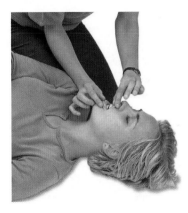

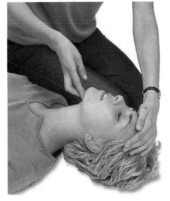

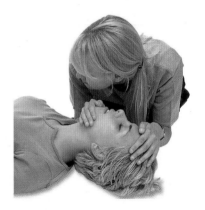

3 Recheck the casualty's mouth for any visible obstructions and remove anything you can see very carefully; do not poke your finger blindly around the mouth.

4 Open the airway by placing one hand on the forehead and two fingers of your other hand under the chin, and tilting the head back gently, as far as possible.

5 Check for breathing by looking, listening and feeling – as muscles relax during unconsciousness the victim may now be breathing again.

6 If you decide that they are not breathing, get someone to call the emergency services. (If you are alone, give CPR for about 1 minute before going for help.) Give 2 rescue breaths. If unsuccessful, reposition the head and try again.

7 If the rescue breaths do not go in, start chest compressions in an attempt to dislodge the obstruction. Do not check for signs of circulation. After 15 compressions, check the mouth for the dislodged obstruction, remove anything you find and then attempt 2 further rescue breaths. Continue to give cycles of 15 compressions followed by 2 rescue breaths. If the breaths go in fairly easily, check for signs of a circulation and continue as for a non-choking casualty. If they do not, repeat the cycle of compressions and breaths until help arrives.

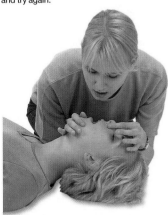

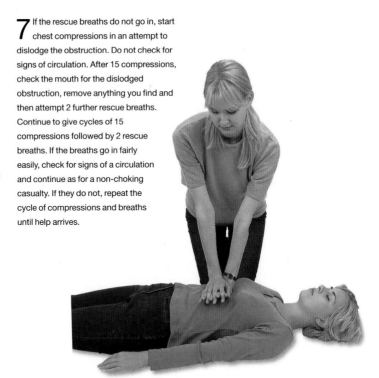

SKILLS CHECKLIST FOR
LIFE-SAVING
PRIORITIES

KEY POINTS

- Every minute is vital ☐

- Don't waste time checking for a pulse unless you are highly trained in this technique ☐

- Always stick to DRSABC procedures when dealing with life-support situations ☐

- Don't attempt CPR unless you have had full training and practice ☐

- Pay plenty of attention to keeping a casualty's airway open ☐

- The technique for helping a choking victim depends on whether the person is conscious or unconscious ☐

SKILLS LEARNED

- Rescue breathing, also known as mouth-to-mouth respiration, artificial ventilation, or the "kiss of life" ☐

- Cardiac compression (heart massage) ☐

- The correct sequence of resuscitation ☐

- The recovery position ☐

- Back slaps to treat choking ☐

- Abdominal thrusts to treat choking ☐

- Chest thrusts to treat choking ☐

CHILDREN'S LIFE SUPPORT

Children are notoriously accident-prone and both babies and children can get dangerously ill very rapidly, so every second counts and you must get help for a collapsed child as fast as possible. The whole story is not entirely depressing, however – children often have remarkable powers of recuperation. It is essential for first-aiders to appreciate the differences between dealing with an older child or adult and dealing with a baby or young child. Many of the basic principles remain the same as for adults, but the techniques used must be tailored to smaller, more fragile bodies.

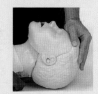

CONTENTS

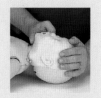

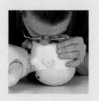

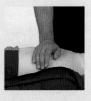

Basic life support

Young children are not mini-adults, but the basic life-support rules of checking airway, breathing and circulation still apply. Babies under 1 require different treatment to older children. Children over 8 can be treated as adults. One important issue to bear in mind is that adult first-aiders may feel more emotionally affected by a young casualty, and this can sometimes cloud their judgement – you must avoid this and act decisively. The elements of life support are shown below, and are then put together as a full routine on the following pages.

As in adults, basic life support in babies and children involves rescue breaths and chest massage, and is given to ensure that air continues to enter the lungs and blood to circulate around the body in an emergency. The techniques of rescue breathing and chest compressions are used, but the methods are slightly different depending on the age of the child.

The causes of cardiac arrest in children are very different to those in adults. Children rarely have problems with their hearts, but a healthy heart will stop if insufficient oxygen reaches other vital organs, such as the brain.

Children are anatomically different to adults, hence the need for different life-support techniques. They have narrower air passages and these are more prone to blockage. Their windpipe is more flexible and, if the neck is bent back too far, the airway may become blocked. A child's tongue is bigger than an adult's relative to their mouth and throat, and it is more likely to block the airway, particularly if the child is unconscious.

MANAGING THE AIRWAY

Open the airway in the same way as in an adult. In children, be careful not to over-tilt the head and block off the airway. Children breathe mainly by using their diaphragms, rather than their chest muscles. Look for their stomach rising and falling when checking their breathing.

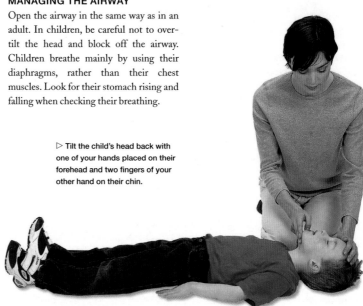

▷ Tilt the child's head back with one of your hands placed on their forehead and two fingers of your other hand on their chin.

REMEMBER DRSABC

Remembering and acting on these priorities will save lives:

D for DANGER
R for RESPONSE
S for SHOUT
A for AIRWAY
B for BREATHING
C for CIRCULATION

RESCUE BREATHING

If you are alone with a baby or child who is not breathing, give rescue breaths for 1 minute before calling for an ambulance. Ideally, take the child with you when you go to make the call, but do not stop the rescue breathing. Don't blow an adult-sized breath – use just enough air to make their chest rise and then fall, as if they have taken a deep breath. In a baby, it is easier to put your mouth over both their nose and mouth. Use the following guidelines when you are administering CPR in children:

• Babies and children up to 8 years – 1 breath per 5 compressions.
• Older children (8+ years) – 2 breaths per 15 compressions.

It might be that you cannot get any air into the casualty's chest, even after trying to do so with their head in several different positions. In this case, they may have choked, and you must follow the appropriate choking procedure.

FINDING AND USING THE CPR COMPRESSION SITE IN A BABY (UNDER 1 YEAR)

1 Hold the index finger of one hand horizontally between the baby's nipples, in such a way that the centre of your finger is at the sternum, or breastbone.

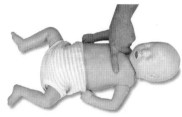

2 The correct compression site is located one finger's width beneath this line between the nipples. Position two fingertips over this site, ready to press down.

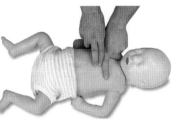

3 Using these two fingertips, compress the breastbone to a depth of approximately one-third to one-half of the infant's chest. Release. Give 5 compressions over a period of about 3 seconds (a little over 1 compression per second, or 100 per minute). For every 5 compressions performed, give 1 effective rescue breath. Continue to give the infant chest compressions and rescue breaths, at a ratio of 5:1.

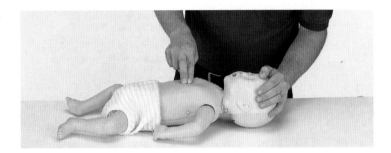

FINDING AND USING THE CPR COMPRESSION SITE IN A CHILD (1–8 YEARS)

1 First, find the child's xiphisternum – the small protrusions at the base of the breastbone, where the ribs join.

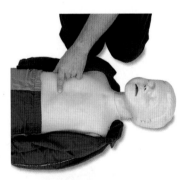

2 Place the heel of your other hand on the lower half of the child's breastbone. Make sure that you do not press on or below the xiphisternum.

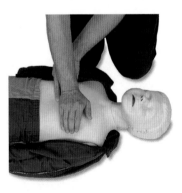

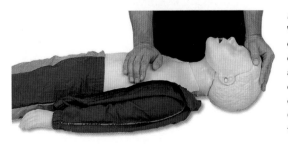

3 To give a chest compression, press down vertically with the heel of one hand to a depth of roughly one-third to one-half the depth of the child's chest. Do this 5 times in about 3 seconds (a rate of 100 chest compressions per minute). After every 5 compressions, give 1 effective rescue breath. Continue with this ratio of 5 compressions followed by 1 effective rescue breath.

Resuscitating a baby or child

SEE ALSO

➤ Responsiveness and
   the airway, p32
➤ Rescue breathing, p34
➤ Basic life support, p48
➤ Recovery position, p52
➤ Choking, p54

Every second is vital when resuscitating a baby or child. If their heart stops, their chances of a full recovery are greatly reduced. Taking quick, effective action may prevent brain damage and save life. Resuscitation of a baby differs slightly from that of an older child, so familiarize yourself with both techniques. Also, your approach will vary depending on whether you are alone or have helpers. When checking for an initial response, remember that you cannot rely on a verbal response from babies and very young children, so look for other responsiveness clues.

RESUSCITATING A BABY (UNDER 1 YEAR)

DANGER, RESPONSE, SHOUT
• Make yourself and the baby safe.
• To test responsiveness, shout, tap the baby gently, or flick the soles of their feet. Never shake them – this can cause brain damage and may even prove fatal.
• Shout out to any passers-by for help.

AIRWAY
• Open their airway: remove any obvious obstructions from the mouth and tilt the head back by lifting their chin with one finger, placing your other hand on their forehead, and tilting back gently.

BREATHING
• Look, listen and feel for breathing and for any signs of life, for up to 10 seconds.
• If they are unconscious but breathing, hold them in the recovery position and call an ambulance.

• If there are no signs of breathing after checking for up to 10 seconds, make up to 5 attempts to give 2 effective rescue breaths. Seal your lips tightly around the baby's mouth and nose, and breathe lightly into the lungs until the chest rises. If the airway is blocked and your breaths do not make the chest or stomach rise, you should treat as for choking.

CIRCULATION
• **Look, listen and feel** for signs of circulation for up to 10 seconds.
• If there are no signs, give 5 chest compressions, using two fingers.
• Making sure that the chin is up and the head back, give 1 effective breath.
• Continue in cycles of 1 effective breath to 5 compressions.

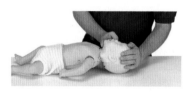

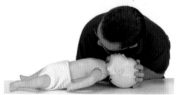

1 Having checked for a response and shouted for help, remove blood, vomit or other visible obstructions, as already explained. Tilt the head back to open up the baby's airway.

2 Look, listen and feel for signs of breathing, and vital signs such as warmth and colour, for up to 10 seconds. If they are breathing, place in the recovery position and get help.

WHEN TO CALL AN AMBULANCE

➤ If you are alone with a baby or child who is not breathing, perform resuscitation (breaths and compressions) for about 1 minute before going for help.

➤ Take the child with you if possible; if you can continue CPR as you go, so much the better.

➤ If you have help, one of you should start resuscitation while another goes to call for emergency assistance.

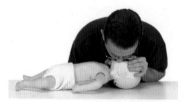

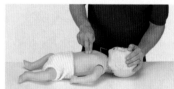

3 If breathing seems to be absent, place your mouth over the baby's mouth and nose. Make up to 5 attempts to give 2 effective breaths. If you have any helpers, send one to call for an ambulance as you start the rescue breathing. If your rescue breaths aren't going in, then treat as for choking.

4 Check for a circulation. If absent, start chest compressions. Give 1 breath for every 5 compressions. If there is a circulation, continue rescue breaths at a rate of one breath every 3 seconds. If breathing starts, hold the baby in the recovery position and monitor and record their breathing, circulation and response.

RESUSCITATING A CHILD (1–8 YEARS)

Follow the same rules about when to call for an ambulance (depending on whether you are alone or have helpers) as for a baby.

DANGER, RESPONSE, SHOUT
- Make yourself and the child safe.
- To test the child's responsiveness, shout or tap firmly on the shoulder.
- Shout out to any passers-by for help.

AIRWAY
- Open the airway: remove any obvious obstructions and gently tilt back the head with two fingers under the chin and the other hand on the forehead.

BREATHING
- Look, listen and feel for breathing and for any signs of life, for up to 10 seconds.
- If the child is unconscious but breathing, place them in the recovery position and call an ambulance.
- If there are no signs of breathing after checking for up to 10 seconds, make up to 5 attempts to give 2 effective rescue breaths. If the child's airway is blocked and your breaths do not make the chest or stomach rise, treat as for choking.

CIRCULATION
- Check for signs of circulation: look, listen and feel for normal breathing, coughing and movement for up to 10 seconds.
- Give 5 chest compressions, using the heel of one hand, as previously explained.
- Making sure that the chin is up and the head back, give 1 effective breath.
- Continue in cycles of 1 effective breath to 5 compressions.

CHILDREN OVER 8 YEARS
For older children, it may be necessary to use two-handed compressions (as for an adult), to get sufficient depth of compression. Follow the same rules about going for help, whether you are acting alone or with helpers, as you would for a baby or younger child.

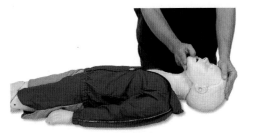

1 Having checked for a response and shouted for help, remove blood, vomit or any other visible obstruction, as already explained. Tilt the head back to open up the airway.

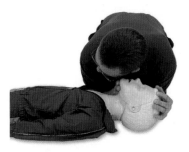

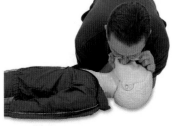

2 Look, listen and feel for signs of breathing, and vital signs such as warmth and colour, for up to 10 seconds. If the child is breathing, place in the recovery position and get help.

3 If breathing seems to be absent, place your mouth over the child's mouth. Try up to 5 times to give 2 effective breaths. If you have help, send someone to call for an ambulance as you start the rescue breathing. If your rescue breaths aren't going in, treat as for choking.

4 Check for a circulation. If absent, start chest compressions. Give 1 breath for every 5 compressions. If there is a circulation, continue rescue breaths at a rate of one breath every 3 seconds. If breathing starts, hold the baby in the recovery position and monitor and record their breathing, circulation and response.

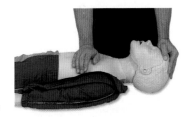

WARNING
If you have no helpers and a child known to have heart disease collapses suddenly (and this was not caused by an accident or poisoning), go for help straight away, before starting CPR.

CONTINUE RESUSCITATING UNTIL:
➤ The baby/child shows basic signs of life (breathing or circulation).

➤ Someone else takes over.

➤ Qualified professionals arrive at the scene.

➤ You are completely exhausted.

The recovery position

SEE ALSO

➤ Rescue breathing, p34
➤ The recovery position, p40
➤ Basic life support, p48
➤ Choking in babies and children, p54

An unconscious child who is still breathing should be placed in the recovery position (essentially the same as for an adult). This simple procedure can be a life-saver. It keeps the airway open, allows the tongue to fall forwards so it does not block the airway and lets any fluids that could cause choking drain out of the mouth – most specifically lessening the likelihood of inhaling and choking on vomit while unconscious. This vital position should be learned by anyone who cares for or works with babies and children.

PLACING A CHILD IN THE RECOVERY POSITION

The purpose of the recovery position is to minimize the possibility of the child choking on their tongue or the contents of their stomach while you wait for professional help to arrive. The position is secure enough for you to leave the child for a short time to summon help. The sequence shown here starts with the child on their back; the technique is shorter if the casualty is found on their side or front.

1 Kneel near the head of the unconscious child. With one hand on their forehead and the fingers of the other hand under the chin, tilt the head back to keep the airway open.

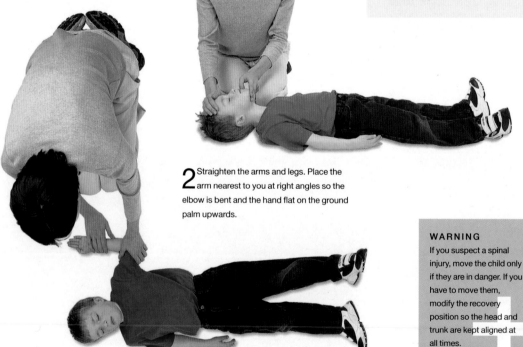

2 Straighten the arms and legs. Place the arm nearest to you at right angles so the elbow is bent and the hand flat on the ground palm upwards.

TIPS FOR DEALING WITH UNCONSCIOUS CHILDREN

➤ A child's windpipe is flexible, and it may close up if you over-extend their head when opening their airway.

➤ Keep an eye on their breathing and circulation and start resuscitating if either has stopped.

➤ Place the child in the recovery position before you go for help.

WARNING

If you suspect a spinal injury, move the child only if they are in danger. If you have to move them, modify the recovery position so the head and trunk are kept aligned at all times.

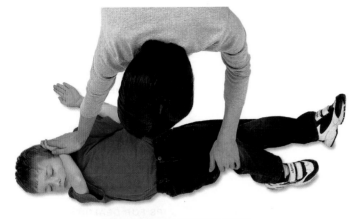

3 Move the other arm across the child's chest. Position the back of the hand against the cheek that is on the same side of the body as the bent arm. Bend the knee furthest from you and hold the leg at the thigh. Try to keep the foot of the bent leg on the ground as you do this.

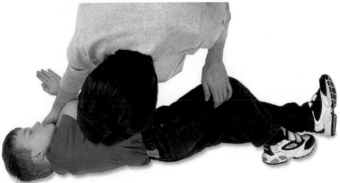

4 Hold the child's hand in position against their cheek. Pull them towards you using the bent leg to gently roll them over. The child should end up lying on their side.

PLACING A BABY IN THE RECOVERY POSITION

Infants under 1 year are too small to place in the conventional recovery position, but by keeping them on their side and with the head tilted down, the principles remain the same. Hold the baby with one hand under their head and the other under their lower back and bottom. Place their head lower than the rest of their body. Try not to press against their stomach as this may make them vomit.

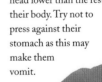

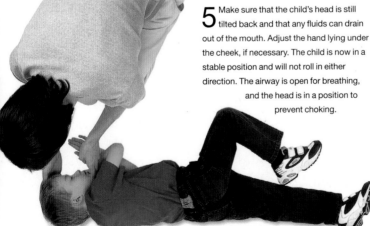

5 Make sure that the child's head is still tilted back and that any fluids can drain out of the mouth. Adjust the hand lying under the cheek, if necessary. The child is now in a stable position and will not roll in either direction. The airway is open for breathing, and the head is in a position to prevent choking.

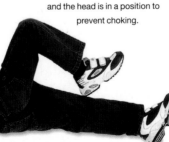

▷ Try to remember to keep the baby's head lower than their body. This is so that, if they vomit, they will not inhale it and choke.

Choking in babies and children

SEE ALSO

➤ Rescue breathing, p34

➤ Basic life support, p48

➤ Safety in the home, p228

A few common-sense measures will do much to prevent choking incidents in the young. These include avoiding foods such as nuts, boiled sweets and popcorn in children under four, and making sure children don't run around with objects such as pens in their mouths. However, if choking does occur, you must act decisively as there may not be enough time to wait for the emergency services. The sad fact is that significant numbers of small children die each year from choking, but the good news is that it is often easy to prevent.

SIGNS AND SYMPTOMS

➤ Unable to speak or cough.

➤ Blue lips.

➤ Pale/blue/ashen skin.

➤ Loss of consciousness/collapse.

TREATMENT FOR A CHOKING BABY (UNDER 1 YEAR)

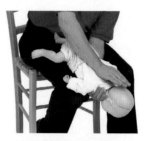

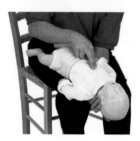

◁ Left and bottom left: to give a baby back blows (top), lay the baby face down on your forearm, with their head down low. For chest thrusts (bottom), use two fingertips placed on the lower half of their breastbone, a finger's width below the nipples.

FIRST AID FOR A CHOKING CONSCIOUS BABY (UNDER 1 YEAR)

1. **Check the mouth and breathing** and remove any obvious obstruction.

2. **Give up to 5 back slaps** with them face down on/along your arm.

3. **Re-check their mouth and breathing.** Carefully turn them face up, and remove any obvious obstruction.

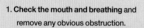

4. **If this is unsuccessful, use 2 fingers to give 5 sharp chest compressions** (1 thrust per 3 seconds).

5. **Repeat 1–4** until the baby starts breathing spontaneously or becomes unconscious. Calling an ambulance: do this immediately if the first set of chest thrusts fails.

SOME BASIC ISSUES

There are certain differences between treating choking babies and choking children. There are also differences in their treatment depending on whether they are conscious or unconscious. One of the most important points to appreciate is that, whether you are dealing with a child or a baby, rescue breathing is started only once the child or baby becomes (or already is) unconscious. The airway may become clear as the muscles relax with loss of consciousness, in which case the rescue breathing will cause the chest to rise, and you should move on to basic life support measures.

FIRST AID FOR A CHOKING UNCONSCIOUS BABY (UNDER 1 YEAR)

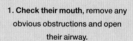

1. **Check their mouth,** remove any obvious obstructions and open their airway.

2. **Make up to 5 attempts to give 2 effective rescue breaths.** If there are no chest movements, move on to number 3. If the chest rises with rescue breaths, move on to the "C" of DRSABC.

3. **Give up to 5 back slaps.**

4. **Give 5 chest compressions.**

5. **Check their mouth,** remove any obvious obstructions and open the airway.

6. **Repeat the sequence 2–5.**

TREATMENT FOR A CHOKING CHILD (1–8 YEARS)

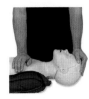

△ Unconscious child – open the airway.

△ Unconscious child – check for breathing.

△ Unconscious child – rescue breaths.

△ Unconscious child – chest compressions.

FIRST AID FOR A CHOKING CONSCIOUS CHILD (1–8 YEARS)

1. Get the child to cough.

2. If unsuccessful, **give the child up to 5 back slaps. Check their mouth.**

3. If unsuccessful, **give up to 5 chest thrusts:** standing behind the child, place your fist against the lower part of their breastbone. Grasp it with the other hand and pull sharply inwards and upwards, once every 3 seconds. Re-check the mouth.

4. If unsuccessful, **send for help. Repeat back slaps and re-check the mouth.**

5. If still unsuccessful, **give up to 5 abdominal thrusts. Re-check the mouth.**

6. If still unsuccessful, alternate **chest thrusts with abdominal thrusts between back slaps.** Even if the obstruction is removed, take the child to casualty – the airway lining may be damaged.

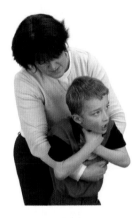

△ Abdominal thrusts on a conscious child who is choking are done from behind the victim, employing the same technique as for adults, but using less force.

IMPORTANT POINTS

➤ Never blindly sweep a finger inside anyone's mouth as it may make the obstruction worse.

➤ If the baby or child is still passing some air in and out of the lungs, and you know or suspect that an obstruction remains, do nothing and quickly call the emergency services.

➤ If a child has collapsed and is unconscious and not breathing they may have choked. Start the "ABC" of resuscitation and if the chest does not move with up to 5 rescue breaths, treat for choking.

➤ Abdominal thrusts are not used at all in babies as they may damage their internal organs.

FIRST AID FOR A CHOKING UNCONSCIOUS CHILD (1–8 YEARS)

1. **Check their mouth and open their airway.** Remove any obvious obstructions.

2. **Make up to 5 attempts to give 2 effective rescue breaths.** If there are no chest movements, move on to step 3. If the chest rises, then move on to "C" in the ABC of basic life support. Start CPR if necessary.

3. **Give up to 5 back slaps.**

4. If still choking, give 5 **chest compressions.**

5. **Check their mouth, and open their airway.**

6. **Give 5 rescue breaths.** If these are unsuccessful, and the chest does not rise, move on to number 7.

7. **Give 5 back slaps.**

8. If they are still choking, **give 5 abdominal thrusts.**

9. **Recheck the mouth and airway**, and if still not breathing, repeat the sequence from 2 to 8 until help arrives or the chest starts rising, when you should move on to "C" in the ABC of the basic life support sequence. Start CPR if necessary.

SKILLS CHECKLIST FOR
CHILDREN'S
LIFE SUPPORT

KEY POINTS

- Resuscitation is carried out differently in babies and young children from adults ☐

- Following the correct sequence of resuscitation is of the utmost importance ☐

- Speedy action is particularly important where young casualties are concerned ☐

SKILLS LEARNED

- Basic techniques of life support for babies and young children ☐

- Cardiac compressions for babies and young children ☐

- The correct sequence of resuscitation techniques for babies and children ☐

- The recovery position for babies and children ☐

- Coping with a choking baby or child ☐

LUNGS AND BREATHING

Breathing is vital for each of us to stay alive, and two of the most important components of first aid are airway and breathing – the A and B of ABC (C being circulation). A basic knowledge of the parts of the respiratory system and how they work can help if you have to deal with an emergency involving breathing problems. While serious accidents can cause breathing to stop, a number of diseases and accidents directly affect the working of the breathing apparatus. These include certain respiratory conditions (such as asthma), inhalation of noxious fumes or smoke, drowning, hanging and strangulation.

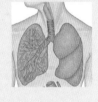

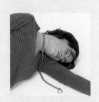

Understanding the respiratory system

SEE ALSO

➤ Understanding
  resuscitation, p30
➤ Responsiveness and
  the airway, p32
➤ Rescue breathing,
  p34

The technical term for breathing is respiration. With each breath, air enters the lungs and oxygen passes into the blood through the delicate tissues of the lung. Every cell in our bodies needs oxygen to work properly. Without oxygen, muscles cannot contract, nerves cannot send impulses, the heart stops and the brain cannot function. The end product of respiration is carbon dioxide, which leaves the blood as oxygen enters it. If the lungs did not expel carbon dioxide as we breathe out, confusion, coma and death would follow.

THE BREATHING APPARATUS

The lungs form the main part of the respiratory system – two spongy organs lying within the chest cavity. They are surrounded and protected by a bony cage comprising the ribs, spine and sternum. The diaphragm is a dome-shaped muscle attached to the lower ribs lying under the lungs and is the main muscle of breathing control. Other muscles that help with breathing, especially during exercise, or in times of stress or illness, are the intercostal muscles lying between each rib. Together these structures form an airtight, protective cage around the lungs.

Air reaches the lungs through a series of branching airways, which become progressively more numerous and smaller, like the branches of a tree. Air enters the body through the nose and mouth, and down the throat. It then passes the larynx, or voice box, which contains the vocal chords. The epiglottis is a flap of cartilage that covers the larynx when we swallow food, in order to prevent food from entering the trachea, or windpipe.

The air then reaches the trachea, which soon divides into two branches called bronchi – one going to the left lung and the other to the right. These branch into smaller vessels called bronchioles. The bronchioles taper into smaller and smaller branches, until they end in tiny sacs of lung tissue called alveoli. This is where gas exchange takes place. Tiny branches of veins and arteries are wrapped around the alveoli, and through their walls, oxygen and carbon dioxide are transferred in and out of the blood.

THE RESPIRATORY SYSTEM

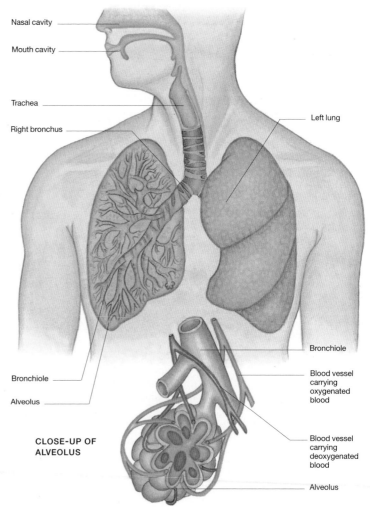

Nasal cavity

Mouth cavity

Trachea

Right bronchus

Left lung

Bronchiole

Alveolus

Bronchiole

Blood vessel
carrying
oxygenated
blood

Blood vessel
carrying
deoxygenated
blood

Alveolus

**CLOSE-UP OF
ALVEOLUS**

HOW DO WE BREATHE?

We breathe automatically. Apart from being able to control how fast or deeply we breathe over a short period, our breathing is beyond our voluntary control. The respiratory centre in the brain stem controls the basic rhythm of breathing. It is from here that messages are sent to and from the nerves supplying the diaphragm and intercostal muscles. This leads to a continuous cycle of relaxation and contraction of the breathing muscles.

As the diaphragm contracts and moves down, the intercostal muscles pull the ribs up and out. This causes an increase in chest volume, which in turn results in expansion of the lungs, and the reduced pressure causes air to be sucked in – this is called inspiration. In the reverse process, the diaphragm relaxes, the ribs move down and in, and air is pushed out – this is called expiration.

In an adult, the normal rate for breathing at rest is 13–17 breaths per minute. This rate increases during exercise, which is a normal response to the body's increased demand for oxygen. An increased rate at rest or during only mild exertion can be a sign of physical illness. Psychological problems, such as extreme anxiety and panic attacks, can also increase breathing rate.

In babies and young children, breathing rate is much higher, ranging from around 50 breaths a minute in a baby under 1 year to 30 breaths a minute in children over 5 years.

PROBLEMS WITH BREATHING

All kinds of different diseases and situations can adversely affect breathing. As soon as the delicate balance between air on one side and blood on the other is upset, problems start to arise. Part of a lung may fill with fluid from a tumour or infection. A lung may collapse or burst and then become squashed due to air escaping into the space between the lungs and the chest wall. The airways may go into temporary spasm as in asthma, or become permanently narrowed, as in the chronic lung disease, emphysema.

Breathing problems may be caused by:
• Heart disease.

BREATHING IN AND OUT

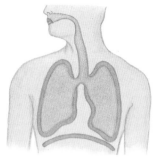

1 In between breathing in or out, the powerful diaphragm muscle found below the lungs rests in its relaxed position – in a pronounced dome shape.

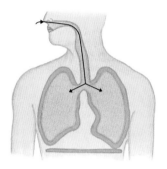

3 As the chest cavity and lungs expand, pressure in the cavity and lungs drops and air rushes in to equalize it – breathing in. At full contraction, the diaphragm lies flat.

2 The diaphragm muscle now starts to contract, moving downwards as it does so. The intercostal muscles also contract, expanding the rib cage.

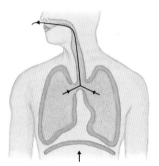

4 The diaphragm relaxes and moves up again. The intercostal muscles relax and the rib cage contracts. Pressure rises in the lungs, so air starts to rush out – breathing out.

• Chest infection.
• Lung tumour or lung disease.
• Collapsed or punctured lung.
• Asthma.
• Smoking.
• Fear, panic and anxiety.
• Inhalation of fumes.
• Choking.
• Chest injury.
• Head injury.

A person who develops breathing problems suddenly must be seen by a doctor without delay. While you are waiting for help to arrive, give any necessary first aid.

SIGNS AND SYMPTOMS OF BREATHING PROBLEMS

➤ Pale or blue face and lips.

➤ A rapid respiratory rate (this will vary with age, but the rate should be less than 20 breaths per minute in a healthy adult).

➤ Noisy breathing.

➤ Cough.

➤ Shortness of breath.

➤ Confusion and aggression.

Dealing with breathing difficulties

SEE ALSO

➤ What is first aid?, p16

➤ Coping with choking 1 and 2, pp42, 44

➤ Coping with a heart attack, p76

Breathlessness occurs in healthy people as a normal response to exercising, but it can also be a symptom of many diseases, including chronic conditions such as asthma and emphysema. Breathing difficulty should always be taken seriously, especially if it starts suddenly. Even young, fit people can be affected by conditions that cause breathing difficulty, such as a collapsed lung (pneumothorax), or a clot in the lung (pulmonary embolus). These conditions can be life-threatening, so prompt recognition and medical treatment are very important.

ACTION FOR BREATHING DIFFICULTY

Even if you do not know the cause of the breathing difficulty, act as follows:
• Sit the sufferer upright and supported.
• If they are on medication for breathing problems, get them to take it.
• Loosen clothing around the neck.
• Try to keep the sufferer calm.
• If the breathing does not return to normal, seek medical attention.

ASTHMA

At least 5 per cent of people suffer from chronic, lifelong asthma. Asthma is a condition in which the airways become narrowed and blocked with secretions. Asthmatics typically suffer from repeated attacks of wheezing and breathlessness. People with diagnosed asthma may use a "relieving" inhaler (usually blue) for immediate relief, and a "preventive" inhaler (usually brown or red) for longer-term treatment and prevention. There are also combined inhalers. Other inhaler colours include green and orange. A casualty should know which inhaler to use during an attack.

Causes of asthma

Asthma tends to be triggered by factors that differ between individuals. Sufferers are often allergic to pollen, animals, dust, smoke, air pollution, foods or drugs. Asthma attacks may also be triggered by viral infections, exercise, certain chemicals, stress or intense emotions.

FIRST AID FOR ASTHMA

People with long-term asthma may carry medication – look for this first. Children and people having their first attack will probably need expert help. Never delay seeking help if in doubt, or if you can't find medication.

Most asthmatics will sit upright, often grasping the arms of a chair, to help them breathe. Leave them in whatever position is comfortable, as long as it is sitting up.

The casualty should use an inhaler that will relieve symptoms, ideally with a spacer device so more drug reaches the lungs. Let the casualty take the medication themselves. Help them if necessary. If no spacer is available and they are not overly distressed, tell them to hold each inhaled puff for a few seconds. After a few puffs, wait for 5 minutes or so, and then try again. If this does not relieve the wheezing, or there are signs of a serious attack, call the emergency services.

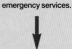

If hospital admission is necessary, more medication may be given, plus oxygen via a mask or tube. This treatment usually eases the attack within 12 to 24 hours.

RECOGNIZING AN ASTHMA ATTACK

As asthma can be life-threatening, it is important that symptoms are recognized and action taken as early as possible.

Signs of worsening asthma that needs medical attention:

➤ Wheezing or coughing occurs during exercise and at night.

➤ Inhaled medications are less effective at controlling symptoms.

➤ Peak-flow measurements start dropping. (An instrument that many asthmatics have at home, a peak-flow device measures the maximum volume of air that a person can breathe out.)

Signs of a very serious attack (always call the emergency services for these):

➤ Inability to finish sentences in one breath.

➤ Exhaustion from the effort of breathing.

➤ Confusion and irritability caused by lack of oxygen.

➤ Blue lips, and pale, clammy skin.

Signs of imminent respiratory arrest:

➤ Complete inability to talk.

➤ A silent chest (no wheezing) – the blocked airways cannot let air in.

➤ Weak, fast pulse.

DEALING WITH AN ASTHMA ATTACK

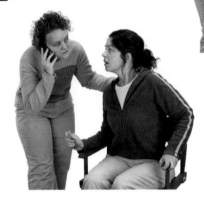

1 Make sure that a person having an asthma attack is sitting upright. They may be distressed and tense, as shown here. Comfort them and get them to relax back into their chair if possible, as relaxing conserves vital oxygen.

2 In the first instance, get the casualty to take the reliever medication themselves, ideally through a spacer device. If one is not available, get them to use their inhaler (shown). If absolutely necessary, help them to take it.

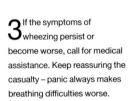

3 If the symptoms of wheezing persist or become worse, call for medical assistance. Keep reassuring the casualty – panic always makes breathing difficulties worse.

DEALING WITH HYPERVENTILATION

Rapid breathing or over-breathing, also known as hyperventilation, is often caused by anxiety. It differs from breathing difficulty in that the sufferer has some control over the situation, although they may not feel this. Hyperventilation causes tingling in the extremities and around the mouth, dizziness, chest pains and cramps. These symptoms make the sufferer feel even more anxious, and so they over-breathe even more.

The symptoms are caused by a lack of carbon dioxide, which the sufferer is breathing out at a very fast rate. A vicious circle ensues, with more anxiety developing as the hyperventilation worsens. Eventually, if the sufferer does not stop over-breathing, they faint, and the body resumes a normal breathing pattern. Hyperventilation can be a feature of phobias and panic attacks, both of which can be treated by psychologists.

WHAT TO DO
Calm the sufferer and get them to breathe into and out of a paper bag. This allows them to breathe in exhaled carbon dioxide and will ease symptoms. For recurring attacks, treatment should be sought.

PANIC ATTACKS

Hyperventilation may be a sign of a panic attack, a sudden and shortlived bout of exteme anxiety. The victim may also experience tension causing headache or pressure in the chest, trembling, sweating and palpitations.

➤ Try to identify the cause of the fear and escort the victim to a quiet place.

➤ Reassure them and stay with them until they are calm. Advise them to consult a doctor to address the underlying cause of the attack.

Tackling fume inhalation

SEE ALSO
➤ Dealing with breathing difficulties, p60
➤ Coping with headache, p90
➤ Managing dizziness and fainting, p92

Fumes inhaled into the lungs have the potential to do serious damage to the respiratory system. If you find a casualty you suspect has inhaled fumes, you must move them from the source, provided it does not put you at risk. Dangerous fumes include car exhaust, smoke, fumes from faulty domestic appliances, such as boilers, or blocked chimneys, fumes from smouldering foam-filled upholstery, such as sofas, and tobacco smoke. Dry-cleaning solvents and some other chemicals also give off toxic fumes.

DAMAGE FROM FUMES

Accidental or deliberate inhalation of fumes – whether from a cigarette or the smoke in a burning building – is very damaging. The extent of the damage depends on the length of exposure and the type of fume. The likelihood of fume inhalation increases dramatically if the fire or leakage is in an enclosed space. It is important to know that people are usually overcome by the fumes of a fire well before the flames reach them.

Children and the elderly are the groups most vulnerable to fumes; children because of their size, and the elderly because they are generally less robust. Another problem is that injury to the casualty may not be obvious until up to 36 hours after exposure to the fumes, by which time irreparable damage to the lung tissue may have occurred.

Why are fumes harmful?

Fire eats up oxygen, as do the materials that burn in a fire, which means little is left for a casualty to breathe. The burning materials give off toxic gases such as carbon monoxide and cyanide. These poison the casualty as they breathe in and irritate the lining of their lungs, making them wheeze and cough. The heat of the fire burns the mouth, throat and upper airways, which then swell and obstruct entry of air even more.

What to do in an emergency

As serious damage can be done by fumes, always assess the situation before rushing in to a potentially lethal scene. You should not make a rescue attempt if it puts your own life at risk; do not go into a fume-filled building or room unless you are sure you are safe. Unless you are well protected yourself, you are likely to meet the same fate as the person you are rescuing. Never enter a room filled with smoke from a fire. If you are attempting a rescue, call the emergency services first.

If you can do so safely, get any trapped people away from the fumes as quickly as possible. Sit them upright, and if they are not too distressed, get them to take deep, slow breaths. If distressed people try to take deep breaths, they will simply become more distressed and breathless. Check for signs of fume inhalation, and also burns and any other injuries that may have been sustained in the accident. While waiting for the emergency services, check the casualty's vital signs and begin resuscitation if necessary.

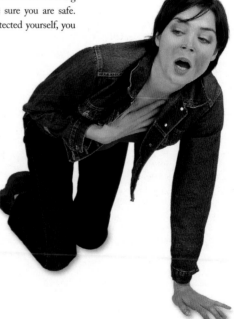

SIGNS AND SYMPTOMS OF SMOKE FUME INHALATION

➤ A hoarse voice or no voice at all.

➤ Drooling or dribbling.

➤ Soot in the nostrils or phlegm.

➤ Singed hairs around the nostrils.

➤ Wheezing.

➤ Noisy breathing on inhaling.

➤ Burns around the mouth and neck.

➤ A large area of burns on any part of the body.

➤ Confusion.

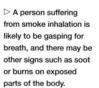
▷ A person suffering from smoke inhalation is likely to be gasping for breath, and there may be other signs such as soot or burns on exposed parts of the body.

IS YOUR HOME SAFE?

Many cases of fire and fume inhalation occur in the home, but with a few simple safety measures the risk of an accident can be greatly reduced. Follow these guidelines to safeguard your family, friends and home-based employees:

- Fit smoke detectors. These reduce the number of deaths from fires by 60 per cent. They should be fitted on every floor of your home, including any areas, such as hallways, shared with other people. Check regularly that they work.
- Boilers and central heating systems should be serviced by a professional boiler engineer/plumber once a year.
- Gas appliances should be checked on a regular basis.
- Motor engines should not be left on in an enclosed space, for example a car engine running in a garage or a petrol-powered mower running in a garage or shed.
- Tobacco smoke is a lethal cocktail containing over 4000 chemicals, all of which can injure the lungs in both the short term and the long term. Emphysema and lung cancer are the well-known conditions associated with smoking, but tobacco also causes many other disorders, such as chronic bronchitis. Giving up smoking is one of the most effective steps that you can take to improve your health. Passive smoking is also a health risk, so avoid smoky atmospheres. Smoking has been implicated in the causes of sudden infant death syndrome (cot death).

- All upholstered furniture made today must by law be fire retardant. Until the end of the twentieth century, when these laws were introduced, upholstered furniture could give off cyanide fumes in a fire. These fumes kill within 40 seconds of exposure and have caused many hundreds of deaths. Take extra care with old upholstered furniture, such as sofas, armchairs and beds, as they are unlikely to have been made under the latest rigorous safety standards.
- Never use aerosol sprays and dry-cleaning products in a confined area.
- Solvents burn at low temperatures, and are easily ignited. Store them away from ignition sources, properly labelled, and never smoke near them.
- Purchase a carbon monoxide monitor and keep a regular check on emissions from heating appliances.

Outside the home, make sure that there are smoke detectors at your place of work and at your child's nursery or school, childminder's premises, and anywhere else where they spend any length of time.

How to avoid fume damage

If you are in a situation where you have to escape from fumes, you need to employ a coordinated set of actions that, ideally, has been discussed previously with other members of the household. This should include a place for you to meet and be accounted for outside the building. If you are away from the house during the day and your children are cared for by someone else, make sure that they know what to do in an emergency.

ESCAPING FROM FUMES

Leave as fast as possible. Do not stop too long to find the source of the smoke – you will put yourself and others at risk of inhaling a toxic level of fumes.

As you escape, lie low on the floor and crawl below the level of the heat and fumes. Otherwise, you may be overcome by fumes before you have time to act.

Smoke inhalation causes confusion and disorientation. If the smoke is so thick that you cannot see, work your way towards a safe exit by sticking to familiar walls. Always feel a door before you open it; if it is hot, leave it shut. It will provide a barrier to fire and fumes for as long as it is closed and standing.

CARBON MONOXIDE POISONING

Carbon monoxide is one of the most toxic fumes. It has no taste or smell so is hard to detect. It is present in exhaust fumes, most types of smoke and can escape from defective gas or paraffin heaters and blocked chimney flues. A large amount of carbon monoxide is quickly fatal, but most cases occur more gradually as a result of a slow leakage from a faulty appliance. Simple gauges are available that indicate whether there is a leakage near a heater.

Symptoms of long-term exposure

➤ Irritability, confusion and bizarre behaviour.

➤ Headache, nausea and vomiting.

Symptoms of sudden exposure

➤ Lips and tissues lining the mouth turn cherry red.

➤ Distressed breathing pattern leading very quickly to a loss of consciousness.

Action in suspected carbon monoxide poisoning

➤ Get the victim out into the fresh air without delay.

➤ Loosen any tight clothing worn by the casualty.

➤ Call an ambulance immediately. The casualty may need special hyperbaric oxygen treatment, so it is essential that you act quickly to obtain professional help.

Drowning: what to do

Drowning is the third most common cause of accidental death. It can happen not only in the sea and rivers but also in swimming pools and garden ponds, and even in the bath. Falling asleep in the bath through tiredness or being drunk can cause a fatal accident. A toddler can drown in just a few inches of water, so you must never leave a young child alone in the bathroom or anywhere near water, even if it is very shallow. Knowing what to do in a drowning incident, and doing it as effectively and quickly as possible, can save someone's life.

Many of those who die through drowning are children and teenagers. It is not only non-swimmers who drown. Someone may have a heart attack while in the water, a boating accident may cause head injury, or a normally good swimmer may panic in a strong current or if they have cramp.

WHAT IS DROWNING?

Drowning is submersion in water causing death by suffocation. Most people die from "wet drowning", where water enters the lungs and rapidly causes respiratory failure and death. Sometimes a casualty may survive but deteriorate later from damage caused by fluid in the lungs ("secondary drowning"). "Dry drowning" occurs when a small amount of water makes the upper airways go into spasm, causing suffocation. Dry drowning can also cause cardiac arrest.

The effect of cold water

Cold water can be a blessing or a curse. Sometimes, especially in children, the cold water shuts the body down; the heart rate drops and blood vessels constrict in major organs and muscles, so that heart and brain function are prioritized. Hypothermia sets in and the body's demand for oxygen drops dramatically. In this state of "hibernation" people have survived for up to 40 minutes under water.

However, a more common reaction to cold water is for the casualty to take an automatic and involuntary gasp as they hit the water, and then start hyperventilating. They may then drown before they have a chance to swim to safety. This is known as cold shock.

> **SIGNS AND SYMPTOMS OF NEAR DROWNING**
>
> ➤ No breathing or laboured breathing.
>
> ➤ Confusion, irritability or loss of consciousness.
>
> ➤ Cold, blue skin.
>
> ➤ Cough with frothy pink sputum.

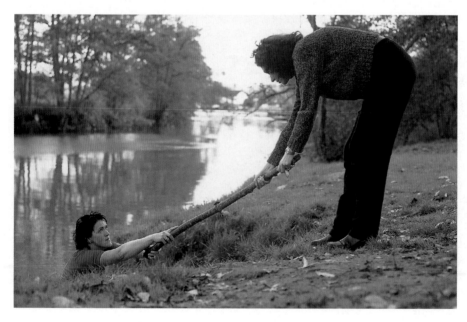

◁ Never jump in the water when dealing with a potential drowning. Hand the person something to hold on to. If nothing is available, lie down and extend your arms so that they can haul themselves up to the safety of the bank.

FIRST AID FOR DROWNING

Remember that the casualty may have swallowed a lot of water, as well as inhaling it. If they vomit, they may inhale the swallowed water into their lungs. To avoid this occurring, try to keep their head lower than the rest of their body when you take them out of the water.

If the casualty is not breathing, do as follows. If the water is shallow enough for you to stand, start rescue breaths in the water. Never attempt rescue breaths in deeper water unless you are trained and practised in lifeguard skills. If the casualty's heart has stopped, remove them from the water and start CPR.

Follow DRSABC until help arrives.

Do not try to empty their lungs and stomach of water.

Keep them warm, as they may be suffering from hypothermia. Take off the wet clothes – but only if you have dry ones to use in their place. Cover the ground under them, as heat is lost via this route.

If they start breathing; place in the recovery position, protecting their neck and spine. As there is a risk of secondary drowning, they must go to hospital, even if they appear to have completely recovered.

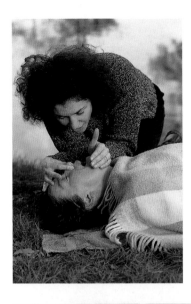

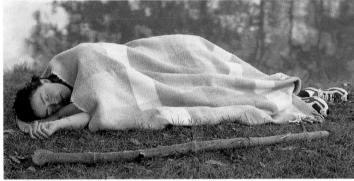

RESCUE SAFETY TIPS

➤ Do not enter the water if you can avoid it (never dive in). Water rescue is a skilled operation for which you need training.

➤ Throw the person a rope attached to a buoyancy aid and tow them ashore, or use a rowing boat to get them ashore.

➤ Remember that, in cold water, hypothermia may make it difficult to detect signs of a circulation.

◁ Lose no time in resuscitating. If you are alone, act as you would when resuscitating a child and perform CPR for 1 minute before going for help.

▽ If breathing, place the casualty in the recovery position, keeping them warm and well covered until the emergency services arrive.

PREVENTION OF DROWNING

To minimize the chances of an accidental drowning, follow these guidelines:

➤ Children should be supervised when they are near water – at the beach, by a lake, a pond or paddling pool. Even competent swimmers should be watched. Toddlers have drowned in minute amounts of water. Any water in the home should be kept covered – even fish tanks and toilets.

➤ Avoid alcohol if going for a swim. Many drownings are linked with excessive alcohol intake, especially in teenagers.

➤ Fence off swimming pools and ponds. Make sure the gate is self-shutting and the catch too high for a child to reach.

➤ Keep away from unfamiliar rivers, lakes or ponds, and never dive into unexplored or shallow waters.

➤ Ask the lifeguard on the beach about swimming conditions such as hidden currents or other hazards.

➤ Never swim outdoors if there is a storm brewing, as the risk of lightning striking the water is high and lethal.

Hanging and strangling: what to do

SEE ALSO

➤ What is first aid?, p16

➤ Responsiveness and the airway, p32

➤ The recovery position, p40

Both hanging and strangling involve compression of the windpipe and major blood vessels in the neck, which eventually causes death. In hanging, when the body is suspended by a noose around the neck, the neck is often broken. Strangling is constriction around the neck. Babies and young children are very vulnerable to strangulation by items such as cot rails, banisters or railings. Such accidents occur with adults too, for example if clothing is caught in machinery. However, deliberate hanging as a form of suicide is also a possibility.

Although most cases of strangling in babies and children are accidents, hanging is a common method of suicide in men, and strangulation is often the method used in homicide. Death occurs because constriction of blood vessels in the neck stops oxygen reaching the brain, rather than because the airway is blocked. In hangings, the situation can be complicated because the neck is often broken.

It is essential to remove the constricting item and give first aid as quickly as possible to give the best chance of restoring breathing. If you are dealing with a hanging casualty you must handle them very carefully to avoid aggravating a spinal injury.

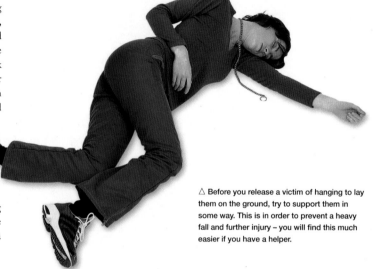

△ Before you release a victim of hanging to lay them on the ground, try to support them in some way. This is in order to prevent a heavy fall and further injury – you will find this much easier if you have a helper.

SIGNS OF HANGING OR STRANGLING

➤ Numerous tiny haemorrhages above the constriction line, including the whites of the eyes.

➤ Bruising, scratches and swelling around the neck – even finger marks may be obvious.

➤ If the casualty is still conscious, their neck will be very tender.

➤ Very noisy breathing, due to the swelling around the airway, as well as a muffled voice and cough.

REDUCING THE RISKS

Babies under three months old are vulnerable to accidental strangling on cot bars, other railings or dummies on a string around their necks. They are not strong enough to physically push themselves out of trouble. Toddlers may lie with their neck over an object, and their body weight is enough to cause strangulation. Never leave babies and children alone in the house and be vigilant for hazards.

Older children, particularly boys, tend to take great risks when they are playing, and climbing trees and making dens are especially treacherous sources of potential danger. Children should always be made aware of the possible consequences – preferably without spoiling their fun and without making them terrified of anything and everything around them. Play with younger siblings should be supervised if at all possible.

Automatic doors in shops and public buildings, and electric car windows, are responsible for significant numbers of accidental stranglings. Getting dangling clothing caught in escalators is another potential hazard. Always watch children very carefully whenever they are around such devices.

FIRST AID FOR HANGING

You need to act swiftly in an incident of hanging or strangling as the combination of a compressed airway and a possible neck injury can lead to a very rapid death. Your aim is to remove the constriction, restore breathing and summon the emergency services.

If the casualty is still hanging, try to support their body as you lift them down (call for help with this if you can).

Cut off the rope or constricting object as quickly as you can.

Lay them flat and assess their ABC. Be aware that there may be spinal injury at the neck, and so you must not over-flex the neck during any resuscitation efforts.

If they are breathing, place them in the recovery position while protecting their spine. You can then go for help.

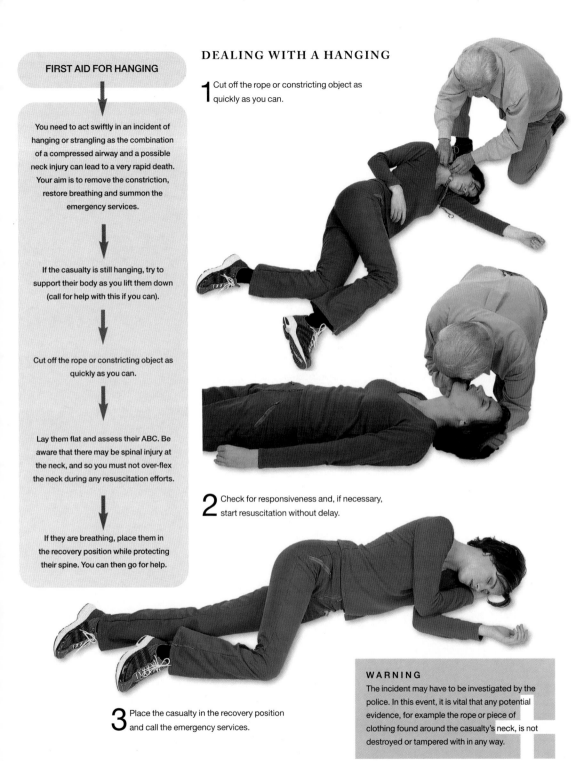

1 Cut off the rope or constricting object as quickly as you can.

2 Check for responsiveness and, if necessary, start resuscitation without delay.

3 Place the casualty in the recovery position and call the emergency services.

WARNING

The incident may have to be investigated by the police. In this event, it is vital that any potential evidence, for example the rope or piece of clothing found around the casualty's neck, is not destroyed or tampered with in any way.

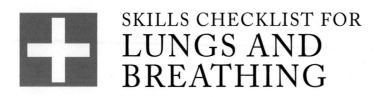

SKILLS CHECKLIST FOR
LUNGS AND BREATHING

KEY POINTS

- Always take any breathing difficulty seriously, and watch closely for deterioration ☐

- Swiftly follow basic guidelines for dealing with breathing difficulties, even if you don't know the root cause of the problem ☐

- Never put yourself at risk when dealing with noxious fume or drowning scenarios ☐

- Use common sense vigilance to prevent all kinds of strangling and hanging accidents ☐

SKILLS LEARNED

- Recognizing the signs and symptoms of breathing problems ☐

- How to help an asthma sufferer during an attack ☐

- Recognizing the severity of an asthma attack ☐

- How to treat hyperventilation ☐

- How to help casualties who have inhaled toxic fumes ☐

- Preventing and dealing with drowning ☐

- Dealing with hanging and strangulation ☐

5

HEART AND CIRCULATION

The heart and circulation are together responsible for providing every single cell in the body with blood – without blood there is no life. When things go wrong with this system, the outcome can quickly be catastrophic, so it is important to be prepared. This chapter describes the first aid to be given in conditions that affect the circulation, such as shock and anaphylaxis. Appropriate first-aid techniques are also given for heart attack and other abnormal heart conditions, including angina, heart failure and cardiac arrest. However, calling an ambulance is the single most important piece of action that can be taken to save life.

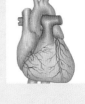

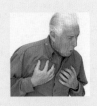

Understanding the cardiovascular system

SEE ALSO
➤ What is first aid?, p16
➤ Cardiac compressions, p36
➤ Full resuscitation sequence, p38

The cardiovascular system is made up of the heart ("cardio") and the blood vessels ("vascular"). The heart – which is essentially a large, powerful muscle about the size of your clenched fist – pumps blood at an average rate of 60–80 times a minute for a person's entire lifespan. The heart and the circulatory system can develop a range of disorders, due to the great demands placed on them. A number of these problems call for prompt emergency first-aid techniques in order to save the casualty's life.

THE HEART

Situated between the lungs, the heart is slightly to the left side of the body. The hollow area inside the heart muscle is made up of two separate compartments: one on the left and one on the right.

In healthy people, these separate heart compartments have no communication with each other. However, some babies are born with a communication between the two – a condition known as having a "hole in the heart".

Each of the compartments has two chambers, an upper atrium and a lower ventricle, giving four compartments in total: the left ventricle and atrium, and the right ventricle and atrium.

THE BLOOD VESSELS

The ventricles send blood to all parts of the body through the arteries, which branch out all over the body into smaller vessels called arterioles. These then become minute vessels called capillaries, which form a network that bathes all body tissues allowing easy exchange of oxygen, nutrients, carbon dioxide and other waste products. The capillaries then join with tiny vessels called venules, which form larger and larger veins, until the vena cavae arrive back at the right side of the heart.

THE CIRCULATION

The blood arriving at the right side of the heart has been around the body and therefore has a low oxygen content. This deoxygenated blood is a dark red colour, rather than the bright red colour it will turn when it has been through the lungs and has filled up with oxygen. This blood arrives back at the heart through the veins. The two veins that lead into the heart are the vena

STRUCTURE OF THE HEART

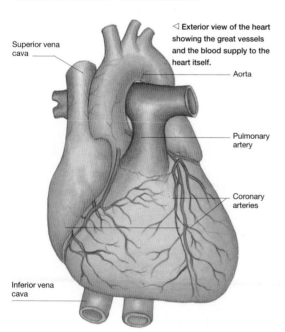

◁ Exterior view of the heart showing the great vessels and the blood supply to the heart itself.

Superior vena cava

Aorta

Pulmonary artery

Coronary arteries

Inferior vena cava

▽ Cross-section through the heart showing the four chambers surrounded by a thick muscular layer around the outside.

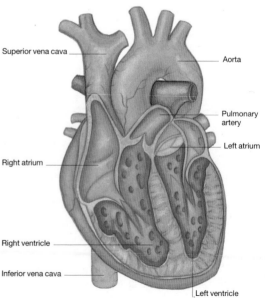

Superior vena cava

Aorta

Pulmonary artery

Left atrium

Right atrium

Right ventricle

Inferior vena cava

Left ventricle

CIRCULATING OXYGEN IN THE BLOOD

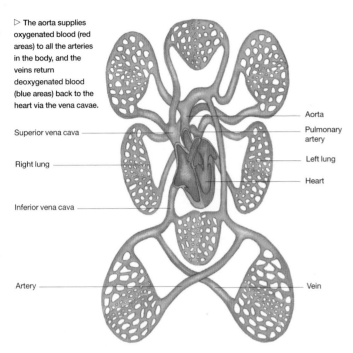

▷ The aorta supplies oxygenated blood (red areas) to all the arteries in the body, and the veins return deoxygenated blood (blue areas) back to the heart via the vena cavae.

- Superior vena cava
- Right lung
- Inferior vena cava
- Artery

- Aorta
- Pulmonary artery
- Left lung
- Heart
- Vein

ARTERIES AND VEINS

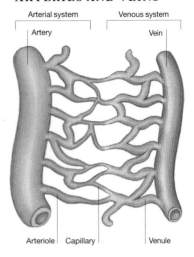

Arterial system — Artery

Venous system — Vein

Arteriole | Capillary | Venule

△ Close-up of a section of the circulatory system. The arterial system, which carries oxygenated blood (red), runs into smaller and smaller arteries until it reaches the tiny veins in the venous system, which carries deoxygenated blood (blue). The veins gradually enlarge until the blood reaches the vena cavae.

cavae. Deoxygenated venous blood arrives in the right atrium, moves down into the right ventricle, and is then pumped through the lungs and back into the left atrium. This fresh, oxygenated blood passes into the left ventricle and then exits the heart via the aorta (the body's biggest vessel), starting its journey round the body. The whole process – including the time taken for the chambers to fill with blood and then contract and circulate the blood – takes about 0.8 seconds at rest, or less when the pulse is rapid.

THE BLOOD

Blood carries nutrients around the body, as well as taking oxygen from, and carbon dioxide to, the lungs. It protects against blood loss through its clotting ability, and infection through its white blood cells.

Fifty-five per cent of blood is made up of a straw-coloured clear fluid called plasma, which is also rich in proteins. When bleeding occurs, we lose plasma, and the blood volume drops. Eventually, there is not

enough blood for the heart to pump, and the circulatory system collapses. Death swiftly follows. Within the plasma float red and white blood cells, plus substances (such as platelets) that are needed for clot-forming. White cells are mainly involved in fighting infection, while red cells carry oxygen.

WHAT IS THE PULSE?

Our pulse is caused by the aorta springing back down to its normal size, having been filled with blood from the heart. This drives

▽ The "carotid" pulse in the neck is often a good one to find. Use two fingers to feel in the groove on either side of the windpipe.

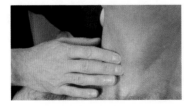

oxygen-rich blood around the body, and the force of the aorta recoil travels along the large arteries – it can be felt wherever an artery lies close to the surface of the skin. Use two fingers to feel for an adult's or child's pulse at the thumb side of the wrist, at the neck or on the front of the arm at the elbow joint. A baby's pulse is best felt on the inside of the upper arm.

It can be much trickier than most people imagine to determine whether someone has a pulse, so this check is often best left to those with medical experience. Remember that vital signs such as coughing, gasping, twitching or blinking also indicate a circulation, and anyone can check for those.

▽ Practise feeling for a pulse. Try on an adult and also on a child.

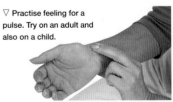

Dealing with shock

SEE ALSO

➤ What is first aid?, p16

➤ Full resuscitation sequence, p38

➤ Managing anaphylactic shock, p74

Shock is a serious condition caused by a sudden and dramatic drop in blood pressure. Without swift medical attention, shock can be life-threatening. It can be caused by any illness or injury that causes too little blood to circulate around the body, such as a heart attack or serious bleeding. This deprives the body of oxygen, leading to the pale, cold, collapsed state that typifies shock. This so-called physiological or circulatory shock must not be confused with the psychological or emotional shock that often occurs after a traumatic event.

Normally, the circulation provides a perfect balance between delivering oxygen and other nutrients to all cells in the body and removing toxic waste products. If this system fails and the amount of blood circulating around the body drops, the combined effect of a lack of oxygen reaching vital organs and a build-up of toxins leads to circulatory shock. If untreated or not attended to quickly enough, shock can be fatal.

WHAT CAUSES SHOCK?

Any trauma or illness that reduces blood circulation is capable of causing shock. Blood circulation can fail for many different reasons. If the heart is unable to pump effectively, after a heart attack for example, shock will follow. Abnormal heart rhythm can lead to shock. Electrocution can cause the heart to stop pumping blood.

Another common cause of shock is excessive loss of body fluids, which may be due to blood loss after a serious accident or fluid loss caused by extensive burns or prolonged diarrhoea and vomiting. A person can lose up to 0.5 litre (1 pint) of blood without any effect; after a loss of 2 litres (3.5 pints), symptoms of shock become apparent; and after losing 3 litres (5 pints) of blood, which is half the body's normal capacity, the end stages of shock, including loss of consciousness and heart failure, appear.

A severe head or spinal injury might affect control of the body's blood flow. The blood vessels may widen abnormally in severe infections and some types of poisoning. A severe allergic reaction in susceptible people may lead to the same symptoms – a very specific and rapidly life-threatening condition known as anaphylactic shock.

SIGNS AND SYMPTOMS OF CIRCULATORY SHOCK

➤ Pale or grey skin that feels cold and clammy.

➤ Fast, weak pulse.

➤ Profuse sweating.

➤ Fast, shallow breathing.

➤ Dizziness and faintness.

➤ Nausea and vomiting.

➤ Blurred vision.

➤ Thirst.

➤ Yawning, sighing, and gasping for air.

➤ Restlessness.

➤ Anxiety and/or confusion.

➤ Loss of consciousness.

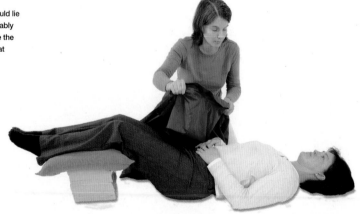

▷ If the casualty is conscious, they should lie down with their legs supported comfortably on an object that raises their legs above the level of their heart. (Do not raise legs that may be fractured, however.) The knees should be bent, as shown, to prevent straining the hamstring tendon at the back of the knee. You might want to pad the object with a folded blanket, garment or cushion. Do not raise their head up on cushions, as this restricts the airway – place on a blanket or similar if needed. Once in position, cover the casualty to keep them warm.

FIRST AID FOR CIRCULATORY SHOCK

If the casualty is unconscious, check DRSABC. Start resuscitating, if necessary. Get someone to control heavy bleeding, if possible.

If the casualty is unconscious but breathing, put them in the recovery position. Stop any heavy bleeding.

If the casualty is conscious, lie them down and calm them. Staunch any heavy bleeding.

Call the emergency services, if you have not already done so.

Check the body for fractures, wounds, and burns. Deal with these as necessary; make sure any heavy bleeding is controlled.

Unless you think their legs may be fractured, place their legs on a low, padded support (with legs higher than heart).

Cover the casualty with a blanket, and try to keep them calm and reassured.

Do not give the casualty anything to eat or drink. Moisten an uncomfortably dry mouth with a wet flannel or towel.

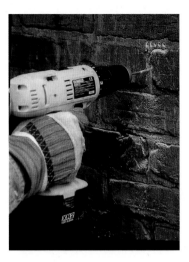

△ Electrocution is one of the traumas that can lead to circulatory shock. A common cause of electrocution around the home is using electrical DIY or gardening equipment.

SYMPTOMS OF SHOCK

In reaction to the reduced circulation of blood, the body directs blood to vital areas such as the heart and lungs, and away from the skin. This makes the skin cold and pale. The body releases adrenaline as an emergency response and this causes a rapid pulse and sweating. As the blood flow weakens further, the brain begins to suffer from lack of oxygen, leading to nausea, dizziness, blurred vision, and confusion. If blood circulation is not restored rapidly, the casualty will start gasping for breath and will soon lose consciousness.

WHAT YOU CAN DO TO HELP

If you think you have come across a casualty in shock, it is crucial to call the emergency services because medical help is always necessary. First-aid measures can help maintain the limited blood circulation to the brain, heart and lungs while waiting for expert help. Should the casualty slip into unconsciousness, you must assess them (ABC) and then administer life-saving techniques as necessary, for as long as you are able or until expert help arrives at the scene.

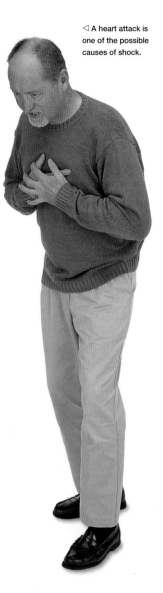

◁ A heart attack is one of the possible causes of shock.

WARNING

Do not try to warm the casualty by any means other than by covering with a blanket. Avoid hot water bottles, electric blankets, fan heaters or any other form of direct heat, as overheating the body will increase the danger.

Managing anaphylactic shock

SEE ALSO

➤ What is first aid?, p16

➤ Full resuscitation sequence, p38

➤ Dealing with bites and stings, p108

Anaphylactic shock is a massive allergic reaction that can develop a short time after contact with a trigger substance. This is a potentially fatal condition caused by the body's inappropriate response to a substance that usually has no serious effect: a food, a drug or an insect sting, for example. It is a form of circulatory shock, but the effects are so sudden and so dramatic that a susceptible person needs to carry an injection of adrenaline in case of accidental exposure. Once the condition has developed, the risk of anaphylaxis lasts for life.

What causes anaphylactic shock? The body's immune system overreacts to what it sees as a foreign body, even though, in most cases it would not cause any reaction. People become sensitized to a substance, often at an early age, and may not initially have any reaction to the substance – it will be the second and subsequent exposures that lead to anaphylaxis. From that time on, such people will remain at risk for the rest of their lives.

Even a tiny amount of the substance can set off a reaction – a trace of peanut oil in a sandwich might be enough for a person sensitive to nuts. Their body releases a massive amount of histamine; this makes their blood vessels dilate and leak fluid, and the lungs go into spasm, causing the symptoms of asthma. The most common causes of anaphylaxis are peanuts, sesame oil, fish, shellfish, dairy products, eggs, wasp or bee stings, rubber, penicillin, other drugs or injections.

People known to be allergic to peanuts, for example, must be very vigilant when buying processed foods, ensuring that they check the ingredients label to check for nut traces. They must also take great care when ordering food in restaurants and even more so if buying food from street markets and stalls.

RECOGNIZING ANAPHYLAXIS

Anyone who has reacted to any substance – even to a mild extent – should be referred to an allergy specialist, because subsequent reactions can be sudden and severe. The specialist cannot always identify exactly

SIGNS AND SYMPTOMS OF ANAPHYLACTIC SHOCK

➤ Intensely itchy rash, often with white raised areas.

➤ A sudden drop in blood pressure (difficult to determine and not visible).

➤ Extreme anxiety, including a sense of imminent death.

➤ Swollen face, lips, tongue and throat.

➤ Rapid pulse.

➤ Puffy eyes.

➤ Difficulty speaking or swallowing.

➤ Wheezing, tight chest and breathing difficulty.

➤ Abdominal pain, feelings of nausea and vomiting.

➤ Faintness.

➤ Loss of consciousness.

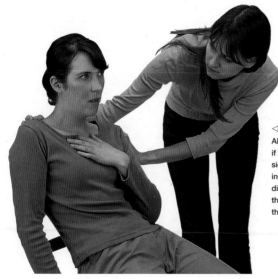

◁ Check through the ABC of resuscitation if necessary. Look for signs of shock, including breathing difficulty, swelling of the mouth, tongue or throat and pale skin.

what has caused the reaction, but skin prick and blood tests may be useful. In some cases of food allergy, a challenge test will be carried out in which minute quantities of the suspect allergen are ingested. This is the only certain way to confirm the allergen. Such a test is done only in a hospital setting under very strict guidelines and only if the patient and their family are happy to undergo it.

In some countries, desensitizing injections are given to reduce a person's sensitivity to a substance. However, this can induce anaphylaxis, and many people feel the risk is too great.

FIRST AID FOR ANAPHYLAXIS

People with a history of anaphylaxis should carry adrenaline injections with them. Search in their bag for the medicine if they are too ill to do so themselves. Get them to inject themselves. Only administer these injections yourself if you are highly trained and practised in this skill – incorrect practice can cause very serious damage. If they continue to suffer severe symptoms, with mouth and lip swelling or breathing difficulties, they should have a second injection.

If the casualty is carrying an asthma reliever inhaler (usually in a blue container), this may help to relieve any wheezing or breathing difficulty.

Dial the emergency services. Make the casualty sit up and keep them comfortable until the ambulance arrives.

Insist that the sufferer go to hospital, even if their reaction was mild and they feel better. Anaphylaxis can recur several hours after contact with the agent and it may be more serious next time around.

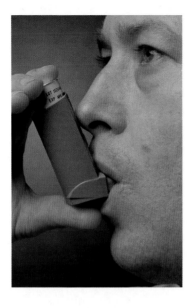

△ If the casualty is having difficulty breathing and they carry a reliever inhaler (usually blue), get them to use this to ease their breathing. Always try to get them to take this themselves – only assist if absolutely necessary.

TIPS FOR ANAPHYLAXIS SUFFERERS

➤ If you are allergic to a food, be extra careful when eating out. Ask for ingredients details of any dishes you might order, and avoid anything that could contain the allergen.

➤ Read food ingredients labels – look out for lists hidden under sticky price tags. You may miss something vital otherwise. If in doubt, avoid it.

➤ Practise using adrenaline jabs – on an orange, not on other people. Be comfortable with using it before an emergency occurs.

➤ Tell family, friends and work colleagues what happens when you have an allergic reaction, and ensure that key people around you are properly trained in giving adrenaline. If your child is a sufferer, make sure their teachers and friends' parents know about the allergy and understand the importance of getting adrenaline administered.

➤ Wear a medical ID tag of some kind (often worn as a bracelet).

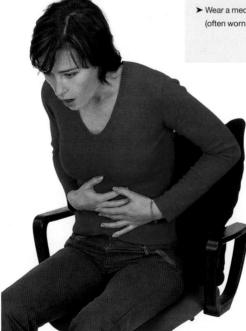

◁ Abdominal pain, nausea and vomiting are among the common symptoms of anaphylactic shock.

Coping with a heart attack

SEE ALSO
➤ What is first aid?, p16
➤ Cardiac compressions, p36
➤ Full resuscitation sequence, p38

Heart attack is one of the leading causes of death in developed countries. For the best chance of survival, immediate hospital admission is necessary. To ensure that this happens you need to recognize when a person is possibly having a heart attack and phone for an ambulance without delay. The cause of a heart attack is nearly always a blockage in one of the major arteries supplying the heart muscle. There may be warning signs, such as angina, or a heart attack may occur suddenly, particularly in people at high risk.

A heart attack is also called a myocardial infarction or coronary thrombosis. This literally means the death of an area of tissue due to an interrupted blood supply. The coronary arteries, which supply the heart muscle, can become furred up with a fatty substance, a condition known as atherosclerosis. Eventually, one or more of these arteries becomes entirely blocked and part of the heart muscle dies as a result. This is a heart attack.

WHO HAS HEART ATTACKS?

Heart attacks become more common as we get older. However, some people are at greater risk of having a heart attack at an early age. These include:

- People with a family history of heart attacks – a close relative who has had a heart attack under the age of 60.
- Anyone with a high blood level of cholesterol. High levels of this fatty substance are linked to an increased risk of atherosclerosis, leading to heart attack.
- Smokers.
- People who are overweight.
- Anyone with high blood pressure.
- People with diabetes.

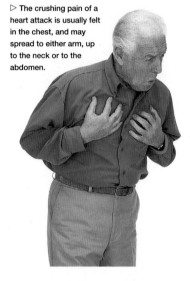

▷ The crushing pain of a heart attack is usually felt in the chest, and may spread to either arm, up to the neck or to the abdomen.

- Female hormones give pre-menopausal women some protection against heart attacks, but after the menopause they are just as much at risk as men.

HOW TO AVOID HEART ATTACKS

If you are in a high-risk group, your doctor will monitor your condition on a regular basis and prescribe drugs. You may also be put on a special diet aimed at reducing the chances of your having a heart attack. For the majority of other people, the risk of heart attack can be reduced by the following guidelines:

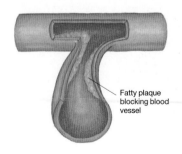

◁ This shows a cross-section of the junction between two arterial blood vessels. A fatty plaque has gathered and is constricting blood flow – atherosclerosis. If this occurs in arteries that supply the heart, a heart attack can occur.

Fatty plaque blocking blood vessel

SIGNS AND SYMPTOMS OF A HEART ATTACK

➤ Chest pain: "crushing" or "tight" pain, usually felt behind the breastbone. The pain may spread to an arm, up to the jaw, neck and teeth, or to the upper or middle part of the abdomen. (Note: some heart attacks are painless.)

➤ Pale/grey colour or blue lips.

➤ Nausea.

➤ Sweating and clammy skin.

➤ Feeling restless.

➤ Rapid, weak pulse.

➤ Breathlessness.

➤ Loss of consciousness.

- Keep within the healthy weight range for your height and build.
- Take regular exercise (it is often best to check with a doctor before starting any exercise regime).
- Give up smoking.
- Eat a balanced diet that is low in animal fat, salt and processed/convenience food.
- Learn to manage stress.

WARNING

Beware a persistent pain that is like indigestion, which is not relieved by remedies for indigestion. Many people have died from a heart attack, having put up with what they thought was a bad bout of indigestion for a few days. If in any doubt, go to see a doctor.

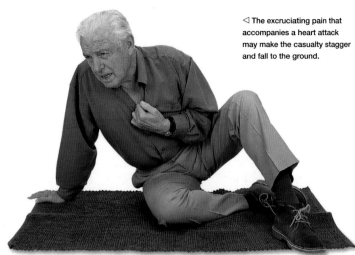

◁ The excruciating pain that accompanies a heart attack may make the casualty stagger and fall to the ground.

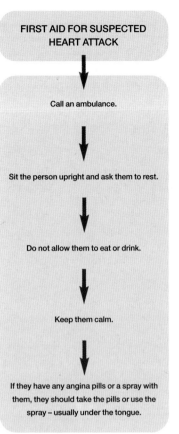

FIRST AID FOR SUSPECTED HEART ATTACK

↓

Call an ambulance.

↓

Sit the person upright and ask them to rest.

↓

Do not allow them to eat or drink.

↓

Keep them calm.

↓

If they have any angina pills or a spray with them, they should take the pills or use the spray – usually under the tongue.

ANGINA PECTORIS

Usually shortened to angina, the term angina pectoris literally means pain in the chest. Angina is caused by temporary blockage of one or more of the coronary arteries. The blockage causes pain that is usually relieved by resting, or special medication that dilates the arteries, or it may settle spontaneously. Angina may lead on to a full-blown heart attack. People at risk of angina are the same group as those at risk of heart attack. Those at risk should avoid the triggers that can bring on angina, which include excessive exercise, cold weather, heavy meals and anxiety.

ADVICE FOR DEALING WITH ANGINA

➤ Ensure that the person is sitting down and resting.

➤ If they have had angina before and have an angina spray, let them administer it themselves, or if necessary, help them to use it.

➤ If the pain is worse than normal or lasts for more than 20 minutes, or if the sufferer's condition starts to deteriorate, call for an ambulance.

▷ Sit the casualty upright and get them to rest until the emergency services arrive.

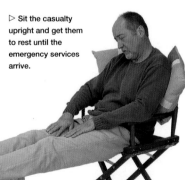

HEART FAILURE

A condition that often develops slowly over several weeks or months, heart failure occurs because the heart fails to pump efficiently enough to keep up with the body's demands. This results in gradually increasing shortness of breath on exertion, and fluid building up in the feet, ankles, legs and abdomen.

However, an acute type of heart failure can develop when fluid suddenly builds up in the lungs, causing a sharp shortness of breath. This may occur alongside a heart attack or on its own. Such a situation requires emergency treatment. Sit the person upright, preferably with their legs over the side of a bed. Keep them calm, and do not let them move out of the bed. Call the emergency services immediately.

SIGNS AND SYMPTOMS OF HEART FAILURE

➤ Breathing is fast, shallow and laboured.

➤ Skin is cold, clammy and sweaty.

➤ Blue lips, skin and nails.

➤ Sense of confusion and acute anxiety.

Dealing with an abnormal heart rate

SEE ALSO

➤ Cardiac compressions, p36

➤ Full resuscitation sequence, p38

➤ Coping with a heart attack, p76

Abnormal heart rate or rhythm, also known as arrhythmia, can cause palpitations and breathlessness. Occasional awareness of one's heartbeat is a normal reaction to fear or excitement, or it may be a sign of too much coffee or alcohol. Frequent palpitations may indicate disease, so this should always be investigated by a doctor. Arrhythmias are common after a heart attack, when the heart muscle is in a state of irritability; this is what often causes the heart to stop working altogether, otherwise known as cardiac arrest.

Everyone occasionally feels their heart "leap" – hopefully from love rather than fear, and sometimes for no apparent reason at all. That sudden thump or feeling that the heart has missed a beat is called a palpitation. This is only worrying when it becomes more than an occasional symptom. Frequent palpitations may be an indication of an illness, such as an overactive thyroid or heart disease. However, panic attacks and anxiety may also be the cause of palpitations, as may be over-indulgence in coffee, cigarettes, alcohol or illegal drugs.

WHAT CONTROLS HEART RATE?

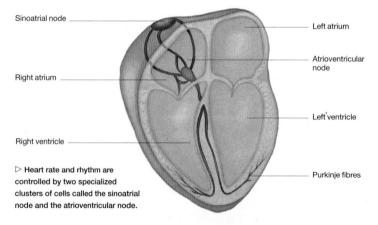

Sinoatrial node

Right atrium

Right ventricle

Left atrium

Atrioventricular node

Left ventricle

Purkinje fibres

▷ Heart rate and rhythm are controlled by two specialized clusters of cells called the sinoatrial node and the atrioventricular node.

HOW THE HEART RATE IS REGULATED

The heart is a muscle that contracts and relaxes continuously and rhythmically between 60 and 80 times a minute, on average, throughout our lives. Heart muscle is unique because it has its own conduction system so it contracts without any outside control. Chemicals such as adrenaline or caffeine can alter the heart rate, as can anxiety, or a drop in blood pressure.

Each contraction of the heart muscle is controlled from within, by the conduction system. This system comprises groups of cells that charge up and fire spontaneously. One group of cells, called the sinoatrial (S/A) node, sets the rhythm for the rest of the heart – it acts as the heart's internal pacemaker. An electrical wave spreads from the S/A node through the atria, until it reaches a second node called the atrioventricular node. It then continues through a right and left branch, until it reaches the outermost parts of the heart. This contains specialized Purkinje fibres – a wiring system that transmits the impulses.

TYPES OF ARRHYTHMIA

Heart rate and rhythm may be either too high or too low. The most serious type of arrhythmia is ventricular fibrillation, which is caused by too high a heart rate in the ventricles (the lower heart chambers). This is the most common cause of death after a heart attack. In ventricular fibrillation, the heart "quivers", rather than beating in a coordinated fashion. The heart cannot pump blood efficiently in this state, and the casualty rapidly loses consciousness and will die as a result of cardiac arrest (when the heart stops) unless the heart can get back into a normal rhythm.

CARDIAC ARREST

A life-threatening emergency situation, cardiac arrest occurs when the heart stops beating. The most common cause is a heart attack, but there are many other causes. After a car accident, cardiac arrest may occur because of massive blood loss, or a collapsed lung. Cardiac arrest may occur in a pulmonary embolism, a condition in which blood clots form in the lungs. Electrocution or a lightning strike injury may cause a cardiac arrest. Asthmatics may have a cardiac arrest during a severe asthma attack.

Cardiopulmonary resuscitation is not a definitive life-saving treatment for cardiac arrest, and can only keep the blood pumping around the body until specialized help is available. The only effective treatment is "defibrillation", in which a high-energy electric shock is applied to the chest wall. The sooner this is done after cardiac arrest, the more likely that the

FIRST AID FOR PALPITATIONS

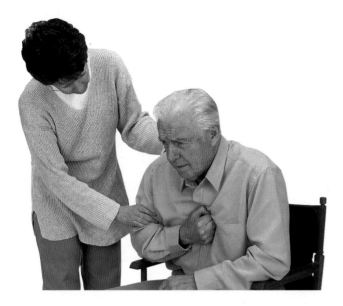

1 Sit the casualty down and reassure them if they are anxious. This may be all that is needed to settle the palpitations. Talk to them to find out whether they have experienced an abnormal heart rate before and whether they have a diagnosed heart condition.

2 Get them to cough, or hold their nose and blow as if popping their ears. If the palpitations do not settle after a few minutes but there are no other symptoms, phone a doctor. If the casualty feels breathless, faint or has chest pains, call an ambulance.

AUTOMATED EXTERNAL DEFIBRILLATOR (AED)

If someone suffers cardiac arrest in a public place, a defibrillator may be available on site. It should be used only by a trained operator.

➤ If you are already carrying out CPR, stop when the defibrillator and its operator are ready.

➤ Make sure you and any other helpers are not touching the victim while the machine is analysing the heart or administering shocks.

➤ The prompts from the defibrillator should be followed until the paramedics arrive.

heart will return to a normal rhythm and resume pumping blood around the body.

Until recently defibrillators could only be used by trained paramedics and doctors. However, a new development has been launched in some areas. This is the automated external defibrillator, which requires some training but is much more user-friendly than the hospital types, and prompts the correct sequence of actions for its use. The rescuer needs to recognize that cardiac arrest may have occurred, and then to attach two sticky pads to the chest wall and switch on the machine. Such equipment is already kept at some busy public places, such as sports stadia, leisure centres and airports. This new technology means that the average citizen, with minimal training, will be able to save a life.

FIRST AID FOR CARDIAC ARREST

The main rule is to assess the casualty according to DRSABC procedure, as follows.

Make sure the casualty's airway is clear and open. Check whether the casualty is breathing. If not, call an ambulance and start giving rescue breaths, 2 at a time.

Assess for signs of circulation. If signs are absent, begin resuscitation, alternating 2 rescue breaths with 15 chest compressions.

Repeat this 2:15 ratio of breaths and compressions until the emergency services arrive.

SIGNS OF CARDIAC ARREST

➤ Loss of consciousness.

➤ Pale, blue skin.

➤ No sign of breathing.

➤ No pulse or heart sounds (for those with medical experience only).

➤ Dilated pupils that do not constrict when a light is directed at the eye (for highly trained first-aiders only).

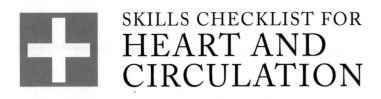

SKILLS CHECKLIST FOR
HEART AND CIRCULATION

KEY POINTS

- Effective blood circulation is essential for an individual to survive ☐

- Always call the emergency services out promptly to shock cases ☐

- Always call the emergency services out promptly if you suspect heart problems – they can quickly become life-threatening ☐

- Frequent heart palpitations must be investigated by a doctor – they are a symptom of various health problems ☐

SKILLS LEARNED

- An understanding of how the circulatory system works ☐

- Recognizing and dealing with circulatory shock ☐

- Recognizing, treating and avoiding anaphylactic shock ☐

- Recognizing and dealing with a heart attack ☐

- Recognizing and dealing with heart failure and angina ☐

- Dealing with palpitations and cardiac arrest ☐

BRAIN AND NERVOUS SYSTEM

The brain is the control centre of the central nervous system, an extraordinarily complex set of mechanisms that is behind every function in the body and mind. Electrical and chemical signals rush around the body causing millions of actions every minute. However, the system is very delicate and easily damaged by injury or disease. Knowing what to do in the event of an accident affecting any part of the nervous system is of prime importance to the outlook for the casualty, and may even save their life. Even something as apparently minor as a headache may warn of a serious condition that must be investigated by a doctor.

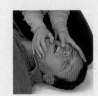

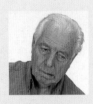

Understanding the nervous system

SEE ALSO

➤ What is first aid?, p16
➤ Dealing with head injury, p84
➤ Coping with headache, p90

The importance of the brain and the central nervous system to the rest of the body cannot be overstated. Every part of the body, and every bodily function, is under its control. For this reason, head and spinal injuries may prove particularly serious and have effects on many parts of the body at some distance from the injury. First aid is of the ultimate importance, particularly maintaining the vital functions of breathing and circulation. Alert the emergency services without delay if you are in any doubt about the casualty's condition.

Human beings have a highly developed and sophisticated nervous system. The brain and nervous system are organized into many parts that serve specific and important functions – together they make up the body's main control centre. All body sensations, muscle contractions, gland secretions and a host of other complex interactions vital to life are relayed through the central nervous system.

HOW THE NERVOUS SYSTEM IS ORGANIZED

The nervous system is divided into two main sections – the central nervous system (CNS), which comprises the brain and the spinal cord, and the peripheral nervous system (PNS), which is made up of all the nerves that branch off the CNS. Nerves from the brain are called cranial nerves and those from the spinal cord are spinal nerves. The PNS is further broken down into nerves under voluntary control, such as those that control the muscles used for conscious movements, and nerves under involuntary control, such as those governing our internal systems – our heart rate and the changing size of our pupil in response to light, for example. The part of the system that regulates actions over which we have no voluntary control is known as the autonomic nervous system (ANS).

We take in information through our five senses – sight, smell, hearing, touch and taste – and the brain acts on this information through the motor system. For example, when a toddler touches a hot oven, the brain receives a message via the senses and acts through the motor system to make the muscles move. The toddler pulls the hand away from the painful stimulus. Although this is a reflex action, the brain remembers the pain and the toddler will be wary of touching the oven in future.

THE CENTRAL NERVOUS SYSTEM

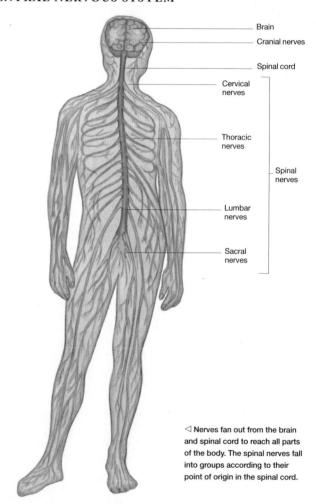

Brain
Cranial nerves
Spinal cord
Cervical nerves
Thoracic nerves
Lumbar nerves
Sacral nerves
Spinal nerves

◁ Nerves fan out from the brain and spinal cord to reach all parts of the body. The spinal nerves fall into groups according to their point of origin in the spinal cord.

CROSS-SECTION THROUGH THE BRAIN

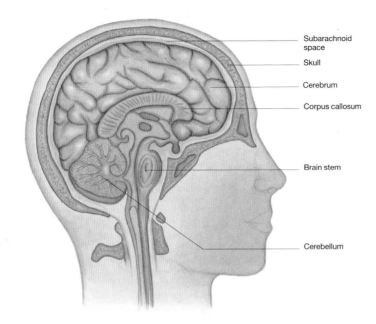

Subarachnoid space

Skull

Cerebrum

Corpus callosum

Brain stem

Cerebellum

MULTIPOLAR NEURONE

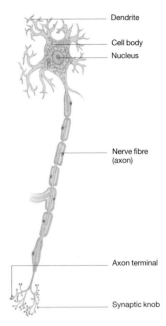

Dendrite

Cell body

Nucleus

Nerve fibre (axon)

Axon terminal

Synaptic knob

THE BRAIN

Our brain controls our thoughts, memories, speech, movements and all the functions of the organs. Divided into three parts, the brain comprises the cerebrum, the cerebellum and the brain stem.

The cerebrum forms the bulk of the brain: it controls sensation, movement, emotion and intellect. The cerebrum is divided into two hemispheres, the left and the right. One of these hemispheres controls speech, and this is called the dominant hemisphere. In right-handed people, this is the left hemisphere, but left-handed people have their dominant hemisphere on the right. The effects of a stroke can, therefore, be very different depending on which hemisphere is affected. Damage to the left hemisphere will cause speech problems in a right-handed person, while a left-hander's speech will be unaffected.

The cerebellum controls coordination of movement, balance and posture. People with damage to their cerebellum sometimes appear drunk and they may

stagger, slur their words and suffer from severe dizziness.

The brain stem regulates the heart rate and breathing, as well as coordinating activities such as coughing, sneezing and swallowing. Life is impossible to sustain if the brain stem is damaged.

NERVES AND NEURONES

The nuts and bolts of the nervous system are cells called neurones and neuroglia. The neurones conduct electrical activity from one part of the body to another, while the neuroglia support and protect the neurones. Billions of these highly specialized cells are joined together to form nerves, which stretch from the brain or spinal cord to every part of the body.

Neurones in the brain are very densely packed and number around 1000 billion. Neurones in the spinal cord and around the body are very long and form an extensive communication system. The cell bodies of neurones are linked together by nerve fibres (axons), and the many projections coming off the cell bodies are called dendrites.

Nerve impulses in the form of electrical signals travel along the neurones at rapid speeds of up to 275 km/h (125 mph). With chemicals called neurotransmitters, signals from the brain are translated into effects at the target cell, for example in a muscle.

PROBLEMS WITH THE NERVOUS SYSTEM

Although peripheral nerves will regenerate if they are sewn back together fast enough, the central nervous system has no such ability. If the spinal cord is severed, it cannot heal or grow back. If nervous tissue is damaged, whether due to a stroke or multiple sclerosis, it is gone forever.

Problems with the nervous system can manifest themselves in a multitude of ways, but they are largely determined by the parts of the brain that are affected. Abnormal electrical activity causes epilepsy, degeneration of nervous tissue may cause dementia or Parkinson's disease, and processes that affect neurochemicals can trigger psychiatric conditions such as depression and schizophrenia.

Dealing with head injury

SEE ALSO

➤ What is first aid?, p16

➤ Full resuscitation sequence, p38

➤ Tackling skull and facial fractures, p156

Serious head injury is a medical emergency, particularly if the casualty loses consciousness. The first-aider should protect the casualty's airway, start resuscitation if necessary and alert the emergency services without delay. A cut or bump on the scalp will lead to a suspicion of head injury, but serious internal injury is often not evident from external signs. It is worth remembering also that the very young and the elderly are especially susceptible to developing delayed reactions to relatively minor head injuries – so such cases may need checking out.

Head injuries are potentially serious because they can damage the brain and surrounding blood vessels. Although the bony skull protects the brain, it also provides an enclosed space in which the brain can be easily shaken and damaged, and where there is little room for any swelling or bleeding following injury.

The main causes of head injuries are road traffic accidents, falls and assaults.

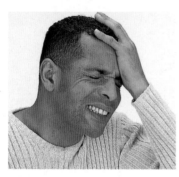

△ A sudden, crushing headache should always be investigated, particularly if it comes on at some point after a blow to the head.

TYPES OF HEAD INJURY

There are five main types of head injury, and casualties may have several simultaneously:

Cuts

Large cuts to the scalp look alarming, but are only likely to be serious if caused by a major blow. A large blow may cause brain damage.

Concussion

Symptoms such as loss of consciousness, short-term memory loss or headache after a head injury are termed concussion. The loss of consciousness may last up to six hours, and the loss of memory 24 hours, with little or no internal damage being suffered.

Contusion

Bruising, or contusion, may occur to the brain after an injury, and this causes swelling of the brain tissue. This may lead to much longer periods of unconsciousness

SIGNS AND SYMPTOMS OF SERIOUS HEAD INJURY

➤ Deep cuts or tears to the scalp, or goose egg swelling over the scalp.

➤ Nausea and/or vomiting.

➤ Severe headache.

➤ Drowsiness or difficulty being roused.

➤ Unequal sized pupils, or pupils that do not respond to light.

➤ Visual disturbance.

➤ Fluid flowing from eyes and/or mouth.

➤ Paralysis, numbness or loss of function over one half of the body.

➤ Problems with balance.

➤ Behaving as though drunk.

➤ Fits, confusion or unconsciousness.

CONTRA-COUP INJURY

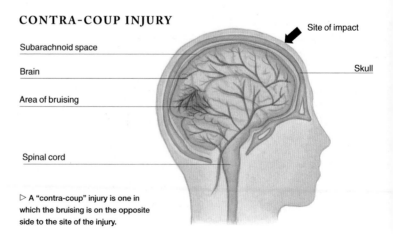

Subarachnoid space

Brain

Area of bruising

Spinal cord

Site of impact

Skull

▷ A "contra-coup" injury is one in which the bruising is on the opposite side to the site of the injury.

POSSIBLE SITE OF BRAIN INJURY
FOLLOWING BLOW TO BACK OF HEAD

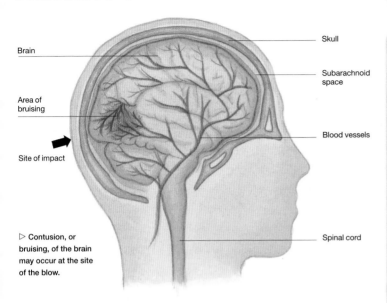

Brain

Area of
bruising

Site of impact

▷ Contusion, or
bruising, of the brain
may occur at the site
of the blow.

Skull

Subarachnoid
space

Blood vessels

Spinal cord

Breathing in vomit while unconscious is the
most common cause of death after a head
injury. The first priority is to protect the
victim's airway by tilting back the jaw.
Always assume that they may have spinal
injuries and protect their neck while trying
to keep their airway open: if trained to do
so, use the jaw thrust to open the airway. If
they are not breathing, start resuscitation.

Carefully apply direct pressure to any
scalp wounds that are bleeding.

Watch for vomiting.

following an accident, and possibly much
longer periods of amnesia after regaining
consciousness. In addition there may be
signs of brain injury in other parts of the
body, such as paralysis, numbness or
changes in breathing.

The bruising may be directly at the site
of the injury, or it may be on the opposite
side of the skull as the brain bounces away
– this is called a contra-coup brain injury.

Haemorrhage

Bleeding within the skull, or haemorrhage,
is a common consequence of head injury.
The tough sheath (dura mater) attached to
the inside of the skull is well supplied with
blood vessels. These may be damaged and
cause bleeding; sometimes the effects are
delayed for several weeks after the injury.

Compression

The skull is an enclosed space, and if there
is any swelling or bleeding within it, a
point is reached when there is no more
room for expansion. Compression of the

SIGNS AND SYMPTOMS OF RISING PRESSURE WITHIN THE SKULL

➤ Intense headache, worse when lying
flat and/or with physical exertion.

➤ Vomiting.

➤ Unequal or dilated pupils.

➤ Weakness on one side of the body.

➤ Noisy, irregular breathing.

➤ Irritable or aggressive behaviour.

brain can lead to quite severe damage and a
wide range of symptoms. In extreme cases,
it can cause brain tissue to squeeze out of
the base of the skull – a condition known
as coning. This is fatal so it is absolutely
vital that any rise in pressure within the
skull is recognized before this happens.

Even after seemingly minor head
injuries, always be very vigilant for signs of
increased cerebral pressure and get help
promptly if you spot any.

If they are conscious, lay them on the floor
with head and shoulders slightly raised. If
unconscious, place them in the recovery
position while protecting their neck.

Call the emergency services.

See how alert they are using AVPU.
Reassure them if they are alert.

Continue to watch their breathing,
circulation and level of consciousness
until help arrives and be prepared to
resuscitate if necessary. Even if they
regain consciousness, insist that they
go to hospital to be checked out.

Coping with epilepsy

SEE ALSO
➤ Responsiveness and the airway, p32
➤ The recovery position, p40
➤ Recognizing a stroke, p88

Epileptic fits, or "seizures", are caused by an instability of electrical activity in the brain. Such fits can be alarming, but there is usually no physical damage to the brain itself. There are over 40 types of seizure, which may be partial (affecting part of the brain) or generalized (affecting the whole brain). These many types range from an "absence" seizure (once called *petit mal*), where the sufferer simply seems to be daydreaming briefly, to a full-blown "tonic-clonic" fit (once called *grand mal*), where the sufferer writhes uncontrollably.

The nature of epileptic seizures depends on which part of the brain is affected. At one end of the scale, there is a brief "absence" of attention; at the other, the major jerking and total unconsciousness (tonic-clonic fit) traditionally associated with epilepsy. Partial seizures may develop into generalized ones. So, for example, someone might start off with one hand affected and progress to a complete tonic-clonic fit. It is reassuring to know that many people only ever have one fit during their lifetime.

WHAT CAUSES SEIZURES?

All kinds of things can cause a seizure:
• Brain damage caused by:
- Head injury;
- Difficulties at birth;
- Reduced brain oxygen (for example, suffocation);
- Brain problems (tumours, bleeding, swelling).
• Certain diseases (diabetes, liver failure).
• Certain poisons (such as pesticides).
• An inherited low "seizure threshold".
• A large intake of alcohol. Also, alcoholics commonly have seizures if they suddenly stop drinking alcohol.

• A high temperature (in children). Children up to the age of five years often have convulsions, typically as part of a feverish illness. They usually grow out of these in middle childhood. Feverish convulsions do not indicate that a child may develop epilepsy later on.
• The cause often remains unknown.

CHARACTERISTICS OF SEIZURES

In an absence seizure, the person typically stops what they are doing and stares into space for 10–15 seconds. They have actually lost consciousness briefly and are unaware of their surroundings. They will then continue as if nothing had happened, and will have no memory of the event.

In a tonic-clonic seizure, the person is fully unconscious for up to 10 minutes and may be very sleepy for an hour or two after the seizure. The main features include:
• A change in mood/behaviour several hours or days before a fit – known as a prodrome.
• Immediately before the fit an imaginary smell or vision may be apparent, or a sense of déjà vu – called an aura.
• Sudden unconsciousness, followed by stiffening of the arms and legs – the tonic

phase. Then jerky movements of the limbs and face – the clonic phase.
• There may be loss of bladder control and the sufferer may bite their tongue.

HOW TO RECOGNIZE EPILEPSY

Someone who has fainted may jerk slightly – this is not epilepsy. There are many other non-epileptic causes of "funny turns".

A person who has had an epileptic seizure will come to in a confused state. It will help them to hear from a witness what has happened, particularly on the first occasion, as this can then be reported to the emergency services or the hospital.

Epilepsy is diagnosed by neurological tests. These include electroencephalography (EEG), in which brain activity is measured by attaching electrodes to the scalp, and a computerized tomography (CT) scan to exclude brain tumour and stroke. A person recently diagnosed with epilepsy needs reassurance and support to build up their confidence for leading a normal life.

COMMON TRIGGERS

➤ Excess alcohol.

➤ Tiredness.

➤ Emotion (stress/excitement).

➤ Failure to take medication regularly.

➤ Certain foods/not eating properly.

➤ Illness.

➤ Hormonal changes.

➤ Flashing lights.

▽ Do not try to restrain someone having an epileptic fit but move any obstacles, such as chairs, out of the way to prevent injury.

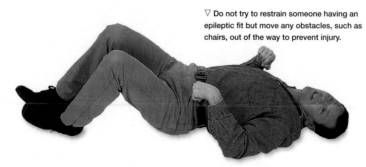
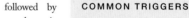

DEALING WITH AN EPILEPTIC FIT

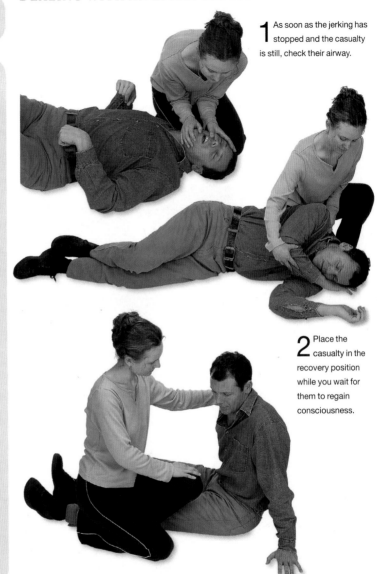

1 As soon as the jerking has stopped and the casualty is still, check their airway.

2 Place the casualty in the recovery position while you wait for them to regain consciousness.

FIRST AID FOR AN EPILEPTIC FIT

You may want to look quickly to see if the casualty is wearing a medical ID tag, or is carrying a card that says they suffer from epilepsy and tells you what to do.

During the seizure: prevent any avoidable injury. Move chairs and other obstacles that might hurt the sufferer out of the way. Never restrain them or put anything in their mouth.

After the seizure: put them into the recovery position and make sure that they have a clear airway – remove any obstacles if you can do so easily.

CALLING THE EMERGENCY SERVICES

If this is their first fit, dial the emergency services, as a hospital assessment is necessary. There is usually no need to call an ambulance for a routine seizure suffered by a diagnosed epileptic. However, you should call an ambulance if:
• They do not stop fitting after 20 minutes.
• The fit is worse than usual: more prolonged or violent.
• They suffer a series of fits with short gaps.
• Serious injury has occurred.
• The person remains unconscious for more than 2–3 minutes.

HOW IS EPILEPSY TREATED?

Epilepsy is usually controlled with anticonvulsant drugs, taken until the sufferer has been seizure-free for 2–3 years. Women with epilepsy considering pregnancy should speak to their doctor first as they may have to be put on a different anticonvulsant drug.

3 Explain to the casualty what happened. Find out whether this has occurred before, and if not, send them to hospital. Ask whether they would like you to contact anyone.

WARNING
People with epilepsy should not swim alone or cycle in traffic-dense areas. Driving is not allowed for a year or even longer after diagnosis, depending on the individual case. The situation is reviewed regularly, and driving may be permitted again if the epilepsy is well controlled and there is no risk of a seizure.

Recognizing a stroke

SEE ALSO

➤ Dealing with an
   abnormal heart rate,
   p78
➤ Coping with
   headache, p90
➤ Managing dizziness
   and fainting, p92

Strokes are caused by a sudden stoppage of the blood supply to part of the brain. They are usually the result of a blood clot or a ruptured artery, and vary in severity: some leave no lasting effects, others cause paralysis on one side of the body, and some prove instantly fatal. Although more common in elderly people, people who smoke, have high blood pressure, or take the combined oral contraceptive pill are at increased risk of having a stroke. First-aid treatment aims to maintain breathing and circulation until the emergency services arrive.

A stroke occurs when the blood supply to a part of the brain is cut off. This may be caused by a blood clot in a vessel in the brain or by bleeding into the brain. A stroke's short- and long-term effects depend on which part of the brain is affected.

A stroke tends to occur very suddenly with very little warning. If you find yourself having to administer first aid to a probable stroke victim, it is important to act swiftly and ensure the emergency services are called without delay.

WHAT CAUSES A STROKE?

Generally, strokes tend to affect older people, and people with high blood pressure or a circulatory problem.

There are also a number of other factors that can increase a person's risk of having a stroke. These include taking the combined oral contraceptive pill, having a high blood cholesterol, being diabetic, smoking, and being overweight.

Atherosclerosis

Atheroma is a thick, fatty substance that builds up in the arteries over the years, gradually narrowing them and eventually blocking them altogether. This condition, known as atherosclerosis, slows the flow of blood around the body and encourages the formation of blood clots. If a blood clot occurs in one of the cerebral arteries, it will cause a stroke.

Embolism

A fragment of material travelling through the bloodstream, often a piece of blood clot, is called an embolus. An embolus may

CROSS-SECTION OF BRAIN AFTER A STROKE

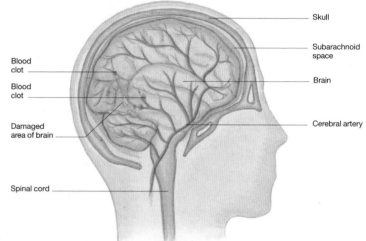

Skull

Subarachnoid space

Brain

Cerebral artery

Blood clot

Blood clot

Damaged area of brain

Spinal cord

△ A common cause of stroke is a blood clot in a cerebral artery, which supplies blood to the brain. This will starve nearby tissue of oxygen and other nutrients, which will cause temporary or permanent loss of function.

arise in the heart, travel to the brain and cause a stroke. Anyone with a heart valve abnormality or an abnormal heart rhythm is more likely to develop an embolus.

Aneurysm

Some people are born with a weakness in one of the arteries at the base of the brain; this is called an aneurysm. It may leak, causing warning headaches, but often it will suddenly burst, causing a severe and often fatal stroke.

HOW TO RECOGNIZE A STROKE

Sometimes there may be prior warning signs of an imminent stroke, with the person feeling very unwell and suffering a severe headache and copious vomiting. The initial symptoms usually happen quickly over minutes or hours, and the situation may deteriorate progressively over several days.

Usually, the part of the body affected is on the opposite side to the side of the brain affected. If the person is right-handed then a left-sided stroke will usually affect their speech. If left-handed, the opposite is true. Occasionally a person may be totally unaware that they have a right or left side at all. For example, they might only eat food on the side of the plate that they are aware of.

CAN STROKE BE PREVENTED?

Although none of us can escape the increased risk of having a stroke that comes with growing older, there are a number of measures we can take to reduce the risk.

Smoking increases the risk of a stroke occurring by several hundredfold, and high blood pressure is also closely linked to a higher chance of having a stroke. People with high levels of cholesterol and other fats in their blood will develop atherosclerosis; this causes a build-up of a fatty substance that blocks the arteries and may cause a stroke, amongst other diseases. All these factors can be controlled by diet, exercise, abstension from smoking and, if necessary, with drugs.

SIGNS AND SYMPTOMS OF A STROKE

➤ Sudden, severe headache.

➤ Dizziness.

➤ Loss of consciousness.

➤ Confusion and slurred speech that could be mistaken for drunkenness.

➤ Dribbling when trying to smile, speak or swallow.

➤ Inability to speak or understand words.

➤ Weakness or complete loss of the ability to use one side of the body.

FIRST AID FOR STROKE

Assess according to DRSABC, and be prepared to resuscitate if necessary.

If you know it is a stroke, call an ambulance – prompt aid is vital.

If unconscious (or unable to keep upright), but breathing, put in the recovery position. This is so that, if they vomit, they do not inhale it into their lungs, which can be fatal (stroke victims often lose their gag reflex).

If conscious, lay them on their back with head and shoulders comfortably raised.

Look quickly for a medical ID tag. The casualty may be suffering from another condition, such as diabetic hypoglycaemia.

Call an ambulance if not called already. Do not give food or water at any stage.

▷ In many stroke casualties, the side of the face droops and they may be unable to speak, smile or swallow without dribbling. There may be loss of sensation in one arm. These symptoms often don't appear until a little while after the initial stroke.

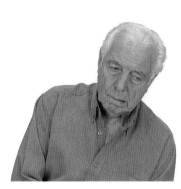

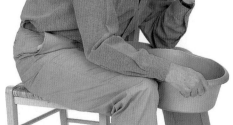

◁ Stroke casualties may vomit copiously. Make sure they are not in a position where they might inhale their vomit, as this can prove fatal.

TRANSIENT ISCHAEMIC ATTACKS

A transient ischaemic attack (TIA) is like a mini-stroke. Symptoms last briefly and totally disappear within 24 hours. TIAs are often a warning sign of a full-blown stroke, there being about a 10 per cent risk that a stroke will happen within a year. The sufferer should be investigated urgently for the cause of the TIA in order to prevent either a recurrence or a full stroke. They will probably be put on aspirin by their doctor, to thin the blood and make clotting less likely.

Coping with headache

SEE ALSO

➤ Dealing with head injury, p84

➤ Recognizing a stroke, p88

➤ Tackling skull and facial fractures, p156

Headaches are such a common complaint that very few people will go through life without experiencing one. Usually a headache is associated with stress, tension, overwork or too much alcohol; it quickly passes with self-help remedies and there is no need for concern.

However, it is important to be aware that severe, persistent or recurrent headaches may have a more serious underlying cause and should be investigated by a doctor. A person experiencing a migraine attack for the first time should also seek the advice of a doctor.

Everybody suffers from headaches at some time in their life and their cause is usually obvious. Persistent headaches that do not ease with simple painkillers, or severe ones that start suddenly, may mean you should see a doctor. Headaches have many different causes, including alcohol, caffeine-withdrawal, lack of fresh air, dehydration (a very common cause, often arising from excess alcohol), stress, menstruation and sinusitis, but very few causes are in any way life-threatening.

Headache following head injury is common and may last for months and even years after the accident. Seek medical attention if there are other symptoms, such as fever, fainting, fits or any discharge from the ears or nose.

TYPES OF HEADACHE

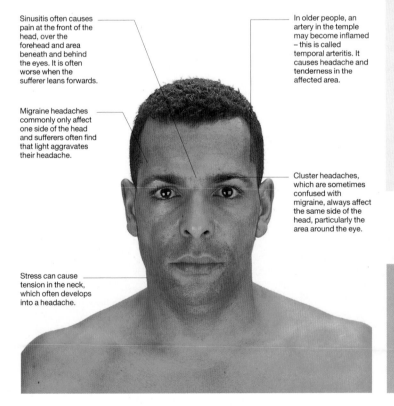

Sinusitis often causes pain at the front of the head, over the forehead and area beneath and behind the eyes. It is often worse when the sufferer leans forwards.

Migraine headaches commonly only affect one side of the head and sufferers often find that light aggravates their headache.

Stress can cause tension in the neck, which often develops into a headache.

In older people, an artery in the temple may become inflamed – this is called temporal arteritis. It causes headache and tenderness in the affected area.

Cluster headaches, which are sometimes confused with migraine, always affect the same side of the head, particularly the area around the eye.

WHEN TO SEE A DOCTOR
A person with any of the following types of headache should be seen by a doctor:

➤ Sudden onset.

➤ Persistent headaches.

➤ Associated with a fever and neck stiffness.

➤ Accompanied by a rash.

➤ Following head injury.

➤ Feels like "the worst headache ever".

➤ Accompanied by persistent or severe vomiting.

➤ Worse when lying flat or straining.

➤ Accompanied by confusion, drowsiness or loss of consciousness.

➤ Accompanied by numbness, tingling of the limbs or any other neurological problem.

➤ Regular headaches starting after the age of 50.

WARNING
Any severe headache that persists for several days should be investigated promptly by a doctor. There may be a serious underlying cause, although in most dangerous conditions, such as a brain tumour or stroke, additional symptoms usually accompany the headache.

MIGRAINE

Migraines are a problem often passed down through generations of a family. Migraine is believed to be caused by blood flow changes in the brain, which lead to chemicals being released that act on the blood vessels in the brain. This causes severe pain, vomiting, and visual problems. The root of these changes is as yet unknown, although the neurotransmitter serotonin may play a big role, as does the food enzyme, tyramine (see "Triggers" box).

Recognizing migraine

Migraines are usually felt on one side of the head, and they might last up to three days. In some people, a migraine attack is preceded by a warning called an aura. This is primarily visual, such as seeing zigzag lines or spots in the field of vision. There may be other symptoms present such as dizziness, tingling, temporary speech difficulties and

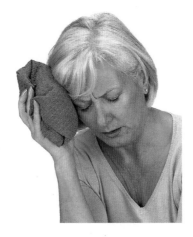

△ Wrapping a bag of frozen vegetables in a cloth and placing it against the headache site may ease the pain a little. Heat applied in the same way may also work.

blurred vision. Since visual problems often accompany migraine it is not advisable to attempt to drive during an attack.

Treating migraine

A large selection of drugs is available to prevent and treat migraine. Both over-the-counter and prescription drugs are available, and it is best to discuss the options with your doctor. You need to consider the frequency of attacks, how long each attack lasts and the extent to which the debility affects everyday life.

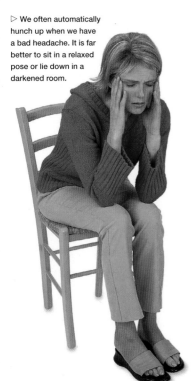

▷ We often automatically hunch up when we have a bad headache. It is far better to sit in a relaxed pose or lie down in a darkened room.

HOME REMEDIES FOR ROUTINE HEADACHES

➤ Over-the-counter painkillers.

➤ An ice pack or heating pad over the site of the headache.

➤ Bed rest, preferably in the dark.

➤ Relaxation techniques.

➤ Complementary remedies, including herbal remedies such as feverfew, valerian, lavender and betony. Never take feverfew with any blood-thinning drugs and always check the safety of a herbal preparation in case you have a condition that makes its use unsafe.

➤ Massage and acupressure.

There are over-the-counter drugs that combine paracetamol with an anti-sickness treatment, and some people find that ibuprofen helps.

Some people find complementary treatments, such as lavender or betony and homeopathic remedies, very effective.

▽ Nausea and vomiting are very common in migraine – try taking an anti-sickness drug.

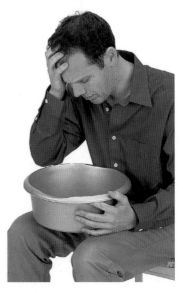

MIGRAINE TRIGGERS

➤ Stress, or relaxing after stress.

➤ Strong smells, loud noises, flickering screens.

➤ Premenstrual hormonal surge.

➤ Contraceptive pill.

➤ Missing meals.

➤ Foods, such as: chocolate, ripe cheese, cured/pickled foods, citrus fruit, monosodium glutamate, yeast extract, cola drinks, red/fortified wine, caffeine. (The enzyme tyramine plays a part here.)

Managing dizziness and fainting

SEE ALSO

➤ What is first aid?, p16

➤ Dealing with head injury, p84

➤ Coping with headache, p90

Dizziness, or a feeling of unsteadiness, is a common complaint and is usually a momentary sensation of no consequence. Dizziness may lead to fainting, which is a short-lived loss of consciousness that usually resolves the giddiness. A brief dizzy spell, with or without fainting, can be caused by a hot, stuffy atmosphere, fatigue, anxiety, emotional shock, lack of food, blood loss, or standing still for too long. Vertigo, or the sensation that your surroundings are spinning for no apparent reason, may have a more serious cause.

The main issue with dizziness is whether or not it is caused by a balance disorder.

CAUSES OF DIZZINESS

Non-vertigo dizziness might be felt as wooziness or light-headedness and may be due to anything from low blood sugar (not eating regularly) to high blood pressure, anaemia, or wax in the ears. If this type of dizziness occurs regularly, you should see your doctor, who will determine whether an underlying condition is to blame. The dizziness will have to be controlled, so that activities such as driving can be continued.

One common trigger for dizziness is standing up suddenly. This is often caused by your blood vessels not adjusting fast enough to accommodate a changed body position. It can also happen if you bend down or turn around very quickly. If this persists, see a doctor.

CAUSES OF VERTIGO

Balance is controlled by a part of the inner ear called the labyrinth, and also centrally in the brain. A problem with any part of this system might cause dizziness. The dizzy sensation in this case is more dramatic and is known as vertigo – the person feels their surroundings spinning around them alarmingly (for example after drinking too much alcohol or going on a fairground ride).

Vertigo is often due to a viral infection of the labyrinth, known medically as labyrinthitis, which may last a few weeks but from which complete recovery is usual. It responds well to medication that controls the dizziness and nausea that often accompany true vertigo.

Another reasonably common, but unfortunately life-long, illness that causes dizziness is Ménière's disease. In this instance, typical symptoms that accompany the vertigo include intermittent deafness and tinnitus (noises heard in the ear that are similar to an aircraft taking off). This condition usually develops in middle age and is treated with drugs.

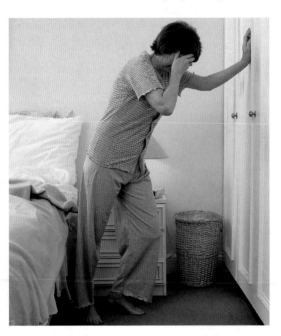

▷ If you get dizzy on standing up suddenly, for example when you first get up in the morning, lean against the wall in case you faint and then kneel or sit down till the dizziness clears. When you get up again, do so more slowly than you did first time round.

WHEN TO SEE A DOCTOR
Most types of dizziness are short-lived but you should see your doctor if any of the following apply:

➤ Dizziness happens regularly.

➤ You have vertigo rather than light-headedness.

➤ Other symptoms, such as deafness, earache, ear popping, tinnitus, nausea or vomiting accompany the dizziness.

➤ There is a family history of Ménière's disease.

➤ You are taking any medication that could be causing the dizziness.

Your main concern should be to stop the sufferer from hurting themselves or others, for example if they are driving a car when dizziness strikes.

Sit the sufferer down. If the dizziness continues, lie them flat so that if they faint they won't hurt themselves.

Unless they have sustained a head injury, raise their legs higher than their head.

Ask whether this has happened before, and whether they have any anti-dizziness medication that you could give them.

FAINTING

This occurs when there is a temporary lack of oxygen to the brain. It may happen for many reasons, including hunger, a sudden change of atmosphere from cold to warm, or standing still for a long time. If a person stands still without regularly clenching their calf muscles, the blood pools in their legs and they may faint as the brain does not receive enough oxygen. By fainting, the body is able to get blood and oxygen back up to the brain again – and so the person "comes to" as the brain recovers its function.

Fainting can often cause a lot of worry about more serious complaints such as brain tumours or epilepsy. The following features distinguish simple fainting from other causes of brief unconsciousness:

• There may be certain brief sensations that warn of a fainting episode: a sense of narrowed vision or of voices becoming distant, for example.

• The victim's skin looks very pale and feels clammy to the touch.

• The victim's pulse becomes slow.

• When they recover, there is no prolonged drowsiness (as there is with epilepsy).

• They may jerk slightly after they pass out, but there is no epileptic-type fit.

Check airways and breathing. If OK, lie the casualty flat on their back and raise their legs higher than their head (unless they have a head injury/pains).

Loosen their clothing – especially around the neck – and if the atmosphere is hot and stuffy, open doors and windows.

If they don't wake up after a few minutes, re-check their ABC, place in the recovery position, and call the emergency services. Monitor their airways and breathing until help arrives.

Tell the casualty exactly what happened when they fainted; this witness information may be vital in distinguishing a simple faint from something more alarming. The casualty should see their doctor if there were any unusual signs, such as loss of bladder control or drowsiness, after the faint.

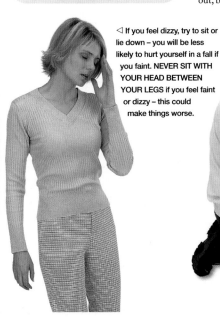

◁ If you feel dizzy, try to sit or lie down – you will be less likely to hurt yourself in a fall if you faint. NEVER SIT WITH YOUR HEAD BETWEEN YOUR LEGS if you feel faint or dizzy – this could make things worse.

◁ In fainting cases, support the casualty's legs above the level of their head so that blood returns quickly to the brain and resolves the dizziness. If possible, keep their knees slightly bent. Do not raise their legs if they have sustained a head injury or have sudden/persistent head pains, or if you suspect bad leg injuries.

BRAIN AND NERVOUS SYSTEM

KEY POINTS

- After someone has sustained any blow to the head, be very vigilant for further problems ☐

- Never try to restrain someone who is having an epileptic fit ☐

- Get emergency aid to a stroke casualty as fast as possible ☐

- Persistent or unusual headaches or dizziness should be investigated by a doctor ☐

SKILLS LEARNED

- Recognizing the signs of a serious head injury ☐

- Dealing with a head injury ☐

- What to do if someone has an epileptic fit ☐

- Recognizing and dealing with a stroke ☐

- Knowing when to consult a doctor about headaches ☐

- Giving first aid for dizziness and fainting ☐

- Knowing when to consult a doctor about dizziness and fainting ☐

OTHER MEDICAL EMERGENCIES

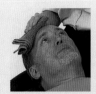

This chapter describes what to do in the event of a range of potentially critical situations. In some of them, including antenatal emergencies, emergency childbirth and diabetic crisis, the emergency services are needed, but there is action you can take to minimize risk before the ambulance arrives. Others are conditions that can usually be dealt with by home first-aid action but that might develop into more serious conditions requiring expert help; these include allergies, bites and stings, and heat and cold disorders. More common symptoms, such as abdominal pain, nausea and vomiting, and fever, are also covered.

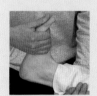

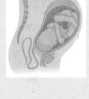

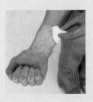

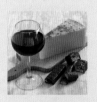

Coping with antenatal emergencies

SEE ALSO

➤ CHILDREN'S LIFE
   SUPPORT, p47
➤ Helping with
   emergency
   childbirth, p98
➤ Bleeding from
   orifices, p146

Situations sometimes arise in pregnancy that call for immediate action. These include bleeding, severe abdominal pain, headache, continuous vomiting, breaking of the waters, and lack of fetal movements. The first priority is to call for the emergency services and explain what has happened so they can warn the hospital. While waiting for specialist help, keep the mother calm and reassure her that help is on the way and that the baby will be fine. You should be prepared to monitor her condition and take appropriate action if it changes.

Problems in pregnancy may occur that require getting to hospital quickly, and occasionally rapid action is needed prior to reaching hospital. You should familiarize yourself with what constitutes an antenatal emergency, but always seek medical advice if you are in any doubt at all about a pregnant woman's symptoms.

COLLAPSE IN PREGNANCY

Any woman of fertile age who suddenly collapses should be considered possibly to be pregnant. The main concern is that the collapse may be due to a tubal pregnancy, also known as an ectopic pregnancy.

A heavily pregnant woman should not be laid on her back if she collapses. Keep her on her left side and perform CPR at a 30-degree angle. The pregnant uterus lies on the vessels that feed blood back to the heart, so resuscitation and cardiac compressions will only be effective if the woman is turned slightly on to her left side, in order that these vessels are not constrained in any way.

BLEEDING IN EARLY PREGNANCY

Any bleeding during the first eight weeks of pregnancy could be due to an ectopic pregnancy, in which the baby develops in one of the Fallopian tubes. There is often, but not always, low pelvic pain before the bleeding starts. In this case, the pregnant woman should see her doctor urgently, even if the bleeding is very light.

If there is any abdominal pain with the bleeding, or if the woman feels unwell, particularly if she is pale, dizzy or prone to fainting, it is important to seek a doctor's advice urgently.

Miscarriage

Another possible cause of bleeding in early pregnancy (up to 23 weeks) is miscarriage, and the woman should see her doctor

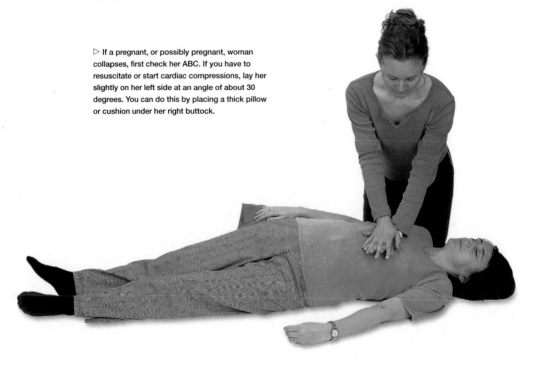

▷ If a pregnant, or possibly pregnant, woman collapses, first check her ABC. If you have to resuscitate or start cardiac compressions, lay her slightly on her left side at an angle of about 30 degrees. You can do this by placing a thick pillow or cushion under her right buttock.

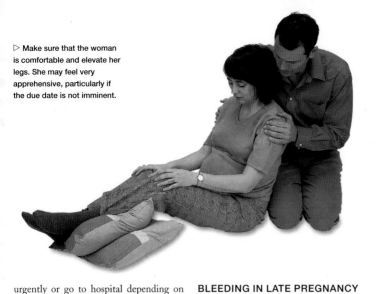

▷ Make sure that the woman is comfortable and elevate her legs. She may feel very apprehensive, particularly if the due date is not imminent.

WARNING

You must seek urgent medical help if any of the following occur during pregnancy:

➤ Vaginal bleeding.

➤ Severe abdominal pain, particularly if accompanied by bleeding.

➤ Continuous and severe headache, with or without blurred vision and with or without swelling of hands and ankles.

➤ Excessive vomiting.

➤ Breaking of the waters.

➤ Fewer than 10 fetal movements in 24 hours.

urgently or go to hospital depending on the severity of symptoms. Sometimes there is only a very small amount of blood and very little abdominal pain. This is usually called a threatened miscarriage, and bed rest and avoidance of sex may be the only advice from the doctor.

In other cases, the bleeding from a miscarriage may be extremely heavy and accompanied by cramp-like pains in the lower abdomen. There may even be signs and symptoms of shock when the miscarriage has become inevitable, and there may also be visible parts of the placenta and fetus in the blood. Such severe symptoms require admission to hospital, where it is likely that an operation will be performed under anaesthetic to ensure that the entire contents of the uterus are removed.

▽ In case a pregnant woman passes out, put her in the recovery position, as lying on the left side is best while waiting for the emergency services to arrive.

BLEEDING IN LATE PREGNANCY

Any bleeding after 23 weeks should be taken very seriously, and the woman should be taken to a doctor immediately. It may only be a harmless "mucous plug", which sits in the cervix until near the end of pregnancy. However, it may also be a sign that the placenta is bleeding, or has started to rupture away from the wall of the uterus. These placental conditions are known as placenta previa (in which there is painless bleeding) and placental abruption (in which there is severe pain). Both conditions can threaten the baby's life.

BREAKING OF THE WATERS

The membranes surrounding the baby in the uterus normally rupture at the onset of labour. This may release a gush of amniotic fluid or a more gentle leakage. Sometimes, however, the waters can break before the baby is ready to be born and the woman will have to be admitted to hospital to protect the baby from infection.

ACTION FOR BLEEDING IN PREGNANCY

In early pregnancy with painless bleeding:

➤ Make the woman as comfortable as possible.

➤ Make sure that she is wearing a sanitary towel.

➤ Get her to see a doctor the same day.

In early pregnancy with heavy bleeding and the passing of clots:

➤ Lay her flat and elevate her legs.

➤ Monitor her breathing and circulation every few minutes in case she collapses.

➤ Seek medical advice urgently.

In pregnancy after the 23rd week:

➤ Lay her on her left side.

➤ Keep a close eye on her breathing and circulation.

➤ Call an ambulance.

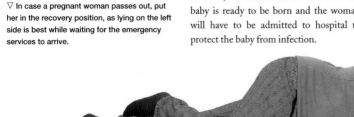

Helping with emergency childbirth

SEE ALSO

➤ Full resuscitation sequence, p38
➤ CHILDREN'S LIFE SUPPORT, p47
➤ Coping with antenatal emergencies, p96

It is not usually first-time mothers who deliver on the kitchen floor but the more experienced second- and third-timers, whose labours are less predictable and occur at a faster pace. Knowing what to do if a woman goes into labour is essential first-aid knowledge.

Although the mother does most of the work during labour and birth, there are a number of things you can do to help. Newborn babies sometimes struggle to breathe, and you might have to provide crucial help. Bringing a new life into the world is an unforgettable experience.

Although there may be few signs that labour is imminent, sometimes the baby's movements are less frequent a day or two before labour begins. As a general rule, a mother should feel her baby move at least ten times a day even just before labour starts. However, there is much variation and she need only be concerned if she feels a significant drop in fetal activity: she should see a midwife or doctor about this.

LABOUR

There are three stages of labour. The first stage starts with contractions and ends when the cervix is fully dilated. The second stage begins as the baby descends through the birth canal and ends when the baby is born. The third stage is when the placenta or afterbirth is delivered.

First stage

During this stage the cervix dilates to allow the baby's head through at the second stage. The first labour signs come on at this stage – the contractions. These are regular pains that start like a much more intense version of period-type pain, felt across the lower abdomen. They come and go every 5-20 minutes, lasting up to 30 seconds. The mother may also feel the "waters breaking", as the amniotic fluid around the baby gushes out. If the fluid is brownish, rather than clear yellow, the baby may be in distress, and hospital delivery becomes a top priority.

Second stage

At this stage, the mother has an overwhelming urge to push with each contraction. She may involuntarily open her bowels. Try to clear away the faeces without contaminating the vulval area and risking infecting the baby.

Let the mother get into whatever position feels comfortable for her. The baby is ready to be born when you can see the head sitting behind the vulva at the vaginal entrance. At this point, the mother should pant through the urge to push, to prevent the baby shooting out too fast.

As the baby's head arrives, it will normally be facing the floor. Support the head with your hand beneath it – the head naturally turns 90 degrees at this stage. Let it come naturally and do not pull. As soon as the baby's head is out, check to see if the umbilical cord is around the neck. If it is, then slip it carefully over the baby's head. If you cannot, then put two sterile string ties

FIRST AND SECOND STAGES OF LABOUR

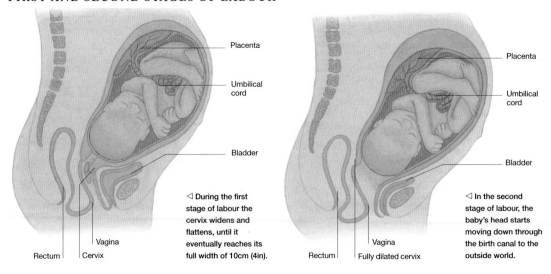

Placenta

Umbilical cord

Bladder

◁ During the first stage of labour the cervix widens and flattens, until it eventually reaches its full width of 10cm (4in).

Rectum | Cervix | Vagina

Placenta

Umbilical cord

Bladder

◁ In the second stage of labour, the baby's head starts moving down through the birth canal to the outside world.

Rectum | Fully dilated cervix | Vagina

wherever you can on the cord and cut the cord somewhere between the ties. The shoulders should appear next. If not, you may have to help by pulling them down.

The rest of the body arrives quickly after this. The emerging baby will be slippery, so be careful not to drop it. Wait for the cord to stop pulsating (about 20 seconds), then use sterile string ties to tie the cord, at 10, 15 and 20cm (4, 6 and 8in) from the baby's navel. Keep the baby level with the mother's vagina until the cord is cut. Cut between the two ties that are furthest from the baby.

The baby should start to cry. If it does, wrap it in clean sheets and a warm blanket and place it on the mother's stomach. If there are no signs of breathing, flick the baby's toes with your fingers. If there is still no breathing, remove obvious obstructions from the mouth and give 2 rescue breaths with your mouth over the baby's mouth and nose. Continue as per the standard basic life support routine for a baby.

Third stage

The placenta may not be delivered until up to an hour after the baby's arrival. It should arrive naturally without any action by you. Keep the placenta to take to the hospital. Gently massage the uterus to reduce the chance of haemorrhage. The uterus can be easily felt just above the pubic bone.

DELIVERY OF THE BABY

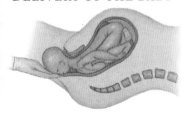

1 Most babies come out with the back of their heads facing upwards and their faces pointing downwards.

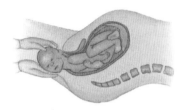

2 Support the head rather than pulling on it, to avoid causing any damage to the nerves supplying the neck and shoulder area.

3 When most of the body has emerged, keep it at the same level as the mother. Make sure you hold the baby carefully as it will be covered in blood and amniotic fluid and will be very slippery.

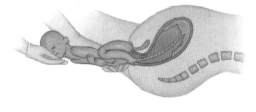

4 Hold the baby in a tilted position with its head slightly lower than the rest of its body in case it vomits.

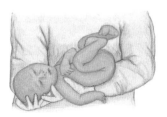

HOW TO PREPARE FOR AN EMERGENCY DELIVERY

If a pregnant woman is having continuous contractions, or is trying to push, there will be no time to get her to hospital and you must prepare for an emergency delivery. First, call for an ambulance. The ambulance controller can give you step-by-step instructions while the paramedics are on their way. Listen carefully. What they say may well contain the following advice, but always stick to their instructions.

Cleanliness is vital. Mother and baby are vulnerable to infection, so take all possible precautions to prevent its spread.

Use a large plastic sheet to cover the lowest and firmest bed in the house, or clear a space on the floor. Find two or three clean sheets.

Find three clean string ties about 30cm (12in) long. Boil the strings, and a pair of scissors in water for 10 minutes to sterilize them.

Find a nappy or something you can use as one for the baby. Arrange towels, flannel and warm water for the mother.

Wear gloves, and ideally change them whenever you have been in contact with potentially contaminated material, such as blood or faeces.

Managing diabetic conditions

SEE ALSO

➤ Responsiveness and
  the airway, p32

➤ The recovery
  position, p40

Diabetes is a condition in which the body cannot control sugar levels in the blood. This can create all kinds of symptoms, from excessive thirst to loss of consciousness. There are over 120 million people with diabetes worldwide. However, most of them are able to live normal lives because their diabetes is carefully controlled with insulin, drugs, and in some cases with diet alone. Since a diabetic crisis can be life-threatening it is important to recognize the signs of an impending episode and to take appropriate first-aid action.

People with diabetes mellitus have a problem with control of blood glucose. The body obtains glucose from sweet and starchy foods such as biscuits, bread and potatoes. The glucose is absorbed into the blood through the gut and provides fuel for all our body cells.

In people without diabetes, blood glucose levels are regulated by insulin, a hormone produced by the pancreas. Diabetes means the pancreas produces too little or no insulin. A diabetes sufferer's blood sugar levels are not controlled properly, which may cause symptoms that can develop into a crisis.

WHAT ARE THE TYPES?

There are two main types of diabetes mellitus – insulin-dependent (Type 1, which accounts for 10–25 per cent of cases) and non-insulin dependent (Type 2, the remainder of cases). Type 1 usually develops before people reach 40; Type 2 tends to begin after the age of 40, often in people who are overweight.

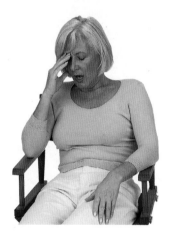

▷ Feeling very tired
most of the time is a
common sign of
untreated diabetes.

SIGNS AND SYMPTOMS OF DIABETES

Type 1 diabetics become ill very quickly over several weeks. Type 2 diabetics may be symptom-free for many months or years before the condition is discovered. Symptoms include:

➤ Passing urine often, in large amounts.

➤ Exceptional thirst.

➤ Tiredness.

➤ Blurred vision.

➤ Weight loss, despite healthy appetite.

➤ Recurrent boils.

➤ Abscesses.

➤ Genital thrush.

LOCATION OF THE PANCREAS

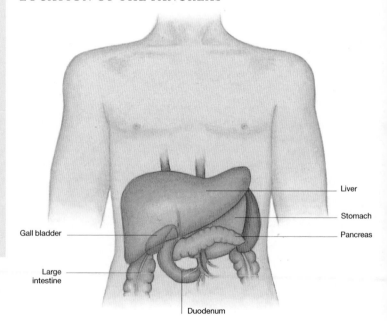

Liver

Stomach

Pancreas

Gall bladder

Large
intestine

Duodenum

▷ The pancreas is an elongated gland that secretes insulin. It actually lies just behind the stomach, but has been shown in front here so that it can be seen clearly.

WARNING
If you have to deal with an unconscious or unwell person, always consider the possibility of diabetes. If you don't suspect it from other clues, they may be wearing a medical ID tag of some kind, which tells you they have diabetes, or they may be able to tell you themselves.

FIRST AID FOR HYPOGLYCAEMIA AND HYPERGLYCAEMIA

IF UNCONSCIOUS:
Follow DRSABC and call an ambulance. Do not try to give them anything to eat or drink. If breathing, place in the recovery position and monitor breathing while waiting for the ambulance.

IF CONSCIOUS:
Loosen tight clothing. In hypoglycaemics, give a sweet drink such as cola, lemonade, fruit juice, or some squares of chocolate. Do not give "diet"/diabetic drinks of any kind. Call emergency services if condition seems at all worrying. Continue giving these until help arrives or casualty recovers. In hyperglycaemics, give sweet drinks if help is delayed.

Do not administer insulin, if you find it on the casualty. If properly alert, they will know to take it themselves. Look for clues about their condition so you can inform emergency services: medical ID tags/cards, an insulin "pen", glucose tablets, medication or a blood-testing kit.

CAUSES OF DIABETES

Both types of diabetes can sometimes run in families. Conditions that may lead to diabetes include obesity and disorders of glands such as the pancreas (pancreatitis, for example), the adrenals and the thyroid. However, very little is really known about the causes.

HOW IS DIABETES TREATED?

In both types of diabetes diet is crucial, with plenty of complex carbohydrates (e.g. brown rice, wholemeal bread) and low in sugar and fat. It may help to lose weight, exercise regularly and stop smoking, but always consult your doctor about diet and exercise first. Type 1 requires daily injections of insulin; Type 2 can often be controlled by diet alone, but sometimes tablets and occasionally insulin are needed.

WHAT CAN GO WRONG?

There are some long-term health risks associated with diabetes, but the only likely emergencies are hypoglycaemia or, less commonly, hyperglycaemia.

Hypoglycaemia

This crisis, often called a "hypo" or "low", results from too little blood sugar. It can be caused by lack of food, too much exercise, shock or stress, and can be so sudden that the person is unable to take the necessary action, (generally, eating some form of sugar). See Signs and Symptoms box.

Hyperglycaemia

This results from too high a level of blood sugar, sometimes caused by too much food, forgetting to take tablets, or by a virus. It develops more slowly than hypoglycaemia, except in children or with viruses, but is more difficult to treat and likely to need medical attention. A viral illness unsettles the blood sugar balance, making a person with diabetes dehydrated, with abnormal levels of sodium and potassium and acid in the blood. This makes them very ill and may even lead to a coma. See Signs and Symptoms box.

SIGNS AND SYMPTOMS OF BLOOD SUGAR PROBLEMS

Hypoglycaemia

➤ Rapid onset of symptoms.

➤ Hunger.

➤ Weakness/hand tremors/staggering.

➤ Feeling faint or dizzy.

➤ Sweating.

➤ Pale colour.

➤ Strong. rapid pulse.

➤ Confused/aggressive/uncooperative/ uncharacteristic behaviour that may be mistaken for being intoxicated.

➤ Slurred speech.

➤ Drowsiness; may become unconscious.

➤ Dry skin.

➤ Convulsions/fits are possible.

Hyperglycaemia

➤ Extreme thirst.

➤ Dry skin.

➤ Rapid pulse.

➤ A pear-drop or nail-varnish remover smell (acetone) on the breath.

▽ Cola or lemonade, a few squares of chocolate or a milky sweetened drink are good first-aid choices for hypoglycaemia.

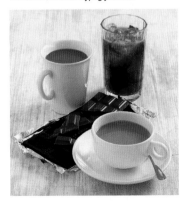

Dealing with nausea and vomiting

SEE ALSO
➤ Dealing with head injury, p84
➤ Coping with headache, p90
➤ ACTION ON POISONING, p189

Nausea and vomiting are common symptoms that are usually short-lived with no serious consequences. They arise from all kinds of causes, notably food poisoning, travel sickness, migraine, viral infection, allergic reaction, a drug side-effect or pregnancy. Nausea and vomiting may also have more serious causes, such as appendicitis, which will need to be investigated at your nearest hospital accident and emergency department. Prolonged vomiting can lead to dehydration, which can quickly become a medical emergency.

There are many causes of nausea and vomiting. Most of them are "self-limiting", which means they will settle without the need for further treatment or investigation. However, nausea and vomiting may be the beginning of a serious illness, and if they persist or dehydration sets in, the patient should be seen by a doctor.

CAUSES OF NAUSEA

Common reasons for nausea and vomiting include:
• Motion sickness.
• Migraine.
• Food poisoning.
• Viral gastroenteritis.
• Pregnancy.
• Drug side-effect.

More serious causes of nausea and vomiting, such as head injury, appendicitis, hepatitis, urinary tract infection and bowel obstruction, will usually be accompanied by other symptoms such as headache, abdominal pain, yellow conjunctiva (whites of eyes), fever, frequent and burning urine or abnormal bowel movements, which may range from loose and frequent to entirely absent for a few days.

TREATMENT FOR VOMITING

Urge the patient to drink small sips of iced fluid, every 30 minutes or so, and to refrain from eating for 12 hours. When vomiting stops and the appetite returns, stick to bland foods, such as rice. If there are signs of dehydration, they need to see a doctor.

▷ Encourage the patient to drink a little plain water every half an hour in order to prevent any danger of dehydration.

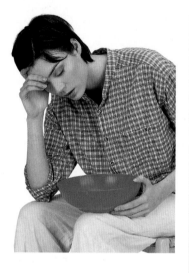

△ Seek immediate medical assistance if vomiting is accompanied by a headache that might be due to head injury.

SIGNS AND SYMPTOMS OF DEHYDRATION

Mild
➤ Headaches.
➤ Thirst.
➤ Dark urine.
➤ Dry, scaly-looking lips and tongue.

Moderate
➤ A fast pulse.
➤ No urine passed in over 24 hours.
➤ Breath smells of nail-varnish remover.
➤ Sunken eyes.

Severe
➤ The skin remains in folds even after letting go of a pinch.
➤ Drowsiness.

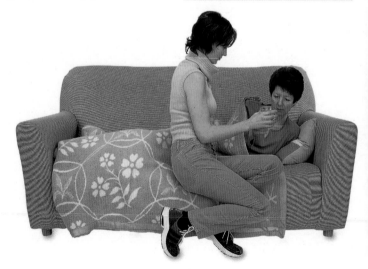

Tackling diarrhoea, fever and cramp

SEE ALSO
➤ Dealing with nausea and vomiting, p102
➤ Dealing with abdominal pain, p104

Diarrhoea is a common complaint that usually clears up on its own, although persistent cases should be investigated. Fever is usually a symptom of infectious illness. If the temperature is very high or persists, see a doctor. With fever and diarrhoea, replacing fluid is all-important.

Cramp is another common problem, and one that may be exacerbated by fever (or any other factor that raises body temperature). Cramp spasms occur when muscle fibres over-contract. This often happens after exercise, due mostly to a build-up of lactic acid in the muscles.

DIARRHOEA

Characterized by loose, frequent bowel movements, diarrhoea usually gets better without treatment. It may be accompanied by vomiting, and is commonly caused by gastroenteritis, which may be viral or caused by contaminated foods – especially shellfish, meat, milk or egg products – that have not been cooked properly or kept cool enough in storage. Diarrhoea may occur in many other illnesses, from harmless conditions such as earache to bowel cancer. Even constipation can lead to diarrhoea, as loose stools start to overflow the blocked-up bowel. Seek medical help if:

• Diarrhoea persists beyond 7–10 days.
• The stools are blood-stained.
• Dehydration is developing.
• There is fever.
• There is persistent abdominal pain.
• It occurs in babies or young children.

FEVER

A raised temperature is a sign that the body is fighting infection or illness. It makes people tired and shivery, and they may have cold-like symptoms, feel sick or even vomit. Other symptoms that often accompany fever include diarrhoea and a burning sensation when passing urine.

It is useful to have a thermometer in your medicine cabinet, particularly if you have children. The most common methods for taking a temperature are: oral or under arm, using a mercury or a digital thermometer; and a digital strip that is placed on the forehead. Rectal thermometers are also available but are more difficult to use.

Paracetamol brings down a temperature. Keep the casualty cool by sponging with lukewarm water or using a fan. Increase fluid intake to make up that lost in sweating and to protect against possible dehydration.

TAKING TEMPERATURE

Normal body temperature varies slightly depending on where, and at what time of day, it is taken:

Method	°C	°F
Under arm	36.5	97.7
Oral	37.0	98.6

CRAMP

Cramp is usually felt at night when we are most immobile, and it happens most commonly in the calf muscles. Getting out of bed and walking around is the best way of relieving cramp, or try massaging the affected muscle or pulling the toes towards you as far as they will go.

Cramp occurs more often during pregnancy, and may also be a sign of serious circulation problems, particularly in older smokers. Anyone experiencing regular cramp when exercising, which is relieved by rest, should see a doctor.

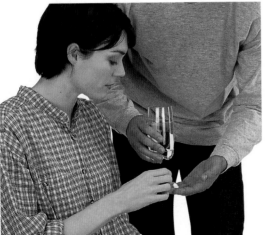

◁ Paracetamol tablets or capsules taken with water will bring down a raised temperature.

▷ In order to relieve calf muscle cramp, extend the leg through the pain and the cramp will disappear.

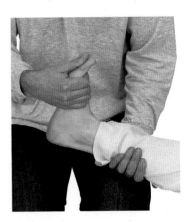

Dealing with abdominal pain

SEE ALSO
➤ Coping with antenatal emergencies, p96
➤ Dealing with nausea and vomiting, p102

Abdominal pain is one of the most common symptoms, with causes ranging from menstruation to appendicitis or even pneumonia. In helping the casualty with abdominal pain, you need first to ascertain the likely cause. You need to find out when the pain started, where it is sited and how severe it is. Accompanying symptoms, such as vomiting or vaginal bleeding, will help your assessment. Call a doctor if the pain is severe and prolonged, and if there is unexpected vaginal blood, or blood in the motions, vomit or urine.

Of all the areas in the body, apart from the chest, the painful abdomen probably causes the most worry. Abdominal pain is very common in all age groups, and even recurrent pain may be due to completely benign and treatable causes.

In attending a person with abdominal pain, it is important to be able to make a distinction between a minor episode that will pass without any problems and a serious, possibly life-threatening, condition such as an ectopic pregnancy.

WHERE AND WHY ABDOMINAL PAIN ARISES

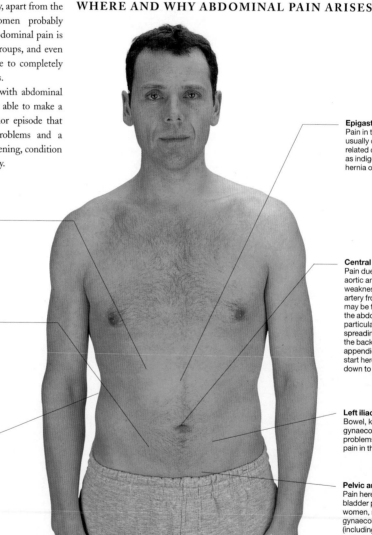

Epigastrium
Pain in this area is usually due to stomach-related conditions, such as indigestion, hiatus hernia or peptic ulcer.

Right upper quadrant
The gall bladder, liver and pancreas lie in this area. Pain here is often due to gallstones or pancreatitis.

Right iliac fossa
This is typically where the pain of appendicitis is felt, although bowel, kidney and gynaecological problems can cause pain here.

Right and left loin
This is where the kidneys lie, and pain from them is often felt here, spreading down to the lower pelvic areas.

Central abdomen
Pain due to a rupturing aortic aneurysm (a weakness in the main artery from the heart) may be felt all over the abdomen, but particularly in this area, spreading through to the back. Pain from appendicitis may often start here and then move down to the right.

Left iliac fossa
Bowel, kidney or gynaecological problems can cause pain in this region.

Pelvic area
Pain here is often due to bladder problems or, in women, may have gynaecological causes (including ordinary period pain).

ASSESSING ABDOMINAL PAIN

Before you start to consider what might be causing the abdominal pain, you should bear in mind the following considerations:

• Remember that the pain may not just be over a specific organ as it can be "referred" to other areas. This is especially true in appendicitis.

• Any woman of childbearing age with abdominal pain might be pregnant.

• Very ill or old people do not necessarily have a high temperature with serious causes of abdominal pain.

• People taking regular anti-inflammatory medication for arthritis or muscular pain can suffer perforation of their stomach with no pain at all. The first sign may be shock as they start bleeding internally.

CAUSES OF ABDOMINAL PAIN

It is not only the site of the pain that gives clues to its origins. Hollow organs such as the gut and renal tract tend to cause pain that comes and goes rather like labour pains, and this is often called "colicky" pain. Pain due to peritonitis, where the membrane that lines the abdominal cavity becomes inflamed, is a constant, uninterrupted ache. Pains that occur around the time that the bowels open are usually due to a bowel-related problem.

There may be other clues to the origin of the pain, such as symptoms relating to the kidneys (including a burning when passing urine and passing urine often or not at all).

The duration of the pain is important. Regular bouts of pain that settle after a few days may be due to irritable bowel syndrome or diverticulitis. Severe pain of sudden onset is more likely to be a serious condition such as appendicitis.

SIGNS OF POTENTIALLY SERIOUS ABDOMINAL PAIN

➤ Nausea and vomiting.

➤ Diarrhoea or constipation.

➤ Back pain.

➤ Shallow, fast breathing.

➤ Fever.

➤ Signs of developing shock – rapid pulse and sweaty, cold skin.

➤ A bulging or rigid abdominal wall.

➤ Tenderness on pressing the abdomen.

➤ A lump or mass in the abdomen.

➤ Any bleeding from the rectum, in the urine, or non-menstrual vaginal bleeding.

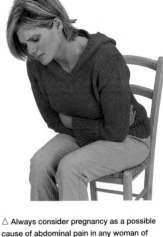

△ Always consider pregnancy as a possible cause of abdominal pain in any woman of childbearing age.

FIRST AID FOR ABDOMINAL PAIN

Have a vessel nearby in case of vomiting.

GENERAL, NON-ACUTE STOMACH/ABDOMINAL ACHES:
Keep the sufferer comfortable and give them fluids little and often, rather than a glassful that may be vomited straight back. A hot-water bottle or heating pad placed on the painful area may ease the pain. If the pain does not settle with simple painkillers and rest, call a doctor.

ACUTE STOMACH/ABDOMINAL PAIN:
If there is severe or sudden acute pain, or pain accompanied by fever, call the emergency services. Give nothing to eat or drink with acute abdominal pain, and never apply heat if there is fever or acute pain (for example, applying heat to an inflamed appendix would be very dangerous).

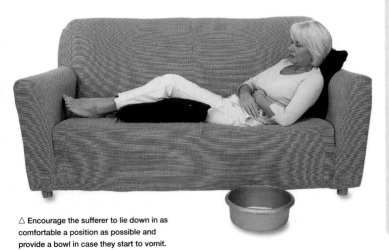

△ Encourage the sufferer to lie down in as comfortable a position as possible and provide a bowl in case they start to vomit.

Coping with allergy

SEE ALSO

▶ LUNGS AND
   BREATHING, p57
▶ Managing
   anaphylactic shock,
   p74
▶ Dealing with bites and
   stings, p108

Allergic responses may be minor or they may be severe. At worst, an allergen can cause anaphylactic shock, which demands immediate medical help to prevent serious illness and even death. People with allergic illnesses, such as asthma and eczema, are likely to develop allergic responses to other allergens. A relatively minor response on the first exposure may be followed by a much more dramatic response the next time. You should be familiar with the first aid necessary to assist the casualty and know how to prevent exposure in future.

The immune system is designed to protect us, but in allergy it works against us. Normally harmless substances, such as pollen or cat fur, are called allergens, because they can cause an allergic reaction if they come into contact with the immune system of a susceptible person. The immune cells act as if the allergens are dangerous invaders and the cells release damaging chemicals, such as histamine, in order to eradicate the invader. This causes allergic symptoms in the sufferer.

Once sensitized to a particular allergen, the immune system will react to it in every future contact. This may cause inflammation of the eyes, nose, throat, lungs, skin or digestive system causing a wide variety of symptoms from wheezing and running eyes to vomiting. The respiratory allergens such as pollen, dust and animal hairs tend to lead to fairly mild

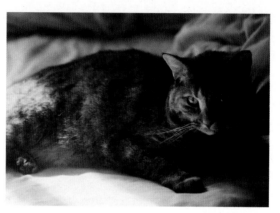

◁ Cats are well-recognized causes of allergic reaction, causing the sufferer to wheeze and sneeze within minutes of entering the same room.

reactions, while allergens such as penicillin or bee stings may be much more severe.

At its worst, an allergic reaction can cause anaphylactic shock, with the risk of serious illness and death.

HOW TO SPOT AN ALLERGY

Allergic reactions vary depending on which part of the body is reacting. Respiratory allergies tend to cause hay fever and asthma. Intestinal allergies cause diarrhoea and vomiting as well as stomach pain. Skin allergies may cause a rash called hives or urticaria that looks like a nettle sting but is often more widespread.

You may start to recognize a seasonal pattern to certain symptoms, or that they only happen when there is a cat in the house or when mowing the lawn. Certain blood tests can help identify if a reaction is allergic or not, but they cannot tell you reliably what the allergen is. Skin prick tests are not very reliable, especially for food allergies.

FOOD ALLERGY OR INTOLERANCE?

Many people believe they have allergies to foods when, in fact, they have a food intolerance. A food intolerance is due to a lack of one or more of the digestive enzymes

COMMON ALLERGENS

Almost any substance can be an allergen but these are the most common culprits:

➤ Foods – fish, shellfish, milk, nuts, eggs, chocolate, wheat and soya.

➤ Antibiotics – penicillin, tetracycline.

➤ Other drugs, for example insulin.

➤ Venoms – wasp, bee, snake.

➤ Dust, pollens and moulds.

➤ Chemicals in plants.

➤ Iodine-containing dyes used in certain X-ray investigations.

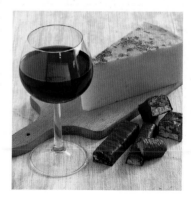

▷ These foods can produce a food intolerance reaction rather than an allergic reaction.

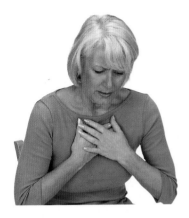

△ Coughing, a tight chest and breathing difficulty may be potentially worrying signs of an allergy that is affecting the respiratory system.

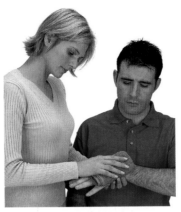

△ Try using a wrapped ice pack or bag of frozen vegetables to reduce the pain and inflammation of an insect sting or bite.

that break down food, such as those that digest lactose or monosodium glutamate.

A true food allergy should be suspected if the person has repeated symptoms, such as abdominal pain, diarrhoea, nausea, vomiting, and cramps after eating a particular food. The only way to test for a food allergy is to follow an exclusion diet and reintroduce the excluded food to see if there is a recurrence of the symptoms.

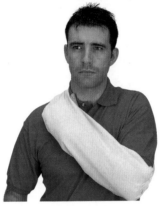

△ If you are dealing with an insect sting, elevate the affected part of the body in a sling if this is possible.

KEEPING HOUSE-DUST MITES UNDER CONTROL

➤ Try not to have too many carpets in the house – floorboards, tiles, vinyl flooring or linoleum are healthier.

➤ Keep the house well ventilated and dust-free.

➤ Buy dust-resistant pillows and mattresses or mattress covers, or vacuum the mattress daily.

➤ Put soft toys into the freezer every six months to kill the house-dust mite.

➤ Avoid sheepskin underlays, as they attract house-dust mite.

➤ Use damp cloths rather than dusters for cleaning around the house.

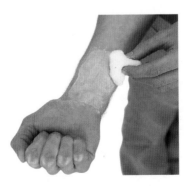

△ Calamine lotion is a cooling first-aid remedy for itchy rashes and insect bites.

FIRST AID FOR ALLERGIC REACTION

If there is any swelling around the face or neck, any difficulty breathing or symptoms threatening loss of consciousness, such as dizziness, get medical aid urgently. With any severe reaction, follow DRSABC and look for any allergy information or medication that the sufferer may carry. If conscious, help them into a position that eases breathing. If unconscious, check ABC; be prepared to resuscitate if necessary.

Try ice on swellings due to insect bites; scrape off the stinger and elevate the affected part in a high sling if possible.

Antihistamines can be bought over the counter and may help with a nettle-type rash common in skin allergies. Use only on advice from a chemist.

Calamine lotion and ice are useful for itchy rashes or insect bite reactions.

Anti-allergy nose drops can be bought over the counter and can be useful for hayfever-type reactions.

In the long term, avoiding the allergen is the best option, as in not having pets or mowing the lawn early in the morning or in the evening when pollen is less troublesome.

Dealing with bites and stings

SEE ALSO

➤ What is first aid?, p16

➤ Dealing with breathing difficulties, p60

➤ Coping with allergy, p106

Animals, insects, snakes, and sea creatures may all present a hazard either at home or when travelling. Any bite or sting is potentially dangerous, and however careful you are to avoid them, accidents happen. Dogs can inflict very nasty wounds, and in certain countries they may be carrying rabies; jellyfish and other sea creatures may inject poison; parrots and cats can produce unpleasant wounds; and some people are allergic to bee and wasp stings. Knowing the correct first aid to administer in the event of an accident gives peace of mind.

Many countries, such as Australia and the US, are home to a variety of poisonous snakes and insects, and knowledge of how to treat any problems arising from contact with them is useful. Although some bites and stings may not be venomous, they can cause infection or an allergic reaction.

HUMAN AND ANIMAL BITES

Human bites often become infected. The most common way of sustaining a bite is "in reverse", when someone punches someone else in the mouth and teeth break the skin of their knuckle. The joint underlying this knuckle area usually becomes infected, and may need surgery to open it up and clean out the infection. Cat bites and scratches often lead to infection, especially on the hand and face.

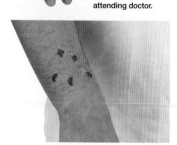

◁ Human bites need antibiotics, and possibly surgery, to clear any infection.

▽ A dog bite must be thoroughly cleaned and the question of tetanus (and rabies in certain countries) resolved with the attending doctor.

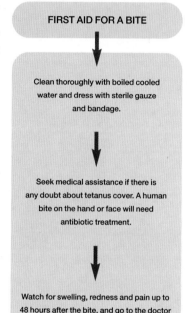

FIRST AID FOR A BITE

⬇

Clean thoroughly with boiled cooled water and dress with sterile gauze and bandage.

⬇

Seek medical assistance if there is any doubt about tetanus cover. A human bite on the hand or face will need antibiotic treatment.

⬇

Watch for swelling, redness and pain up to 48 hours after the bite, and go to the doctor for antibiotics if these symptoms develop.

SYMPTOMS AND SIGNS OF A VENOMOUS BITE

➤ Puncture marks in the skin.

➤ Feeling generally unwell.

➤ Lack of appetite.

➤ Abdominal pains.

➤ Rash, headache or fever.

➤ Muscle spasms.

➤ Joint pains.

WASP AND BEE STINGS

In a susceptible person, wasp and bee stings can cause an allergic reaction. Infections also commonly occur after stings. Suspect an allergy if there is much swelling, dizziness, fainting, difficulty breathing, nausea or vomiting, hives and a tight throat or chest. If an allergic reaction develops, take the sufferer to a doctor.

A bee may leave behind a sting attached to a venomous sac. If you squeeze it, more venom will be released. Instead, scrape it off carefully with a fingernail or blunt knife, and wash the area with soap and water. Place ice over the sting to reduce swelling and pain. Taking an oral antihistamine may be advised, in case an allergic reaction develops.

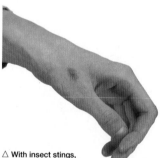

△ With insect stings, watch out for swelling, redness or pain, as this may indicate bacterial infection. Never squeeze a sting left in the skin. Use a clean fingernail, blunt knife or credit card to scrape it off – carefully but decisively.

SNAKE BITES

Poisonous snakes release venom when they bite, which can cause pain and swelling, abdominal pain, vomiting and diarrhoea. Dizziness due to blood pressure dropping may also occur, and the skin may become pale, cool and increasingly sweaty, indicating that shock has occurred.

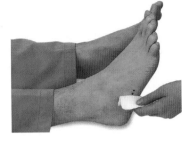

△ Stem bleeding from a bite using firm pressure with an absorbent dressing, ideally a gauze swab.

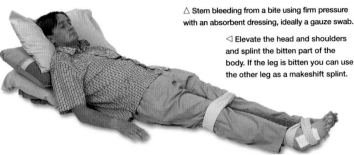

◁ Elevate the head and shoulders and splint the bitten part of the body. If the leg is bitten you can use the other leg as a makeshift splint.

SEA CREATURES

Some marine animals can inflict damage, either by puncturing the skin with spines, or by injecting venom. Many of them are invisible as they blend with the sand and rocks, such as the weaver fish in cool waters or the stonefish in the tropics. If you step on a sea urchin, the spines break off in the foot, causing pain. Spines must be removed and wounds disinfected.

Lethal jellyfish are found in some parts of the world, notably in Australia. They inject a neurotoxin that stops muscles working, which leads swiftly to respiratory arrest and suffocation.

FIRST AID FOR SNAKE BITE

Follow DRSABC. Do not bite, cut, squeeze, suck or apply ice or a tourniquet to the bite.

Calm the casualty and keep them as still as possible, so the poison does not spread.

Call the emergency services/get the sufferer to medical help quickly so that anti-venom can be given. Follow any instructions given over the phone by the emergency services.

If you cannot get medical help or advice within 30 minutes, bandage the bitten part firmly, but not so tightly that it stops blood reaching or leaving the affected part. Splint the bitten part to rest it.

FIRST AID FOR A MARINE STING

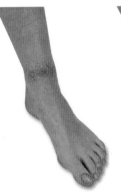
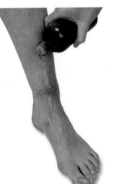
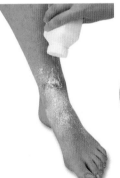
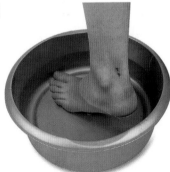

1 Get the victim out of the water as quickly as possible. You may need to summon help to do this.

2 Pour liberal amounts of vinegar on to a jellyfish sting to stop any further venom from being released.

3 Apply talcum powder to make any stinging cells stick together. Watch for any problems with breathing, and start resuscitating if necessary.

4 Place the injured part in hot water for at least 30 minutes. Call the emergency services in case anti-venom is needed for symptoms of poisoning.

Managing heat and cold disorders

SEE ALSO

➤ Dealing with breathing difficulties, p60

➤ Dealing with shock, p72

➤ Dealing with nausea and vomiting, p102

It takes time for our bodies to get used to a different temperature. The brain controls our response to hot and cold conditions mainly by altering sweat production and the amount of blood circulating in our body. If it is not given sufficient time to adapt to excessive temperature change, we may become ill – sometimes dangerously so. Temperature disorders in which the sufferer overheats include heat stroke, heat exhaustion (which may lead to heat stroke) and heat cramps; extremes of cold can cause frostbite and hypothermia.

HYPOTHERMIA

Caused by cold conditions, hypothermia occurs when the body's core temperature drops below 35°C (95°F).

It most commonly occurs:

- In a poorly heated home, particularly with the elderly or undernourished.
- In cold outdoor conditions, such as moors and mountains and at some road traffic accidents. Temperatures do not have to be freezing. It is more likely in wet and windy conditions.
- During or after immersion in cold water.

The elderly are particularly vulnerable to hypothermia in the winter months: they may sit still for long periods, they may not eat properly or be unable to heat their home sufficiently, and their metabolism is slower than that of a younger person.

Diagnosis can be difficult, and unconscious hypothermia sufferers may be mistaken for dead. However, due to the body's reduced need for oxygen when very cold, even prolonged resuscitation efforts have been successful.

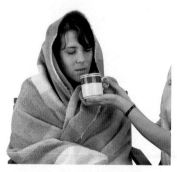
△ Give the shivering casualty a warm drink, such as sweetened tea. Do not give alcohol.

FIRST AID FOR HYPOTHERMIA

BASIC PRINCIPLES:
• Prevent further heat loss • Get urgent help • Rewarm the casualty – gradually • Follow DRSABC

Keep movement of the casualty to a minimum, and very gentle. Sudden movement can cause heart problems.

IF OUTDOORS
Keep casualty in shelter. Replace wet clothing with dry, ideally warmed (e.g. from dry, warm bystanders). Cover the casualty's head and insulate them against cold from the ground. Wrap them in something warm such as a sleeping bag or plastic bags (leave face uncovered), or ideally a survival bag.

IF INDOORS
Rewarm gradually in a generally warm room. Replace any cold, damp clothing.

If alert enough to eat/drink, give hot, sweet fluids (no alcohol) and a little high-calorie food. Do not: heat up the body too fast, apply direct heat (hot-water bottles, sitting someone against a radiator), massage or rub the skin, get the casualty to exercise.

SIGNS AND SYMPTOMS OF HYPOTHERMIA

Mild – body temp. 35°C (95°F) or less

➤ Casualty feels very cold.

➤ Uncontrollable shivering.

➤ Stumbling, poor coordination, slurred speech, mild confusion, odd behaviour.

Deep – body temp. 33°C (91.4°F) or less

➤ No sensation of cold.

➤ Shivering stops.

➤ Drowsy, becoming unconscious.

➤ Breathing slows.

➤ There may be no detectable pulse.

HEAT EXHAUSTION

Due to excessive loss of water and salt from profuse sweating, heat exhaustion often occurs after heavy exercise and on hot days. If not treated promptly, heat exhaustion can prove fatal or develop into heat stroke.

SIGNS AND SYMPTOMS OF HEAT EXHAUSTION

➤ Occurs gradually over several hours.

➤ Body temperature may be normal, but may rise to 38–40°C (100.4–104°F).

➤ Headache, dizziness, tiredness, nausea.

➤ Cold, pale, clammy skin and sweating.

➤ A rapid, weak pulse.

➤ Feeling faint or actually fainting.

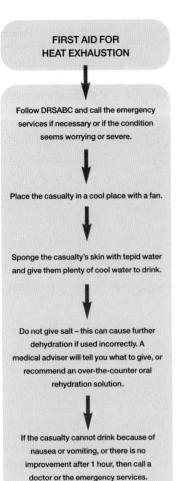

FIRST AID FOR HEAT EXHAUSTION

Follow DRSABC and call the emergency services if necessary or if the condition seems worrying or severe.

Place the casualty in a cool place with a fan.

Sponge the casualty's skin with tepid water and give them plenty of cool water to drink.

Do not give salt – this can cause further dehydration if used incorrectly. A medical adviser will tell you what to give, or recommend an over-the-counter oral rehydration solution.

If the casualty cannot drink because of nausea or vomiting, or there is no improvement after 1 hour, then call a doctor or the emergency services.

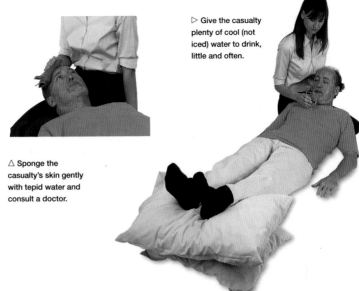

△ Sponge the casualty's skin gently with tepid water and consult a doctor.

▷ Give the casualty plenty of cool (not iced) water to drink, little and often.

HEAT STROKE

A very serious condition, heat stroke is often fatal. It may start as heat exhaustion, but if the body does not cool down, its heat-regulating mechanism fails, and body tissues start to heat up. Muscles and major organs begin to break down. Heat stroke tends to happen mainly in a very hot environment or with a fever.

Certain people are more vulnerable to heat stroke, such as the elderly, the disabled and infirm, those with diabetes, the obese and alcoholics. Some drugs, especially anti-depressants, diuretics and sedatives, can increase susceptibility.

Dealing with heat stroke

A person suffering from heat stroke needs urgent medical attention. Call the emergency services without delay and, while waiting for them, follow these steps:
- Having followed DRSABC, move the casualty out of the sun to a cool place. Remove excessive clothes.
- Lie the casualty flat. If they have heart problems, keep them sitting up.
- Watch for breathing problems.
- Cool the casualty down but do not immerse them in water – this makes blood vessels in the skin shrink and so delays cooling. The best way to cool down

SIGNS AND SYMPTOMS OF HEAT STROKE

➤ Similar to heat exhaustion but with no sweating.

➤ Pulse is strong and rapid.

➤ Temperature is over 41°C (105.8°F).

➤ Sudden delirium, with confusion and agitation.

➤ Convulsions, coma and death.

a hot person is to spray their skin with water and then put them near a fan.

HEAT CRAMPS

These may happen after excessive exercise, or exercising in very hot weather. The muscle cramps occur as a result of loss of salt and water from sweating. People may also feel sick and dizzy. First-aid treatment involves moving the sufferer to a cool place and giving them fluids with added sugar.

PREVENTING HEAT PROBLEMS

Follow these important tips whenever you are in hot conditions:
- Stay in the shade and use air conditioning when it is available.
- Drink 5–6 litres (9–10½ pints) of fluid per day if sweating a lot in a hot climate or because of exercise or fever, and avoid excessive alcohol. (Normal daily fluid intake is 2–3 litres/3½–5 pints; dark urine will tell you that you must drink more.)
- Avoid over-exertion and take frequent cool showers.
- Ensure adequate ventilation indoors.
- Wear a hat at all times.
- Avoid going out when the sun is at its hottest – between 11 a.m. and 3 p.m.

SKILLS CHECKLIST FOR
OTHER MEDICAL EMERGENCIES

KEY POINTS

- Unusual symptoms in pregnancy should always be dealt with urgently ☐

- Always consider blood-sugar problems when the cause of collapse is unknown ☐

- Although usually self-limiting, nausea and vomiting can point to serious conditions ☐

- Consult a doctor for persistent or severe abdominal pain ☐

- Always seek rapid medical help in the event of a serious allergic reaction or snake bite ☐

SKILLS LEARNED

- What to do for collapse and bleeding in pregnancy ☐

- Assisting at the birth of a baby ☐

- Coping with a diabetic crisis ☐

- Dealing with sickness, diarrhoea, fever, cramp and dehydration ☐

- Recognizing severe abdominal pain ☐

- Coping with allergic reactions and bites and stings ☐

- Dealing with temperature-related conditions: hypothermia and heat stroke ☐

CHILDHOOD PROBLEMS

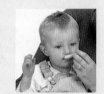

Babies and young children can deteriorate alarmingly quickly when they are ill. It is therefore wise to take seriously any symptoms they may have. Symptoms such as fever, vomiting, diarrhoea, breathing difficulties, coughs, abdominal pain and headache may be signs of routine, non-threatening childhood complaints, but they could signal something more serious. As a preventative measure, you should leave your child only with trusted and experienced childminders or at registered nursery schools where you can be sure that your child will receive good care in the event of developing an illness.

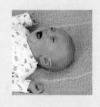

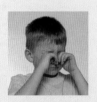

CONTENTS

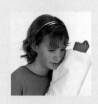

Recognizing childhood illness

SEE ALSO

➤ CHILDREN'S LIFE SUPPORT, p47

➤ Dealing with problems in babies, p116

Babies and young children can become seriously ill within a very short space of time. It is vital that the parents and any other carers are familiar with what is normal for that particular child and, therefore, know when something is wrong. Very often children are unable to articulate exactly what the problem is and so you have to be prepared to make an informed guess about the cause. Whenever you are in any doubt about the health of a child you should consult a doctor or go to hospital immediately, no matter what time of day, or night, it is.

Children are not simply miniature adults – their bodies are different and respond differently to illness and trauma. The responses of a baby will differ to that of a toddler, and the responses of a 7-year-old or a teenager will differ too. Children may not be physically or emotionally able to articulate how or why they feel ill, or where it hurts. This is why it is always important to listen to their parents. Parents may not be certain of what the problem is either, but they know that "something is not right" with their child.

Doctors always find time to see children, as they know how difficult it can be to judge childhood illness, and that problems may develop rapidly. At the same time, being able to deal with the common, short-lived childhood illnesses and with emergency situations yourself may allow you to avoid seeking unnecessary medical help or to improve matters until further medical help is available.

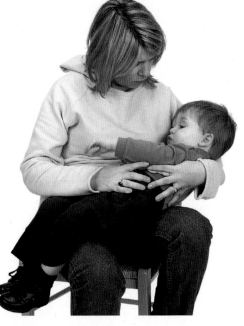

◁ The young sick child will probably be clingy and tearful. Look closely for any signs of illness.

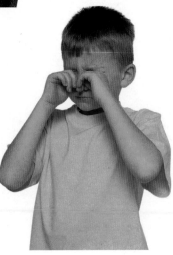

▽ The sick child is usually unhappy and subdued, although they may be unable to explain exactly what is wrong.

ASSESSING AN ILL CHILD

Children react differently to illness at different ages. So, a baby's small nasal passages and inability to mouth-breathe make a cold a very distressing experience that affects sleep and feeding, whereas an older child tolerates the symptoms more easily. There are, however, a few pointers to illness that apply more generally:

➤ How alert is the child? If they show interest in their toys and in people around them, this is a good sign. If they are slumped, silent and inert in their parent's lap, you should be concerned.

➤ Look for rashes or abnormal skin colour, for example a greyish pallor may indicate a very sick child.

➤ Identify any areas of pain. You can ask an older child where the pain is, but in babies and younger children you may have to use your intuition.

➤ Is there any restricted movement in the arms or legs? The child may be protecting an injured limb.

➤ Babies' cries can offer clues – a high-pitched cry is often a sign of illness.

RECOGNIZING A SERIOUSLY ILL CHILD

Children get seriously ill very quickly, and tend to recover as suddenly. Potentially worrying signs include:

➤ Altered consciousness: not engaging with people, unusually agitated or apathetic, drowsy or unrousable.

➤ Breathing quickly, noisily or not at all.

➤ Grey/white/blue skin colour.

➤ Sunken eyes, caked and dry lips and tongue that suggest dehydration.

➤ Weak pulse.

➤ Hot trunk and head but cold limbs.

➤ Pupils are unequal/do not react to light.

➤ Aversion to light.

➤ Stiff neck.

➤ Weak, high-pitched cry.

➤ No spontaneous movement.

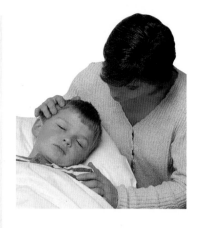

△ If the child is extremely apathetic and drowsy, consult a doctor immediately.

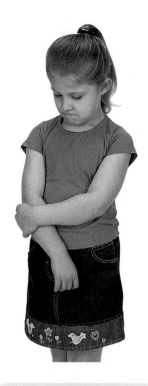

▷ If the child exhibits no sign of illness other than not being her usual self, then she may be unhappy. Childhood depression often goes unrecognized.

A REASSURING MANNER

Always try to calm a sick child – children soak up, and respond to, mood and atmosphere very readily. Being reassuring and friendly lessens their fear, which may, in turn, lessen their pain and distress. If you come across a situation where you are dealing with distraught parents as well as an ill child, the key thing is to put both the parents and the child at ease before attempting to examine the child. Chat calmly to the parents before addressing their child at all, and try to gather as much information about the situation as possible. Then keep the child occupied by playing and chatting quietly with them.

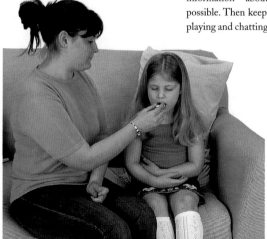

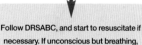

◁ Giving your child paracetamol syrup is a good first line of treatment for any type of pain or feverish illness.

FIRST AID FOR A SERIOUSLY ILL CHILD

Follow DRSABC, and start to resuscitate if necessary. If unconscious but breathing, put in recovery position (hold those under 1 year in the babies' recovery position). Emergency services must be called.

If the ABC is adequate but the child is struggling to breathe, you must still call the emergency services. Sit the child up and keep them as calm as possible while waiting for the ambulance.

If breathing is adequate but your child is feverish, then give them paracetamol syrup and call your doctor for further advice.

Dealing with problems in babies

Young babies commonly suffer from a number of problems, most of which are perfectly normal. Crying is a baby's main method of communication so a change in the pattern or type of crying may indicate that something is wrong. Parents soon become attuned to their baby's crying. Problems that commonly affect babies include feeding and sleeping difficulty, colic, nappy rash and teething. Symptoms such as fever or diarrhoea should never be attributed to minor baby problems, and you should seek your doctor's advice if such symptoms develop.

New babies arrive after a long and sometimes seemingly endless nine months. It seems that there is ample time to prepare for their arrival, and yet so often these tiny, innocent beings arrive in their expectant households like miniature missiles. This is especially true for first-time parents, who before the birth can rarely see past the labour to the daily care routine beyond.

New babies don't know that they are meant to sleep at night and be more awake during the day. They have no routine – but their parents are often used to rigid schedules that they have stuck to for many years before their child's arrival. In the first few weeks, babies seem to do nothing but sleep, feed and cry, in an entirely random way. It helps to know what to expect.

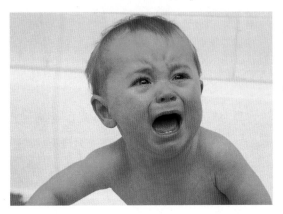

◁ The cry of a sick child is noticeably different to their normal cry. Parents can usually recognize a cry that is simply asking for cuddles or food.

CRYING

A baby's cry has a remarkably unsettling effect on its parents, especially the mother. Other people may hardly notice the noise but the mother will find it very hard to ignore. There is a good reason for this, rooted in evolution. When a mother is breastfeeding, she is the only person who can feed the baby, and if their cries do not make her run to them, they would starve. Crying is a baby's only means of communication.

Most parents quickly recognize that their baby has different cries. Sometimes it will be the weak, "don't leave me" cry of the tired baby left to fall asleep in their cot; at others, the alarmed and heart-rending cry of the hungry baby. A very sick baby may have a high-pitched cry that sounds odd and frightening, or may be too weak to cry at all. Some babies hardly seem to cry while others never seem to stop.

Babies cry for many reasons including hunger, tiredness, pain, colic and dirty nappies. Babies differ in their tolerance of discomfort: some can have a filthy nappy and not fret at all, while others cannot bear even to be just a little wet.

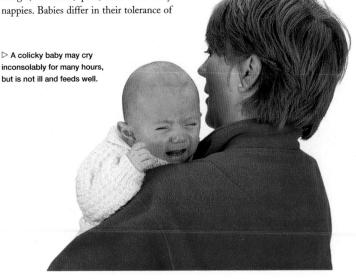

▷ A colicky baby may cry inconsolably for many hours, but is not ill and feeds well.

SIMPLE WAYS OF DEALING WITH COLIC

➤ Rock your baby gently or walk around with your baby either in your arms or in a baby sling.

➤ Put your baby into the pram or buggy and wheel it to and fro inside the house, or, if convenient, go out for a walk with the baby.

➤ Rub or massage your baby's abdomen and feet, following the path of the digestive system.

➤ Try giving your baby dimethicone drops 20 minutes before a feed.

➤ Dill, fennel and chamomile are age-old traditional herbal remedies for colic – look out for the special herbal preparations for babies that are now available.

➤ If you are breast-feeding, then you should try to rest during the day if at all possible – this will help to replenish your supply of milk, ready for the evening feeds.

➤ Making sure that you always drink plenty of fluids, and eat good, nutritionally balanced meals, will help to keep your milk supply going well.

▽ Nappy rash can be alleviated by regularly leaving the baby on a towel with no nappy, allowing the circulation of air.

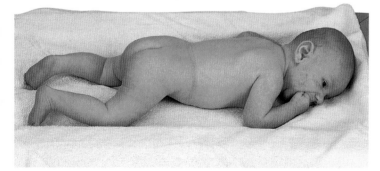

COLIC

Characterized by very sudden attacks of stomach pain, colic causes the baby to draw up their legs and cry inconsolably for several hours, day after day. No one knows what causes colic, which makes it rather difficult to treat. Colic often follows a definite pattern: it occurs at specific times of the day, usually in the evening, and it peaks at two to three months of age, improving or disappearing altogether by around six months.

Parents of colicky babies need to be reassured that there is nothing at all wrong with their baby; and they will often need emotional support, or someone else to look after the baby for a while.

RASHES

Babies often have blotchy skin when they arrive, and a few weeks out of the womb, their skin often becomes dry and spotty.

Milia

These little white "milk spots" appear round the nose of a newborn baby's face. They usually disappear after a few weeks.

Nappy rash

Babies have very sensitive skin, and so it is not surprising that their bottoms become sore from contact with urine and faeces.

To reduce the likelihood of nappy rash occurring, always change your baby if the nappy is dirtied or wet. Using a liberal application of a barrier cream at each change helps protect the skin. Also, give your baby some time, after a bath or during the day, when they are bare-bottomed.

When a baby is teething or ill, especially with diarrhoea or fever, they are much more susceptible to nappy rash. Be aware of this and make sure you do not delay changing their nappy.

If there are little red and white spots either within or outside the general rash area, then the baby may have thrush. Over-the-counter creams are available for this condition.

PREVENTING NAPPY RASH

➤ Use a barrier cream on their bottoms all the time – zinc and paraffin oil creams are best.

➤ Try to use only water and cotton wool in the early weeks, as they may react to wipes or lotions.

➤ Change their nappies regularly, rather than wait for them to start leaking through clothes.

➤ If a baby's bottom is beginning to look a little red, try leaving them on a towel without a nappy for a while. This will allow some air to circulate around their bottom.

TEETHING

Some babies cut their teeth with very little fuss, whereas others seem to have a lot of trouble. The incisors at the front of the mouth usually arrive fairly painlessly around 6 months, but the bigger teeth at the back (molars), which arrive later, can cause a lot of upset.

Rubbing the gums with special teething gel and giving liquid paracetamol may help. For some babies, biting on a hard object, such as a special teething ring or hard biscuits, can relieve the pain.

Coping with fever

SEE ALSO
➤ Recognizing childhood illness, p114
➤ Dealing with problems in babies, p116

Fever is usually a sign of infection – although it can be caused by immunization or being overdressed or in an overheated room – and there is a risk that it can lead to fits in young children. Try simple ways of bringing the temperature down first – such as removing clothing and bedding and reducing the room temperature. Sponge the child's skin with tepid water and perhaps give your child paracetamol. Keep a look-out for other symptoms that might give a clue as to the cause of a fever, and always call a doctor if you are concerned.

For many of us, the fear of fever in a child stems from the worry that the child will have a fit if we cannot bring the fever down. There is also the worry about what might be causing the fever.

A child's temperature often rises for up to 24 hours or even longer with no other obvious signs of infection, such as an earache, a sore throat or a common or garden cold. In many ways, it is reassuring when the first signs of a runny nose and cough appear as the cause of the temperature is then obvious.

NORMAL TEMPERATURE

Under arm/forehead	36.5°C (97.7°F)
Oral	37.0°C (98.6°F)

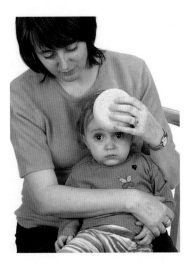

△ A feverish child will benefit from gentle sponging with lukewarm water.

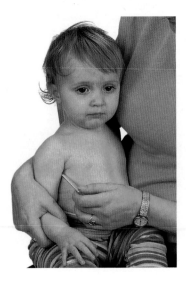

△ In a baby, a digital strip thermometer on the forehead is the easiest way to take a temperature.

▷ You can take a child's temperature using a conventional thermometer under the arm.

FIRST AID FOR A CHILD WITH A FEVER

Turn down the central heating or any other source of direct heat, and keep covers and clothes to a minimum.

Give your child paracetamol syrup (never aspirin) at the correct dose for their age, to bring down their temperature. Babies under three months should not have paracetamol unless the doctor advises it.

Sponge their body and forehead with tepid water. Avoid using a fan – it may make them shiver, which will generate even more heat.

DANGER SIGNS AND SYMPTOMS

➤ Baby under 3 months old.

➤ Fever over 40°C (104°F).

➤ Baby refusing feeds.

➤ A rash that does not disappear when a glass is pressed on it.

➤ Fever persists for more than 48 hours without there being any obvious source of infection present.

Dealing with vomiting and diarrhoea

SEE ALSO
➤ Recognizing childhood illness p114
➤ Dealing with problems in babies p116

Extremely common symptoms in babies and children, diarrhoea and vomiting usually clear up quickly without any special treatment. Viral gastroenteritis and food intolerance are common causes. If diarrhoea and/or vomiting is profuse and persistent there is a danger of dehydration, particularly in babies and very young children. It is important to make sure the child drinks plenty of clear fluids for the duration of the illness. If other symptoms develop or there is no improvement after 48 hours, you should seek a doctor's advice.

DEHYDRATION DANGER

What cannot be stressed enough with these childhood complaints is that babies and children are more prone to dehydration than adults because they are less able to replace fluid losses.

BABIES

Vomiting and diarrhoea without a serious cause occur quite often in babies because their digestive systems are still immature.

A little vomiting after feeding is normal and is called "posseting". Some babies are prone to bringing up a lot of their feeds, which is worrying only if the baby is not gaining weight. Babies may vomit as a sign of a general infection.

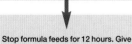

FIRST AID FOR A BABY WITH VOMITING AND/OR DIARRHOEA

Stop formula feeds for 12 hours. Give rehydration fluids from the pharmacist, then try half-strength formula feeds.

If breast-feeding, do not stop, but include bottles of water between feeds.

Continue to give regular feeds, and seek medical help if the problem persists for more than 48 hours or if you are worried.

You should ask for medical advice with:
• Sudden onset of vomiting.
• Unwell baby with a fever.
• Green-stained vomit.
• Projectile vomiting.
• Signs of dehydration.
Breast-fed babies have runny, bright yellow stools that smell like cottage cheese; babies on formula often have dark green, liquid bowel motions. Diarrhoea is different – watery, frequent, and often foul-smelling stools.

OLDER CHILDREN

There are many causes of vomiting and diarrhoea in children, but the most common is viral gastroenteritis. Although this gets better without treatment, dehydration may develop if the child does not drink enough. Encourage your child to drink clear, diluted fluids and avoid fizzy and milk-based drinks. An alternative is rehydration sachets that can be bought from the pharmacist.

▽ A child who is vomiting may be drowsy and listless. Take the child's temperature and consult your doctor if you are worried.

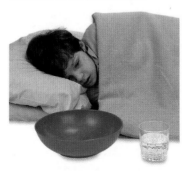

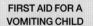

FIRST AID FOR A VOMITING CHILD

Give sips of fluid to the child in small amounts, and at frequent intervals. This way, the fluid is more likely to stay in the stomach.

If they feel feverish, try giving them some paracetamol.

Keep them off food while they are vomiting. Once it settles, try bland foods such as rice, soup and bread.

SIGNS AND SYMPTOMS OF DEHYDRATION

➤ The soft spot on top of a baby's head becomes sunken.

➤ The eyes become sunken and hollow looking.

➤ The lips are parched and the tongue is dry.

➤ Urine production falls. A baby's nappy may remain dry all day.

➤ They may be drowsy and listless.

➤ Pulse is raised.

Managing abdominal pain

SEE ALSO
➤ Coping with fever, p118
➤ Dealing with vomiting and diarrhoea, p119

Abdominal pain is a very common symptom in young children, and it is usually short-lived. It can occur for a wide range of reasons, which may or may not affect the digestive tract. Children tend not to suffer from indigestion, but anxiety and even migraine can cause stomachache. However, there are a few serious conditions that require immediate medical attention, and you should be alert for other symptoms that might signal such a situation. If you have any doubts, you should always consult a doctor immediately.

Children often complain of stomachache, but the pain will usually disappear spontaneously. Even children admitted to hospital with stomach pain are often sent home with no definite diagnosis. Children often experience physical symptoms as a result of unhappiness or anxiety. For example, a child who complains of recurring stomach pain may have problems at school or at home.

CAUSES OF ABDOMINAL PAIN

In children, abdominal pain is often not connected with the digestive system and may have causes such as a twisted testis or migraine, which in young children tends to affect the stomach rather than the head.

Urinary tract infections, which are particularly common in girls, can cause abdominal pain. Even a general infection, such as a cold or flu, might give a child a stomachache – this is due to the glands swelling in their abdominal cavity as well as the head and neck area.

The type of pain and its location often give valuable clues to what might be causing it, but it is often difficult for a child to describe the pain accurately or to tell you exactly where it is situated. Accompanying symptoms, such as fever, diarrhoea or vomiting, can help to narrow down the possible causes but you should never hesitate to contact your doctor if you are at all concerned.

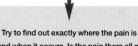

FIRST AID FOR A CHILD WITH ABDOMINAL PAIN

Try to find out exactly where the pain is and when it occurs. Is the pain there all of the time or does it relate to opening the bowels or urinating?

Give your child paracetamol syrup (never aspirin), at the correct dosage for their age, to ease the pain.

A wrapped hot-water bottle placed on their stomach can be extremely comforting.

If the child is vomiting or is suffering from diarrhoea, then they should avoid solid foods for 12–24 hours. Give them little amounts of fluid often.

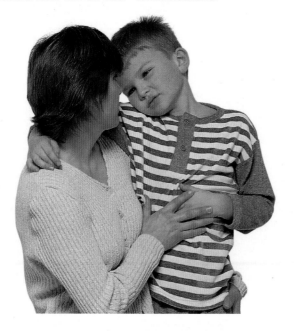

◁ Talk to your child to try to assess whether the abdominal pain has an emotional rather than a physical cause.

PAINFUL CONSTIPATION

If you have never seen the distress that constipation – passing infrequent hard stools – causes in a baby, this may seem an odd condition to discuss in a first-aid book. However, it is one of the commonest causes of abdominal pain in children, and it is very useful to be aware of this fact.

A baby who screams and strains at the same time, while drawing up their knees, may be constipated. They may pass very hard, pellet-like stools or not have any bowel movements for a few days. It often happens briefly when bottle-fed babies change from the "first milks" to the more filling "second milks". A baby who has had bowel difficulties from birth may have a problem with the nerves that supply the gut – this is known as Hirschsprung's disease. It is a serious condition that always requires surgical treatment.

Constipation may begin to be a problem during potty training. Parents should be aware that this can impede the learning process, as it is obviously unpleasant for the child – a situation to look out for and handle carefully. A child might also pass one large, hard motion that tears their anus. If they then start holding on to their stools to avoid pain, this could set up a vicious cycle which may eventually lead to the child being unable to control their bowel motions and soiling themselves. Plenty of fluids and gentle laxatives are needed to stop this scenario from developing – the earlier the better.

WHEN TO CALL THE DOCTOR

Call the doctor if a child's abdominal pain is accompanied by any of these symptoms:

➤ Sudden, severe pain that does not settle if you give your child paracetamol.

➤ If the abdomen is swollen.

➤ Vomiting.

➤ If there are signs of dehydration, for example dry lips and mouth, no urine passed for several hours or noticeably sunken eyes.

➤ If there is a lump in the stomach.

➤ If the pain has lasted intermittently for 24 hours and is getting worse.

APPENDICITIS

The appendix is a tiny tube of gut attached to the intestine that may become blocked and inflamed. Children of all ages can develop appendicitis. Pain often starts around the navel, and after a few hours shifts to the lower right-hand side of the abdomen, where the appendix is sited. They may vomit, lack appetite, or have a fever and bad breath. There is a danger of perforation, so if you think appendicitis is a possibility you should seek a doctor's advice or go to hospital without delay.

INTUSSUSCEPTION

A condition that occurs between the ages of 3 months and 2 years, intussusception must

FIRST AID FOR A BABY WITH CONSTIPATION

Try giving them plain water in a bottle or on a spoon between milk feeds.

Try a teaspoon or syringe of prune juice or orange juice diluted 50/50 with water.

A small amount of petroleum jelly applied around the anus can help move a hard stool that may have formed.

Your health visitor is a good source of advice but you must see the doctor if the baby passes blood, starts to vomit or fails to gain weight.

be treated as an emergency. The cause is unknown, but the result is that a section of intestine folds into itself, rather like the sleeve of a jersey. The child will be in severe pain and highly distressed. Vomiting may occur and a red, jelly-like stool may also be passed. If any of these symptoms occur, you must call an ambulance straight away.

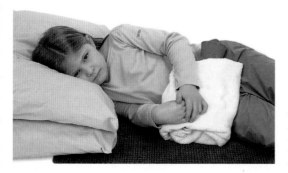

◁ A wrapped hot-water bottle placed on the child's stomach can be comforting and may also relieve the pain.

WARNING

Call an ambulance if your child has any of the following symptoms:

➤ Pain that has lasted continuously for over 6 hours.

➤ Pain in the groin or testes.

➤ Greenish-yellow vomit.

➤ Red material in the faeces.

Coughs and breathing difficulty

SEE ALSO

➤ CHILDREN'S LIFE SUPPORT, p47

➤ Dealing with breathing difficulties, p60

➤ Recognizing childhood illness, p114

Colds and coughs are very common in young children but they are not usually a cause for concern, and home remedies can generally provide relief. Occasionally, however, a child may experience severe difficulty in breathing: this constitutes an emergency and you should call an ambulance immediately. Causes of breathing difficulty range from asthma to choking, and some childhood infections, such as bronchiolitis. Breathing difficulty can be life-threatening and is alarming for both parent and child; never hesitate to call for help.

Children's air passages are smaller than adults', and so they are more likely to become blocked. A child can be unwell with a cough and a runny nose, but this is seldom likely to lead to any serious breathing problems. However, some conditions can lead to sudden breathing problems that may require first aid or emergency medical treatment.

COUGH

All too common in childhood, coughs and colds are rarely serious. Sometimes the type of cough may give clues to what is causing it. A barking cough and hoarse voice is characteristic of croup, a viral infection affecting the larynx and vocal chords. The noise can be very alarming, sounding somewhat like a seal barking.

Humidifying the atmosphere with steam can help.

A cough that comes in paroxysms so that at the end of the coughing fit, the child has to take such a deep breath that they make a "whooping" noise, is characteristic of whooping cough. Vomiting with the coughing is common with whooping cough. However, this condition is less common since the advent of the whooping cough vaccine.

NOISY BREATHING

Children may make all sorts of noises when they breathe, but noisy breathing does not necessarily indicate difficulties with breathing. The type of noise they make may help to pinpoint what the problem is likely to be.

Wheezing

Usually heard when a child breathes out, wheezing is a rather musical noise, often said to be similar to a seagull's cry. Most people associate wheezing with asthma, but wheezing can also be due to viral infections, principally a viral infection called bronchiolitis. This is mostly seen in infants under 1 year and may require hospital admission if they have feeding problems, but is usually self-limiting. They may go on to develop asthma, but many do not.

Noisy in-breaths

A harsh noise made as a child breathes in ("stridor") comes from the upper airways. It is caused by the airways being blocked or narrowed. Croup causes this type of noise, but it may also be due to inhaling a foreign body or very rarely due to a bacterial infection called epiglottitis.

TIPS FOR TACKLING CHILDREN'S COUGHS

➤ Use a humidifier or boil some pans of water to create a steamy atmosphere. Do this twice an hour if necessary.

➤ Place a wet towel on a warm radiator to moisten the air.

➤ Give your child paracetamol syrup regularly while they are unwell. It will ease any fever and aching that accompany the cough.

➤ Menthol and eucalyptus oil added to a bowl of warm water, or on the pillow or sheets, can help to ease a cough caused by an infection.

➤ Never smoke in the house.

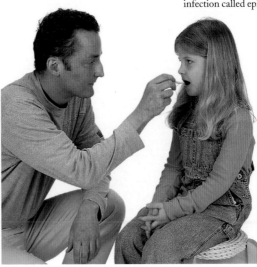

◁ Giving your child liquid paracetamol can help reduce a fever and may help to make them feel much better.

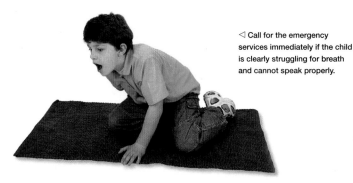

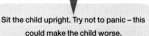

◁ Call for the emergency services immediately if the child is clearly struggling for breath and cannot speak properly.

Grunting

This noise can indicate serious breathing difficulties in a baby, and often pneumonia in an older child.

Snuffling

Babies will often snuffle when they have a cold. They then find it difficult to sleep and feed, which disturbs both them and their parents. However, most babies manage to find a way over this temporary problem without too much difficulty.

▽ If your child is on asthma medication, and they start to cough or wheeze, they must take some of the "reliever" drug (often in a blue case), preferably using a "spacer device", which assists uptake. You may need to help them take the drug.

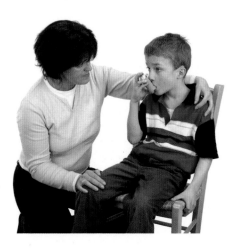

ASTHMA

Childhood asthma can be hard to recognize – for example, it often shows itself as sudden coughing fits or night-time coughing rather than wheezing. Children with asthma may cough, wheeze and, in severe attacks, have extreme breathing problems that require hospitalization. As asthma is potentially life-threatening it is essential to recognize the symptoms that need hospital treatment.

A child who has been diagnosed with asthma will have one or more inhalers, which normally keep the condition well controlled. Occasionally, maybe in the summer when the pollen count is high or if the child has a bad cold, the asthma does not respond to the normal treatment and breathing difficulties develop. This may mean that it is necessary to make a reassessment of the medication that the child is taking.

An asthmatic child who is having breathing problems can become seriously ill very rapidly, so never hesitate to call for an ambulance or take them to a hospital.

FIRST AID FOR SEVERE BREATHING DIFFICULTY

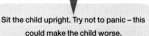

⬇

Sit the child upright. Try not to panic – this could make the child worse.

⬇

Known asthmatics should take several puffs of a reliever inhaler (usually blue) through a spacer device, if available.

⬇

Call a doctor/emergency services, depending on the severity of the problem.

WARNING

Call an ambulance immediately if:

➤ Breathlessness and noisy breathing start suddenly, especially after choking.

➤ Breathing is so laboured that a baby or child is unable to feed/eat or drink.

➤ The child cannot speak in proper sentences or even utter sounds.

➤ The child is drowsy or confused.

➤ There is a visible "sucking in" of the ribcage as they breathe in and out.

➤ The child stops breathing altogether for more than a few seconds.

➤ The lips turn blue.

Specific asthma danger signs:

➤ Too breathless to speak or feed/eat.

➤ Breathing rate over 50 breaths/minute.

➤ Pulse over 140/minute.

➤ Blue lips.

➤ Very wheezy chest turning into no wheezing – no air is getting through.

➤ Fatigue/exhaustion.

➤ Drowsiness/agitation.

Tackling headaches

SEE ALSO

➤ Recognizing childhood illness, p114

➤ Coping with fever, p118

Headaches are a very common complaint in childhood. Usually, the headache passes quickly without the need to consult a doctor. Often a headache can signal the beginning of a childhood infectious illness, so look out for other symptoms. Occasionally, a headache can be a sign of a serious condition, such as meningitis, that requires urgent medical help. On the other hand, a headache may have its root in something as simple as a child having stayed out a little too long in the sun or not having drunk enough fluid.

Because most children often complain of having a headache, the difficulty is knowing when to worry about it and seek help, and when to assume it has a self-limiting cause and will settle down by itself. Younger children obviously may not be able to articulate that they have a headache, but their actions may suggest it, for example they may dislike having their head moved, or be very irritable when moved at all, or they may be very sensitive to bright light or noise.

COMMON TYPES AND CAUSES OF HEADACHES

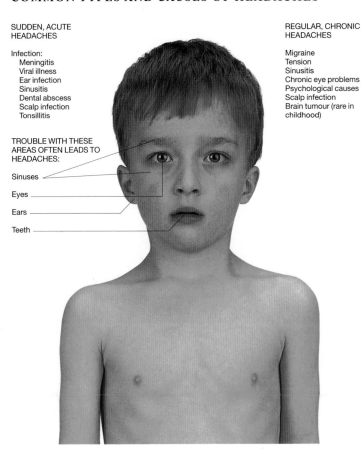

SUDDEN, ACUTE HEADACHES

Infection:
  Meningitis
  Viral illness
  Ear infection
  Sinusitis
  Dental abscess
  Scalp infection
  Tonsillitis

TROUBLE WITH THESE AREAS OFTEN LEADS TO HEADACHES:

Sinuses

Eyes

Ears

Teeth

REGULAR, CHRONIC HEADACHES

Migraine
Tension
Sinusitis
Chronic eye problems
Psychological causes
Scalp infection
Brain tumour (rare in childhood)

FIRST AID FOR A CHILD'S HEADACHE

Remove your child from any noisy, bright or disturbing environment.

Give them the appropriate amount of paracetamol for their age. Children should not be given aspirin.

Make sure they drink plenty of clear liquids and try placing a cooled, damp flannel on their forehead to soothe the pain.

If pain persists, take their temperature. If it is at all raised, it is even more important to give them plenty of clear fluids.

Look all over the body for a rash – this might signify a childhood infectious disease.

If they vomit, are drowsy, are very sensitive to light, have neck stiffness or any other worrying symptoms, or if the headache does not shift, call a doctor immediately.

WHEN IS A HEADACHE SERIOUS?

Your child's behaviour and distress level can indicate how serious the headache is, but you should always seek medical advice in the following circumstances:

➤ If it comes on suddenly.

➤ If it is accompanied by vomiting, irritability, fever, drowsiness, rash and/or neck stiffness.

➤ If the headache lasts longer than 24 hours.

➤ If the headache is recurrent and starts early in the morning.

➤ If the headaches are becoming increasingly severe and more frequent.

➤ If the headache pain is not relieved by simple, over-the-counter painkillers.

➤ If the headache immediately follows an accident.

➤ If the headache occurs some hours after the child has suffered a bump on the head.

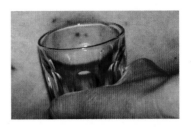

▷ The meningitis rash caused by meningococcal bacteria has a dark red/blue, paint-speckled look. Test for it by pressing a clear glass against the rash to see if it fades. If you can still see the rash through the glass, call for an ambulance.

MENINGITIS

A headache can be a sign of meningitis – an infection of the linings covering the brain that is caused by either a bacterium or a virus. It is very worrying for all parents, and difficult to recognize, as it may resemble other, lesser infections.

While a headache is often a principal symptom of meningitis, other signs – such as high fever, drowsiness, neck stiffness, light sensitivity and/or profuse vomiting – may be more obvious. A child who has been mildly unwell and then worsens should be examined by a doctor. In bacterial meningitis, there may be a characteristic rash, but this is one of the later symptoms. (In babies with any kind of meningitis, they may just be non-specifically unwell and do not generally have neck stiffness.)

A WORD ON RASHES

Children often develop rashes when they are unwell. As well as meningitis, infections such as chicken pox, measles and German measles have a specific rash that helps diagnose the condition. Many unspecific viral infections cause a child to have a rash, often as their temperature settles and they improve. Drug allergies may cause rashes that resemble nettle stings.

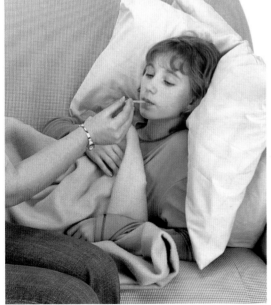

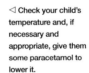
◁ Check your child's temperature and, if necessary and appropriate, give them some paracetamol to lower it.

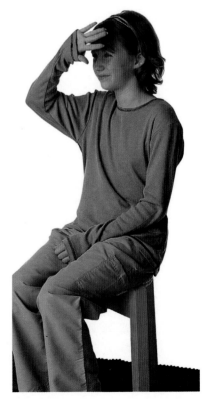
▷ A strong aversion to bright light of any kind can accompany various headaches – from migraines to those caused by meningitis.

Managing other problems

SEE ALSO

➤ Recognizing childhood illness, p114

➤ Coping with fever, p118

➤ Managing abdominal pain, p120

Children's immature immune systems make them very susceptible to a range of minor infections, such as earache and sore throat. It is not uncommon, particularly during the winter, for children to have endless colds and other infections but these are rarely of an emergency nature and can be dealt with safely at home. Toothache tends to affect older children; it is important to look after teeth from babyhood to prevent tooth decay later. If your child is feeling feverish and generally unwell, do not overlook the possibility of a urinary tract infection.

Children are more prone than adults to mild infectious illnesses, probably because their immune systems are still developing and they have countless opportunities to pick up infections from other children. Sometimes these illnesses have serious consequences, such as short-term deafness or lots of time off school, but for the most part, they are minor, self-limiting problems that can be treated at home.

EARACHE

Practically every child has an earache at some stage during a normal year. It often starts after a cold, the pain from the earache being caused by a build-up of infection behind the eardrum – a condition called otitis media. Pus builds up behind the drum, causing an unbearable increase in pressure that may be relieved when the eardrum finally bursts and lets the pus out. Antibiotics are prescribed for such severe cases. Earache may be caused by an infection in the outer ear canal, a toothache that is radiating out to the ear or a foreign body in the ear. It can also accompany tonsillitis.

Sometimes a thick, gluey substance remains behind in the ear after otitis media and makes the child temporarily deaf for

FIRST AID FOR A CHILD WITH EARACHE

Try giving your child paracetamol syrup – it is very effective at relieving earache pain.

Give small amounts of fluids to stave off any mild dehydration that can worsen the pain.

Give the child a wrapped hot-water bottle to hold against the ear – it is comforting and pain-relieving.

Prop up the child with pillows or cushions – this may be more comfortable.

up to six months; this is called glue ear. Your doctor may examine the ear six weeks after the otitis media, and refer the child to a specialist if glue ear has developed.

WHEN TO SEE A DOCTOR IF YOUR CHILD HAS EARACHE

These are the main pointers for when to seek expert advice:

➤ If the child has a high fever, especially if the fever lasts for longer than about 24 hours.

➤ If there is fluid or blood coming out of the ear.

➤ If the child is not drinking, or is generally unwell.

➤ If there is any deafness.

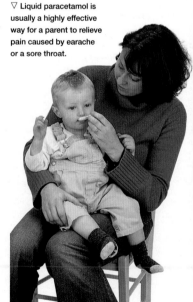

▽ Liquid paracetamol is usually a highly effective way for a parent to relieve pain caused by earache or a sore throat.

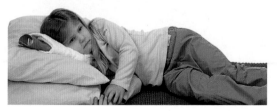

◁ Lying with the affected ear against a wrapped hot-water bottle may help to ease earache pain.

TOOTHACHE

Toothache may be due to an infected tooth, in which case the pain is often throbbing and there may be obvious swelling around the gum area. It may settle by itself, but if it lasts longer than 24 hours the child should see a dentist.

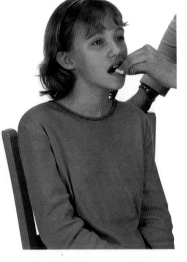

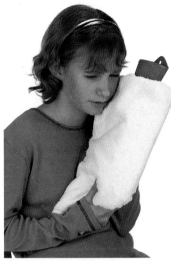

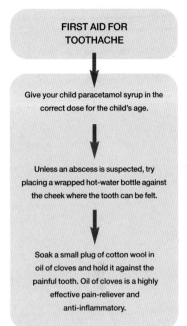

FIRST AID FOR TOOTHACHE

↓

Give your child paracetamol syrup in the correct dose for the child's age.

↓

Unless an abscess is suspected, try placing a wrapped hot-water bottle against the cheek where the tooth can be felt.

↓

Soak a small plug of cotton wool in oil of cloves and hold it against the painful tooth. Oil of cloves is a highly effective pain-reliever and anti-inflammatory.

△ Try soaking a small piece of cotton wool in oil of cloves and placing this on the offending tooth – it can be surprisingly effective at relieving pain.

△ Another good way to relieve the pain of toothache is to hold a wrapped hot-water bottle against the offending cheek (but not if an abscess is suspected).

SORE THROAT

Most sore throats in children are caused by self-limiting viral infections and can be helped simply by giving your child paracetamol syrup and plentiful fluids. Unless the child cannot swallow fluids or is very hot and unwell, they will usually get better after a few days without needing to see a doctor. However, do keep watch for a high temperature.

URINARY TRACT INFECTIONS

Children can also develop an infection in their urinary tract. The problem with a urinary infection is that it could be a sign of an abnormal kidney system. If it is not detected and treated immediately with antibiotics, the infection may also cause scarring of the kidney system and, ultimately, over a long period of time, kidney failure.

Babies and young children may not seem to have any urine-related symptoms but just be unwell with a fever, vomiting, diarrhoea, and feeding difficulties. If a child is hot and unwell for a few days with no other obvious cause for the fever (such as a cold, cough or runny nose), they may have a urinary tract infection. Simple dip-stick tests carried out in the GP's surgery can usually tell if there is any infection.

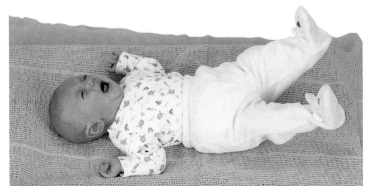

◁ Sore throats can be hard to diagnose in babies. A doctor may be able to tell by shining a light into the back of the throat while the baby is crying.

SKILLS CHECKLIST FOR
CHILDHOOD PROBLEMS

KEY POINTS

- Babies' and children's bodies function differently from those of adults ☐

- A baby or child can become seriously ill very rapidly – within the space of a few hours ☐

- Always be on the look-out for dehydration ☐

- If in doubt about a baby's or child's health, consult a doctor immediately ☐

- If abdominal pain, headache or breathing problems in a young child do not resolve quickly, get help; always seek help urgently if you suspect meningitis ☐

SKILLS LEARNED

- Recognizing a seriously ill child ☐

- Managing babies' crying, nappy rash, teething and colic ☐

- Treating fever, vomiting and diarrhoea ☐

- Dealing with abdominal pain and recognizing appendicitis ☐

- When to seek medical assistance for a child with breathing difficulties ☐

- When to seek medical assistance for headaches in a child ☐

- How to recognize meningitis ☐

- Action for earache, toothache, sore throats and possible urinary tract infections ☐

WOUNDS AND BLEEDING

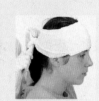

Minor wounds can be carefully cleaned and dressed at home. Any large wound, or a wound that is severely bleeding or contains foreign matter, must be professionally cleaned and treated at a hospital. If you are in any doubt about whether or not a wound needs stitching, take the casualty to hospital – the more promptly this is done, the better the outcome is likely to be. Protecting the first-aider from infection is another important issue when discussing wounds – you will find dealing with blood and other body fluids covered elsewhere.

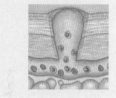

CONTENTS

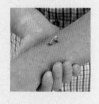

Types of wound

SEE ALSO

▶ Tackling embedded objects, p134
▶ Coping with severed body parts, p140
▶ Miscellaneous foreign bodies, p148

Even minor wounds can become infected and cause real problems with the casualty's health. However, most bites, grazes and cuts heal without too much trouble and can easily be treated at home. It is important that you are aware of the type of wound sustained so that you can carry out the appropriate first aid, described in detail on the following pages. Some wounds, such as puncture wounds, are more likely to cause damage to the underlying tissues and organs, and so they need professional assessment by medical personnel.

There are two main types of wound: closed and open. Closed wounds are usually caused by a blunt object, and vary from a small bruise to serious internal organ damage. A bruise the size of the casualty's fist would cause substantial blood loss. Open wounds range from surface abrasions to deep puncture wounds. Identifying the wound type helps first-aiders decide whether damage to underlying structures is likely.

ABRASIONS

Abrasions tend to be caused by a blunt object applied at an angle, or by falling on to, or sliding along, a hard or rough surface. A knee, ankle or elbow is a common place for an abrasion arising from a fall or slide.

LACERATIONS

A laceration is a wound with jagged edges. These are often seen in car accidents, and may cause heavy bleeding (although some large lacerations show little bleeding). As the object causing the wound may be very dirty, the risk of subsequent infection is high.

INCISIONS

These are clean-edged cuts, such as those caused by a knife or broken glass, and they may be deep. Incision wounds may look relatively harmless, but there can be considerable damage to underlying tendons, nerves, blood vessels and even organs. Deep incisions may be life-threatening, especially if the injury is around the chest or abdomen. Bleeding from incisions can take some time to stop. Superficial incisions often heal quickly and well as the edges come together cleanly.

PUNCTURE WOUNDS

Often caused by long, needle-like objects, these can be tricky to assess, as the size of the external wound gives no clue to how deep it goes (and the extent of tissue damage). Professional assessment may be needed.

BITES

All bites carry a high risk of infection, with human bites almost invariably becoming infected – a doctor should see any human bite at all, in case antibiotics are needed.

BRUISES

A bruise is discoloration of unbroken skin, caused by blood escaping from a vessel. This may be minor, as from a small area of broken capillaries after a bump, or may indicate internal bleeding. Most look more alarming than they are, and gradually disappear. A new bruise is usually red or purple; older ones are brown, yellow or greenish.

SCARRING

The extent of scarring after an injury will vary depending on the individual.

▶ Children's skin is usually flawless and so any scarring will show up more clearly than in an adult. However, children also heal much more quickly and more effectively. A childhood scar will often fade completely over time.

▶ Some people are unlucky and their skin forms what are known as keloid scars. Here, cut or wounded skin heals over-enthusiastically, forming huge, often unsightly, scars.

GRITTY WOUNDS

Dirty or gritty wounds must be cleaned in hospital to remove foreign bodies from the wound and prevent infection.

GUNSHOT WOUNDS

Guns can inflict many types of wound, and bleeding can be external and internal. Handguns, low-calibre rifles and shotguns fire fairly low-velocity projectiles, which usually stay in the body, while high-velocity bullets from military weapons often leave entry and exit wounds. High-velocity bullets create powerful shock waves that can break bones and cause widespread tissue damage.

AMPUTATIONS

The cutting or tearing off of body parts needs urgent help. Keep the severed part dry and cool and take it straight to hospital along with the casualty, as reattachment may be possible.

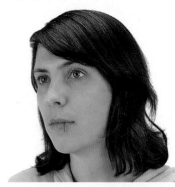

△ A cut that extends beyond the outer edge of the lip should be professionally treated. The cut edges need to be matched up exactly so they heal with minimal scarring.

TYPES OF WOUND

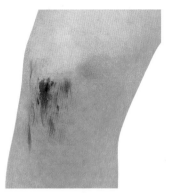

△ Abrasion

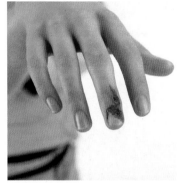

△ Lacerated wound

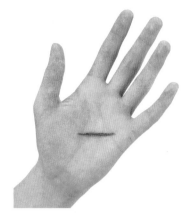

△ Incision wound

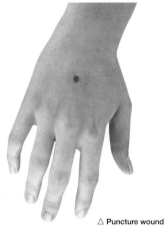

△ Puncture wound

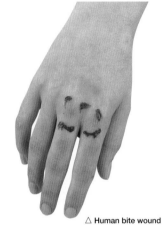

△ Human bite wound

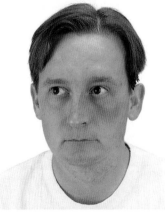

◁ Dog bite wound

△ Gritty wound

△ Gunshot wound

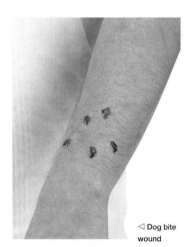

△ Bruising

Wounds and wound healing

SEE ALSO
➤ Dealing with major wounds, p138
➤ Controlling severe bleeding, p142
➤ Recognizing internal bleeding, p144

It is very useful for a first-aider to understand both how wounds affect our body as a whole, and how the body heals itself. Remember that any major loss to the body's constantly circulating blood supply is a potential emergency, as it can lead progressively from a drop in blood pressure through to fainting, unconsciousness, loss of breathing and heartbeat, and death. It is also vital to grasp the basic issues of wound care – including stemming blood loss and preventing infection – and also to be able to tell a minor from a major wound.

Our skin has many important functions. Nerves in the skin let us feel temperature, pain, touch and pressure. We get rid of water, salts and toxins through our skin, and changes to the flow of blood to the skin also help us to control our body temperature. The skin produces vitamin D, which helps to keep our bones strong and healthy. Our skin protects the tissues lying beneath it from infection, trauma, dehydration and the harmful rays of the sun. The skin is our first line of defence and is easily damaged.

THE HEALING PROCESS

A superficial wound, such as a surface burn, only involves the topmost layer of skin, called the epidermis. This heals very quickly, in one to two days. A deeper wound takes longer to heal.

As blood rushes into the wound, it clots and effectively seals the wound. The wound then fills with white cells which kill any bugs and absorb foreign matter. However, in a large or dirty wound, the

INSIDE A BLOOD VESSEL

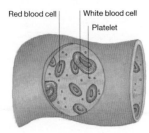

Red blood cell | White blood cell | Platelet

△ Important constituents of wound-healing: white and red blood cells and platelets.

HOW A WOUND HEALS

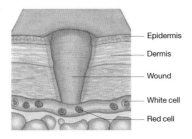

Epidermis
Dermis
Wound
White cell
Red cell

1 A large wound in the skin penetrates both the epidermis and the dermis.

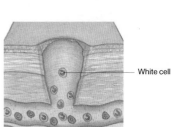

White cell

2 Blood rushing into the wound forms a clot as it exits. White cells fight infection.

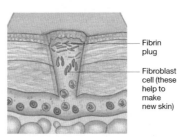

Fibrin plug
Fibroblast cell (these help to make new skin)

3 Strands of fibrin form a plug that slowly shrinks. New tissue forms underneath.

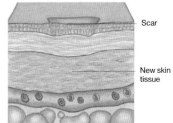

Scar
New skin tissue

4 The plug forms a scab, which eventually drops off. A scar remains.

white blood cells may be outnumbered and so infection begins. The wound may also be too big to allow clotting to stop the bleeding, resulting in continual blood loss (and, potentially, shock).

The body does all it can to reduce the bleeding from a wound. Damaged blood vessels within the wound go into spasm, and may stay in spasm for anything up to several hours. At the same time, platelet cells from the blood help to form a "plug" that may be enough to stop bleeding in a small wound. The body also uses a complex series of processes in the blood to produce strands of a substance called fibrin. These stick together to form a substantial protective plug, beneath which new skin tissue forms.

CLOTTING PROBLEMS

When someone's blood clots too easily, a clot may form in an unbroken blood vessel. This condition – "thrombosis" – is more

CLEANING AND DRESSING A WOUND

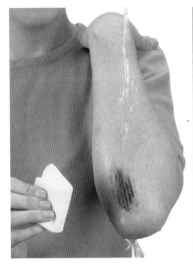

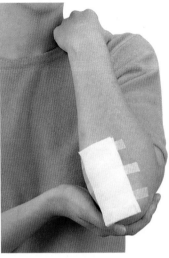

1 Expose the wound and clean it well (grit and dirt can cause infection and slow healing). Staunch any bleeding with direct pressure.

2 Cover small wounds with a plaster. Larger wounds: ideally a non-adhesive dressing and then a sterile dressing and bandage.

likely in people who have had major surgery, in smokers and after long-distance travel. If the blood is slow to clot – as in people taking blood-thinning medication or those who have the inherited condition haemophilia – severe bleeding may occur after relatively minor injuries.

WARNING

➤ Any penetrating injury that could have pierced a body cavity, for example an injury in the chest or abdomen, should be treated very seriously, even if it looks small and insignificant.

➤ If broken glass was involved, the wound will need to be X-rayed.

➤ Wounds caused by sharp implements, such as knives and glass, may have caused damage to tendons or nerves under the skin.

➤ It may well be relevant whether the casualty has tetanus protection; they may need to get this from a doctor.

MINOR AND MAJOR WOUNDS

A minor wound is a small wound that stops bleeding easily and is neither too deep nor infected. A brief look at the wound, and finding out how it occurred, will help you to make your assessment and proceed accordingly. You should treat it as a major/serious wound, and seek qualified medical aid, if:

• The bleeding is not stopped by an adhesive dressing (plaster).
• The wound looks as if it could be deeper than 1–2mm, or appears to need stitching.
• You think that there might be damage to underlying structures such as nerves and tendons – for example, if there seems to be any loss of function or numbness.
• There is potential for infection.
• The wound may leave ugly scarring, as in facial wounds.
• The wound covers a large area.

Stitching is needed on some wounds, to stop bleeding or prevent infection. Never use steri-strips (paper stitches

designed for smaller wounds) unless you are medically qualified, as incorrect use can lead to abscesses.

KEEPING WOUNDS DRY

A wound must stay fairly dry in order to heal. Wounds kept enclosed and damp are more likely to become infected and can take longer to heal. If the pad of a plaster becomes wet, it should be carefully changed for a dry one. Some small, minor wounds, grazes and open blisters respond well to exposure to the air – provided dirt or dust are unlikely to get into them.

FIRST AID FOR MINOR WOUNDS

Wash your hands thoroughly. Avoid touching the wound, in order to prevent infection. Wear gloves if you have them.

Take a brief look and find out how and where the wound was caused.

Wash the wound under running tap water, or bottled drinking water/boiled and cooled water if you are somewhere where the tap water is unsuitable for drinking.

Dry the wound and apply a sterile adhesive dressing (plaster). For wounds over a larger area, it may be better to use a non-adhesive dressing, sterile dressing and bandage, if you have these to hand.

The casualty must keep the wound clean and dry for the next few days.

Tackling embedded objects

SEE ALSO
➤ Dealing with major wounds, p138
➤ Miscellaneous foreign bodies, p148

A "foreign body" that has lodged within a wound can cause infection. The object may be relatively easy to remove, as is usually the case with a splinter. However, if you are in any doubt about your ability to remove it safely and cleanly, leave it until you can get professional help. This is essential if the object is large or deeply embedded. A foreign body will usually set up an infection around the site within hours so this problem should be promptly resolved. An embedded object left in the wound could cause an infection of the bloodstream.

Even tiny embedded objects can be very painful, and they may travel and cause further problems – such as pressure on a nerve or an annoying lump. Only remove an embedded body (or any foreign body) if the injury is minor and it is easy to do so; otherwise, get medical help. Sometimes doctors decide to leave an embedded object in place, because it is more risky to remove it than to leave it where it is.

SMALL SPLINTERS

A small splinter of wood, metal or glass may come out if you gently squeeze the skin on either side. If it is protruding from the skin, it may be easy to remove with a pair of sterile tweezers. Sterilize them in boiling water for a few seconds, or hold them in a gas flame, and allow to cool before using. Pull the splinter out at the angle it went in. (Soft wood may need expert aid, as it falls apart easily.) Small splinters that are visible just under the skin may be taken out very carefully with sterile tweezers and a sterile needle, but never dig around – you could cause great harm.

WARNING

If you cannot see a splinter, be very wary of trying to remove it. Small objects under the skin often become surrounded by pus after a few days, and then pop out easily. Glass is very difficult to find and does not always show up on X-rays. Even a foreign body that does show up on an X-ray can be hard to locate, so removal is best left to experts. Whether or not a casualty has tetanus cover may affect your assessment.

FISH HOOKS

These can be very sharp and often get stuck in people's fingers. The barb means you can't pull them back out the way they went in.
• Your first priority is to get medical help.
• Ask if the casualty has tetanus cover; if not, medical aid is particularly important.
• Remove a hook only if no help is available, especially if you can't see the barb.
• If the barb is visible, use pliers to cut the barb off and then pull the hook out.
• If you know that there is a barb, but cannot see it, only try to pull the hook out if no medical help is available. The person may require an anaesthetic before this is done, so it is best to take them to a doctor. If you do have to remove it, still get them to a doctor as fast as possible to be checked out.

DEALING WITH FISH HOOKS

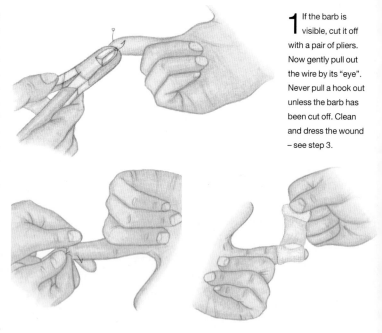

1 If the barb is visible, cut it off with a pair of pliers. Now gently pull out the wire by its "eye". Never pull a hook out unless the barb has been cut off. Clean and dress the wound – see step 3.

2 If the barb is not visible, and no medical help is available, push the hook firmly but carefully through the wound until the barb emerges. Cut the barb off and remove the wire.

3 When the wire is out, clean the wound with tap water, or sterile water (boiled and cooled) where tap water is suspect. Pad the wound with gauze and bandage it up. Seek medical help.

DRESSING ARM WOUNDS WITH EMBEDDED OBJECTS

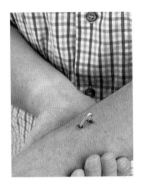 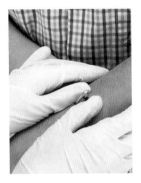 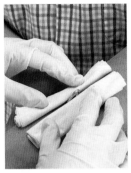 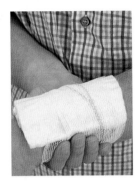

1 Do not try to remove this kind of embedded object as you may cause further damage. Your aim is to deal with bleeding and protect the area from infection, and to get aid promptly.

2 If the wound is bleeding, apply pressure to the surrounding area with your hands. Never apply pressure directly on to an embedded object. Elevating the wounded part will also help.

3 Place padding around the object. If possible, as it would be here, build this padding up until it is as high as the embedded object, ready to bandage over smoothly.

4 Bandage over the padding (or on either side of the object if it is a long one and still protrudes). Apply no direct pressure at all to the object. Now keep the wound elevated until help arrives.

LARGE EMBEDDED OBJECTS

If a large object is embedded in the wound, you should not try to remove it but should seek urgent medical help. This is especially important if the injury is to the chest or abdomen. The object may have cut through large blood vessels or even be embedded in the heart, but while it remains in the wound, it may act as a plug and prevent further bleeding. You could do just as much damage pulling it out as occurred as the object went in.

If someone is impaled, on a railing for example, do not try to get them off it. Only do this is if the person needs to be resuscitated, in which case this takes priority. Instead, help the person to stay still and try to support their weight in as comfortable a position as possible. Cover them with a coat or blanket to keep them warm, and call the emergency services immediately, or ask a helper to do so. Tell the operator that the casualty is impaled, as the fire brigade will be required with cutting equipment. Reassure the casualty that help is on its way, and keep talking to them to keep them calm.

▷ Small children playing with pencils or crayons is one of the many everyday situations that can turn into an embedded object incident – children frequently embed pencils in their face or staples in their fingers. Keep a careful eye on children.

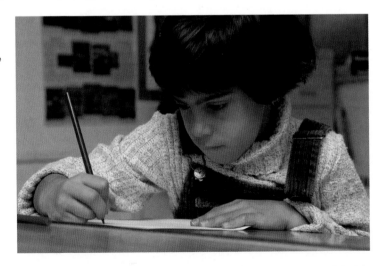

Treating infected wounds

SEE ALSO

➤ Types of wound, p130

➤ Tackling embedded objects, p134

When a wound becomes infected, it will need very careful monitoring and handling. If not treated correctly, the wound may become increasingly infected, spreading to a larger and larger area of the body. An infected wound can also lead to poisoning of the bloodstream, a serious condition known as septicaemia. Bites, whether inflicted by a human or a dog, cat or other animal, are all likely to cause infection unless the site of the wound has been professionally cleaned and treated. The person will often need to take antibiotics.

Sometimes a wound becomes infected despite having been cleaned and dressed correctly, and kept clean and dry. Certain types of wound are prone to infection – bites, for example, and particularly human or cat bites. If there is a lot of blood under a wound and this is not cleared out and its reappearance prevented, or if a wound is deep and dirty, then infection is more likely. Some people are more vulnerable to infection. These include those with diabetes, those with a compromised immune system (due to drugs or illness), and alcoholics.

There are usually many warning signs that a wound has become infected, giving plenty of time for it to be treated with antibiotics and drainage if necessary.

SIGNS AND SYMPTOMS OF INFECTION

➤ An infection may start to show itself within a few hours of the injury, or may not appear for several days.

➤ Be aware of pain around the site of the wound – often an early sign of infection.

➤ Watch for any redness, tenderness, swelling under the wound or pus, or for the start of a fever.

➤ Swollen glands (armpit/groin).

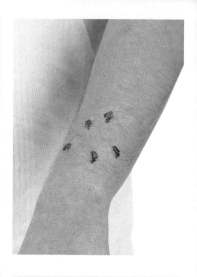

▷ This wound, caused by a dog, will need to be assessed by a doctor. Antibiotics may be given as a preventative measure.

FIRST AID FOR INFECTION

⬇

Cover the wound with a sterile bandage. Leave the surrounding area visible, so that you can monitor signs of spreading infection – vital information for the doctor.

⬇

Elevate and support the infected area if possible. For example, if a forearm is infected, the raised arm could be placed so that its elbow rests on some books topped with a sweater as cushioning.

⬇

Get the casualty to a doctor as soon as possible.

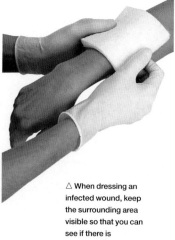

△ When dressing an infected wound, keep the surrounding area visible so that you can see if there is spreading infection.

WOUNDS THAT ARE PRONE TO INFECTION

Any wound can become infected, but certain kinds are more at risk:

➤ Bite wounds: animal or human.

➤ Wounds/scratches from human nails or the claws of animals.

➤ Stab (penetrating) wounds.

➤ Wounds sustained while working: in soil or manure; in or around waste or excrement; with animals.

➤ Wounds from dirty tools or objects, such as garden injuries or dirty nails in the foot while working on building sites.

➤ Wounds with embedded objects, especially softwood splinters, grit and plant thorns.

SIGNS OF INFECTION

You may notice the first signs of infection in and around a wound within hours but it frequently takes longer to manifest itself. The infection may not surface until a day or two after the injury when the casualty may have more or less forgotten the injury.

Pain, redness, tenderness and swelling are all signs of infection. The casualty may also experience fever and notice pus oozing from the wound.

SPREADING INFECTION

Infection may spread under the skin (cellulitis) and/or into the bloodstream (septicaemia). Cellulitis may appear even without an obvious wound, and is often from an unsuspected insect bite.

If the wound is near a joint, infection may spread into the joint. This is particularly true of human bites on the knuckles – these may be "self-inflicted", occurring when someone aims a punch at someone's face and sustains a laceration to the knuckles from their victim's teeth. Some people, such as those with the disease osteoarthritis, may develop a joint infection with no actual wound.

You should suspect cellulitis if there is a spreading redness and swelling beyond the wound site. The glands in the armpits, neck or groins may be sore and tender, and there may be a red line going up the limb towards the glands.

Suspect septicaemia if the casualty feels unwell with a fever, thirst, shivering and lethargy. A joint infection may be present if the joint feels hot or swollen, or if it is exceedingly painful, especially with movement. All these conditions require medical treatment – as a first-aider, your priority is to recognize the likely symptoms and get the person professional medical assistance.

TETANUS

A bacterium commonly found in soil and animal faeces, tetanus can contaminate the tiniest of wounds. In general, the dirtier the wound, the greater the chance of infection, but some 20 per cent of people with tetanus infection have no obvious wound through which the infection could have entered. It may take three months for signs of the disease to develop, although it is usually obvious within two weeks.

Tetanus is a particularly vicious disease. The tetanus bacterium produces a neurotoxin that causes painful muscle spasms (lockjaw) as well as having a detrimental effect on the heart. People still develop this infection worldwide, and it is a huge killer. However, you can be vaccinated against the disease – both as general preventative and if an injury is sustained that puts you at greater risk of developing it.

Tetanus immunization

The usual tetanus immunization programme in Western countries starts at about three months, is boosted around four years old and in adolescence, and then every ten years. If a casualty has not had a booster for ten years, they will require another booster to ensure that they do not develop the infection. If they are elderly or from abroad, they may need the whole three-dose course, and if the wound is very dirty, they may be given an extra tetanus booster or even some anti-tetanus protein if they have never had any tetanus immunization.

If there is any doubt about tetanus cover, it is best to assume the person is not covered and get them seen in hospital.

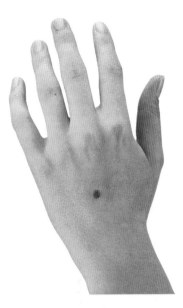

△ Penetrating wounds caused by needle-like objects or cats' teeth are prone to infection.

TETANUS-PRONE WOUNDS

The following wounds are particularly prone to infection with tetanus.

➤ Those contaminated with soil or faeces.

➤ Old wounds (more than six hours).

➤ Puncture wounds.

➤ Wounds with a poor blood supply.

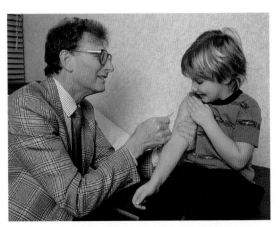

◁ A child is given the tetanus vaccine (combined with diphtheria and pertussis vaccines). When dealing with anyone with a wound, no matter how clean it looks, always try to check if their immunization against tetanus is up to date. Elderly people in particular may never have had any routine tetanus boosters.

Dealing with major wounds

SEE ALSO

➤ Controlling severe bleeding, p142

➤ Recognizing internal bleeding, p144

➤ Managing rib fractures, p164

The two main priorities when treating major wounds are to stop the bleeding and get help as fast as possible. You must call the emergency services as fast as possible because large blood loss is very serious, and because the wound may conceal further internal injury. Try to dress the wound effectively if you can, although large wounds will usually need professional cleaning and stitching in a hospital's accident and emergency department. While you wait for paramedics to arrive, keep the casualty warm and reassure them that help is on the way.

Large wounds may bleed profusely and signify greater problems internally. When wounds are over the abdomen or chest, particular care must be taken to avoid exacerbating the situation. You should not attempt to remove an object embedded in a wound (see page 134), nor should you try to stop the bleeding by applying a tourniquet (see page 140).

If possible, wear protective gloves before treating the bleeding; otherwise wash your hands well both before and afterwards. Once you have stopped the bleeding, brushed any debris off the wound (do not wash it) and dressed it, call for an ambulance if this has not already been done by a helper.

The casualty may lose consciousness and may also develop symptoms of shock. Do not leave them alone except to call for help. Keep the person warm while you wait for the emergency services to arrive.

BASIC FIRST AID FOR MAJOR WOUNDS

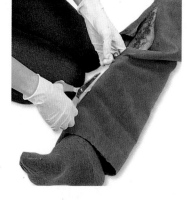

1 Wear protective gloves. Expose the wound. Do not drag clothing over the wound, but cut or lift aside the clothing.

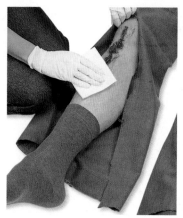

2 Using a gauze pad, clear the wound surface of any obvious debris such as large shards of glass, lumps of grit or mud.

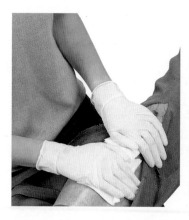

3 Control bleeding with direct pressure and then by elevating the limb.

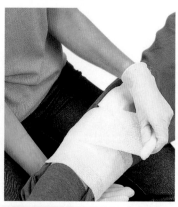

4 Once bleeding is controlled, apply a bandage to the wound.

5 Keep the casualty warm and rested until help arrives. (If the casualty is suffering badly from shock, keep both legs raised above heart level, comfortably supported.)

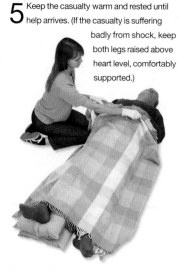

ABDOMINAL WOUNDS

There are many organs within the abdominal cavity, all of which may become injured and bleed profusely with little sign of external damage. Any penetrating injury to the abdomen could damage the internal organs, and might also introduce infection into the abdominal cavity, leading to peritonitis. If a penetrating object – such as a knife or a piece of metal – remains in the wound, it should be left where it is, or even more damage may be inflicted.

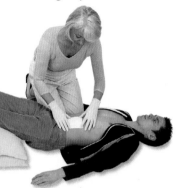

△ When dealing with abdominal wounds, try to keep the casualty's legs elevated at about this height or slightly higher, with knees bent.

CHEST WOUNDS

Take great care when dealing with any injury in the chest area. Look out for breathing difficulty, a penetrating wound, or a "flail chest" (multiple rib fractures causing unusual movement). These conditions can indicate life-threatening damage that needs emergency attention.

In many cases, especially after a high-speed car accident or a fall, the casualty may have fluid or bruising in the lungs, which will make them very short of breath. You can do little in this kind of scenario except keep your casualty sitting up and supported, and reassure them, until emergency aid arrives.

First-aid efforts are potentially life-saving where a casualty has an injury that penetrates the chest wall. This may occur as a result of a rib fracture (even a person with a simple rib fracture may perforate a lung if they bend at an awkward angle), a stabbing or a gunshot injury, for example. The casualty may end up with air entering the lung cavity as they breathe in, and this will eventually lead to lung collapse. If the lung is perforated, air escapes out of the lung into the space between the lung and the chest wall, and will again cause the lung to collapse. These cases need urgent help.

FIRST AID FOR AN ABDOMINAL WOUND

Lay the casualty flat and raise their legs.

Call the emergency services.

If there are organs visible, cover them with plastic food wrap to stop them drying out or sticking to dressings.

Dress other wounds with a large sterile dressing.

Stabilize any penetrating objects by using your hands.

If the casualty starts to vomit or loses consciousness, place them in the recovery position. Support the wound during coughing or vomiting.

FIRST AID FOR A CHEST WOUND

FOR ALL CHEST WOUNDS:
Sit casualty on the floor, upright and supported, without bending forward.

Summon emergency help urgently, using a bystander if possible.

Monitor the casualty's ABC; be prepared to resuscitate if breathing or pulse stops.

FOR PENETRATING CHEST WOUNDS:
Leave any penetrating object in place and keep it still with your hand(s).

Seal the wound by hand, either:
• Pinching the flesh together both sides of the penetrating object.
• With your hand over the casualty's hand, placed flat on to the hole.

If you need to attend to other injuries, or the casualty seems to be losing consciousness: seal the wound completely with something plastic, then a flat pad on top, all held in place with very tight bandages.

IMPORTANT NOTES:
• Do not let further air enter the wound while applying bandages.
• Do not use sticky tape – it may not stick to the shocked person's sweaty skin; taped dressings may leak or let further air in if applied slowly or incorrectly.
• The priority is to seal the hole completely and get help rapidly.

Coping with severed body parts

SEE ALSO

➤ What is first aid?, p16
➤ Full resuscitation sequence, p38
➤ Dealing with shock, p72
➤ Controlling severe bleeding, p142

When a person loses a finger, hand, toe, ear or limb as the result of an accident, there may be considerable bleeding and the person is likely to suffer shock. Your priorities are to stop the bleeding and to get the person to hospital or summon the emergency services immediately.

It is vital that you take the body part with you as it may be possible for it to be reattached. Keeping it cool improves the chances of this, but you should not freeze or place ice directly next to the body part. It is also important that you do your best to keep the casualty calm.

A severing of a body part by whatever means, whether accidental or surgical, is known as an amputation. Accidental amputations are most commonly the result of occupational injuries inflicted by power tools or industrial machinery; they also can often occur during a road accident. The body part may be torn, crushed or sliced off. The smaller parts of the body such as fingers and toes are most likely to be involved.

The main priority in the case of an amputation is to stop the bleeding, but also to remember to take the amputated body part to the hospital with the casualty. If a body part is kept at 4°C (39.2°F), there is still a chance that it can be sewn back or "re-implanted" within 12–24 hours.

If you have to take a severed body part to hospital, keep it dry and cool – wrapped in plastic, then protected with padding and placed in ice (see flowchart). **Do not**:

- Let ice or water come into direct contact with the part – this causes tissue damage.
- Use dry ice or chemical additives.
- Freeze the part.
- Use cotton wool or fluffy dressings, as the fibres may stick to the part.
- Wash the part, especially with soap or disinfectant.

WARNING

Tourniquets are emergency devices for stemming bleeding – the simplest form is a very tight bandage. Tourniquets risk making the tissue damage even worse by cutting off its blood supply, and thus necessitating even more of the limb being amputated. They also lessen the chances of successful re-implantation. This is why they should never be used in first aid, except by highly trained professionals under specific circumstances.

FIRST AID AFTER AN AMPUTATION

Follow DRSABC and if necessary, administer basic life support.

↓

Control bleeding by applying pressure directly to the wound using gauze cloths, and elevation.

↓

Call the emergency services. Tell them that the case involves amputation.

↓

If pressure does not stop the bleeding, press harder and elevate higher. Do not consider using a tourniquet unless you are a trained professional (see Warning box).

↓

Keep the amputated part dry, protected and cool: double-wrap it in plastic, then add padding and place in a container or bag of ice.

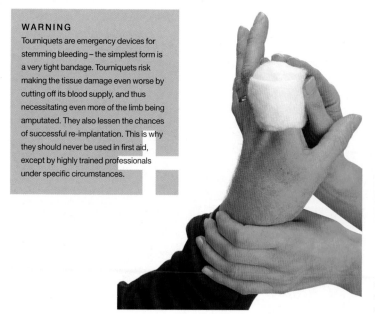

◁ Pressure and elevation are the key things for a first-aider to remember when trying to stop bleeding after an amputation.

Managing crush injuries

SEE ALSO
▶ Full resuscitation sequence, p38
▶ Dealing with shock, p72
▶ BONE AND MUSCLE INJURIES, p151

A casualty who has suffered a crush injury requires the urgent attention of paramedics, and ambulance transfer to hospital. Crush injuries occur in road accidents, for example when someone becomes crushed against the steering wheel, in buildings that suffer structural damage, and in industrial and agricultural accidents when someone is crushed by heavy machinery. The injury may result in serious complications, so it is essential to call the emergency services as quickly as possible, and to control any external bleeding.

In all cases involving trapped casualties or crush injuries, call the emergency services immediately. As well as paramedics, the fire service may be needed to release the casualty. Generally it is safer all round to leave the release of a casualty to the professionals.

CRUSHED HANDS, FINGERS, FEET AND TOES

If these are caught in machinery or tricky to release, leave this to the professionals. If the crushed part has already been released:
• Deal with any bleeding, and apply a sterile dressing.
• Treat as for fractures, with padding, immobilization and elevation.

CRUSHED LIMBS

The offending object may be just bulky enough to cut off the blood supply, or a hard impact or very heavy object may have caused fractures and severe tissue damage.

If left for too long, toxins, waste products and blood clots can develop in crushed limbs. When released, these may lead to fatal kidney and heart failure. However, this usually takes over 30 minutes to occur, by which time emergency helpers will hopefully be in control. Where a crushed limb has been released, treat it as a fracture.

CRUSHED ABDOMEN AND PELVIS

Any crushing or blunt impact to the abdomen can cause severe internal bleeding and damage. The casualty may show no outward signs at first, so the accident history could be your only clue to a potentially severe condition.

The ideal first-aid position here is the "shock" position, with legs raised – unless this might worsen damage, in which case keep them still. If they need to vomit, you may need to turn them on their side. Do not sit them up. Treat a crushed pelvis as a fracture, and get help very quickly.

CRUSHED CHEST

A heavy weight on the chest can cause a casualty's breathing to stop. Check that nothing under the object is penetrating the chest and then carefully lift the object off, if you can. If breathing has stopped, prepare to resuscitate. Conscious casualties may find it easier to breathe sitting up, but keeping them in their current position until help arrives will often prevent further damage.

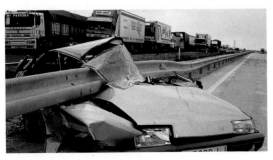

◁ Road accidents are a major cause of crush injuries. Such accidents also have great potential for further disaster. Never step into a dangerous environment or try to release anyone if you are risking your own safety or could cause them further harm.

FIRST AID FOR CRUSH INJURIES

Make any threatening structures/objects safe/stable, but only if this will not endanger yourself or the casualty.

Check the casualty's RABC and contact the emergency services.

Only try to release the casualty if vital (e.g. crushed chest) or if it will be 30 minutes or more before emergency aid arrives. Only do this if you will not endanger yourself or further endanger the casualty.

If injuries involve the head or neck, make sure that these are kept still (to avoid worsening any possible spinal injury).

Treat any bleeding or fractures.

Treat for shock, but only raise the legs if pretty certain there are no leg fractures.

Keep the casualty warm and still. Continue to monitor their RABC until help arrives.

Controlling severe bleeding

SEE ALSO
➤ Dealing with head injury, p84
➤ Dealing with major wounds, p138

Stemming blood flow from a large wound is a life-saving procedure. The main method used combines pressure and elevation. Apply direct pressure to the site of the blood loss with your hand or the casualty's hand, unless the wound contains foreign matter such as glass. In this case, squeeze the edges of the wound together. Elevating the wounded area also helps to stem blood loss – even if a limb is fractured, your priority is to stop the bleeding, especially if it is heavy, and then worry about the fracture. However, try to handle fractured limbs gently.

Injury to an artery can lead to a life-threatening loss of blood in a very short time. Stemming the blood flow may save the casualty's life and is your main priority as a first-aider (once you have dealt with the casualty's ABC, that is).

With more superficial wounds, bleeding may sometimes seem profuse without, in fact, being too dangerous. Head wounds are a good case in point here. The scalp has a very rich blood supply, so head wounds often bleed profusely, even if they are quite superficial. Do not, however, automatically go to the other extreme and assume that it is not serious. Also, always try to assess any underlying damage – especially important with head wounds.

CONTROLLING BLEEDING ON A HEAD WOUND

Dealing with heavy bleeding from a head wound varies slightly in some details from tackling heavy bleeding from other sites (see text elsewhere on other types of wound).

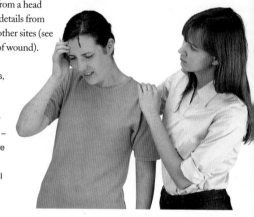

1 If the casualty is unconscious, follow DRSABC before dealing with the wound – airway and breathing are top priority. Try to find the source of the bleeding – remember that there may be more than one site. If the casualty is conscious, ask them to tell you all they can about what happened, to help your assessment.

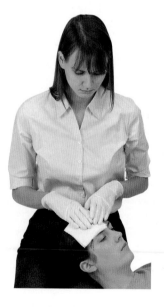

2 To control bleeding, place firm pressure directly over the wound using a clean pad (a sterile first-aid dressing or a towel, sanitary towel, tea towel or T-shirt). Use gentle pressure if you suspect a fracture. Getting the casualty to lie down with head and shoulders raised (and supported) helps to reduce pressure within the head. Send for emergency help, if you have not already done so.

3 Secure the dressing with a roller bandage or equivalent. If the casualty's general condition seems good, sitting them up may reduce bleeding, but don't get them sitting up and lying down like a yo-yo. Make sure that the dressing covers the whole wound. If blood starts oozing through the dressing, don't take the original dressing off but place another one on top.

Note: It isn't always easy to find the exact site of a head wound. If you are not sure, cover the bloodiest area on the scalp with a dressing.

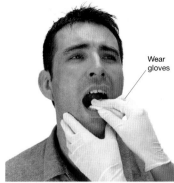

Wear gloves

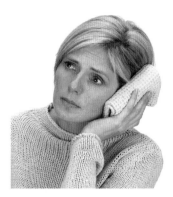

△ Bleeding from the mouth: place a wad of sterile gauze in the mouth and ask the casualty to bite down on it to soak up the blood.

△ Nosebleed: the casualty should breathe though the mouth and pinch the soft end of the nose. If it still bleeds, they should pinch harder.

△ Bleeding from the ear: place a sterile pad or clean towel over the ear and tilt the head to drain out the blood. Call a doctor immediately.

BLEEDING FROM THE MOUTH

This may arise from biting the inside of the mouth, or after a tooth has fallen out or been extracted. It can occur after violent impact, along with concussion and jaw fracture. The main concern should be keeping the airway clear of blood, especially if the person is unconscious.

BLEEDING FROM THE NOSE

Nosebleeds usually start at the lower end of the nose, although in older people with very high blood pressure, they may come from the back of the nose and be harder to stop. Nosebleeds often occur during or after a cold when the lining is inflamed. Other causes are a direct impact (which may also have caused concussion and head or facial fractures), violent nose-blowing and nose-picking. Watery blood from the nose may arise from a fracture at the base of the skull.

BLEEDING FROM THE EAR

Like a nosebleed, watery blood from the ear may be a sign of a fractured base of the skull if it happens after a head injury. However, it is usually due to local causes – often a hairgrip or other foreign body has been inserted into the ear and has perforated the eardrum. Other causes of a perforated eardrum are loud explosions, blows to the head and, most commonly, an infection in the middle ear. The person always has severe ear pain when this happens, after which those with middle ear infections will often feel a relief of their symptoms. Ear infections often need antibiotics.

FIRST AID FOR BLEEDING FROM THE MOUTH

Wear gloves. If the person has lost a tooth or had one extracted, place a wad of sterile gauze against the tooth socket and get them to bite down on it. Change it if it becomes soaked. With a mouth wound, ask the person to apply pressure with their finger and thumb until bleeding stops.

Tell the person to spit out the blood – it may make them vomit if they swallow it. They should avoid hot drinks.

If bleeding persists, take the casualty to hospital. They may need to see a dentist.

FIRST AID FOR A NOSEBLEED

Casualty must lean forwards, breathe through the mouth and pinch the soft end of their nose. If bleeding persists, they must pinch harder. Pinch for at least 10 minutes, then check to see if the bleeding has stopped. Place a bag of frozen peas (wrapped in a towel or similar to prevent burning the skin) over the nose.

Get the person to rest for several hours, and avoid sniffing, blowing or picking their nose. If bleeding continues for 30 minutes, take them to hospital (lots of swallowing may indicate blood still going down the back of the throat). If it is very heavy and shock symptoms set in, call for an ambulance.

FIRST AID FOR BLEEDING FROM THE EAR

Put a pad over the ear, and get the sufferer to tilt their heads to allow the blood to drain out.

Give them pain relief (but only if there is no head injury) and seek medical attention.

Miscellaneous foreign bodies

SEE ALSO
► Tackling embedded objects, p134
► Treating infected wounds, p136
► Bleeding from orifices, p146

As well as becoming embedded in wounds, foreign bodies of all kinds – from an insect flying into the ear to a piece of grit caught under an eyelid – can become lodged in the body's orifices. Such objects may cause injury, bleeding, infection and other problems. Children are notorious for putting things in their mouths and ears and up their noses, as they explore the world around them, when they are too young to realize the potential danger. Foreign bodies must be removed safely and cleanly, to avoid the risk of damage or infection.

It is usually children and people with psychiatric problems who place foreign bodies inside their orifices deliberately. But foreign bodies can become lodged in part of the body accidentally as well.

SWALLOWING OBJECTS

Children often put things in their mouths and then swallow them – plastic toys, pen lids, money and paper clips, to name a few. If this occurs, the child may have a choking episode and then fully recover – but with a noticeable absence of the object that was in their hand. Adults may also accidentally swallow small, whole items of food, such as peanuts or sweets, if they are eating while talking or laughing.

If, instead of being swallowed, the object sticks in the windpipe, it may cause partial or complete choking. Because this will impede breathing, it is an acute emergency. If the object sticks in the oesophagus, the upper gullet leading down to the stomach, the person may drool, gag or be unable to eat or drink anything – also a medical emergency.

Once in the stomach, inedible objects usually pass through the gut and out in the faeces with no problems. Unless a child develops acute stomach pain or vomiting, or stops opening their bowels, nothing needs to be done. However, if they have swallowed a battery or a sharp object such as a pin, these can damage the digestive tract and must be removed; they will show up on an X-ray.

GENITALS AND RECTUM

People may end up with objects lodged in the penis, the female urethra, the vagina or the rectum. In any of these cases, never try to retrieve the object, as this can cause damage to these delicate areas. Take the person to an accident and emergency department for treatment by a doctor or nurse.

NOSES

Children often put small objects up their noses. The child may develop a foul-smelling discharge from one nostril after a few days. Blocking the other nostril and getting the child to blow their nose often brings out the foreign body. There is a danger that the child will inhale the foreign body into their airway, so if you do not succeed in removing it, take them to hospital immediately.

EYES

People often get things in their eyes – dust on a windy day, a bit of ash from a bonfire or even a fragment of metal hammered off a metal object. They can often feel the object in the eye, or the eye may feel irritated and painful, and it will usually water profusely and look red. An X-ray may be needed if any metal hits the eye at speed, as it may end up at the back of the eye.

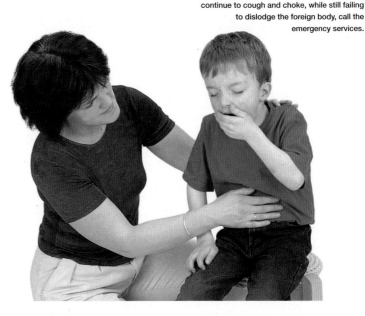

▽ If a swallowed object makes a child or adult continue to cough and choke, while still failing to dislodge the foreign body, call the emergency services.

HOW TO EXAMINE THE EYES

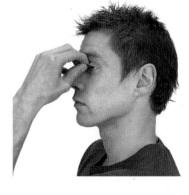

1 Examine the person's eye either in natural daylight or under a direct ray from a lamp. Stand behind them, so that you are looking down on them. Keeping their head very still, ask them to look from side to side and then up and down. In each direction, have a good look at the white of the eye, called the conjunctiva, then look at the coloured part of the eye, the iris.

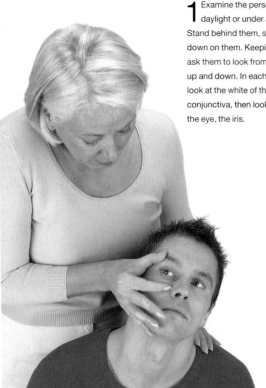

2 Ask them to look down and then gently pull out the lower lid by the lashes. Look on the underside of the upper lid – specks of grit often stick here.

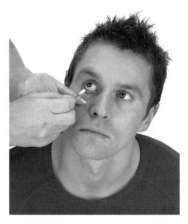

3 To remove an object, try to brush it off with a cotton bud moistened in water (on the eyeball, only touch the white area, and only once). Or flush the eye with clean, luke-warm water or an eye-wash solution. If all this fails, cover the eye with an eye pad and take them to a doctor.

EARS

Insects flying into ears is a fairly common occurrence, and this can be alarming. Deafness is the main symptom of a foreign body in the ear, or there may be a loud buzzing from a trapped fly. Whatever the culprit, do not attempt to prise it out. Try filling the ear with olive oil. This will kill any insects, and small foreign bodies may float out. Ask the person to turn their head so that the ear containing the foreign body points downwards – this may lead to the foreign body dropping out. If all fails, take them to a doctor.

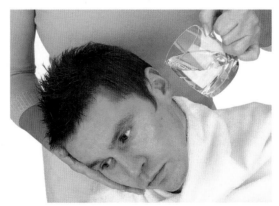

◁ Flush out a foreign body in the ear with lukewarm water or with olive oil. Never try to dig or poke it out as you may cause damage to the eardrum.

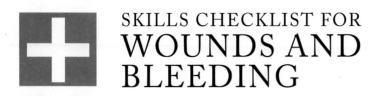

KEY POINTS

- The basic issues of wound-care are stemming blood loss and preventing infection. For major wounds, the priorities (after assessing ABC) are stopping bleeding and getting help. ☐

- Heavy blood loss leads rapidly to body shut-down. ☐

- Foreign objects can cause severe damage and infection and must be dealt with promptly. ☐

- Any infected wound must be closely monitored. ☐

- Wounds may mask underlying damage – which is why getting help fast is so vital. ☐

- It is usually best to leave the release of crushed/trapped casualties to the professionals. ☐

- Stem heavy blood loss by using pressure and elevation. ☐

- Internal bleeding often shows few clear outward signs. Urgent medical help is vital. ☐

SKILLS LEARNED

- How to recognize different types of wound and follow appropriate treatment. ☐

- How to control bleeding and deal with infection. ☐

- What to do with severe wounds and injuries. ☐

- When to suspect internal bleeding. ☐

- How to tackle embedded and lodged foreign bodies. ☐

BONE AND
MUSCLE INJURIES

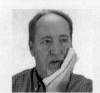

It is not always easy to distinguish a fracture from a dislocation or a sprain. This chapter explains how to help a casualty in the event of various types of fracture, sprains, dislocations and back pain. It is essential if there is any possibility of a neck or spinal injury that the casualty is not moved, unless not moving them would put them in further danger. The main priorities in dealing with bone and muscle injuries are to immobilize the affected limb, cover any open wounds and alert the emergency services.

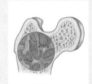

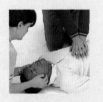

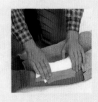

Understanding the skeleton

SEE ALSO

➤ Removing clothing and helmets, p22

➤ Moving and handling safely 1 and 2, pp24, 26

➤ Dealing with broken bones, p154

The body's bones come in all shapes and sizes, and it is the muscles that are attached at multiple points all over the skeleton that enable us to move about. If any of the 206 bones in the body are injured through fracture (a clean break, a messy break, a chip, a splinter, or a crack), our ability to move properly can be substantially diminished, and pain and swelling may occur around the site of the injured bone. Initial first aid, followed by professional treatment in hospital, is vital for optimum healing of all such bone injuries or fractures.

Bone is a living tissue that continuously builds, degrades, and rebuilds itself throughout life. The skeleton's bony framework has many functions: bones protect the organs from damage; muscles attach to bones so that we can move; many types of blood cell are produced in the bone's marrow; and bone acts as a store of the minerals calcium and phosphate.

As we grow older, the strength of our bones – bone density – declines as bones lose calcium, so they become easy to break. Many elderly people break bones after minor bumps or falls.

WHAT IS BONE MADE OF?

Bone is made of a meshwork of a protein (collagen) into which calcium is deposited to give hardness and strength. Although bone is extremely strong it is not completely solid. The outer layer is hard and compact, but beneath it lies a centre of spongy bone. The spaces within the spongy bone allow room for the skeleton's immense blood supply and nerves.

INSIDE A TYPICAL BONE

▽ The circle section shows a close-up view of the internal meshwork of the spongy bone.

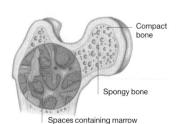

Compact bone

Spongy bone

Spaces containing marrow

THE SKELETON

▷ The many bones of the skeleton give the body shape and structure. Bones that are commonly fractured are named on this illustration.

Scapula (shoulder blade)

Humerus

Radius

Ulna

Calcaneus (heelbone)

Skull

Mandible (jaw)

Sternum (breastbone)

Clavicle (collarbone)

Rib

Vertebral column

Ilium

Pubis
Ischium

(all three together known as the pelvis)

Femur (thighbone)

Tibia

Fibula

WHAT HEALTHY BONES NEED

➤ Calcium – Your diet should include plenty of calcium-rich foods such as milk, cheese and yogurt. At certain stages of life, such as childhood and during pregnancy and breastfeeding, a higher calcium intake may be needed so that your body doesn't raid the skeleton's stores of this mineral.

➤ Vitamin D – The body makes vitamin D in the skin when it is exposed to sunlight. This vitamin allows the body to absorb calcium and phosphorus from food.

➤ Exercise – Weight-bearing exercise, such as walking or skipping, promotes bone growth and bone density.

HOW BONES CAN FRACTURE

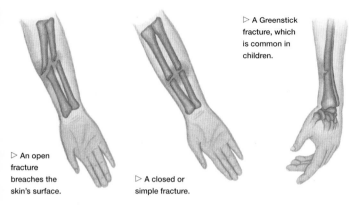

▷ An open fracture breaches the skin's surface.

▷ A closed or simple fracture.

▷ A Greenstick fracture, which is common in children.

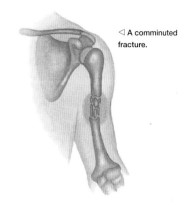

◁ A comminuted fracture.

WHAT CAUSES A FRACTURE?

A bone may break because of a direct blow, such as a punch or kick, or from indirect forces. Bones fracture indirectly when, for example, a person falls on to a hand that they have stretched out to break their fall. The forces from the fall travel up the arm (which remains unharmed) and cause the collarbone to break. Bones may also fracture from rotating movements – when someone twists an ankle, for example.

OPEN OR CLOSED FRACTURES?

There are two basic types of fracture known as open and closed. Open fractures (also called compound fractures) occur when the broken ends of bone stick out through the skin. In open fractures, the risk of developing an infection is much higher, as are the chances of nerve or blood vessel damage. Closed fractures (also called simple fractures) are fractures in which the skin is not broken over the fracture site.

HOW BONES HEAL

Different bones heal at different rates, so while a fractured collarbone may heal fully in six weeks, a broken thighbone (femur) may take up to six months before it is mended completely. The rate of bone regeneration in children is much faster than in most adults, and so broken bones in children tend to heal much more quickly.

Bone-healing has several stages:
• Six to eight hours after injury – In this inflammatory period, blood seeps out of the broken bone ends and forms a clot.
• After two days – Bone-making cells migrate to the blood clot and start to form new bone, called callus, to bridge the gap between the bones.
• A few weeks to several months – The original shape of the bone is restored.

COMMON FRACTURE TYPES

Bones fracture in different ways in different people and depending on how an incident came about. Common types of fracture are:

➤ Greenstick fracture – Children sometimes fracture only one side of a bone. The other side bends like a new tree branch.

➤ Comminuted fracture – The bone is splintered at the fracture site, and smaller fragments of bone are found between the two main fragments.

➤ Fracture-dislocation – This type of fracture occurs when a bone breaks or cracks near an already dislocated joint.

➤ Avulsion fracture – When a ligament or muscle attached to a bone is ripped off, it often takes a piece of bone with it.

➤ Pathological fractures – Certain medical conditions, such as osteoporosis and osteogenesis imperfecta, make bones more likely to break.

WHAT DELAYS HEALING?

Although infection increases the blood supply to a fracture site, it brings the wrong kind of cells, so healing is delayed. Also, if the bones are not in alignment with one another, they are not going to heal well. This is one reason why splinting, or at least immobilization, of a fracture is vitally important for proper and speedy bone healing.

HOW BONE HEALS

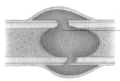

Blood clot fills the gap between the broken bones

△ Six to eight hours after the injury.

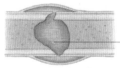

New spongy bone (callus) starts to form

△ Two days after the injury.

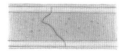

△ A few weeks or months afterwards.

Dealing with broken bones

SEE ALSO
➤ What is first aid?, p16
➤ Dealing with shock, p72
➤ Fixing slings, p210

Bones tend to break as the result of a huge impact or force. A fracture casualty may be able to tell you that they heard or felt a crack when the accident occurred and that they can feel bones grating over one another when they try to move. Such clues are important information for the first-aider. Bear in mind that the casualty could be in great pain, and also watch for signs of shock – this may develop, for example, if the fracture causes heavy internal bleeding. Never move a casualty unless you have to in order to remove them from other serious dangers.

When managing a fracture casualty, always monitor ABC before dealing with possible fractures and always assess the person as a whole – there could well be other injuries.

In the short term, the various methods used to deal with fractures focus on preventing the fracture from becoming worse, and they all achieve this by immobilization – keeping the fracture still. The general idea is to immobilize the fracture and the joints above and below the fracture. Movement of a fracture can cause increased pain, damage to surrounding tissue and structures and possibly even severe complications such as shock from increased bleeding or from bone penetrating through skin, nerves or blood vessels. In the long term, a broken bone needs to be left clean and undisturbed for proper healing.

SHOULD SPLINTS BE USED?

Using splints (rigid supports) for a fracture is little used by most first-aiders today, unless in very remote locations, or where the first-aider is forced to transport the casualty to help. Improvised examples of splints include umbrellas and broom handles. Except for simple, undisplaced arm fractures, transporting a splinted fracture casualty is not recommended unless you have proper training and practice, and a suitable vehicle.

IMMOBILIZATION STRATEGIES

There are two major types of immediate first aid for fractures:
• Basic hand immobilization. Try to imagine the break that has occurred in

BASIC CARE FOR A CLOSED OR SIMPLE FRACTURE

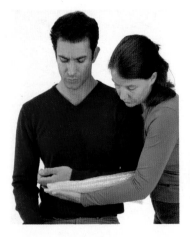

1 Having assessed the casualty, ask them to keep the fracture area still. Support the fracture and apply light padding, such as some folded bubble wrap or a small towel or tea towel (nothing too bulky).

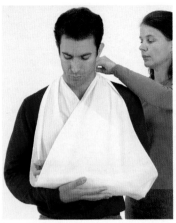

2 Depending on the part of the body involved, you should usually attempt to immobilize the area. Do this here by applying a broad arm sling, as shown, keeping the light padding in place within the sling.

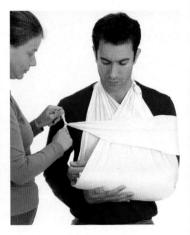

3 Immobilize the arm further by tying a triangular bandage (folded into a long strip), or equivalent, across the chest. This will prevent movement when the casualty is in transit to hospital. Phone for medical help.

the normally rigid bone. Use your hands and arms to cradle the limb in order to stop all movement. This method is most appropriate when help will arrive fairly quickly, or where no other equipment or materials of any kind are available.

- Using padding and boxes. These first-aid props are used mostly for leg fractures or for arm fractures where bending the elbow to put the arm in a sling would cause further damage. For this method, hold the limb still. Roll large, loose sausages from objects such as blankets, coats or towels and place these carefully against the fractured limb. Any gaps beneath the limb, such as from a bent knee, should be carefully filled with just enough padding material to provide support under the area without moving the limb at all. Boxes or other weighted items are now placed either side of the limb to hold the padding in place.

The padding and boxes method is ideal in most populated areas with good ambulance response times. It frees the first-aider to concentrate on taking care of the casualty and on simply minimizing any movement. It also means that paramedics arriving on the scene do not need to waste time removing a first-aider's bandages in order to replace them with their own, superior, equipment.

COMMON SIGNS AND SYMPTOMS OF A FRACTURE

➤ There may be a history of impact or trauma at the site.

➤ Swelling, bruising or deformity at fracture site.

➤ Pain on moving.

➤ Numbness or tingling in injured area.

➤ Wound site at or near fracture site.

➤ The casualty may have heard the bones grating on one another.

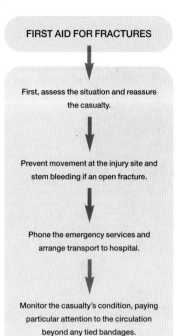

FIRST AID FOR FRACTURES

↓

First, assess the situation and reassure the casualty.

↓

Prevent movement at the injury site and stem bleeding if an open fracture.

↓

Phone the emergency services and arrange transport to hospital.

↓

Monitor the casualty's condition, paying particular attention to the circulation beyond any tied bandages.

FIRST AID FOR AN OPEN FRACTURE

When you are dealing with an open fracture, it is important to prevent blood loss and infection at the injury site as well as immobilizing the area.

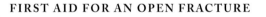

▷ Call the emergency services urgently. Carefully place a dressing or sterile pad over the wound site, and apply hand pressure either side of the protruding bone to control the bleeding. Never press on the protruding bone itself. Build up padding alongside the bone if it is sticking out of the skin. You may want to secure the dressing and padding firmly with a bandage, but do not do so if it causes any movement of the limb, and never bandage too tightly. Monitor the casualty's condition, specifically their ABC, as there may be a risk of shock.

▷ In more extreme circumstances – if you are in a very remote location, emergency help is seriously delayed, or you are forced to take the casualty to a doctor/hospital yourself – you may need to splint the fracture. Add extra padding around the limb and fix with tied bandages or equivalent. Keep any movement to a minimum.

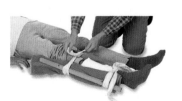

WARNING

In most cases, a first-aider must never straighten or move the fractured limb. If a foot looks blue or bloodless, always tell the paramedics; they may manipulate the fracture in order to restore circulation.

Tackling skull and facial fractures

SEE ALSO

➤ Responsiveness and the airway, p32

➤ Dealing with head injury, p84

➤ Dealing with broken bones, p154

Suspected head injury is always a serious situation. The spinal cord, brain or organs within the head, such as the eye or ear, may also be damaged – not only by the impact of the injury but also by the potential bleeding into the brain that such an injury can cause. It is vital to monitor someone with a suspected skull fracture as they may lose consciousness and/or may have a neck or spinal injury. The main point to bear in mind with any facial fracture is that swollen tissues, blood and saliva may impair breathing by obstructing the airway.

Skull fractures are worrying because an impact large enough to fracture skull bones might also injure the delicate brain beneath. The fracture itself may cause no damage, but if a slab of skull bone is crushed inwards (a "depressed fracture") it may put pressure on the brain. Skull fractures may also cause internal bleeding into the brain area.

Call the emergency services as promptly as possible. Be aware of anything that might suggest a neck or spinal injury – if there is any chance of these injuries, treat the casualty with extreme care and keep them totally still.

SKULL FRACTURES

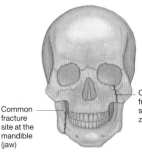

Common fracture site at the mandible (jaw)

Common fracture site at the zygoma

△ The tough skull bones can be fractured; common injury sites are shown above.

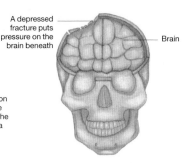

A depressed fracture puts pressure on the brain beneath

Brain

△ A serious skull fracture could mean that the vulnerable tissues of the brain directly beneath are also damaged. If there is also a wound over the fracture site, then the brain may become exposed to the possibility of infection.

SIGNS OF A SKULL FRACTURE

➤ A "boggy" soft swelling or egg-shaped bruise on the head.

➤ Bruising around eye and/or ear area.

➤ A noticeably lopsided appearance to the head – very serious sign.

➤ A deteriorating level of consciousness (remember AVPU) – very serious sign.

➤ Any blood visible in the whites of the eyes – very serious sign.

➤ Clear or blood-stained fluid leaking from the nose or ears – very serious sign.

Signs of possible internal bleeding:

➤ One-sided, worsening headache; headache that worsens with lying flat/making any effort.

➤ Any visual problems.

➤ Change in/loss of consciousness.

➤ Vomiting.

FIRST AID FOR SUSPECTED SKULL FRACTURE

CONSCIOUS CASUALTIES
Call for an ambulance and make sure the casualty is comfortably seated.
Dress any open scalp wounds.
Watch out for drowsiness/loss of consciousness or profuse vomiting and try to keep them awake.
If they have a headache, do not give any medication, or anything else by mouth, until a doctor has assessed them.

UNCONSCIOUS CASUALTIES
Call an ambulance.
Check DRSABC and begin CPR if needed.
If breathing, with signs of circulation, place in recovery position, and dress any open head wounds.

FRACTURES TO THE FACE

Facial injuries are not often fatal, but they are worrying because of their potential to obstruct the airway and result in breathing problems. Compulsory seat-belt wearing has dramatically cut down facial injuries due to road traffic accidents, and the main causes of injuries now are sport, falls and assaults. Heavy force is needed to fracture a bone in the face, and there will often be other injuries of the neck, chest and skull to look out for.

Suspect a facial fracture if:

• The face looks asymmetrical or deformed in any way.

• There is bruising and/or a black eye.

• There is bleeding from the teeth or nose.

• The person cannot clench their teeth.

• There is difficulty breathing, or the casualty is snoring if unconscious.

FIRST AID FOR FACIAL FRACTURES OR INJURIES

↓

Ensure that the casualty's airway is clear. If necessary, remove any debris from the mouth.

↓

If there is a lot of bleeding or you think they may lose consciousness, place them in the recovery position. (Be aware of the risk of neck injury.)

↓

Call the emergency services promptly. Place ice on any swelling of the face.

FIRST AID FOR A FRACTURED JAW

↓

If there is bleeding in the mouth and they have potentially broken both sides of the jaw, lie them down, place them in the recovery position and keep a careful eye on their airway.

↓

Call the emergency services promptly.

↓

If only one side of the jaw is painful and swollen, get them to hold a soft cloth against the area to keep it still.

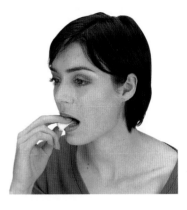

△ The casualty should hold the dislodged tooth in its socket either by keeping the mouth shut or by pressing on it with a pad.

KNOCKED-OUT TEETH

Tooth injuries are especially common in children, and any loose first teeth should be taken out by a dentist, to avoid possible inhalation. Adult teeth can be damaged permanently by fracture or by being dislodged from a socket. If the tooth is not put back into its socket within 24 hours, the tooth dies and the socket shrinks, so that even false teeth cannot be used.

FRACTURES TO THE JAW

The jaw is a common bone to break. Any blow to the chin may break one or both sides of the jaw. If both sides fracture, then the tongue can become unstable and may block the airway. Suspect a fractured jaw if:
• There is pain, nausea and/or swelling of the jaw area.
• The person cannot bite and is dribbling.
• The casualty has difficulty swallowing, breathing or speaking.

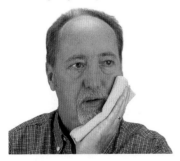

△ In a suspected jaw fracture, ask the casualty to hold a soft cloth against the injured site to protect it, and then transport them to hospital without delay.

NOSE AND CHEEKBONE FRACTURES

Fractures of the nose and cheekbone are generally not serious unless the cheekbone injury involves the eye socket. A direct blow to the eye, especially common in squash games, may cause what is called a "blow-out fracture", making it impossible for the person to look upwards.

If you suspect either a nose or cheekbone (or eye socket) fracture, do not let the person blow their nose. This is because it may cause air to track through broken bones into the skin or into the brain.

Action to take if you suspect a fracture of a cheekbone or nose is to:
• check carefully to see whether the casualty's airway is clear and that it is not obstructed by swollen tissues
• apply a cold compress to the injured site to reduce pain and swelling
• get the casualty to hospital.
If the casualty has a nosebleed, you should try to stop the bleeding; if the liquid is either clear or yellow, then treat as you would for a skull fracture.

FIRST AID FOR A KNOCKED-OUT TOOTH

↓

Pop the tooth back into its socket and ask the casualty to hold the tooth in place.

↓

If they cannot hold it firmly in place, put the tooth in a beaker or a small plastic bag of milk to prevent it drying out.

↓

Take them to a hospital or dentist within 24 hours.

Managing spinal injuries

SEE ALSO

► LIFE-SAVING
   PRIORITIES, p29
► Coping with neck
   injuries, p160

The golden rule with spinal injuries (and neck injuries) is that the casualty must not be moved unless it is vital to do so. People with head injuries of any kind often have spinal injuries as well. The spinal cord, housed within the vertebrae, is commonly damaged at the mobile parts of the backbone such as the neck and lower back. Road accidents, rugby and diving are notorious causes of spinal injuries; other causes include falling from a height, being thrown from a horse, and impact to the head and/or face.

The term spinal injury can refer to damage to the bones of the spine (vertebrae), the spinal cord, the discs between the backbones or any muscles and ligaments attached to the spine. The most serious type of injury is to the spinal cord, as a partial or complete break can result in permanent paralysis. If a splinter of bone or swollen tissue compresses a nerve, a person may suffer a temporary paralysis but sensation and movement return once the injury is treated.

THE BACKBONE

There are 24 moving vertebrae in the spine, and these form a column between the skull and the pelvis. The spinal cord travels down through a channel formed by the vertebral arches. Nerves supplying the arms pass out at the highest level, then those to the trunk, and then those to the legs. Between each vertebra and the next is a disc, which cushions any force or pressure on the vertebrae. Ligaments and muscles also protect and strengthen the spine.

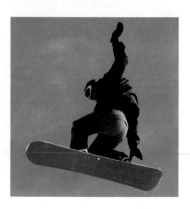

◁ Sport and recreational
pursuits are common
causes of spinal injury.

THE SPINE OR VERTEBRAL COLUMN

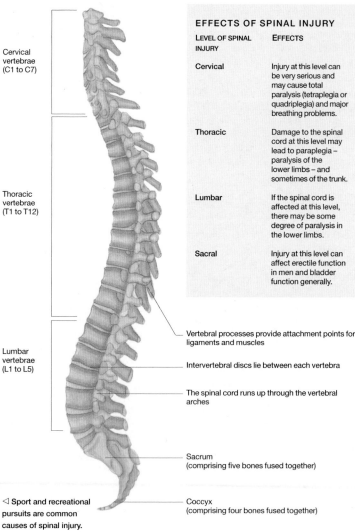

Cervical
vertebrae
(C1 to C7)

Thoracic
vertebrae
(T1 to T12)

Lumbar
vertebrae
(L1 to L5)

Vertebral processes provide attachment points for
ligaments and muscles

Intervertebral discs lie between each vertebra

The spinal cord runs up through the vertebral
arches

Sacrum
(comprising five bones fused together)

Coccyx
(comprising four bones fused together)

EFFECTS OF SPINAL INJURY

LEVEL OF SPINAL INJURY	EFFECTS
Cervical	Injury at this level can be very serious and may cause total paralysis (tetraplegia or quadriplegia) and major breathing problems.
Thoracic	Damage to the spinal cord at this level may lead to paraplegia – paralysis of the lower limbs – and sometimes of the trunk.
Lumbar	If the spinal cord is affected at this level, there may be some degree of paralysis in the lower limbs.
Sacral	Injury at this level can affect erectile function in men and bladder function generally.

FIRST AID FOR SPINAL INJURY IN AN UNCONSCIOUS PERSON

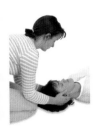

1 Keep the casualty still, in the position in which they are found. Hold the head still, as shown here, in its current position. Ask others to support the rest of the body using hands and blankets, coats or towels. Continue to keep the casualty as still as possible. If the casualty is already on their back, and the airway is clear, with nothing in the mouth and no signs of possible bleeding or vomiting, keep them in that position. If the tongue is falling back and blocking the airway, bring it forward by pushing up at the angles of the jaws, as already explained elsewhere. Do not use a head tilt unless absolutely necessary to clear the airway.

2 With both unconscious and conscious casualties, blood, vomit or other substances in the mouth or throat can block the airway (listen for gurgling). Only if this is a risk, make sure that they are in a position that allows these to drain out of the mouth. If you need to move them for this, be gentle, keep movement minimal, and keep the head still as you do so. Use a "log roll" if turning them from their back to their side.

▽ Using the "log roll" – for draining the mouth or resuscitation.

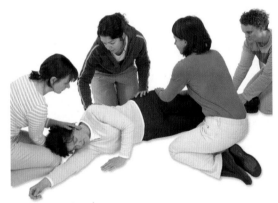

3 If the breathing or heartbeat stops, and the person is not already on their back, you must turn them on to their back to perform rescue breaths or CPR. Use the "log roll" technique, so that there is no change in the spine or head position.

4 To resuscitate, one person holds the head still while another performs resuscitation.

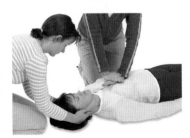

WARNING

Only move a casualty with a suspected or certain spinal injury if you need to: remove them from further serious danger; carry out resuscitation techniques (for which they must be on their back); drain the mouth (for which they need to be on their side). Any moving ideally needs at least three people – to make sure that the spine and the head do not change position.

SIGNS AND SYMPTOMS OF A SPINAL INJURY

Suspect a spinal injury if a person:

➤ Has suffered a significant impact/fall.

➤ Is unconscious after a head injury.

➤ Has fallen from a height and injured their face or head.

➤ Says that their neck hurts.

➤ Holds their neck in an odd position.

➤ Has any paralysis (loss of movement and sensation), loss of sensation or tingling or numbness in their arms and/or legs.

➤ Is confused and uncooperative.

➤ Has lost bowel and bladder control.

➤ Has difficulty breathing, with only small amounts of movement in the abdomen.

➤ Is lying flat on their back with arms stretched above the head, or with arms and hands curled to the chest.

FIRST AID FOR A CONSCIOUS SPINAL INJURY CASUALTY

Reassure the casualty. Unless there is an urgent reason to move them, such as breathing difficulties, do not do so. Call the emergency services promptly.

Ask the casualty to keep absolutely still. Kneel behind their head and hold their head still, in the position in which you found it.

Support the head at all times and ask someone to help monitor their breathing and circulation until medical help arrives.

Coping with neck injuries

SEE ALSO

➤ Removing clothing and helmets, p22
➤ Full resuscitation sequence, p38
➤ Managing spinal injuries, p158

The most important rule for dealing with a casualty with a suspected neck injury is that they are not to be moved, unless they would be in great danger, for example lying in the middle of a road or in the path of a spreading fire. A first-aider's priorities in such accidents are to prevent any further injury and phone the emergency services for urgent assistance. If a casualty has to be moved then the "log roll" technique, which requires at least three people and preferably more, must be used to keep the spine straight and supported at all times.

Fractures of the bones in the neck may be life-threatening because the nerves that supply your main breathing muscle (the diaphragm) pass out of the spinal cord here; if these nerves are damaged by a fractured vertebra, your breathing stops. Unlike other vertebrae in your backbone, the bones in the neck are vulnerable and are easily damaged.

BREATHING IS VITAL

Keeping the neck still is extremely important in a neck injury, but the ability to breathe is even more important. If a person is not breathing, then you must breathe for them. It is perfectly possible to do mouth-to-mouth on a person with a possible neck injury. Ideally, you should get someone else to keep the casualty's head steady and supported, while you perform resuscitation techniques.

FIRST AID FOR A NECK INJURY

In any injury affecting the spine, but especially the neck, it is vital to keep the head still. Another helper should phone for help while you deal with the casualty. You may well find the casualty on their back, as shown here. If not, do not move them on to their back unless you need to in order to deal with ABC problems.

IF YOU ARE ALONE...

If you are a lone first-aider, and have to leave the casualty to get help, immobilize their neck before you go with something like rolled-up towels, held in place by heavier objects. Tell the casualty to stay still and reassure them that you will return as soon as possible.

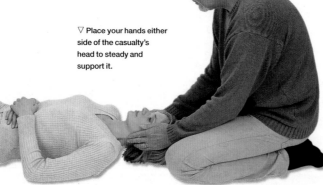

▽ Place your hands either side of the casualty's head to steady and support it.

HOW A NECK INJURY CAN DAMAGE BREATHING

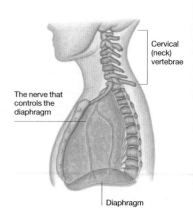

Cervical (neck) vertebrae

The nerve that controls the diaphragm

Diaphragm

▷ The nerve that controls the diaphragm exits the spine in the neck area. If this is damaged by a neck injury, breathing could cease.

THE "LOG ROLL" TECHNIQUE

If you absolutely must move a casualty with a spinal injury you should only use the "log roll" technique. By moving them "as one piece", with everyone in synchronicity, you avoid their head twisting on their shoulders or their body rotating on their pelvis. This minimizes the chances of any of the spinal vertebrae moving and causing more damage. There should be a minimum of four people, ideally six, present to carry out this technique. One person should be in charge of the head and should dictate everyone else's movements. There should always be one helper at the casualty's feet. The other helpers are positioned along the body at close intervals and act as a team. To be absolutely safe, the log roll needs training and team practice.

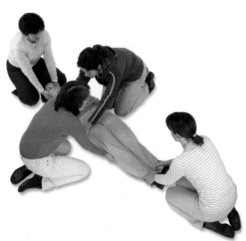

1 To move someone from their back on to their side (if they want to vomit or if blood, vomit or other substances are blocking their mouth/throat): cross their arms over in front. Then, while one person supports the head, the other people stagger themselves along the body, gently straighten out the limbs and prepare to make the "log roll".

**FIRST AID FOR A
SUSPECTED NECK INJURY**

↓

Don't try to straighten or pull on the neck. Keep it in the position found, and as still as possible.

↓

Ask a helper to get some towels or clothing and place these rolled-up items either side of the neck, all the time keeping it still.

↓

Monitor their breathing and pulse and if either start to stop, be prepared to start resuscitation procedures. If they vomit, "log roll" them on to their side.

PREVENTING NECK/SPINAL INJURIES

Most spinal injuries occur in men aged 18 to 30 – the "risk-takers". Certain simple measures can prevent many such injuries:

➤ Always wear proper protective clothing when participating in a sport.

➤ Never dive into water until you know the depth, especially in tidal waters.

➤ Never dive into a swimming pool unless the water is at least 2.7 m (9 ft) deep.

➤ Wear a seat-belt in any vehicle, and a padded jacket on a motorbike.

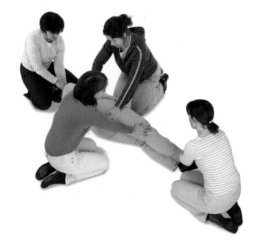

2 The head is supported all the time, and the helpers must hold the body and legs steady. The casualty's head, body and toes must align and all face in the same direction. Once turned on to their side, keep them there, perfectly still, until professional help arrives. Only move them (on to their back again) if they stop breathing or their heart stops and resuscitation becomes necessary.

Tackling upper limb fractures

SEE ALSO
➤Fixing slings, p210

The bones of the shoulder, upper arm, forearm, wrist and hand can all be fractured, and such fractures are relatively common. An outstretched hand or wrist often takes the brunt of forces from a fall but such forces can also travel up the arm and fracture one of the collarbones. With any upper limb fracture, the first-aider's main aims are to immobilize the injured limb (as it may well be unstable) and arrange transport to hospital. Skill in applying various types of slings and bandages is crucial for dealing with such injuries.

When you arrive at an accident scene, watch out for these common signs of a potential fracture:
• Pain and tenderness at the site of injury, which is worse on moving.
• Swelling and deformity.
• Attempts by the casualty to support the injured arm by holding it in a certain way.

A FRACTURED COLLARBONE

The collarbones, also known as the clavicles, are one of the commonest bones to break, especially among young people doing sports. Sometimes the broken ends of the collarbone can pierce surrounding tissues and result in bleeding and swelling.

Most collarbone fractures knit together well simply by fixing the arm in a sling, which uses the weight of the arm to slowly pull the fractured bones back into line.

▽ By immobilizing the arm in a high (or "elevation") sling, pain and discomfort from collarbone fractures can be minimized until arrival at hospital.

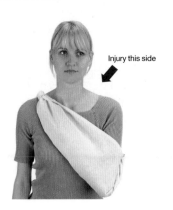

Injury this side

FIRST AID FOR A FRACTURED COLLARBONE

⬇

Ask/help the casualty to sit down.

⬇

Holding the upper arm (on the fracture side) still, carefully raise that forearm until the fingertips just touch the opposite collarbone.

⬇

Place a triangular bandage on top of the affected arm, and tuck it under to form a high (or "elevated") sling. If this causes pain, then secure the arm in whatever position the casualty finds comfortable.

⬇

Arrange transport to hospital.

FRACTURES OF THE UPPER ARM

The long bone that joins the shoulder to the elbow – known as the humerus – fractures most frequently at the top end nearest the shoulder, which is its weakest part. This is a serious form of fracture because it may actually go unnoticed by an observer as it is usually a stable fracture. The casualty may well be feeling some pain but may not seek medical assistance for some time.

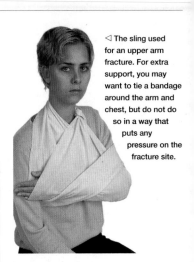

◁ The sling used for an upper arm fracture. For extra support, you may want to tie a bandage around the arm and chest, but do not do so in a way that puts any pressure on the fracture site.

FIRST AID FOR AN UPPER ARM FRACTURE

⬇

Ask the casualty to hold the injured arm across their body with their good hand.

⬇

Place a triangular bandage in between the arm and the chest and tie a sling.

⬇

Tie a broad-band bandage around the chest to secure the sling before transporting the casualty to hospital. Do this very low down the bent arm, so no pressure is put on the fracture site.

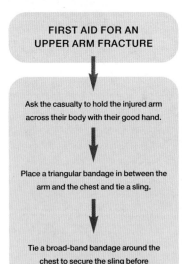

HUMERUS FRACTURE

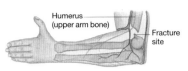

Humerus
(upper arm bone)

Fracture
site

△ Fractures of the humerus above the elbow are common in children. Adults tend to fracture the shoulder end of this bone.

AN INJURED ELBOW

Elbows are highly sensitive when injured, even without fractures, and may be painful and stiff for weeks after an injury.

Dealing with elbow injuries depends on whether or not the elbow can be bent. For elbows that can bend, follow the advice for an upper arm injury. Non-bending elbows need completely different first aid.

FIRST AID FOR AN INJURED FOREARM, WRIST OR HAND

Ask the casualty to sit down and help them if necessary.

Place the arm gently across their body keeping it steady and supported.

Slide a triangular bandage in between the chest and the arm. Surround the forearm with padding, such as a large padded envelope, a very light pillow or a small towel.

Finish tying the arm sling and arrange transport to hospital.

DEALING WITH AN ELBOW THAT CANNOT BEND

1 Help the casualty to lie down. Position soft padding to support and cushion the arm, as shown below. Now add weighted boxes or objects at the side to hold the padding in place. Phone the emergency services. (Note: If you are in a remote location and are forced to transport the casualty to hospital yourself, then use broad bandages tied around the body to secure and immobilize the limb. However, never do this under normal circumstances, as it causes pain and potentially harmful further movement.)

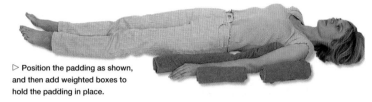

▷ Position the padding as shown, and then add weighted boxes to hold the padding in place.

FRACTURES TO THE FOREARM, WRIST OR HAND

It may be obvious when there is a fracture of the radius and ulna bones of the forearm, as there can be swelling and extreme tenderness. In children, whose soft, new bones often bend rather than break, there may only be a small crack called a greenstick fracture, and minimal swelling in the forearm.

A Colles fracture – a break of the radius bone near the wrist – is a common wrist fracture, often affecting older women.

The most common type of hand fracture affects the knuckle, often from a punch, but the hand can also be crushed, resulting in open fractures with profuse bleeding and swelling. As with any fracture, always compare the suspected injured side with the healthy side.

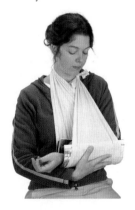

SIGNS AND SYMPTOMS OF A HAND INJURY

➤ An uninjured hand has a natural look called the "cascade" when it rests palm upwards on a flat surface. Each finger curls naturally just under the larger finger next to it. If one finger lies straight or is very bent, serious tendon, bone or nerve injury is likely.

➤ Ask the casualty to make a fist. Do all the fingers work together or do any seem to be out of line? If so, a bone may be broken.

➤ Numbness of any part of the hand beyond a wound is an ominous sign of nerve damage, as is lack of sweating.

FRACTURES TO THE FINGERS

For fractured fingers, apply padding around the hand, elevate in a high sling and take to hospital. Avoid taping fingers together to splint them, as the tape will only have to be removed by hospital staff, causing pain and possible movement. Only splint if help will be delayed for more than 12 hours.

◁ Fractures to the forearm or wrist require supportive padding and a secure sling. Make sure that the support is lightweight – you must not use anything that will strain the neck.

Managing rib fractures

SEE ALSO

➤ Dealing with shock, p72

➤ Dealing with major wounds, p138

➤ Fixing slings, p210

While a cracked rib usually constitutes a relatively minor accident, multiple rib fractures can lead to a collapsed lung (a pneumothorax) or later to pneumonia. If part of the chest wall caves in completely an injury known as a "flail chest" may occur, which may cause severe breathing difficulties and is potentially life-threatening. If ribs lower down the ribcage are fractured they may damage internal organs nearby, such as the liver and spleen, causing internal bleeding, which could cause the casualty to go into shock.

A human ribcage has 12 pairs of ribs. All ribs connect with the spine at the back and all but the lowest pair attach to the breastbone at the front. The ribs are joined together by muscles, which expand and contract in order to move the ribcage. This movement, along with the movement of the diaphragm muscle, allows us to breathe.

The upper ribs protect the heart, lungs and vital blood vessels in this area. The lower ribs help to protect internal organs such as the liver, stomach and spleen.

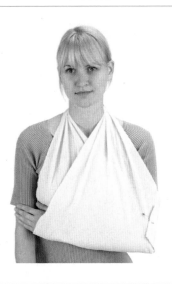

▷ For a fractured rib, use this type of sling to support the arm on the injured side. This prevents certain muscles (ones that are attached to the chest and help to move the arm) from pulling on the ribs.

TYPES OF RIB FRACTURE

There is a difference between a cracked rib caused by a badly aimed kick during a football match, and the sort of fractures that might occur from a steering wheel on the driver's chest after a road traffic accident. Although a single rib fracture can be excruciatingly painful and may remain so for up to ten days after the injury, there is little chance that it could cause serious internal damage. Sometimes, although it is unusual, the jagged edge of a fractured rib

SIGNS AND SYMPTOMS OF A FRACTURED RIB OR RIBS

As fractured ribs can cause a collapsed lung, possible internal bleeding and/or breathing difficulties, it is vital to know which symptoms indicate the severity of the injury so that the right help can be given.

Signs of fractured ribs:

➤ Sharp pain at the site of fracture.

➤ Painful breathing, especially when taking a deep breath in.

➤ Shallow breathing or breathlessness.

➤ Swelling or bruising over the fracture site.

➤ A crackling sensation affecting the chest wall.

➤ "Sucked in" air sounds through an open wound over the fracture site.

Signs of internal bleeding:

➤ Bright red, frothy coughed-up blood in the mouth.

Signs of shock (due to internal bleeding):

➤ Pale skin, and/or a blueness just inside the lips.

➤ Dizziness.

➤ Nausea, possibly vomiting.

➤ Rapid shallow breathing or gasping for air.

➤ Any degree of deteriorating level of consciousness.

FIRST AID FOR A FRACTURED RIB

YOUR AIMS:
For a minor rib fracture you need to prevent further damage, such as from bending forward. For rib injury with possible complications (e.g. lung damage), call the emergency services and sit the casualty up, supported and relaxed, so that they can breathe more easily and oxygen demand is reduced.

For all cases: keep the casualty comfortable and supported and apply a broad arm sling to support the arm on the injured side.

For more minor cases, get them to hospital, keeping the chest supported.

may penetrate a lung and cause it to collapse (a pneumothorax).

Multiple rib fractures are a different story, however. These not only indicate the greater forces involved (and thus an increased chance that internal organs may be damaged) but also pose a potential danger in that the damaged section of the chest wall may lead to a pneumothorax and later to pneumonia. If damaged ribs become detached from the chest wall, part of the chest wall can cave in completely and form what is known as a "flail chest". Such a condition can cause serious breathing problems and is a potentially life-threatening situation.

In cases of rib fracture, especially if the casualty has been crushed, there is increased chance of internal bleeding and, in turn, of developing shock. Be aware of such events, monitor the casualty's ABC and be prepared to give first aid accordingly until medical help arrives.

PARADOXICAL BREATHING

This is a condition that occurs with some flail chest casualties. Usually, as you breathe in, your ribcage moves up and out and as you breathe out it returns to a lower position. If part of the chest wall is damaged, then it will move in on inspiration and out on breathing out – paradoxical breathing.

OPEN CHEST WOUNDS

If there is a deep chest wound at the fracture site, call the emergency services promptly. Apply a totally airtight dressing consisting of plastic first, then a pad and then a bandage. Get the casualty to sit up – they should be supported and preferably leaning towards the injured side. Apply a sling as in a simple rib fracture, keep the casualty supported and await medical help.

FIRST AID FOR FLAIL CHEST

When two or more consecutive ribs on the same side of the chest are fractured in two places, the injured part of the chest wall is known as a "flail segment". The casualty will display all the symptoms of a rib fracture, and may also have paradoxical breathing.

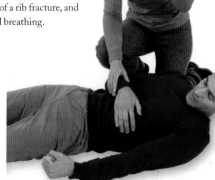

1 First assess the casualty, including their ABC. Whatever their condition, phone the emergency services promptly.

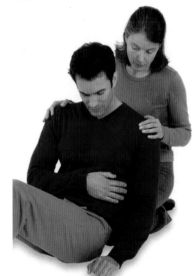

2 ▷ IF THE CASUALTY IS CONSCIOUS: Keep them sitting up as much as possible, relaxed and supported from behind. This means they can breathe more easily and reduces the body's oxygen demand.

▽ IF THE CASUALTY IS UNCONSCIOUS: Place in the recovery position, injured side down. This lets the uninjured side of the ribcage expand. Place padding, in the form of folded blankets, towels or clothes, either side of the flail area, in order to take pressure off the flail site itself. Always try to avoid moving the casualty and then tucking padding underneath. You should place the padding on the floor first and then roll the casualty very carefully on to it.

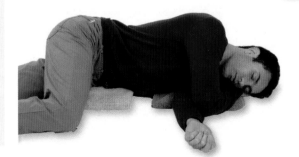

Coping with pelvic and upper-leg injuries

SEE ALSO

➤ Full resuscitation
  sequence, p38

➤ Dealing with shock,
  p72

➤ Recognizing internal
  bleeding, p144

The pelvis, hips and thighbones all have a huge nerve and blood supply; what's more the pelvis contains many vital organs. Damage to any of these regions is an emergency. If fractured, the pelvis and/or thighbone can bleed profusely; multiple pelvic fractures are often fatal. Pelvic fracture may be caused by a crush injury, such as from a steering wheel in a road accident, or by indirect forces of the type occurring during traffic collisions. A horse rider may suffer pelvic injury if they are thrown off, and/or are then kicked by, their horse.

PELVIC FRACTURES

Injuries to the pelvis must be taken seriously. Major blood vessels might be damaged, leading to profuse and even life-threatening internal blood loss. The bladder and urethra may be damaged by the fractured bones, as may the reproductive organs.

Pelvic fractures tend to result from high-speed accidents, and so there will often be other injuries too, including internal damage and spinal injuries. All of these factors may quickly lead to signs of shock developing.

SIGNS AND SYMPTOMS OF A FRACTURED PELVIS

➤ Pain and tenderness in the pelvis, groin or hip especially on moving.

➤ Inability to walk or stand or to lift their legs while lying flat on the floor.

➤ An obviously deformed pelvis.

➤ Blood seeping from the penis or urethra (urinary outlet).

➤ Signs of shock or internal bleeding.

THE PELVIC REGION

▽ The pelvis comprises the ilium, pubis and ischium bones. The head of the femur (thighbone) fits into the pelvis at the hip.

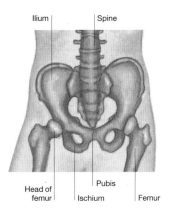

Ilium | Spine

Head of femur | Pubis | Ischium | Femur

WARNING

You should never attempt to move a casualty if you suspect a fractured pelvis unless they are in immediate danger – you could risk further serious damage.

STABILIZING A FRACTURED PELVIS

▷ Place padding as shown. Padding either side of the body should extend above the pelvis and should be held in place by weighted objects. Make sure that the feet cannot rotate in either direction – this rotates the head of the femur in the pelvis.

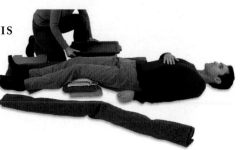

FIRST AID FOR A FRACTURED PELVIS

Call the emergency services urgently.

Move the casualty as little as possible; try to keep their feet in the position found.

Stabilize the pelvis by immobilizing the legs: place rolled blankets or similar under the knees and either side of the legs, held in place by weighted boxes, or similar.

Monitor the casualty's condition, and keep a close eye out for signs of shock.

Only if you are in a very remote location and need to take the casualty to a hospital yourself, tie bandages around the padding and legs at the lower thigh, knees and ankles. However, do not do this if it causes more pain.

FRACTURES TO THE THIGHBONE

The thighbone (femur) forms a large ball and socket joint – the hip – where it meets the pelvis. Any fracture to the thighbone is a serious emergency as it can lead to profuse bleeding if the broken bones pierce the large blood vessels nearby. Shock, then, is a distinct possibility and the casualty should be monitored closely for any such signs that appear.

The thighbone can fracture anywhere but common sites include the long shaft and the neck (top) of the bone, near the hip joint. Fractures to the long shaft would occur after the considerable force involved in traumas such as a traffic accident; fractures of the neck of the bone (that is, at the hip) are common in elderly people simply because their bones become much weaker and more brittle with age. If such a fracture is stable, an elderly person may hobble about on the injured leg. When combined with confusion or dementia, such a fracture may go unnoticed for some time as they may forget that they have fallen or are in pain.

FEMUR FRACTURES

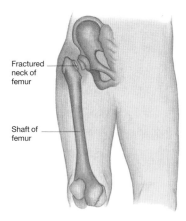

Fractured neck of femur

Shaft of femur

△ The thighbone (femur) commonly fractures at the top and along its shaft.

SIGNS AND SYMPTOMS OF A FRACTURED THIGHBONE

➤ Pain and tenderness at the site of injury or at the knee.

➤ An inability to walk or put weight on the affected leg.

➤ Deformity in the affected leg, making it look shorter than the unaffected one.

➤ An awkward-looking leg that is noticeably bent at the knee and also turned outwards at the ankle.

➤ Signs of shock.

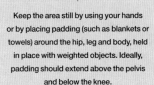

FIRST AID FOR A FRACTURED THIGHBONE

Call the emergency services promptly.

Keep the area still by using your hands or by placing padding (such as blankets or towels) around the hip, leg and body, held in place with weighted objects. Ideally, padding should extend above the pelvis and below the knee.

Monitor the casualty and keep a close eye out for signs of shock.

Only if you are in a very remote location, and need to transport the casualty to hospital yourself, splint the body (ideally from armpit to below the feet) on the injured side and secure the body and limb to the splint with bandages, tied at regular intervals.

FIRST AID FOR A FRACTURED THIGHBONE

▷ If a fractured thighbone casualty is found on their side, keep them in that position (always try to treat in the position found), but support their back in some way. Essentially, a fractured thighbone is treated in the same way as a fractured pelvis, using support and padding. This picture shows an alternative manual method of support, where the first-aider's arm is being used as a splint – suitable for fracture cases where help will arrive quickly or there are few materials to hand.

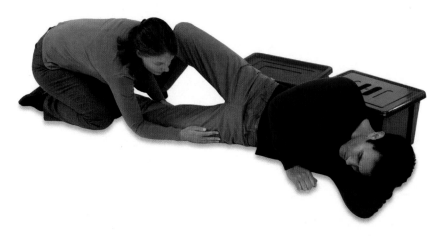

Handling knee and lower-leg injuries

SEE ALSO

➤ Managing sprains and strains, p172

The knee is the body's largest joint. It can perform complex movements and is structured so that it remains stable while bearing the body's weight. The knee has sets of ligaments to hold the bones in place, including the patella (kneecap) at the front. Broken bones, tears or impacts to the knee joint can produce incredible pain and swelling. Any fracture or tear requires immobilization and open wounds should also be dealt with. Your first-aid aims are to immobilize limbs, minimize swelling and arrange for urgent transport to hospital.

INJURIES TO THE KNEE

There are two cruciate ligaments in the knee joint, so called because they cross over each other as they pass diagonally down from the thighbone to the shinbone. These ligaments are most commonly damaged in accidents when the knee is twisted. Other tissues in the knee that can suffer injury include the cartilage and the bony patella (kneecap).

SIGNS AND SYMPTOMS OF A LOWER-LEG INJURY

➤ Pain deep within the knee or localized pain to the injury site, often made worse by trying to move the limb or put weight on it.

➤ Swelling and/or bruising around the knee or injury.

➤ Great pain when trying to straighten the leg (gently) if the knee has "locked".

➤ Broken bones protruding through the skin at the fracture site.

➤ Inability to bear weight on the affected side.

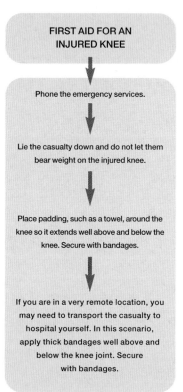

FIRST AID FOR AN INJURED KNEE

Phone the emergency services.

⬇

Lie the casualty down and do not let them bear weight on the injured knee.

⬇

Place padding, such as a towel, around the knee so it extends well above and below the knee. Secure with bandages.

⬇

If you are in a very remote location, you may need to transport the casualty to hospital yourself. In this scenario, apply thick bandages well above and below the knee joint. Secure with bandages.

INJURIES TO THE LOWER LEG

The fibula is a spindly bone that fractures easily without necessarily stopping a person from weight bearing. Fractures of the fibula, therefore, may not be initially obvious. However, if the larger, load-bearing tibia (shinbone) is broken, a person cannot usually stand up or bear weight. A fracture of the tibia may cause bleeding and circulation problems in the area beyond the fracture site. Other injuries include tears to muscles, tendons and ligaments of the lower leg.

LOWER-LEG FRACTURES

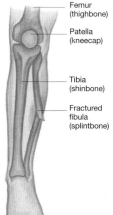

▷ Any of the lower leg bones – patella, tibia or fibula – may be fractured in an accident. This illustration shows a fracture site in the thinner fibula.

Femur (thighbone)

Patella (kneecap)

Tibia (shinbone)

Fractured fibula (splintbone)

FIRST AID FOR AN INJURED KNEE

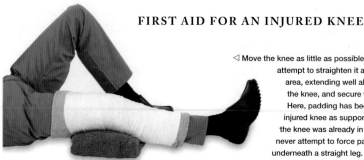

◁ Move the knee as little as possible, and never attempt to straighten it at all. Pad a wide area, extending well above and below the knee, and secure with bandages. Here, padding has been slid under the injured knee as support only because the knee was already in a bent position; never attempt to force padding underneath a straight leg.

FIRST AID FOR A LOWER-LEG FRACTURE

1 Lay the casualty down while supporting the injured leg. Feel the foot and lower leg for warmth and to check that the casualty can sense your touch.

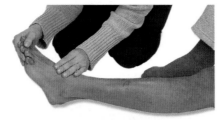

WARNING
Do not try to straighten the knee, as injuries within the knee joint may worsen as a result. For any lower-leg injury, do not let the casualty bear any weight on the affected leg.

2 Phone for the emergency services. Place some soft padding on both sides of the legs, extending well above the knees and held in place by weighted boxes. Ensure that the foot is supported in the position found.

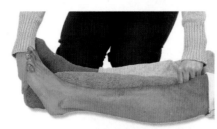

▷ If you are in a remote location and have to take the casualty to a hospital or doctor yourself, then secure the padding with bandages. Place them well above and below the fracture site.

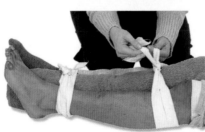

ANKLE INJURIES
By far the most common ankle injury is a sprain, which is dealt with elsewhere using the RICE guidelines (RICE stands for rest, ice, compression and elevation). Any fracture to the ankle bone should be treated as for a lower-leg fracture.

A BROKEN FOOT
There are many small bones in the foot, any of which could be broken during an accident, most often one of a crushing nature. A fracture of the calcaneum (heelbone) is particularly common after a fall from a height on to the feet.

Individual toes may also suffer injury, but unless a toe is twisted right out of its usual alignment, even broken toes generally heal extremely well after professional medical treatment.

FIRST AID FOR A FRACTURE OF THE FOOT

Sit or lay the casualty down. Elevate and support the injured foot immediately to minimize swelling.

Applying a cold compress may further reduce swelling, but do not do if painful.

Get the casualty to hospital by either car or ambulance.

▽ Elevate and comfortably support a fractured foot. Only apply a cold compress (such as ice wrapped in a towel) to reduce swelling if this does not cause pain – extreme temperatures can be very uncomfortable for fracture casualties. Elevate the leg above

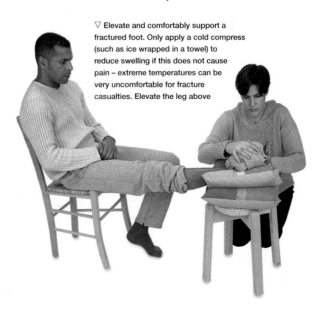

Coping with dislocations

SEE ALSO
➤ Moving and handling safely 1 and 2, pp24, 26
➤ Understanding the skeleton, p152

Any joint may become dislocated due to a violent wrenching action. In dislocated joints, surrounding muscles, ligaments, tendons and blood vessels may be disturbed or damaged as a result. The force of dislocation can sometimes also produce a fracture nearby. Any dislocated joint looks misshapen, and the casualty experiences extreme pain and the joint soon becomes swollen, discoloured and immobile. First-aiders should try to immobilize the injured joint, to prevent further injury and reduce pain, and seek emergency medical help.

Dislocations may occur within any joint, when the end of a bone is pulled or pushed out of place and thus out of the joint. It can be a very distressing experience as the muscles around a dislocated joint often go into spasm, causing intense pain. Nerves and blood vessels around the joint may also be damaged.

It is not always possible to distinguish between a fracture and a dislocation, and both may occur within a joint at the same time. If in doubt, treat a dislocation as if it were a fracture.

The most common joints for dislocation are the shoulder, hip, elbow, jaw and joints of the thumbs and fingers.

WARNING
Never try to relocate the bone of a dislocated joint or attempt any strategies to get the bone to "pop" back in again. It is easy to inflict further serious damage.

SIGNS AND SYMPTOMS OF A DISLOCATED SHOULDER

➤ It may be possible to feel the "popped out" rounded head of the humerus (upper arm bone) in front of the shoulder joint.

➤ Distortion in the shoulder joint; the upper arm may look flat.

➤ Severe pain in the shoulder, which is also difficult to move.

➤ Swelling and/or bruising in the joint.

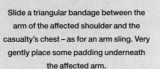

FIRST AID FOR A DISLOCATED SHOULDER

Get the casualty to sit down and make them as comfortable as possible. Let them hold their arm in whatever position is least painful. Calm and reassure the casualty – dislocations can be sudden and acutely painful and so may be highly distressing.

Slide a triangular bandage between the arm of the affected shoulder and the casualty's chest – as for an arm sling. Very gently place some padding underneath the affected arm.

Tie the arm sling so that the affected arm is well supported.

Arrange transport to hospital. In transit, the casualty should stay seated.

SHOULDER DISLOCATION
Some people are unlucky enough to suffer from this common injury recurrently. For these unfortunate few, the condition is often just as painful as for one-off or occasional cases, but the shoulder does "pop" back in much more easily.

IMMEDIATE HELP FOR A DISLOCATED SHOULDER

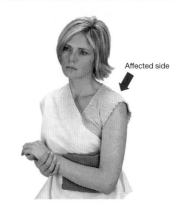

Affected side

1 Carefully place a sling and some soft padding between the arm of the affected shoulder and the body.

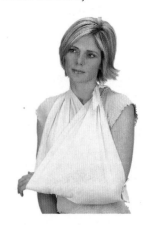

2 Once the padding is in place, tie the sling so that the joint is supported. Get the casualty to hospital straight away.

HOW TO DEAL WITH A DISLOCATED HIP

The hip joint may dislocate, for example, when the knee hits the dashboard in a car accident. This sort of accident often results in a fractured pelvis and damage to nearby nerves as well, resulting in paralysis. The head of the thighbone usually moves backwards, and the leg rotates outwards and is bent at the knee. The bony end of the thighbone may be easily felt or seen sticking out under the skin at or near the hip.

▽ Treatment for a dislocated hip is essentially the same as for a fractured pelvis or thighbone. Treat the casualty in the position found and do not move them if at all possible. Immobilize the immediate and surrounding area by padding and supporting it – using rolled blankets, towels and so on located under the knees and either side of the body and secured by weighted objects such as boxes and briefcases.

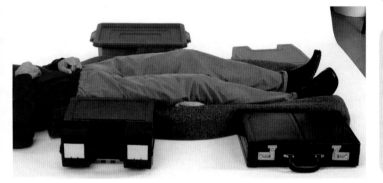

A DISLOCATED ELBOW

Children very easily stretch ligaments. In the elbow, the top of one of the forearm bones (the radius) sometimes "pops out" of the elbow joint, especially if a child's arm is yanked suddenly as might happen in a fall. Suspect a pulled elbow if:
- The child suddenly stops using the affected arm.
- The child cries when the arm is moved or touched at all, especially in the elbow area.

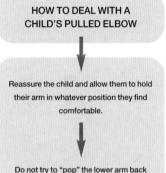

HOW TO DEAL WITH A CHILD'S PULLED ELBOW

↓

Reassure the child and allow them to hold their arm in whatever position they find comfortable.

↓

Do not try to "pop" the lower arm back into place. Phone the emergency services or take the child to hospital.

A DISLOCATED JAW

This is a fairly common occurrence and may be caused by an everyday action of the jaw, such as yawning. In cases of a dislocated jaw, a person will not be able to move the jaw at all so they will be unable to close their mouth or speak properly. The jaw will have to be relocated in hospital, after which it will have to be kept completely immobile for 24 hours.

HAND DISLOCATIONS

Contact sports, such as martial arts, and skiing accidents can often lead to the dislocation of one of the many joints in the hand, especially the thumb. The best action to take is to pad up the hand and elevate it in a high sling before taking the casualty to hospital for medical treatment. Never attempt to change the position of any damaged fingers.

HOW TO DEAL WITH A DISLOCATED HAND

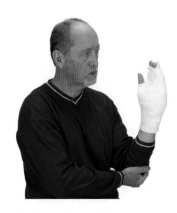

1 Remove any rings before the hand starts to swell, but only if you can avoid bending affected fingers. Ask the casualty to support their arm while you wrap the hand in padding.

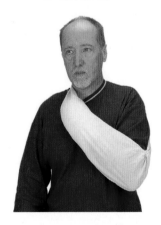

2 Once the casualty is comfortable and the arm supported, immobilize the joint using a high sling (and more padding if necessary). Firmer support could be given by tying another bandage around the sling to attach it to the body. Get the casualty to a doctor.

Managing sprains and strains

SEE ALSO

➤ Moving and handling safely 1 and 2, pp24, 26

➤ Applying dressings & bandages, p204

➤ Applying bandages 1, p206

The soft tissues – muscles, tendons and ligaments – that attach to or support the bones of the skeleton can also be injured or damaged in an accident. Such injuries are generally called sprains and strains and happen most often during sporting activities. The first-aid aims of treating such soft-tissue injuries are to reduce pain and swelling and to seek medical help if necessary. It can sometimes be tricky to distinguish between a sprain and a fracture, and so medical advice should be sought if there is any shadow of a doubt.

For the skeleton to be able to move the body about, it needs the help of essential soft tissues – muscles, tendons and ligaments. Muscles attach to bones via tendons, while ligaments are the tough fibrous cords that hold bones together at joints and allow joints to function properly. Together the bones, muscles and joints are known as the musculoskeletal system.

When there are no broken bones, the injury is called a soft-tissue injury. These are perceived to be less serious than fractures but can still cause a great deal of pain and disability. If they are not dealt with properly in the initial stages, they may lead to long-term weakness and malfunction in a muscle or joint.

"GOING OVER"

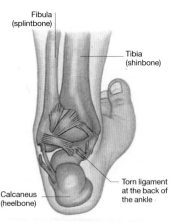

▷ "Going over" on an ankle while running is a common way of spraining this joint.

Sudden movements can easily overstretch ligaments within the ankle

TORN LIGAMENTS

Fibula (splintbone)

Tibia (shinbone)

Calcaneus (heelbone)

Torn ligament at the back of the ankle

△ In a sprained ankle, one or more of the ligaments are partially or completely torn.

SIGNS AND SYMPTOMS OF A SPRAIN OR STRAIN

Bear in mind that it can be difficult to distinguish between a sprain or strain and a fracture. There are a few clues, though, to watch out for.

Symptoms of a sprain or strain include:

➤ Pain and tenderness. (If the casualty heard or felt a crack at the time of the incident, the injury is more likely to be a fracture.)

➤ Inability to use the injured part. (However, an immediate inability to bear weight on the injured part points to a fracture.)

➤ Swelling and bruising. (If the swelling takes several hours to appear it's more likely to be a soft-tissue injury; swelling after a fracture is immediate.)

DIFFERENT TYPES OF SOFT-TISSUE INJURY

➤ Sprain – A common form of ligament injury resulting in tearing or overstretching of the ligament.

➤ Strain – The tearing or overstretching of a muscle. Strains often happen near the junction of the muscle and its tendon, which tethers the muscle to the nearby bone.

➤ Rupture – The complete tearing of a ligament or a muscle.

➤ Bruise – The swelling, pain and bleeding below the skin that result from a direct blow to the body. A large amount of blood that collects as a result of damage is known as a haematoma.

HOW TO TREAT SPRAINS AND STRAINS

After following the RICE guidelines (opposite), you may decide to seek medical attention. After following RICE, minor soft-tissue injuries should be followed by gentle, controlled exercise as soon as symptoms allow. Many sprains remain stiff, swollen and painful even after 48 hours of RICE treatment. This is normal, and it is important to start using the joint or muscle, as it can easily stiffen up and recover slowly. If not properly treated in the first few weeks after injury, a sprain can cause recurrent problems in the long term – even more so than a simple fracture in the same area.

HOW TO DEAL WITH A SPRAINED ANKLE

Follow the RICE guidelines – Rest, Ice, Compress and Elevate.

Rest – Most soft-tissue injuries need to be rested for 24–48 hours while being kept as comfortable as possible.

Ice – Reduce the pain and swelling associated with soft-tissue injuries using ice or a packet of frozen peas wrapped in a cloth. Apply initially and then for short periods of 10–15 minutes at a time for the first 24–48 hours. Do not apply ice or anything frozen directly to the skin; it will be painful and may damage the skin.

Compress – Applying pressure to the injured part may make the casualty more comfortable. Elasticated tubular bandages give the best compression, although crepe bandages over layers of cotton wool also work well.

Elevate – Rest the injured part above horizontal and ideally above the level of the heart, which will reduce swelling.

WARNING
It is always best to get a medical opinion about any sprain or strain. An X-ray may be needed to find out whether it is indeed a sprain, or a fracture has occurred. The casualty may need physiotherapy, or referral to a clinic for regular checks.

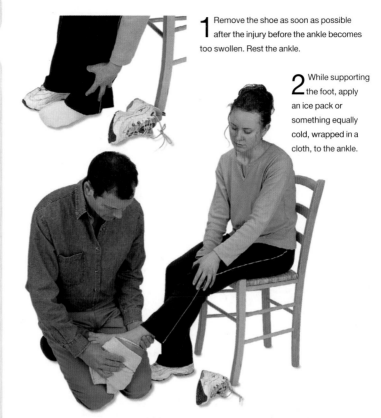

1 Remove the shoe as soon as possible after the injury before the ankle becomes too swollen. Rest the ankle.

2 While supporting the foot, apply an ice pack or something equally cold, wrapped in a cloth, to the ankle.

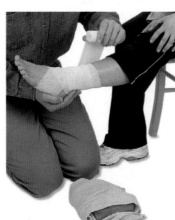

3 Use a crepe or elasticated bandage to apply compression to the injured ankle. Keep supporting the ankle all the time.

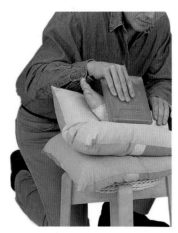

4 Carefully place the injured ankle in a position that keeps it rested, comfortable and elevated. Apply a cold compress regularly.

Controlling back pain

SEE ALSO

➤ Moving and handling safely 1 and 2, pp24, 26

➤ Managing spinal injuries, p158

Back pain varies enormously from person to person. Even an excruciating bout of back pain can resolve itself in a matter of a few weeks. However, anyone who is worried about what is causing the pain in their back should consult their doctor. When approaching an incident where someone complains of back pain, be alert to the danger signs that could indicate some form of spinal injury. Much back pain resolves with painkillers and, contrary to popular opinion, staying active – resting can make the back stiff and immobile.

Most people suffer from back pain at some point in their lives. In the vast majority of cases, the pain is in the lower back, or lumbar region. The lumbar spine has to be strong as it bears the weight of the body as well as any other loads it has to carry.

It is reassuring to know that back pain is not usually due to any serious disease. Most cases of low back pain resolve quickly, although they may take up to 6–8 weeks to settle down completely. Upper back pain is more unusual.

▷ Pain in the mobile regions of the spine – the neck and lower back – is the most common form of back pain.

COMMON PAIN SITES

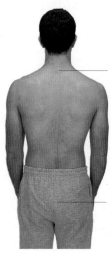

Pain at the top of the spine – the neck – will often cause headaches, and the sufferer may not realize their root cause

Lower back pain that spreads into one or both buttocks and one or both legs is due to impingement of the sciatic nerve

CAUSES OF BACK PAIN

Frustratingly for the sufferer, the exact cause of most back pain is rarely discovered. Back pain tends to originate in the muscles, ligaments and joints of the back, but pinpointing exactly which ones is often impossible. Rarely, there is an underlying cause, such as a tumour, kidney problems, a collapsed vertebra due to the bone-thinning condition osteoporosis, scoliosis (loss of the natural curvature of the spine) or a slipped intervertebral disc.

SPINAL COMPRESSION

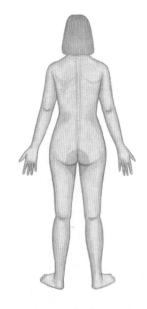

△ People with numbness in this "saddle" area may have spinal compression and should see a doctor immediately. (Sphincter disturbance and lower limb weakness are other signs.)

SIGNS AND SYMPTOMS OF BACK PAIN

Signs of back pain:

➤ Pain, which may vary from dull to severe, across the lower back is particularly common. Sometimes this pain spreads into the buttock and shoots down the leg (sciatica); such pain is due to pressure on the sciatic nerve.

➤ Inability to move the back, especially bending and leaning back.

➤ Muscle spasm in the back muscles, causing a rigid or stiff neck.

➤ Tenderness in the back muscles themselves.

Seek medical help if there is also:

➤ Pain in the buttocks, legs or arms.

➤ Any numbness or tingling in the limbs.

➤ Weight loss.

➤ Fever.

➤ Any loss of sensation or movement.

➤ General feeling of being unwell.

➤ Incontinence or inability to open bowels. Urinary problems such as low output, pain on urinating, unusual colour, smell or cloudiness.

➤ Unremitting/increasing back pain.

➤ If the person is under 20 or over 50.

WHAT YOU CAN DO AT HOME

Most people find it useful to use pain-controlling medication of some kind but your doctor may prescribe a muscle relaxant if your pain is not relieved by painkillers alone. You can also modify your physical activities to avoid potential problems in the first place:

- Lifting – Never twist the back, but turn with your feet instead. Always bend at the knees to grasp the object and use your legs to help you lift rather than relying solely on the strength of your back. Keep the heaviest side of the object close to your body and get help if needed.

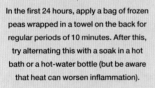

HOW TO DEAL WITH BACK PAIN

↓

You may choose to take your regular painkillers to ease backache. Non-steroidal anti-inflammatory drugs such as ibuprofen, paracetamol-based painkillers and prescription muscle relaxants can all help.

↓

In the first 24 hours, apply a bag of frozen peas wrapped in a towel on the back for regular periods of 10 minutes. After this, try alternating this with a soak in a hot bath or a hot-water bottle (but be aware that heat can worsen inflammation).

↓

Back manipulation – Physical therapies such as osteopathy and chiropractic can help relieve back pain and solve many back-related problems.

↓

Alternative therapies – Acupuncture and reflexology are just two of the alternative treatments available for easing back pain.

PAIN IN THE OVER-50S

The sudden onset of severe and unremitting back pain in anyone over 50 should be taken seriously, especially if it is not in the lower back, but higher up. The bones of the back are a common place for various cancers to spread to, and there are also cancers that develop in the bones of the back.

- Sitting – Sit in an upright chair for no longer than 20 or 30 minutes at a time. Also, a lumbar support helps to keep you sitting "tall" rather than slumping.
- Driving – Travelling of any kind can make back pain a lot worse, especially when undertaking long-distance journeys.
- Sleeping – Get a good night's sleep and lie on a fairly firm, flat surface. Too soft and too hard are both bad for the back.
- Working – Make sure all working surfaces are at a good height for you, so that you are not straining.

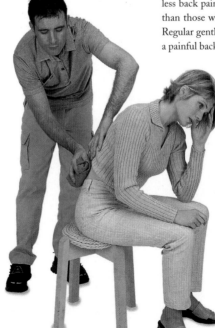

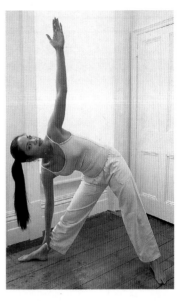

△ When trying out a new activity, such as yoga, take it easy on your back and stretch slowly and gradually.

STAY ACTIVE AND AT WORK

People who are physically fit suffer from less back pain and generally recover faster than those who are unfit and overweight. Regular gentle activity helps to strengthen a painful back, and the sooner this exercise is started the better. Swimming, walking and cycling are all good low-impact exercises that will not damage the back.

◁ One tip that helps to ease back pain, is to ask a friend or partner to apply an ice pack or bag of frozen peas – wrapped in a towel – to the site of the pain.

SKILLS CHECKLIST FOR
BONE AND MUSCLE INJURIES

KEY POINTS

- Take great care over the how and when of moving a casualty with a bone or muscle injury, especially if they have a definite/suspected spinal injury; keeping affected parts still and supported is key ☐

- Splinting is best reserved for extreme situations where you are forced to take the casualty to the nearest doctor/hospital yourself ☐

- Be alert to the possibility of a spinal injury after any accident ☐

- Do not try to relocate a dislocated joint ☐

- Back pain usually resolves itself within six to eight weeks ☐

SKILLS LEARNED

- How to tackle both "open" and "closed" fractures ☐

- How to deal with the many different types of fractures, all over the body ☐

- How to recognize and manage potential spinal problems ☐

- How to "log roll" a casualty ☐

- How to deal with dislocations, strains and sprains ☐

- How to relieve back pain ☐

11

BURNS AND SCALDS

First aid is of paramount importance for the burn casualty. The first-aider can significantly limit the pain, damage and trauma caused by the burn by cooling the area as quickly as possible. Reducing the skin's temperature in this way helps to limit the depth and severity of damage to underlying tissues. Burns range from a straightforward, relatively superficial injury to a very deep injury that penetrates muscles, nerves and bone. Many burns are associated with electrical faults and with smoking and alcohol. Home safety has a major part to play in preventing such accidents. Burns occurring in the home account for 10 per cent of all accidental deaths.

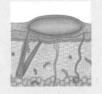

CONTENTS

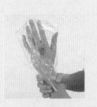

Understanding and assessing burns 1

SEE ALSO
➤ Assessing burns 2,
  p180
➤ Safety in the home,
  p228
➤ Safety in the
  kitchen, p230

Initial action with any burn, however severe, is the same – having dealt with any danger, remove the source of the burn and cool the burnt area. Cooling the skin as quickly as possible reduces any pain and swelling and also helps to prevent damage to underlying tissues.

Burns weaken and damage the skin so when you flood the burnt area with water do not turn on the tap to full power. Remove any constricting articles, such as jewellery. If a burn is larger than 2.5cm (1in) square, the casualty should be seen at a hospital.

The skin is the body's largest organ, covering the entire surface of the body. It forms a barrier against infection and also helps protect against injury and maintain body temperature. Burns to the skin cause instant damage but quick thinking and rapid first-aid action can make all the difference to the outcome. If deep layers of the skin are damaged, they will not heal easily and may even require skin grafts.

COMPLICATIONS OF BURNS

When giving first aid for a serious burn, bear in mind the following life-threatening burn-related complications:
• If the casualty's airway becomes burnt, it may swell, resulting in potentially fatal breathing problems.
• The casualty may have other injuries (if they have jumped to escape a fire or have been in an explosion, for example).
• If the entire circumference of their chest is burnt, they will not be able to move their chest in order to breathe.
• Severe burns lead to large amounts of fluid loss and therefore can lead to shock.

GIVING ALL THE DETAILS

When speaking to the emergency services, it is essential to give them any known information about the cause of the burn. If there was an explosion, for example, the casualty may have other injuries. And, if there was burning material, or the fire was in an enclosed space, there is a risk of inhalation poisoning and airway swelling. Knowing how long the casualty was exposed to the material helps paramedics to assess the extent of any damage.

THE SKIN'S STRUCTURE

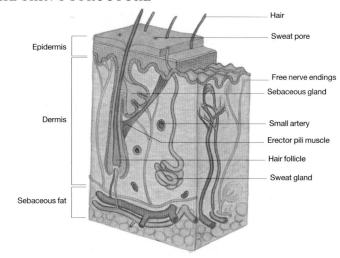

- Epidermis
- Dermis
- Sebaceous fat
- Hair
- Sweat pore
- Free nerve endings
- Sebaceous gland
- Small artery
- Erector pili muscle
- Hair follicle
- Sweat gland

DIFFERENT TYPES OF BURNS

➤ Dry burns – Such injuries are caused by any form of flame or hot surface, such as lighted cigarettes, hot irons and hobs, bonfires and hot barbecue coals.

➤ Wet burns – Also called scalds, these are caused by boiling liquids, steam and cooking fat or oil.

➤ Cold burns – The skin can also be burnt by extreme cold, such as contact with ice-cold metal.

➤ Friction burns – These are the result of a surface (especially of a synthetic material) rubbing against the skin at speed. A moving rope or wire, revolving brushes and machine belts are common culprits.

➤ Radiation burns – Most commonly from over-exposure to ultraviolet light, such as in sunburn.

➤ Chemical burns – Many common household products and work chemicals (such as bleach, ammonia, oven cleaners, drain fluids, caustic soda, wood preserver and treatments for wet and dry rot) contain chemicals that can burn skin. Appropriate safety gloves should be worn when using such products, and appropriate protective clothing should be worn by anyone dealing with industrial chemicals.

➤ Electrical burns – These burns are caused by contact with electricity in any form, including lightning.

ESSENTIALS OF BURN MANAGEMENT

Cooling and covering the burnt area are the major principles to remember when dealing with burns and scalds. Cooling is a vital one – not only will this reduce pain but it will also limit the extent of the burn and any damage.

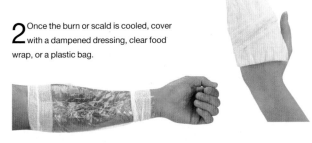

▽ **Loosely wrapped damp gauze placed around a finger burn.**

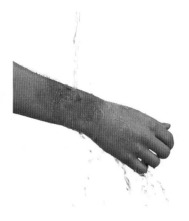

2 Once the burn or scald is cooled, cover with a dampened dressing, clear food wrap, or a plastic bag.

△ To use clear food wrap, discard an initial length of wrap (it will be dirty). Place a piece of wrap around the area fairly loosely, with the ends (the ends running lengthways) folded into a pleat; this allows room in case the burn swells.

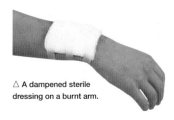

△ **A dampened sterile dressing on a burnt arm.**

1 Cooling the burnt or scalded area is a top priority. Hold the affected area under a stream of cold water for at least 10 minutes. You should only cool the burnt area; do not overcool the casualty.

ASSESSING BURNS

One important aspect of dealing with burns is deciding how severe the problem is. You need to assess whether a burn is minor or major. Factors affecting this include the depth, extent and site of the burns. For example, burns in the neck and head area can compromise the airway, while burns in the genital area may lead to large amounts of swelling and serious problems with passing water.

MINOR AND MAJOR BURNS

Use the following summary when assessing whether a burn is minor or major and deciding what to do. (However, if you are at all unsure, always seek expert help.)

Minor/superficial burns

If the burn seems relatively small and superficial and there is no risk of infection or scarring, then you should simply get the casualty to make an appointment with a practice doctor or nurse.

Superficial/mild partial-thickness burns

(Note: thickness of burns is dealt with in more detail on the following pages.) If the burn is of this type, and there are other symptoms present – such as dizziness, headache or fainting – the casualty should be seen by a doctor or emergency department without delay.

Serious burns

These include:
• Non-superficial burns with an area greater than 2.5cm (1in) square.
• Burns in young children and the elderly.
• Electrical and chemical burns.
• Deep/full-thickness burns of any size.
• Burns that go all around a limb or the chest ("circumferential" burns).

WARNING
Do not touch the burnt area. Do not break blisters or remove loose skin. Never use adhesive, dry or fluffy dressings. Do not apply anything (lotions, ointments or grease) to the burnt area.

• Burns to either the palms of the hands or the genitals.

Potentially life-threatening burns

These include:
• Burns to the airway, face or neck.
• Anyone who has inhaled either smoke, fumes or flames.
• A burn over a large area (more than 1% of the body; see following pages), if deeper than superficial.

You must get these burns seen by emergency medical help immediately.

Understanding and assessing burns 2

SEE ALSO

➤ Understanding and assessing burns 1, p178

➤ Safety in the kitchen, p230

It can be hard to judge exactly how severe burns are, but understanding a little more about burn depth and area will help. If you are in any doubt about the severity of any kind of burn, seek medical help as fast as possible. If the casualty is clearly in distress and some pain, call the emergency services immediately, or get the casualty to a local hospital's accident and emergency department. If the burns are severe or over a large surface area, then the casualty may go into shock, so watch for shock signs and be prepared to resuscitate if necessary.

ASSESSING A BURN'S DEPTH

The depth of a burn depends upon the intensity of, and length of exposure to, the burn agent (such as heat, cold or chemicals). The skin has two layers: a surface layer called the epidermis and a deeper layer called the dermis. How deeply a burn has damaged the skin is an indicator of potential complications – fewer such events occur with superficial burns compared with partial- or full-thickness burns.

SUPERFICIAL BURNS

Formerly known as first-degree burns, this type of burn involves only the very uppermost layer of the skin – the epidermis. Typical features of a superficial burn include:

- Red-looking skin that may be a little puffy but with no blistering; it will feel very sensitive and painful.
- Blanching of the skin when pressed.
- Fairly fast healing – usually within 10 days and without leaving a scar.

PARTIAL-THICKNESS BURNS

Burns of this kind used to be called second-degree burns. They destroy areas of the epidermis and result in blistering. Large amounts of fluid may be lost from partial-thickness burns if they cover a large area of the body.

- The skin is red or white, blistered and extremely painful.
- The burn may heal within 21 days and cause little scarring, but very deep burns may take up to 60 days and leave more extensive scars.

DEPTHS OF BURN

▷ Superficial burns involve only the outermost layer of skin – the epidermis. Underlying layers and the structures they contain, such as nerve endings, are unaffected.

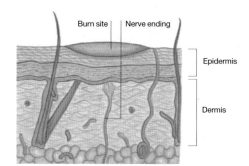

Burn site | Nerve ending

Epidermis

Dermis

▷ A partial-thickness burn is again limited to the epidermis layer. The skin will look red and raw and will be blistered because tissue fluid from damaged tissues accumulates.

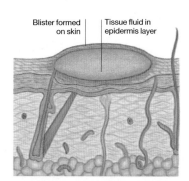

Blister formed on skin | Tissue fluid in epidermis layer

▷ A full-thickness burn affects both layers of the skin. Because of the burn's severity, fat, nerves, muscle and blood vessels may also be damaged.

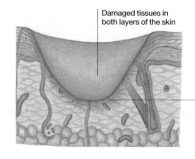

Damaged tissues in both layers of the skin

Pain sensation may be lost as nerve endings are damaged

FULL-THICKNESS BURNS

This type of burn was previously known as a third-degree burn. Such serious burns extend into the skin's dermis and beyond. Hair follicles, nerves and sweat glands, which lie within the dermis, may never recover if they are badly burned. Fluid is unable to ooze through the damaged dermis but is lost internally. In a full-thickness burn:

- The skin is white, black or brown.
- The skin appears leathery or waxy (do not touch it to see how it feels).
- The burnt area is numb and therefore, paradoxically, less painful than a less serious burn.
- The affected skin will never heal on its own and requires a skin graft.

THE EXTENT OF THE BURN

When assessing burns, it is vital to judge how much of the body's surface area is affected, as this will indicate likely fluid losses. When tissue is damaged by burns, tissue fluid leaks from tiny capillaries in the skin as a response and forms blisters or seeps out of the skin blood vessels. The bigger the burn, the bigger the fluid loss and thus the higher the risk of shock.

When trying to assess just how serious a casualty's burns are, it can be helpful to think of the palm of the casualty's hand (including their fingers) as representing 1 per cent of their total body surface. As a good general guide, any partial-thickness burn of 1 per cent or more should be seen urgently by a doctor. Any suspected full-thickness burn, no matter what size, is an emergency and must be seen immediately.

ASSESSING THE BURN AREA

▽ Professional medical personnel have traditionally used the "rule of nines" as a way of accurately assessing the area, and therefore the potential severity, of a burn. Under this rule, parts of the body can be assigned 9 per cent or multiples of 9 per cent. However, the average first-aider should never waste valuable time trying to make such a detailed assessment. Instead, they can quickly compare it to the size of the inner surface of the hand (see right).

▽ Using the burn casualty's hand as a guide is now a common way for first-aiders to assess a burn area. The area of the inner surface of a casualty's hand, including the fingers, represents about 1% of their body area. If a burn is deeper than superficial and has an area of 1% or more, the casualty must be seen urgently at a hospital.

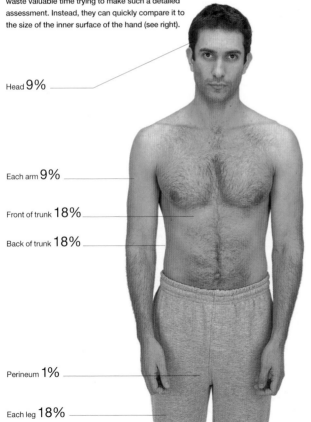

Head 9%

Each arm 9%

Front of trunk 18%

Back of trunk 18%

Perineum 1%

Each leg 18%

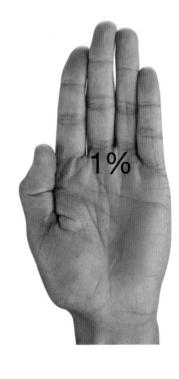

1%

Managing burns

SEE ALSO

➤ Dealing with shock, p72
➤ Understanding and assessing burns 1, p178
➤ Assessing burns 2, p180

Time is of the essence when giving first aid to a casualty with burns. You must ensure that the person is no longer in danger of further burns and then cool the affected area of skin. Do not turn the tap on full force as a powerful jet of water may further damage the delicate skin of the burnt area. Reassure the casualty and phone the emergency services if necessary. If you think the burns are deep or cover a large proportion of the body, watch the casualty carefully and be ready to deal with signs of further problems, such as shock.

As already mentioned, a major priority in all burn cases is to cool the skin. This not only eases much of the pain, but also ultimately reduces the amount of damage done to the skin, so that it heals faster and scars less. However, be careful about making the person too cold and causing hypothermia. If in doubt, cover the casualty with a coat or light blanket.

COVERING BURNS

Skin damage allows potential infection to enter, so burns must be covered. Dry dressings, even non-fluffy ones, tend to stick to burns, so your best options are: wet sterile dressings of various kinds (or dampened clean handkerchiefs or bits of clean cotton pillowcase), clean plastic bags, or clear food wrap film.

PUTTING OUT FLAMES

Dousing a victim in water may be impossible if there is no water nearby or if the flames are too strong. If so, wrap them from head to toe in a heavy, non-synthetic material (for example, a cotton or wool rug, coat or curtain) to exclude the air and smother the flames.

BURNS: BASIC PRIORITIES

Follow the "Danger" step of DRSABC. Protect yourself and the casualty from any further danger and further burns.

⬇

Check the casualty's RABC; monitor for noisy or difficult breathing.

⬇

Cool down the burnt skin. For serious burns, call the emergency services.

⬇

Cover the burn, to prevent infection.

⬇

Minimize shock and check for any other injuries.

WHAT TO DO WITH SMALL BURNS AND SCALDS

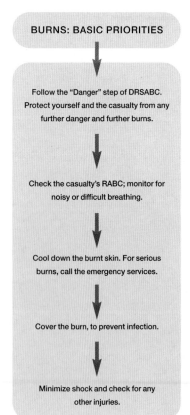

1 Run cold water over the burn site for at least 10 minutes. If the burn is on a hand or arm, remove any watches, rings or bracelets while you are cooling the skin, as the burn may cause some swelling of tissues.

2 After cooling, help prevent infection by wrapping the area with a damp sterile bandage, clear food wrap or a small plastic bag (for hands and feet). When using a plastic bag, fill the bag with air (do not blow into it, as that will introduce germs), gently place the hand or foot in the open bag, then hold loosely in place at the wrist or ankle with a length of dressing, a bandage or similar – never use rubber bands.

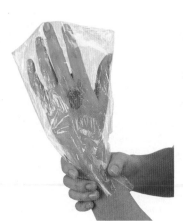

FIRST AID FOR ALL MAJOR BURNS AND SCALDS

1 Having controlled or eliminated any dangers, put the casualty into a safe position. This is usually lying flat, unless there is breathing difficulty, in which case they should sit upright and supported. Send for the emergency services. Now cool the burnt area with cold water for at least 10 minutes. While cooling, remove any constricting items such as rings, watches and bracelets before swelling cuts off the circulation. See box for advice on clothes removal.

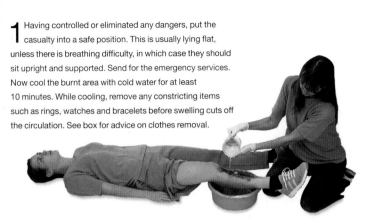

WARNING

Here is a summary of major things to avoid when dealing with burns:

➤ Do not remove anything that is stuck to the burn – you may damage the skin further.

➤ Do not touch the wound and risk introducing infection.

➤ Do not use adhesive, fluffy or dry dressings; these will stick to the burn.

➤ Do not put fats, lotions or ointments on a burn.

➤ Do not burst any blisters. While the skin is still intact it will continue to protect from infection, and provides an element of pain relief.

➤ Do not give the person anything to eat or drink if the burn is severe, unless you are a long way from hospital.

2 If the emergency services have not arrived after 10 minutes of cooling, cover the burnt area to prevent infection. Observe the casualty for breathing problems or worsening shock. Carefully check for other injuries.

▷ Raising a burnt limb may help to minimize swelling; raising both legs may help to reduce any shock symptoms.

REMOVAL OF CLOTHING

Dry burns (from flames, for example):
Douse any smouldering clothes with water to extinguish and cool. Try to cool burns directly onto the skin, but do not remove the clothing unless it is impeding the cooling (in this case, cut around any adhered clothing, leaving the adhered material in place).

Wet burns (scalds from boiling water, for example):
Flood water under the clothing to start cooling and separate it from the skin. Scalded skin is often fragile, so remove clothing carefully by cutting it first some distance away from the scalded area. Continue to cool the affected area gently.

Chemical burns (caustics, acids or alkalis, for example):
Use a shower or hose to drench the area. Remove affected clothing in the shower. In the absence of water, use scissors to remove affected clothing quickly. At any stage, avoid contact with the chemical, the contaminated area, or with "run-off" water used for dousing. Wear suitable protective gloves/clothing – if you can find them quickly.

Chemical, electrical and inhalation burns

SEE ALSO
➤ Understanding and assessing burns, p178
➤ Assessing burns 2, p180
➤ Keeping yourself safe, p224

Chemical and electrical burns are especially hazardous, as further injury is possible both for casualty and helper. With a chemical incident, make the area safe or remove the casualty to safety and then get someone to inform the fire service about the chemical in question. Electrical burns can look deceptively mild at skin level while underlying muscles, nerves and organs may be badly burned. With both chemical and electrical burns, the casualty could go into shock, so monitor their vital signs until medical help arrives.

BURNS FROM CHEMICALS

Corrosive chemicals will continue to damage the skin while in contact with it so dispersing the harmful chemical as soon as possible is a priority. Chemical burns tend to develop more slowly than those from other causes. They may also be particularly hazardous to the first-aider (because you may easily become burnt yourself) and they may give off fumes that could be inhaled. If there is any doubt about the chemical, move everyone away from the casualty and summon expert help.

You may recognize a burn as a chemical burn because:
• The casualty informs you what happened.
• There are containers of chemicals nearby.
• The casualty is suffering intense, stinging pain around the burnt area.
• After some time, blistering and discoloration may develop, along with swollen tissues in the affected area.

▽ While wearing protective gloves, flood the burnt area with cold water to cool the skin and disperse the chemical.

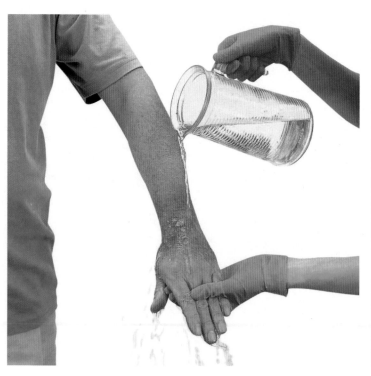

FIRST AID FOR CHEMICAL BURNS

Phone the emergency services or arrange urgent transport to hospital.

⬇

Get the casualty out of the contaminated area as soon as possible, without exposing yourself to danger.

⬇

Protect yourself. Wear appropriate gloves/apron if readily available; open windows and doors for ventilation.

⬇

Flood the injured part with water, for at least 10–15 minutes or until help arrives. Pour the water so that contaminated water neither runs on to other parts of the casualty's body nor on to you.

⬇

Remove any contaminated clothing, unless it is stuck fast to the skin.

WARNING

Do not try to "neutralize" the chemical (by putting alkali on acid or vice versa) as the resulting reaction may produce heat or exacerbate the existing burn.

COMMON CAUSES OF CHEMICAL BURNS

Certain chemicals can irritate, burn or even penetrate the skin's protective layer. Many chemical-related accidents are in industry but the following are all common household chemicals that are corrosive.

➤ Dishwasher products.

➤ Oven cleaners.

➤ Bleach.

➤ Ammonia.

➤ Caustic soda.

BURNS FROM ELECTRICITY

Electrical burns can occur from all kinds of electric current – from lightning strikes and overhead power cables to domestic current. There are three distinct types of electrical burn:

• A flash burn, caused by electricity arcing over a distance, and which leaves a distinctive residue on the skin that is sometimes coppery in appearance.

• Burns from flames caused by electricity.

• Direct burning of the tissues by an electric current.

ELECTRICITY-RELATED DAMAGE

Electrical burns can look deceptively mild. Like chemical burns, the extent of the burn may not be immediately obvious and often looks quite innocuous. There may be entry and exit wounds, which give an idea of the path of the electric current, but these are often hard to find.

Underneath the fairly normal-looking skin, the muscle, blood vessels and nerves may have literally "fried". What's more, the jolt of electricity could have affected the casualty's heartbeat.

If you arrive at an accident scene and find that the casualty is unconscious, first ensure they are not still connected to a live power source, and then check their ABC and be prepared to start resuscitation techniques immediately and to continue until emergency medical assistance arrives.

FIRST AID FOR ELECTRICAL BURNS

Do not touch the casualty unless and until you know they are no longer connected to a live electrical source.

If the casualty is unconscious, check their ABC and start resuscitation if necessary. Call the emergency services.

Treat as for a dry burn.

Watch for any signs of shock, or for any effects on the heartbeat.
Note: Anyone who has suffered more than a mild tingling sensation should be seen at hospital – electricity can affect the heart some time after the initial exposure.

INHALATION BURNS

Breathing in dangerous fumes may affect the respiratory system – the trachea (windpipe), bronchi and lung tissue – and can cause serious damage. Such fumes include car exhaust emissions (including carbon monoxide), smoke from a fire, fumes from faulty domestic appliances (such as a gas heater) and fumes from smouldering foam-filled upholstered furniture. Certain chemicals, including dry-cleaning solvents, may also give off toxic or irritant fumes.

Signs of inhalation burns:
• Soot and singed hairs around the mouth and nose area.
• Breathing difficulties.
• Headache.
• Dizziness.
• Shock.

The best first-aid approach is as follows: Send for the emergency services; get the casualty to a safe place in clean air and do not expose yourself to fire, smoke or fumes; position the casualty sitting up and supported; monitor the casualty for changes in consciousness or breathing; be prepared to resuscitate if necessary (however, if chemicals have been inhaled, then this may be unsafe without special equipment).

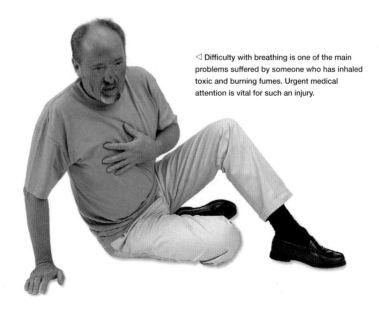

◁ Difficulty with breathing is one of the main problems suffered by someone who has inhaled toxic and burning fumes. Urgent medical attention is vital for such an injury.

Coping with facial burns

SEE ALSO

➤ Dealing with shock, p72

➤ Assessing burns 2, p180

➤ Managing burns, p182

Any type of facial burn is an emergency because it can result in possible blindness, breathing difficulties and obvious scarring. The priorities are to cool the burnt area with cold water and to convey the casualty to hospital. Do remember to reassure the casualty throughout and keep an eye out for any signs of shock. It's a good idea to gather details on what has caused the burn in the first place so that you can relay this information to medical personnel so that they can take prompt and appropriate action.

Burns to the face can have further, highly serious, implications. Because they strongly suggest that there may be other burns – to the casualty's airway, nose and

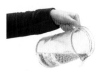
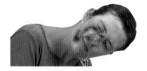

◁ Flood a facial burn with cold water and continue to do so for at least 10 minutes.

mouth – there is a danger they may compromise the casualty's breathing. Also, it is vital to take rapid action in order to minimize any scars from a facial burn, as significant scarring can cause psychological difficulties.

BURNS TO THE EYE

Facial burns to the eye area are especially painful and are prone to significant amounts of swelling, which can make it difficult for the casualty to see and for you to examine the eyeball.

It is vital to get the person to a doctor or hospital very quickly as any burns to the

eyelid or cornea can lead to scarring that may cause blindness. Reassure the casualty throughout as they may think that they are going blind and panic. Keep them calm and remind them that it is just the swelling that is obstructing their vision.

CHEMICAL BURNS TO THE EYE

Chemicals can burn the delicate tissues of the eye and cause scarring, which may lead to blindness. The main first-aid priority is to irrigate the eye to remove as much of the chemical as possible. The casualty's eye may be very painful, red and watery, making it difficult to prise open and flush out.

FIRST AID FOR FACIAL BURNS

↓

Sit the casualty up in case breathing problems develop.

↓

Keep a careful watch on their breathing throughout.

↓

Phone the emergency services.

↓

Apply cold compresses or pour cold water over the burn if this is possible.

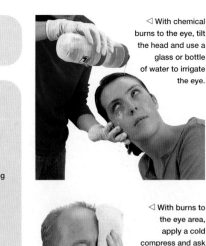

◁ With chemical burns to the eye, tilt the head and use a glass or bottle of water to irrigate the eye.

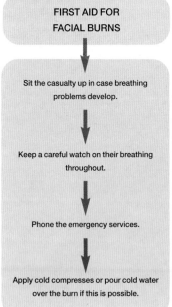

◁ With burns to the eye area, apply a cold compress and ask the casualty to hold it in place.

FIRST AID FOR CHEMICAL BURNS TO THE EYE

↓

Turn the person's head to one side with the affected eye below the good eye so that no chemical runs into the good eye.

↓

Hold the eyelid open under a gently running tap or pour water from a glass or bottle. Flush both sides of the eye; don't splash contaminated water into the good eye.

↓

Cover the eye with a sterile eye pad and secure loosely. Try to find out what chemical has caused the burn and always take the casualty to hospital.

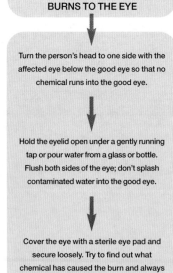

Tackling sunburn

SEE ALSO
► Understanding burns, p178
► Assessing the severity of burns, p180

Burns caused by the ultraviolet rays of the sun can be as dangerous as those caused by anything else. The immune system reacts to the sun's assault to protect the body. First, the skin reddens and starts to itch; then it becomes swollen and painful, eventually blistering and flaking (and sometimes even scarring). Sunbeds and tanning lamps can inflict the same damage as natural sunlight, and so are best avoided. Taking sensible precautions when out in the sun can ensure that a holiday is a happy and healthy one.

Sunburn can not only cause severe skin damage but may also lead to the serious conditions of heat exhaustion or even heat stroke. The sun's ultraviolet radiation can be harmful to the eyes, and sunglasses should be worn when outside, especially in areas where there is a lot of reflected light such as on the sea or in snow. The effects of too much sun are not immediately obvious and can take 12–24 hours to develop.

Many people don't realize that you can get sunburn even on a cloudy day. There are also other factors that make sunburn more likely, including:
- High altitudes – The thinner the atmosphere, the greater the risk of even small amounts of sun causing burning.
- Reflective surfaces – Water, sand, wind, snow and pavements increase the sun's strength by reflecting its rays.
- Sweat and water on the skin – Such moisture increases the chances of burning and stops sunscreens from working properly.

FIRST AID FOR SUNBURN

Remove the casualty from direct sun and keep them in the shade.

↓

Apply cold compresses to the burnt area to cool the skin or immerse the affected area in a cold bath for at least 10 minutes.

↓

As the casualty may be dehydrated, encourage them to take frequent small sips of water.

↓

If the sunburn is mild, apply some soothing calamine lotion; for severe sunburn take the casualty to see a doctor straightaway.

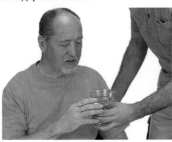

△ To prevent sunburn, wear a T-shirt and a hat and apply some sunscreen.

△ Encourage the sunburnt casualty to sip water frequently as they may be dehydrated.

PREVENTING SUNBURN
A few sensible precautions can prevent sunburn in the first place. Take on board the following advice.

➤ Use a sunscreen on all exposed skin, especially when in open areas with little shade. Reapply regularly.

➤ Wear a wide-brimmed hat ideally with a neck flap.

➤ Always wear sunglasses, especially near snow or expanses of water.

➤ Stay out of the midday sun altogether, especially when in hot countries close to the equator. Make a siesta part of any holiday; resurface at around 3pm when the sun's rays are less damaging.

➤ Remember that no sun tan has to be better than risking skin cancer. If you must sunbathe, build up exposure to the sun very slowly, staying in the sun for no longer than 20 minutes on the first day. Never use low-factor sunscreens.

USING A SUNSCREEN
All sunscreens have an SPF (Sun Protection Factor), which is measured by timing how long skin covered with the sunscreen takes to burn compared with unprotected skin. If your skin normally burns after 10 minutes, then an SPF 15 sunscreen should allow protection for 150 minutes; an SPF8 offers 80 minutes' protection. Even "waterproof" or "water resistant" sunscreens lose their effectiveness once you have been in the water for 40 minutes. The minimum recommended sunscreen is SPF15.

BURNS AND SCALDS

KEY POINTS

- Burns must be cooled – run cold water over a burn site for a minimum of 10 minutes in order to limit the internal damage ☐

- Do not touch burnt skin, to avoid inflicting further injury ☐

- Use non-adhesive dressings (preferably dampened) – never adhesive or fluffy ones ☐

- Many burns occur in domestic house fires that could often have been prevented. These burns account for about 10 per cent of accidental deaths ☐

SKILLS LEARNED

- How to treat minor burns and scalds ☐

- How to treat more extensive burns or scalding ☐

- Assessing the depth, extent and seriousness of a burn ☐

- Recognizing the possibilities of breathing difficulties, shock and internal injury as a consequence of burns ☐

- Avoiding sunburn ☐

12

ACTION ON POISONING

There are some substances that the human body cannot tolerate. These poisons – also known as toxins – include a wide variety of plants and fungi, household products and medicines (both prescription drugs and illicit drugs). The body's defence system recognizes such toxins as threats to survival and tries to get rid of the offending substance – by vomiting and/or diarrhoea, for example. When encountering a poisoning incident, the first-aider is limited to calling for medical emergency services and to gathering any evidence on what the poison could have been. Do not under any circumstances try to make the casualty vomit up the poison.

CONTENTS

Understanding poisoning

SEE ALSO
➤ Managing drug poisoning, p192
➤ Managing poisoning in children, p198

The golden rule in giving first aid for a suspected poisoning is never to attempt to make the casualty vomit until you know what the poison is. Vomiting a poisonous substance back up the oesophagus (gullet) can double the damage if the poison is a corrosive chemical.

Poisons can get into the body in many ways – via the skin, digestive system, lungs or bloodstream. The mode of entry influences the speed of reaction; for instance if a poison is injected into the bloodstream, it can reach all parts of the body within a minute or so.

A poison is any substance that can cause temporary or permanent damage to the body if taken in sufficient quantities. Poisoning may occur accidentally or intentionally. Suicide attempts often involve more than one poisonous agent, and the casualty may resist any help that is offered. Some drugs have no obvious immediate effects when taken in overdose but ultimately are fatal.

Accidental poisoning is most often seen in children and in the elderly. There are fewer deaths from such incidents in children, but some agents may wreak havoc in a child. Elderly people may get confused and take the wrong medicine or the wrong amount.

There are a wide variety of poisons:
• Noxious gases or fumes.
• Cleaning products.
• Toxins in plants and fungi.
• Bacterial and viral toxins (in food).
• Drugs and alcohol.
• Toxins from bites and stings.

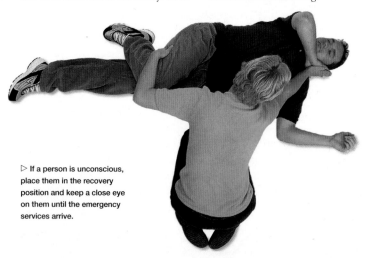

▷ If a person is unconscious, place them in the recovery position and keep a close eye on them until the emergency services arrive.

BASIC GUIDELINES FOR DEALING WITH POISONING

Assess the casualty's ABC (airway, breathing and circulation). If they are breathing but unconscious, put them in the recovery position.

If they are not breathing, start resuscitation techniques once you have checked that there is no poison on the face or in the mouth area.

Phone or get someone to phone the emergency services.

If they start to have a fit, do not restrain them. Keep them out of danger and ensure a clear airway.

Look around to see if you can find any clues to the identity of the poison that has been taken. If the casualty has vomited, take a sample of the vomit to hospital as there is a good chance it will help doctors identify the appropriate treatment.

IDENTIFYING THE CAUSE OF THE POISONING

Once you have dealt with the casualty's immediate needs, gather information to try to identify the poison.

➤ Look for empty pill bottles or loose pills or capsules on the floor. Bag them and give to the emergency services.

➤ Search for codes on containers that will identify any chemical.

➤ Scan the area for a dead insect or snake to bag up and take to hospital.

➤ Cast your eye around for any potentially poisonous foods.

HOW POISONS AFFECT THE BODY

▷ Poisons can have wide-ranging effects on different parts of the body. Effects depend on how the poison gets into the system and how much poison has been taken.

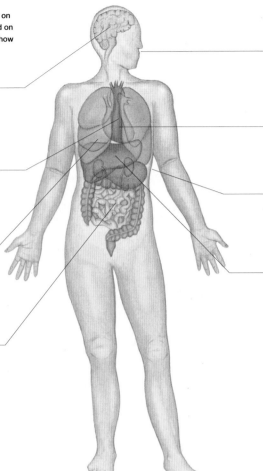

Brain
Once in the bloodstream, drugs can easily reach the brain causing confusion, drowsiness, fits and, at worst, coma. If the part of the brain that controls breathing is affected, a person's breathing can stop altogether.

Blood
Poisonous gases such as cyanide and carbon monoxide react with the blood, so that there is not enough oxygen in the circulation, leading to potentially lethal effects on the body.

Lungs
Inhaled fumes or drugs quickly reach the lungs and then travel in the bloodstream. Such poisons cause breathing difficulties (which can be fatal in people with asthma) and lead to blue skin (cyanosis) – a sign that there's too little oxygen in the body.

Digestive tract
Toxins from bacteria or viruses in contaminated food commonly cause nausea, vomiting and diarrhoea.

Mouth
Corrosive substances such as bleach and dishwashing powder may burn the tissues lining the throat and oesophagus (gullet) and cause nausea and vomiting.

Heart
Injected and swallowed poisons can result in an irregular heartbeat or in the heart beating too fast or too slowly.

Chest wall
Certain snake venom, certain garden fertilizers and botulinum toxin can lead to paralysis of the muscles in the chest wall and therefore cause suffocation.

Liver
This is the body's vital detoxifying centre. Toxins from some wild mushrooms may cause severe liver damage and the everyday painkiller paracetamol can destroy liver cells if taken in excess (even relatively small amounts over the recommended dosage).

COMMON POISONS

Household:

➤ Bleach, caustic soda, household cleaning products, perfume, aftershave, hair spray, nail varnish remover, lighter fuel, turpentine, white spirit and all kinds of solvents, including dry cleaning solvents, mercury-filled thermometer, child's play "putty", shoe creams and polishes, slug pellets, tobacco, weedkiller, glues, wood preservative, lead paint (in old houses), antifreeze, bug and rodent killers.

Drugs and chemicals:

➤ Medicines in excess of stated dose (or if taken by someone who suffers from an allergic reaction to them), large amounts of vitamins A and D, large amounts of Epsom salts, iodine.

Fungi:

➤ Certain types of toadstools and mushrooms can be lethal – even if only tiny quantities have been eaten.

Bites and stings:

➤ From insects, jellyfish and snakes, among others.

Plants:

➤ For example, laburnum, foxglove, holly berries, monkshood and yew.

Gases:

➤ Carbon monoxide may leak from faulty gas heaters, boilers and the vents of air conditioning systems.

Managing drug poisoning

SEE ALSO
➤ What is first aid?, p16
➤ Understanding poisoning, p190
➤ Tackling alcohol and illicit drug poisoning, p194

Each type of drug usually quickly produces specific signs and symptoms when taken in overdose; the exception here is excess paracetamol, which can take a few days to produce recognizable symptoms. The effects of the drugs depend on the type of drug and how it is taken (swallowed, inhaled or injected). The basic first-aid aims when dealing with drug poisoning are to maintain breathing, call the emergency services and look for any information at the scene that could provide vital clues for the medics treating the casualty.

Drug poisoning can result from overdosage of prescription or over-the-counter medicines or from abuse of illicit drugs. Less commonly, it is caused by two or more drugs interacting.

It is often possible to identify what substances have been taken, as they each cause specific signs and symptoms. Such information may be incredibly helpful as the casualty may be unconscious by the time they reach the hospital.

PARACETAMOL-BASED PAINKILLERS

Such painkilling medicine can be commonly bought over the counter and is a basic part of most home medicine cupboards. If paracetamol is taken in overdosage, even just a relatively small amount, destruction of the liver can occur.

The casualty may feel fine for the first few days, until liver (or, less commonly, kidney) damage starts to take effect. Then,

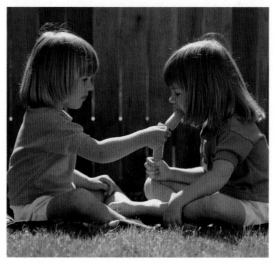

◁ Children love to experiment with tasting things, but if unsupervised, their natural curiosity may result in a poisoning incident. In the same vein, keep an eye on small children going through an adult's bag or a kitchen or bathroom cupboard.

the following symptoms may appear:
• Nausea and profuse vomiting.
• Pain in the upper right-hand abdomen after 24 hours (a sign of liver damage).

Irreversible liver damage can occur within three to four days so prompt recognition and transfer to hospital is vital.

ASPIRIN-BASED PAINKILLERS

If these common painkillers are taken in excessive amounts they can cause the following symptoms:
• Upper abdominal pain.
• Nausea and vomiting.
• Fever, with sweating and dizziness.
• Deep "sighing" breaths.
• Deafness and/or loud noises heard in the ears (tinnitus).
• Restlessness and confusion.
• Deterioration in consciousness or fitting.

◁ Drowsiness followed by loss of consciousness can be a sign of poisoning. Seek immediate medical help.

FIRST AID FOR POISONING

↓

If the casualty is conscious, then let them rest in a comfortable position. Reassure them and ask if they can tell you what they have taken.

↓

Phone the emergency services.

↓

Monitor their breathing and talk to them until help arrives.

↓

Keep samples of any vomit. Look for any clues as to the identity of poisons.

ANTIDEPRESSANT DRUGS

There are many different types of antidepressant medicine available on prescription. If taken in excess, the older type of tricyclic antidepressants, such as amitryptyline, initially cause:

• Blurred vision.
• Dilated pupils.
• Dry mouth.
• An inability to pass urine.

They can then result in:

• Drowsiness.
• Drops in blood pressure and temperature.
• Fits, followed by cardiac arrest.

The newer-style antidepressants, such as fluoxetine and sertraline, have completely different overdosage effects – notably the tendency to cause an erratic heart rate.

TRANQUILLIZERS

Tranquillizing drugs are often prescribed for anxiety and sleeping problems, and commonly include barbiturate and benzodiazepine drugs. If these are taken in overdose, they can result in the following:

• Slurred speech.
• Drowsiness and lethargy, leading to a loss of consciousness.
• Weak, irregular or slow or fast heartbeat.
• Slow breathing rate (breathing may actually stop altogether).

If tranquillizers are taken in combination with excessive alcohol the situation is much more dangerous. Older people often take sleeping tablets; when taken in excess, these may produce hypothermia – a condition to which they are vulnerable.

IRON SUPPLEMENTS

Women often take an iron supplement (commonly as iron tablets) during pregnancy and while breastfeeding. Children can mistake such tablets for sweets and eat them. The signs of iron overdosage include:

• Stomach pain.
• Vomiting and diarrhoea.
• Blood in the vomit or the stool.

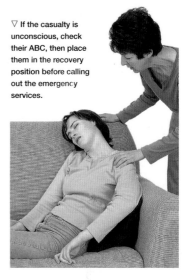

▽ If the casualty is unconscious, check their ABC, then place them in the recovery position before calling out the emergency services.

Excessive iron can cause severe damage to a child's liver and this is one of the few types of tablet that children accidentally take that can turn out to be lethal.

▽ Iron poisoning causes vomiting and severe stomach pain in children. They should be taken straight to hospital.

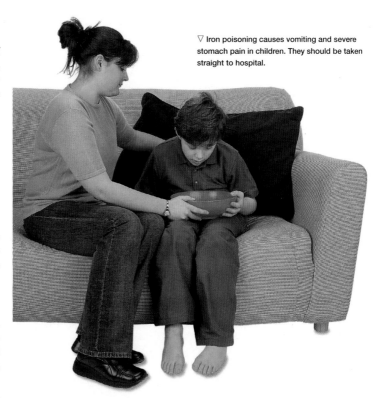

Tackling alcohol and illicit drug poisoning

SEE ALSO

➤ Understanding poisoning, p190

➤ Managing drug poisoning, p192

➤ Managing poisoning in children, p198

Alcohol in moderate amounts is easily detoxified by the liver; but in very large quantities alcohol becomes a poison that the body can no longer deal with – and it can prove fatal. The same doesn't go, however, for many illicit drugs. Even relatively small amounts of a substance such as cocaine or fumes from glue can result in severe effects on the body. Emergency medical treatment is vital, especially if a child has taken alcohol or a drug because children absorb the toxins much more quickly than adults.

Taking illicit substances and drinking large quantities of alcohol is socially acceptable in some parts of society, but such practices are potentially dangerous and lead to medical crises and even fatalities.

ALCOHOL POISONING

Alcohol is a poison when drunk in sufficient quantities. Consumption of half a litre (1 pint) of a spirit, such as vodka, is enough to cause severe alcohol poisoning. Alcohol-related risks include:

• Depression of the central nervous system, most seriously the brain.
• Widening of blood vessels, making the body lose heat and risking hypothermia.
• The inebriated person may choke on their vomit while unconscious.

SIGNS AND SYMPTOMS OF ALCOHOL INTOXICATION

It is usually fairly obvious when someone is intoxicated with alcohol, but similar symptoms may be caused by a head injury or a diabetic hypoglycaemic (low blood sugar) condition.

➤ A smell of alcohol on the breath.

➤ Empty bottles or cans nearby.

➤ Flushed and warm skin.

➤ Actions are aggressive or passive.

➤ Speech and actions are slow and become less coordinated.

➤ Deep, noisy breathing.

➤ Low level of consciousness; they may often slip into unconsciousness.

HOW TO DEAL WITH ALCOHOL INTOXICATION

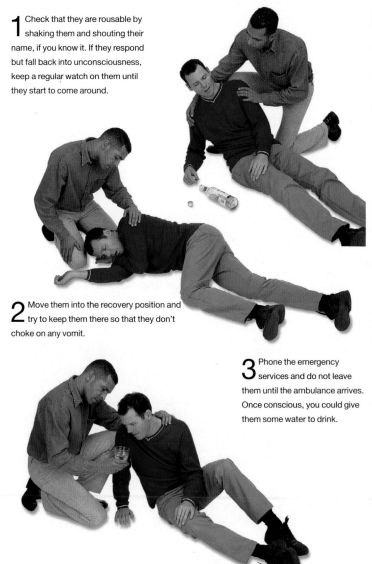

1 Check that they are rousable by shaking them and shouting their name, if you know it. If they respond but fall back into unconsciousness, keep a regular watch on them until they start to come around.

2 Move them into the recovery position and try to keep them there so that they don't choke on any vomit.

3 Phone the emergency services and do not leave them until the ambulance arrives. Once conscious, you could give them some water to drink.

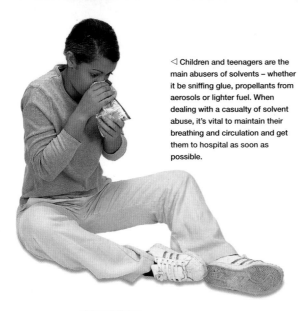

◁ Children and teenagers are the main abusers of solvents – whether it be sniffing glue, propellants from aerosols or lighter fuel. When dealing with a casualty of solvent abuse, it's vital to maintain their breathing and circulation and get them to hospital as soon as possible.

ILLICIT DRUGS

Illicit stimulant drugs include Ecstasy, cocaine, amphetamines and LSD. If you suspect someone has taken any of these drugs, watch out for the following signs:
• Excitable and hyperactive behaviour.
• Sweating.
• Shaking hands.
• Hallucinations.

These drugs can occasionally be fatal. Ecstasy interferes with the brain's ability to control body temperature, which can rise to over 42°C (107.6°F) and cause heat exhaustion. Ecstasy-takers often drink lots of water, which can cause kidney malfunction and abnormal heart rhythms. Cocaine's main effects are on the heart rate – with the potential to lead to abnormal rhythms and even cardiac arrest.

Opiate drugs such as heroin and codeine may depress the respiratory system, causing breathing to stop. Rapid recovery occurs if a particular drug is given intravenously, but this must be done urgently, by trained medical personnel.

POISONING VIA SOLVENT ABUSE

Children and adolescents are the main solvent abusers – they may inhale fumes from glue, paint, lighter fuel, cleaning fluids, aerosols and nail polish to "get high". All such solvents depress breathing and heart activity, and may cause respiratory and cardiac arrest.

FIRST AID FOR SOLVENT ABUSE POISONING

If the casualty has stopped breathing or their heart has stopped beating, start resuscitation immediately.

If unconscious but their ABC (airway, breathing and circulation) is normal, place them in the fresh air in the recovery position.

Phone the emergency services.

Check their ABC regularly.

Often, the casualty starts to "come round" quickly and may seem normal after 20 minutes. Stay with them until help arrives.

SIGNS AND SYMPTOMS OF SOLVENT POISONING

➤ The casualty has a dry throat and cough.

➤ Their chest feels tight and they may be breathless.

➤ They have a headache.

➤ They feel nauseous and may vomit.

➤ They have hallucinations – they "hear voices" or "see things".

➤ Their breathing becomes faster and more laboured as fluid builds up in their lungs.

➤ They become drowsy and confused and eventually may lose consciousness.

➤ They have episodes of fits (convulsions), which may lead to coma and eventually to death.

FIRST AID FOR ILLICIT DRUG POISONING

Do not try to make the casualty vomit.

Place them in the recovery position.

Phone the emergency services.

Check their ABC and monitor their breathing every 10 minutes.

Dealing with food and plant poisoning

SEE ALSO

➤ Dealing with shock, p72
➤ Understanding poisoning, p190
➤ Managing poisoning in children, p198

Potentially poisonous things to eat are all around us: in the garden, the kitchen, the bathroom or a nearby wood. Make your garden safe if you have young children by ensuring that all plants are harmless or that any toxic plants are inaccessible. Never be tempted to try a wild mushroom; it may look harmless but it could give you severe, or even fatal, poisoning. Always practise good food hygiene to avoid food poisoning at home. If you have any worries or doubts at all about a potential poisoning incident, you should always call the emergency services.

Young children are the most likely group to eat poisonous plants as they find brightly coloured seeds and berries attractive. Adults may eat poisonous mushrooms by mistaking them for an edible species. The effects of plant poisoning can be almost anything depending on the plant, while mushrooms tend to upset the digestive system. While many fungi are relatively harmless, the common death cap mushroom, for example, contains a toxin that destroys the liver after a delay of several days.

First-aid priorities for poisoning, whether it is from a plant or a fungus, are to:
• Identify the poisonous agent, if possible.
• Manage any fitting episodes.
• Call the emergency services.

MUSHROOM POISONING

Serious poisoning through eating poisonous mushrooms is rare. Some species of fungus may cause some less serious digestive symptoms, but eating a species such as the death cap can be fatal.

Suspect mushroom poisoning if you notice these signs and symptoms:
• Nausea and vomiting.
• Crampy abdominal pain and diarrhoea.
• Episodes of fitting.
• Deterioration in level of consciousness.

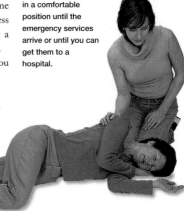

▽ Place the casualty in a comfortable position until the emergency services arrive or until you can get them to a hospital.

SOME COMMON POISONOUS PLANTS

➤ Autumn crocus (*Colchicum*) – all parts are very toxic and can prove to be fatal.

➤ Californian glory (*Fremontodendron*) – little hairs on the stem and leaves can cause skin irritation and itching.

➤ Castor oil plant (*Ricinus communis*) – all parts of this plant – especially the seeds – are very toxic if eaten and could be fatal.

➤ Daffodil (*Narcissus*) – if a bulb is eaten (a child can mistake it for an onion), it causes vomiting, stomachache and diarrhoea.

➤ Deadly nightshade (*Atropa belladonna*) – toxic if eaten and can irritate skin.

➤ Dumb cane or Leopard lily (*Dieffenbachia*) – eating any part of the plant, even a small quantity, can make the tongue, mouth and throat swell and interfere with breathing. Skin contact with the sap causes irritation.

➤ Foxglove (*Digitalis purpurea*) – all parts can be very toxic. As this bitter plant often causes vomiting first, poisoning is rare.

➤ Holly (*Ilex aquifolium*) – red berries are poisonous.

➤ Hyacinth (*Hyacinthus*) – if the bulbs are mistaken for onions and eaten, they will make a person sick and can sometimes cause a skin rash.

➤ Laburnum (*Laburnum anagyroides*) – all parts are toxic, especially the seeds.

➤ Lantana (*Lantana camara*) – all parts of this plant are toxic. The unripe berries, in particular, are attractive to young children.

➤ Lupin (*Lupinus*) – the seeds and pods are poisonous but would have to be eaten in large quantities to do real harm.

➤ Monkshood (*Aconitum*) – all parts are highly toxic if eaten and contact with the sap can cause skin irritation.

➤ Spurge laurel (*Daphne laureola*) – all parts are highly poisonous if eaten.

➤ Umbrella tree (*Schefflera*) – any contact with cut stems or leaves causes skin irritation.

➤ Winter cherry (*Solanum capsicastrum*) – the fruit is poisonous but not fatal.

➤ Woody nightshade (*Solanum dulcamara*) – the berries of this plant are poisonous and when eaten can cause stomachache, vomiting and diarrhoea.

➤ Yew tree (*Taxus*) – all parts of this tree are toxic if eaten.

FIRST AID FOR PLANT OR MUSHROOM POISONING

↓

If the casualty is conscious, ask them what they have eaten.

↓

If they are unconscious, check their ABC (airway, breathing and circulation) and place them in the recovery position.

↓

Try to identify what poisonous plant or mushroom they could have eaten.

↓

Phone the emergency services or take the casualty to hospital. Take a sample of the plant with you to the hospital.

SOME EXAMPLES OF POISONOUS MUSHROOM

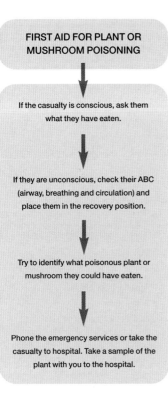

△ Yellow stainer. △ Fly agaric.

△ Death cap. △ Destroying angel.

FOOD POISONING

Symptoms of food poisoning may develop within an hour after consuming the tainted food, although it can sometimes take up to three days. The food often tastes and smells entirely normal. The commonest culprits of food poisoning are bacteria and viruses, including *E. coli*, *Salmonella* and *Staphylococcus*. Foods that often become contaminated and give people food poisoning include shellfish and other protein-containing foods, such as meat or fish, that have been left in the refrigerator or kitchen for a while.

Food poisoning may cause such severe fluid losses, through vomiting and diarrhoea, that dehydration develops. If the lost fluids are not replaced quickly enough, then a further danger is the development of shock.

FIRST AID FOR FOOD POISONING

↓

Encourage the casualty to rest and drink plenty of water.

↓

Do not give them solid food for 24 hours or until their symptoms settle.

↓

If symptoms persist or worsen for more than a few days, call your doctor for medical advice.

◁ Brown roll-rim.

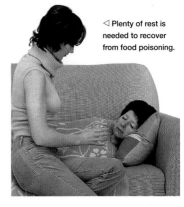

◁ Plenty of rest is needed to recover from food poisoning.

Typical signs of food poisoning are:
• Nausea and vomiting.
• Crampy abdominal pain.
• Diarrhoea, which may be blood-stained.
• Fever and shivering and/or headache.
• Signs of shock.

PREVENTING FOOD POISONING

Take these few sensible precautions to prevent food poisoning altogether.

➤ Fully defrost food before cooking.

➤ Cook meat, fish, poultry and eggs very thoroughly.

➤ Always wash hands thoroughly after using the toilet, and again before food preparation or cooking starts.

➤ Tepid cooked food gathers bacteria fast, so store it in the fridge or freeze it.

➤ Be aware that raw eggs, used in recipes like mayonnaise, have a high risk of containing *Salmonella* bacteria.

➤ When visiting countries where the water supply could be dirty, never eat or drink anything that may be contaminated with local water, such as ice (in drinks), unpeeled fruit or vegetables, ice-cream and salads (which could have been washed in local water).

➤ When in a part of the world where the water is suspect, clean your teeth with bottled water (or sterilized water) rather than using tap water.

Managing poisoning in children

SEE ALSO
➤ What is first aid?, p16
➤ Understanding poisoning, p190
➤ Safety in the home, p228

Young children are naturally interested in searching through cupboards and boxes and generally exploring their environment. They will also put anything and everything into their mouths, including mothballs, dishwasher powder and any variety of potentially fatal household products, liquids and powders. Preventing poisoning in children is an essential part of safety in your home. As with all poisoning incidents, find out what has been taken so that the appropriate medical help can be given and keep a close eye on your child.

Children are naturally inquisitive and have no qualms about touching, inhaling or ingesting anything – all pills are sweets, powders are sherbets and liquids are drinks. Parents are often taken by surprise by what is dangerous for young bodies – alcohol is lethal even in tiny quantities, an excess of iron can kill a child and dishwashing powder can corrode their oesophagus (gullet) in seconds.

Poisons are absorbed faster in children than adults, so their effects can be seen fairly quickly. Suspect poisoning in a child if:
• You observe unusual behaviour such as slurred speech, giggling inappropriately, staggering, drowsiness.
• You find a child playing near an empty pill or chemical container.
• You can see scalds, stains or bits of tablet around their mouth.

FIRST AID FOR ALCOHOL POISONING IN A CHILD

⬇

Place a bowl nearby in case they vomit.

⬇

If unrousable, check their ABC and place in the recovery position.

⬇

If awake, try to keep them awake. Call the emergency services and stay with the casualty until the emergency services arrive.

SYMPTOMS OF ALCOHOL POISONING IN CHILDREN

➤ Strong smell of alcohol.
➤ Flushed skin.
➤ Staggering about.
➤ Slurring of speech.
➤ Nausea.
➤ Noisy breathing.

WARNING
Even a small amount of alcohol can be very harmful to a child.

HOW TO POISON-PROOF YOUR HOME

The best cure is, of course, prevention. Take on board the following advice to ensure your children are never allowed access to potentially deadly poisons.

➤ Never leave unattended glasses full of alcohol around, especially overnight. Children are early risers and may decide to drink up all the dregs while you are sleeping.

➤ Never decant substances from their original containers to empty unlabelled bottles as it may lead to confusion.

➤ Do not use empty food containers such as soft drink bottles to store hazardous substances.

➤ The best place for all potential poisons is out of reach and out of sight in a cupboard that is secured with a childproof catch.

➤ Store food and non-food items in separate cupboards.

➤ Make sure all medicine containers have child-resistant lids on them.

➤ Keep a close eye on your visitors, especially grandparents who may have regular medicines to take and may inadvertently leave such pills in an open handbag or overnight bag. Almost all adult medicines can have devastating effects on a child. For example, diabetic pills that lower blood sugar can reduce a child's blood sugar to such an extent that they fall into a coma and die.

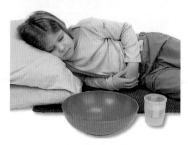

▷ If you suspect alcohol poisoning, place a bowl nearby for any vomit and call the emergency services.

FIRST AID FOR CHEMICAL POISONING IN A CHILD

⬇

Try to find out what chemical has been taken. Look for obvious clues nearby.

⬇

Do not make the child vomit; the chemical may do more damage on its way back up.

⬇

Phone the emergency services.

⬇

If they complain of a sore mouth, moisten the lips only (they should sip/drink nothing).

⬇

To soothe burnt lips, keep moistening frequently with water or milk.

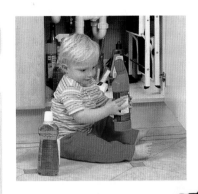

△ All low cupboards should have childproof locks so that household products can be stored safely away from inquisitive children.

FIRST AID FOR DRUG POISONING IN A CHILD

⬇

If the child is unconscious, check they are breathing. If breathing seems normal, place them in the recovery position. If they are not breathing, start resuscitation immediately.

⬇

Phone the emergency services, who may be able to advise you over the phone.

⬇

Look for any signs that the child has swallowed drugs – bits of tablet on the tongue or dye around their mouth.

⬇

Try to work out what drug has been taken and how much and how long ago, if possible.

⬇

Continue to watch ABC until help arrives. Take the drug container with you to hospital or give to the ambulance crew.

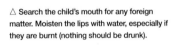

△ Search the child's mouth for any foreign matter. Moisten the lips with water, especially if they are burnt (nothing should be drunk).

FIRST AID FOR PLANT POISONING IN A CHILD

⬇

If the child is unconscious, check that they are breathing. If breathing seems normal, place them in the recovery position. If they are not breathing, start resuscitation immediately.

⬇

Phone the emergency services or take the child to hospital.

⬇

Ask the child what they have eaten.

⬇

Use your finger to search the child's mouth and remove any unswallowed pieces of plant – keep these to hand over to medical personnel.

FIRST AID FOR FUME INHALATION IN A CHILD

⬇

Remove the child from the source of danger, making sure you don't put yourself in danger either.

⬇

Check their breathing. If they are not breathing, start resuscitation immediately. If they are breathing, place them in the recovery position until help arrives.

⬇

Phone the emergency services.

SKILLS CHECKLIST FOR
ACTION ON
POISONING

KEY POINTS

- Never encourage a casualty to vomit back up any poison ☐

- Keep a sample of the suspected poison ☐

- Call the emergency services immediately ☐

SKILLS LEARNED

- Prevention of household poisoning accidents ☐

- How to deal with poisoning in children ☐

- Recognizing the dangers of medicines in excess ☐

- How to deal with food poisoning ☐

- How to cope with illicit drug excess ☐

- How to deal with alcohol poisoning ☐

13

FIRST-AID KIT

It is immediately reassuring to an injured child or any other casualty if you can produce a well-equipped first-aid kit, and it will probably help you to approach any situation confidently if you have certain essential items to hand. A casualty will certainly feel calmer if you show you can dress and bandage an injury professionally and you know how to apply a sling. However, in an emergency, nothing in a first-aid kit is as important as you and your ability to think on your feet and improvise with materials to hand. Communication with the outside world is also very important, so make best use of telephones, neighbours or passers-by, if you are able to.

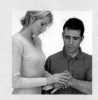

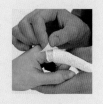

CONTENTS

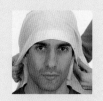

Assembling a first-aid kit

SEE ALSO

➤ What is first aid?, p16

➤ Safety in the home, p228

➤ Travelling safely, p250

A clean and fully equipped first-aid kit in the home, in the car and in the workplace is very important. It should be easily accessible in a kitchen or bathroom cupboard but out of the reach of children. Some items are essential to a first-aid kit but you may find that you'll want to supplement the basic kit with items that you know you use a lot, such as ibuprofen tablets, paracetamol syrup for children or antihistamine cream. Such medicines do not form part of the first aid offered in emergencies and should be for personal use only.

As well as making sure that you have a first-aid kit in the home and the car, you should be aware that every workplace and public recreation establishment and so on is legally required to have a first-aid kit on the premises. So an incident at such a location should prompt a call for their kit. First-aid kits for public use are not supposed to contain any kind of medicine (including ordinary painkillers) or ointments, in case casualties have an adverse reaction to them – what you have in your box at home for private and family use is entirely your affair, of course.

WHAT SHOULD GO IN THE KIT?

The first-aid kit must be kept clean and dry. A large lunch box is ideal for storage, as it is light, durable and easy to open. The following are essential kit items:

• Plasters or adhesive dressings – A good selection of different sizes, shapes and types, for example waterproof, digit-shaped and fabric-backed. Note that very minor cuts and grazes are often better left uncovered.

• Non-adhesive dressings or sterile gauze pads – Usually sealed in protective wrappers, these are easy to use to seal an open wound from possible infection and do not stick to wounds. Have plenty of gauze pads – the best dressing to stop bleeding from a small wound and to dress most small to medium-sized wounds. (Note: in wounds that are bleeding heavily, you may find that a tea towel or towel is the most helpful impromptu dressing.)

• Bandages – Various sizes and types, especially a triangular bandage (for slings/head wounds), elasticated tubular bandages to be used for injured joints, and roller bandages, for securing dressings and stopping bleeding.

• A thermometer, either mercury or digital, to determine body temperature.

• A pair of scissors – Choose a sharp pair in which one side is rounded to allow the safe cutting of dressings and clothing (for example when treating burns or scalds) without the risk of cutting the skin.

• Safety pins – To fix slings and bandages.

• Disposable gloves – Don gloves before attending to cases with blood or open wounds – to ensure that a wound is kept ultra-clean and your hands are protected.

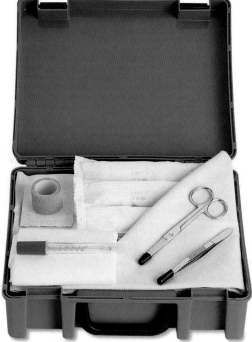

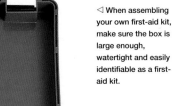

◁ When assembling your own first-aid kit, make sure the box is large enough, watertight and easily identifiable as a first-aid kit.

ESSENTIAL ITEMS FOR A FIRST-AID KIT

Your kit should contain:

➤ Adhesive dressings (plasters in various sizes).

➤ Sterile dressings, various sizes; about 30 gauze dressings and 1 large sterile dressing; plenty of gauze pads.

➤ 1 triangular bandage, tubular bandages and roller bandages.

➤ A thermometer.

➤ A pair of scissors.

➤ Safety pins.

➤ Disposable gloves.

➤ Emergency numbers.

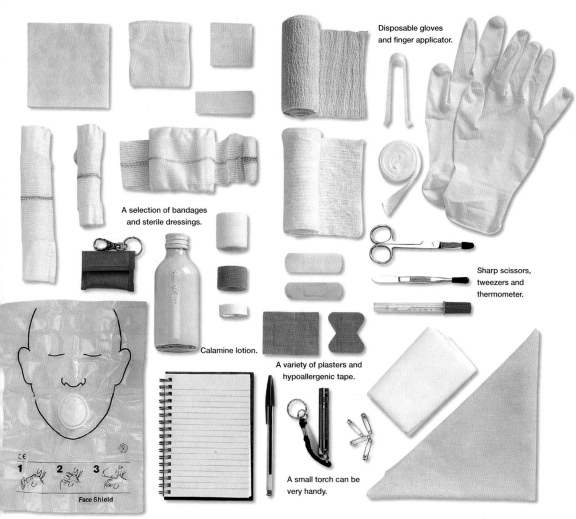

Disposable gloves and finger applicator.

A selection of bandages and sterile dressings.

Sharp scissors, tweezers and thermometer.

Calamine lotion.

A variety of plasters and hypoallergenic tape.

A small torch can be very handy.

Face Shield

A face mask for mouth-to-mouth, stored in a small red pouch.

A notepad and pen with a list of emergency numbers – and to record your observations.

Bandages and safety pins are useful for securing dressings and restricting movement.

- List of emergency telephone numbers – Include your local doctor, chemist, nearest hospital with an accident and emergency department, neighbours and taxi cabs.

Make a note if you use any item from your kit so that you can replace it swiftly.

USEFUL FIRST-AID EXTRAS

In a kit for personal/family use, you may want to keep a small stock of basic medicines such as paracetamol, calamine lotion or antihistamines, and medicine spoons.

- Tweezers – Keep some in your kit for removing splinters of glass and wood.
- Cotton wool or alcohol-free cleansing wipes – Either can be used to clean the skin around a wound but should not be used to dress open wounds, as the fluff will stick to, and clog up, the wound.
- Face protection – A mask or face shield offers protection to you and the casualty when giving mouth-to-mouth.
- Adhesive tape – Waterproof tape can be

△ These are some of the items you may want to keep in your first-aid kit. Select the items you know you may need and that you feel confident about using.

useful when bandaging areas such as the hands, which often get wet. Some people are allergic to such tape; try to check first.

- Cold packs – These gel-filled packs can be warmed up or cooled down. They are useful for easing sprains, cooling a child with a fever, bringing down swelling or cooling superficial burns.

Applying dressings and bandages

SEE ALSO

➤ Assembling a
first-aid kit, p202

➤ Applying bandages
1 and 2,
pp206, 208

All first-aiders should be able to produce a makeshift dressing at the scene of an emergency if none is available. Improvising is a key part of giving first aid, and this can apply to bandages, too. Correct methods of bandaging are easy to learn and are invaluable in many first-aid situations. It can take time to become the perfect "bandager", so practise on friends, or on children (when they are well) if you have them. To be effective, bandages should be applied with a certain amount of pressure and be neither too tight nor too loose.

A dressing is any material held over a wound to stop it from bleeding and to protect it from contamination, whereas a bandage is what holds the dressing in place.

APPLYING DRESSINGS

There are various types of dressing but common basic guidelines apply to the use of any dressing, whichever type is used.

- If possible, always wear disposable gloves when applying a dressing, except if it's an adhesive dressing or plaster.
- Choose the right size dressing so that it covers all of the wound and its edges.

- Avoid touching the dressing where it will come into contact with the wound; hold it at the sides so that it stays sterile and the risk of infection is less.
- Place the dressing on top of the wound and ensure that it sits over its entire surface and the area immediately surrounding the wound. Never slide a dressing around on top of a wound and reposition any dressing that slips off.
- Never take off a dressing, even if a wound continues to bleed through it. Instead, apply more dressing material on top of the first until the bleeding is controlled.

TYPES OF DRESSINGS

Ideally, pre-packed sterile dressings should be used in any incident so that the wound site is free from all germs. However, these dressings are not always to hand and so it's useful to know the other types you can use or how to improvise if you have no first-aid kit whatsoever.

Some different types of dressings include the following:

- Sterile dressings – These dressings are made up from a sterile gauze pad that is covered with a layer of cotton wool and then a bandage. Some sterile dressings come pre-packed and ready to use.
- Adhesive dressings – Also known as plasters, these come in a variety of shapes and sizes (some are specifically designed

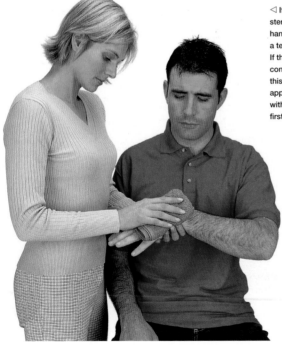

◁ If there aren't any sterile dressings to hand, improvise using a teatowel or similar. If the bleeding continues through this dressing then apply another on top without removing the first one.

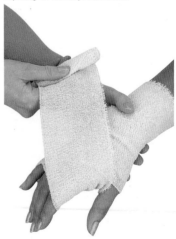

▽ You should aim to wrap a large area of the injured limb in such a way that you are not impeding the casualty's circulation.

to fit a finger or particular body part). Some people have an allergy to certain plasters, so do check with the casualty before you apply one.

- Non-adhesive dressings – These non-fluffy dressings can be applied directly on to a wound and won't stick.
- Makeshift dressings – As is often the case in first-aid situations, improvisation is key. When sterile dressings aren't available, use the cleanest (non-fluffy) material available – teatowels, head scarves or torn-up sheets are all ideal. Sanitary towels make good dressings as they are clean (but not sterile) and bulky.

BANDAGING CORRECTLY

Effective bandaging has several roles – it controls bleeding, aids the return of blood from the wound site, ensures that any dressing stays firmly in place and immobilizes and supports injured limbs. The three basic types of bandage are:

- Roller bandages, for securing dressings and supporting limbs.
- Triangular bandages, for making slings or securing large dressings.
- Tubular bandages, for supporting injured limbs and holding dressings on digits.

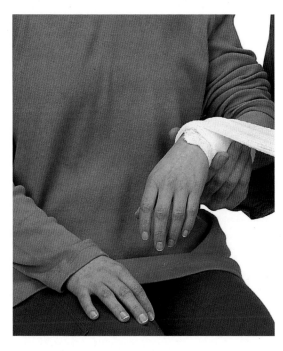
◁ Start from the bottom of the limb and roll the bandage up the arm. Make sure the casualty is comfortable and work from their injured side.

The pressure applied when putting on a bandage is crucial. If a bandage is too tight, fingers or toes will feel cold, the skin will look blue and the limb will be painful. Later on, the skin may look pale and feel cold, and the casualty will tell you that their fingers or toes feel tingly and stiff. Conversely, a loose bandage won't control bleeding or protect a wound site from contamination. Practice makes perfect.

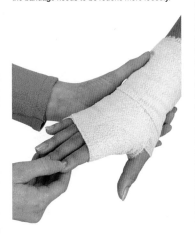
▽ To check that a bandage isn't too tight, press hard on an area downstream of the bandage, a finger in this example. If it takes more than 3 seconds to turn pink again, after being pressed, the bandage needs to be redone more loosely.

THE BASIC RULES OF DRESSING AND BANDAGING

To bandage and apply dressings effectively, follow these simple rules:

DO
- ➤ Start bandaging from the bottom of a limb and work towards the top.
- ➤ Bandage firmly; it shouldn't be too loose, but also not so tight that it cuts off the casualty's circulation.
- ➤ Secure the bandaging with adhesive tape, and guard against loose ends that might get caught when the casualty is being moved.
- ➤ Use uniform pressure when bandaging, and wrap a large area of the limb, which cuts down the chance of impeding the circulation.

DO NOT
- ➤ Use an elasticated bandage to hold a dressing in place, as it may be too tight and cut off the blood flow.
- ➤ Bandage over toes or fingers, unless they are damaged, so that you can check the bandaging is not too tight.
- ➤ Use the wrong-sized bandage – too big and it will be baggy, too small and it will be potentially too tight.
- ➤ Fix a dressing with adhesive tape before first asking the casualty if they have an allergy to such tape.
- ➤ Apply adhesive tape all the way around a limb or a finger or toe as it could cut off the blood flow.

Applying bandages 1

SEE ALSO

➤ Applying dressings and bandages, p204

➤ Applying bandages 2, p208

The only way to become proficient at bandaging is to practise; joints, such as ankles or elbows, can be especially tricky to master. You may find it easiest to watch someone else first and repeat it while you have a chance for some feedback. Make sure that the bandage overlaps on each turn and that you roll it out firmly but not too tightly. If your finished bandage looks floppy within an hour, unwind it and reapply using slightly more pressure. Bandages can become stretched with use but washing quickly restores their elasticity.

The first decision to be made when bandaging is to choose the correct-sized bandage for the affected body part. If it is too small or too big, it won't do its job efficiently and could cause more damage. As a guide, these sizes fit the following body parts: 2.5 cm (1 in) finger; 5 cm (2 in) hand; 7.5–10 cm (3–4 in) arm; and 10–15 cm (4–6 in) leg.

THE BASICS OF BANDAGING

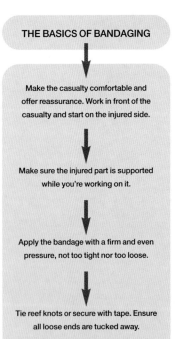

Make the casualty comfortable and offer reassurance. Work in front of the casualty and start on the injured side.

⬇

Make sure the injured part is supported while you're working on it.

⬇

Apply the bandage with a firm and even pressure, not too tight nor too loose.

⬇

Tie reef knots or secure with tape. Ensure all loose ends are tucked away.

⬇

Check the circulation beyond the bandage and check on any bleeding.

HOW TO APPLY A ROLLER BANDAGE

The tip of a roll of bandage is called the "tail", whereas the roll is called the "head". Keep the head of the bandage uppermost, so that if you drop it, it does not fall on to the ground. Think about how the finished bandage will look before starting.

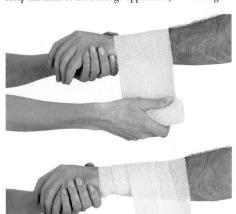

1 Place the tail of the bandage below the injury and work from the inside to the outside, and from the furthermost part to the nearest.

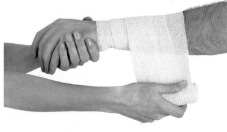

2 Roll the bandage around the limb and start with two overlapping turns. Cover two-thirds of the previous turn with each new one. Finish with two overlapping turns.

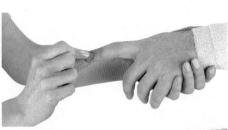

3 Once you've finished, check the circulation; if the bandage is too tight, unroll it and reapply it slightly looser.

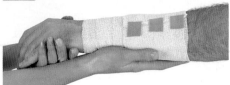

4 Secure the end with adhesive tape or tie the ends of the bandage using a reef knot.

BANDAGING A HAND OR FOOT

The bandaging method below for a hand also applies for a foot, although the heel should be kept clear unless injured. When working on a foot, start bandaging at the big toe.

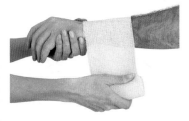

1 Start at the wrist and make two straight turns, working from the inside to the outside of the wrist.

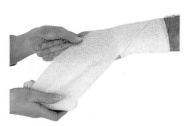

2 From the thumb side of the wrist, take the bandage diagonally across the back of the hand until it is touching the nail of the little finger.

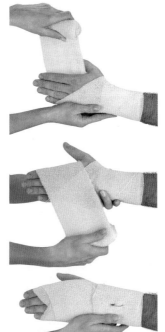

3 Leave the thumb free and take the bandage across the front of the fingers, also keeping the fingertips free.

4 Now, take the bandage across the back of the hand to the outside of the wrist, then around the wrist and back up to the little finger.

5 Repeat these turns, and cover about two-thirds of the previous turn with each new turn.

BANDAGING AN ELBOW OR KNEE JOINT

Bandaging these joints can be tricky, especially if you try to bandage while the joint is fully flexed. So, bandage in a partly flexed position so that it stays in place. For maximum support, these bandages need to be applied using figure-of-eight turns.

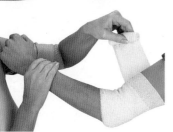

1 Put the tail of the bandage on the inside of the elbow; wind the bandage around the joint twice.

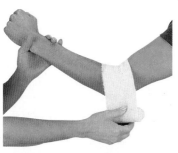

2 Now move the head of the bandage above the joint and wind two turns diagonally, making sure that you have covered half of the previous turn.

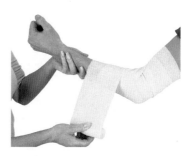

3 Now move the head to below the joint, cover half of the initial straight turns and do two diagonal turns.

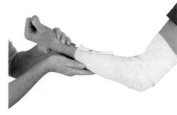

4 Continue doing two diagonal turns above and then below the joint in a figure-of-eight and then finally finish off the bandage with two straight turns.

Applying bandages 2

SEE ALSO

➤ Applying dressings
and bandages,
p204

➤ Applying bandages
1, p206

The head and fingers or toes are probably the trickiest areas to perfect in terms of bandaging technique. Apart from them being difficult areas to make bandages stay in place, they may cause other problems for someone new to bandaging. Tightly wrapped adhesive tape, for example, around a finger can act as a tourniquet. Scalp wounds often bleed profusely and bandages need even but firm pressure to be effective. Here you'll learn how to use a tubular gauze bandage and a triangular bandage, which are included in most first-aid kits.

Tubular bandages come in two types: tubular elasticated bandages for supporting injured joints and tubular gauze for covering a finger or a toe.

Tubular gauze bandages help to staunch the bleeding and also protect a digit from others nearby without impeding its blood flow. If you cannot find a tubular object with which to make the bandage, bend a piece of card in two or, failing that, use a child's sweet tube with the lid removed and bottom punched out.

HOW TO APPLY A TUBULAR BANDAGE TO A FINGER

These elasticated bandages allow sufficient pressure to stop the bleeding but do not impede blood flow. The device shown can be bought from a chemist.

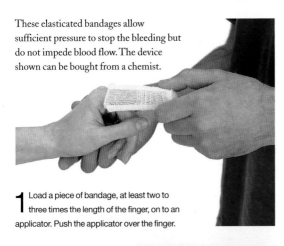

1 Load a piece of bandage, at least two to three times the length of the finger, on to an applicator. Push the applicator over the finger.

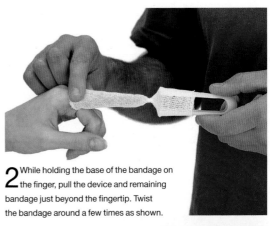

2 While holding the base of the bandage on the finger, pull the device and remaining bandage just beyond the fingertip. Twist the bandage around a few times as shown.

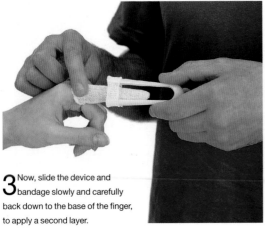

3 Now, slide the device and bandage slowly and carefully back down to the base of the finger, to apply a second layer.

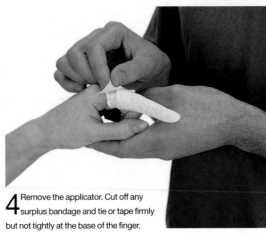

4 Remove the applicator. Cut off any surplus bandage and tie or tape firmly but not tightly at the base of the finger.

HOW TO BANDAGE A HEAD

Initially, apply a gauze wad to a head wound, especially if it is bleeding heavily. The wad helps to apply firm but even pressure across the whole scalp. If blood soaks through the bandage, apply another on top to avoid disturbing any blood clots. A strip bandage could be used, but is harder to keep in place.

1 Apply the triangular bandage with the folded longest edge over the forehead.

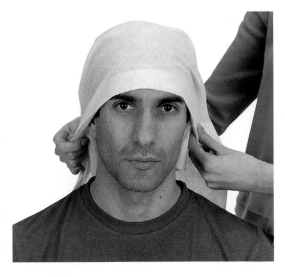

2 Take the two long "tails" at the back of the head and, using firm pressure, cross them over one another.

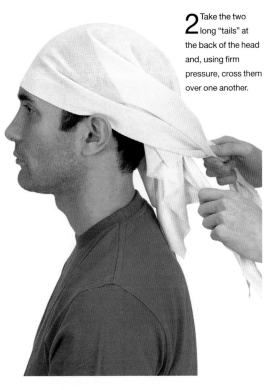

3 Bring the two tails around to the front and tie in the middle of the forehead.

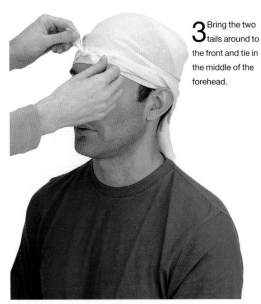

4 Draw up the spare end to the top of the person's head, and then secure with a safety pin or tape.

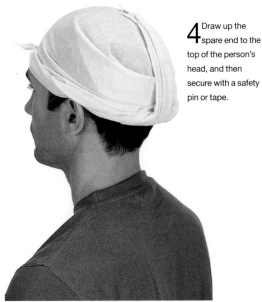

Fixing slings

SEE ALSO

➤ Wounds and wound healing, p132

➤ Treating infected wounds, p136

➤ Dealing with broken bones, p154

Triangular bandages are first-aid kit staples and most kits will contain quite a few. Usually a large triangular bandage is used for making a sling. If there is not one to hand at the scene of an emergency then you can improvise with the upturned hem of a jacket or shirt, or the sleeve of a shirt or jumper. The important functions of a sling are to support and immobilize an injured part of the body, and, in some cases (called high-arm or elevation slings), to stem bleeding from a wound. Here, you'll learn how to tie both types of arm sling.

Slings usually support the arm and can be classed as either a "broad-arm" sling, which supports the arm horizontally, or a "high-arm" sling, which both supports the limb and helps to reduce swelling and bleeding. High-arm slings also support rib fractures.

HOW TO TIE A HIGH-ARM SLING

This high-arm or elevation sling is used to stop the bleeding in a finger or forearm injury and also helps to reduce pain and prevent further injury by immobilizing the limb. This sling can also be used in burn victims to minimize swelling.

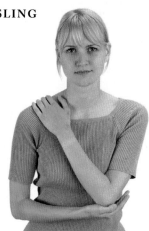

1 Place the injured arm so that the fingers touch the opposite collarbone.

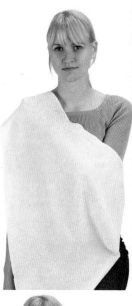

2 Place the triangular bandage to lie over the injured arm with the long edge against the uninjured side and the point to the injured side.

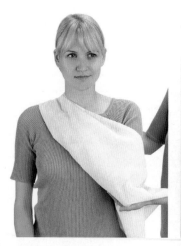

3 Tuck the bandage behind the elbow and forearm. Pass the free end behind the back.

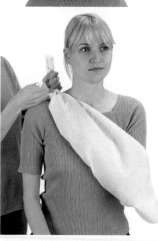

4 At the collarbone, tie the two ends of the bandage together on the uninjured side.

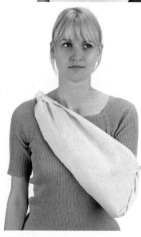

5 To secure the bandage at the elbow, tuck in the fabric or fold and use a safety pin.

FIXING A BROAD-ARM SLING

This type of sling is used for an arm or hand injury, such as a fracture or a sprain. Such a sling immobilizes the limb and can be improvised in many ways.

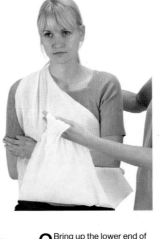

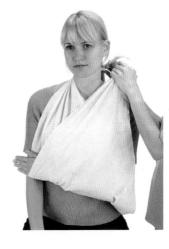

1 Ask the casualty to support their injured arm so that the hand lies just above the uninjured elbow. Now place the bandage in between the body and arm, so that the straight edge lies on the uninjured side.

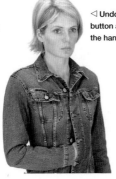

2 Bring up the lower end of the bandage to meet the other end at the shoulder. Tie (or pin) to secure and tuck both ends under the knot.

3 The casualty can let the arm go once you have secured the ends.

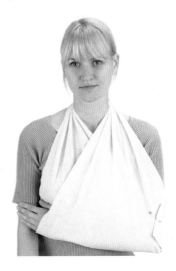

4 Finish the sling by folding over the pointed end of the fabric at the elbow and pinning. This is how the sling should look.

SOME IDEAS FOR IMPROVISING SLINGS

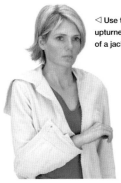

◁ Use the upturned hem of a jacket.

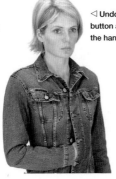

◁ Undo a jacket button and tuck the hand inside.

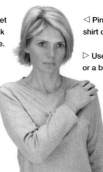

◁ Pin the sleeve of a shirt or jumper.

▷ Use a pair of tights or a belt.

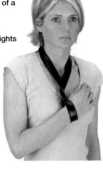

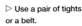

SKILLS CHECKLIST FOR
FIRST-AID KIT

KEY POINTS

- Always have a first-aid kit available at home and in your car ☐

- While a first-aid kit is important the ability to improvise is an essential skill for a first-aider ☐

- Practise your bandaging skills on a friend ☐

SKILLS LEARNED

- How to dress and bandage a wound or injury ☐

- How to improvise dressings and bandages if necessary ☐

- How to bandage an elbow and knee ☐

- How to bandage a finger ☐

- How to cope with scalp bandaging ☐

- How to make slings ☐

14

COMPLEMENTARY THERAPIES

Complementary health therapists believe that their practices encourage the body's natural defences to heal injury – whether that injury be physical or emotional or a combination of the two. Of course, complementary techniques will not be appropriate in many emergencies, where conventional medicine is vital. Where they come into their own is in working alongside conventional medicine, especially for more minor complaints, such as cramps, stings and constipation. As with any first-aid treatment, safety must always be your watchword. Only use safe techniques, sterile dressings and medications you feel really well informed about. Always ask for a medical opinion before using complementary therapies on children.

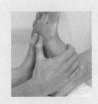

CONTENTS

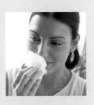

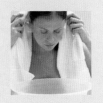

Understanding complementary therapies

SEE ALSO

➤ Complementary first-aid kit, p216

➤ Using complementary therapies 1 and 2, pp218, 220

The complementary therapies frequently referred to when it comes to natural first aid are aromatherapy, herbalism, acupuncture, reflexology and homeopathy. You may find that a number of other therapies – such as Alexander Technique, reiki, massage, colour therapy, meditation or yoga – have a part to play in calming a casualty with minor injuries and in helping them to convalesce. Be sure to seek conventional medical assistance first, and then choose from the many natural therapies to soothe, calm and heal.

It is not that long ago that people had only natural remedies to turn to when dealing with illness or injury. In very recent times, these types of treatment have made a comeback, and new "complementary" approaches have been developed. Many people perceive them to be safer, gentler and more natural than conventional medicines, preferring their holistic approach over modern medicine's emphasis on the disease rather than the person.

Some first-aid scenarios demand life support skills and complementary tactics are not appropriate, but there are many minor cases where alternatives are fine to use. Some of these have been proved effective in clinical trials, while others may not have been formally tested, but are commonly accepted as useful and effective alternatives.

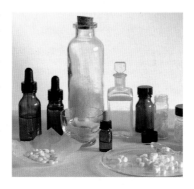

△ A wide range of homeopathic remedies are now widely available at conventional high street pharmacies, where expert help is on hand to advise about their use.

▽ Herbal remedies can be used for all kinds of conditions, but seek advice before using.

BE SAFE!

➤ **Seek conventional advice first**
Before embarking on a complementary therapy, you should have the casualty checked out by a conventional doctor. (Using homeopathy to treat meningitis, or acupuncture for acute asthma, is downright dangerous – sadly, there have been deaths from just such scenarios.) In fact, always seek conventional advice whenever considering complementary treatments. This advice applies especially strongly if you have any medical condition at all.

➤ **Use herbal remedies carefully**
Herbal remedies work because they contain chemicals that interact with the receptors in our bodies. We should be wary of seeing all herbal and related treatments as "naturally safe" – aspirin, for example, was originally a herbally derived drug, and it has both good and bad effects. Herbal remedies can interact with conventional medicines or may contain unknown or toxic substances, or steroids. Unlike prescription medicines, they are rarely tested properly, if at all.

➤ **Using aromatherapy oils**
Always seek expert help before using these. Many natural oils are highly potent, and specific ones can be dangerous if taken by those with certain conditions – pregnant women must be especially careful which oils they use. In most cases, never apply oils directly to skin (lavender and tea tree are notable exceptions), but dilute – for example in a carrier oil. Before applying oils to the skin, always do a patch test.

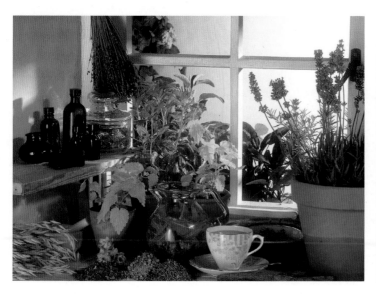

AROMATHERAPY

What is it? This literally means "treatment using scent". The term "aromatherapy" was first used by a French chemist called Gattefosse in 1937. He accidentally discovered the healing powers of essential oils when he burnt his hand and plunged it into a bucket of lavender oil. He was amazed by how quickly and painlessly the burn healed up.

How it works Essential plant oils are used in various ways, including massage, inhalation, baths, cold compresses and vaporizers. The smell of the oils is thought to affect the part of the brain that controls emotions, mood and memory. It may have a calming or an invigorating effect, depending on the aromas used.

Is it harmful? It should be used with caution in pregnancy and in conditions such as high blood pressure, epilepsy and skin conditions. There may be hypersensitive reactions to sunlight. The oils should never be ingested and always kept out of the way of children.

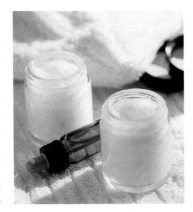

△ Essential oils can be used in many different forms – added to moisturizer, for example.

HERBALISM

Almost all drugs used to be derived from plant parts. Many people like the idea of using herbal remedies, because they feel that they are safer and more natural than conventional drugs.

What is it? Herbalists believe that stress, pollution, poor lifestyle and a bad diet lead to a draining of our life force. They feel that our body's battle to maintain a harmonious balance creates illness. Many people also use herbs to prevent disease by bolstering their immune systems and detoxifying the body.

How are they used? Herbs can be infused, made into tinctures, teas, capsules, creams, compresses and bath products. They can be effective for treating problems such as irritable bowel syndrome, urinary problems, eczema and indigestion.

ACUPUNCTURE/ACUPRESSURE

An ancient Chinese treatment, used for thousands of years, acupuncture involves the insertion of thin needles under the skin at specific points. The points are located along energy channels or "meridians". Acupressure massages these points instead of using needles. No one is certain how this approach works, but it may increase secretions of the body's natural painkillers – endorphins and serotonin.

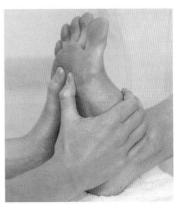

△ Reflexology may prove to be very effective in relieving problems such as back injury.

REFLEXOLOGY

This therapy involves massaging certain areas of the feet and the hands that correspond to different parts of the body and to specific organs.

HOMEOPATHY

Homeopathy fights disease by treating "like with like". In other words, elements that can cause the symptoms of a particular illness can be used to cure it. However, these elements are used in minute doses, to the point where the prescribed substance is so diluted that it is undetectable.

▽ Try "Rescue remedy" and *Arnica* to help recovery from minor bruises and shock.

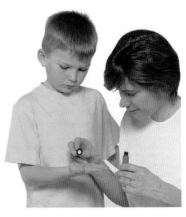

▽ Steam inhalation of certain aromatic oils can soothe anxiety and tension.

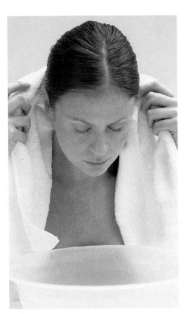

Complementary first-aid kit

SEE ALSO

➤ Understanding complementary therapies, p214

➤ Using therapies 1 and 2, pp218, 220

You can obtain many essential oils and herbs, as well as homeopathic remedies, from high street pharmacies. Choose those that you find appealing or maybe select the remedies that cover most of the common household injuries and the aches and pains that may affect us all from time to time – such as headaches, colds, sore throat, arthritis, insomnia, depression and anxiety. Always check the sell-by dates and bear in mind that it is good to buy in small quantities, until you have established that you find the remedies useful, to avoid wastage.

Recently, a study showed that burning aromatherapy oils on a psychiatric ward had a significantly calming effect on the often disturbed patients. Different oils, homeopathic remedies and herbs work on different ailments, and you could make up a useful first-aid kit of these to use alongside more conventional remedies.

As with many drugs, there are really only a small number of complementary therapies that are definitely safe in pregnancy. It is a good idea to check with an aromatherapist, homeopath or herbalist before trying any therapies – a therapist will be able to advise you on the remedies that will be most useful for you.

▷ Herbal and homeopathic remedies should be stored away from direct sunlight, in dark glass bottles.

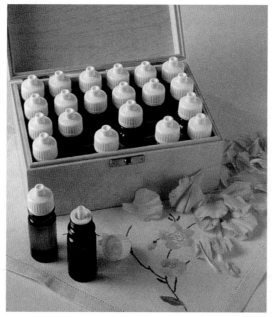

PEPPERMINT

Used as an oil or herb, peppermint has active ingredients that are effective at clearing the upper respiratory tract of mucus, so it is useful as a decongestant in colds and nasal blockage. It is an invigorating herb that can be chosen when you want to feel more awake and alive. Taken as a tea or in capsule form, it is excellent at calming digestive problems, especially trapped wind, heartburn and indigestion. Diluted peppermint oil can also be rubbed into the temples at each side of the forehead and the neck muscles at the top of the spine and around the shoulders to relieve stress headaches.

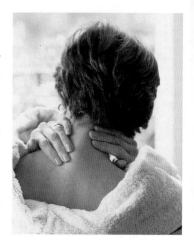

△ Gently massage diluted peppermint oil into the neck muscles to relieve tension headache.

GINGER

This plant is very soothing for digestive disorders and appetite loss. Ginger root is commonly drunk as a tea to ease travel sickness, and it can be used, if advised, to alleviate morning sickness. Effective for muscle spasms and pains, ginger is also useful in rheumatism and arthritis.

CLOVE

Extract of clove is a well-known pain-reliever, and a small amount of clove oil applied to a sore tooth will ease the pain of toothache (note: avoid contact, especially prolonged, with gums or skin, as this can cause some irritation). Clove is also a good insect repellent, so a few drops placed on clothing or bedding will help keep biting insects and mosquitoes away.

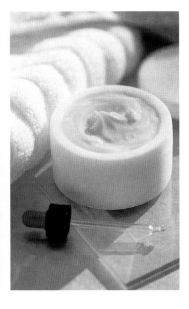

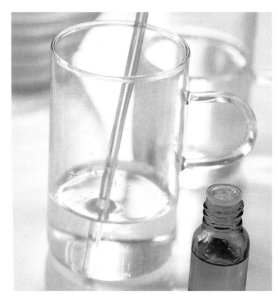

◁ Always check before using essential oils or adding them to your favourite lotions and creams. Some oils are very potent, and must be used in a certain way, or avoided if you have a particular health condition or are pregnant.

▷ If using oils diluted in water, stir very thoroughly.

ARNICA

This flowering herb is poisonous when taken internally, so should be used only in creams and oils topically, or internally as a homeopathic remedy. *Arnica* is useful for bruises, muscle soreness, shock and to promote wound-healing.

LAVENDER

Used as an essential oil, lavender is highly antiseptic and effective when used as a compress for superficial burns, blisters and

▽ Sniff a tissue containing a few drops of lavender oil to relieve insomnia.

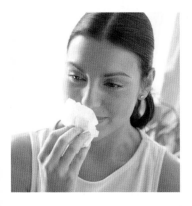

bites. It can be used to help ease depression and insomnia – simply add a few drops to a tissue and sniff, or place the tissue inside your pillowcase, to help you get off to sleep and enjoy a refreshing rest.

TEA TREE

The essential oil of tea tree is used topically as an antibacterial, antiseptic remedy. Diluted in water, a tea tree spray can ease the pain of a sore throat.

CHAMOMILE

Made up as a tea, chamomile is extremely calming and soothing, and is good for insomnia, depression and anxiety. A few drops of the oil in a bedtime bath will also aid peaceful sleep.

GERANIUM

This is a very effective herb when used to treat psychological problems such as anxiety or panic attacks.

CLARY SAGE

This is a useful essential oil for dealing with depression, anxiety and frayed nerves. It can be added, diluted, to a bath, or dispersed in an oil burner.

SOME OTHER IDEAS FOR YOUR NATURAL KIT

➤ Tincture of *Calendula* (pot marigold) – minor burns and scalds.

➤ Comfrey oil/ointment – bruises and sprains. Never use any oil/ointment on open wounds (it encourages infection).

➤ Witch hazel – insect bites and stings, sprains, bruises, mild sunburn.

▽ Oil from geranium leaves is a calming and cooling remedy, ideal for easing anxieties.

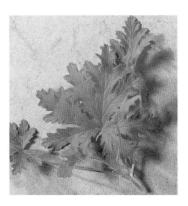

Using complementary therapies 1

SEE ALSO

➤ Refer to index for all other references to these conditions throughout book

Accidents, injuries and trauma may produce a wide range of associated conditions, ranging from nausea and constipation to cramp. These kinds of symptoms can often be eased by complementary therapies. Psychological after-shock and tension are also natural reactions to injury and accident, and you might find that complementary approaches can be effective in these cases, too. However, always remember that your first priority must be to arrange for conventional medical treatment for an individual's injuries.

NAUSEA AND VOMITING

There are many causes of nausea and vomiting. Most of them will be "self-limiting", which means they will settle without the need for further treatment or investigation. It is recommended that you should seek conventional advice first when tackling health conditions, but mild nausea can usually be treated safely with natural remedies. However, as with diarrhoea, if the symptoms are not settling in 1–2 days and dehydration is developing, or the symptoms are mild but persistent, medical help must be sought.

Herbal remedies An infusion of ginger root may settle nausea. Also try chamomile or black horehound (but always avoid the latter in pregnancy).

Acupuncture/acupressure Use the anti-nausea point that is two thumb widths above the wrist crease, between the two prominent tendons passing to the hand. A therapist can treat this area with a needle, or you can use firm pressure at this point for

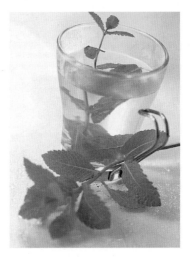

△ A peppermint infusion is a highly effective remedy for nausea and indigestion – and also useful as a general pick-me-up.

one minute. There are also wristbands for sale that exert pressure, and can be used in pregnancy. For travel sickness, press your index finger into the hollow at the back of the jawline for a minute.

Homeopathy *Ipecac* and *Nux Vomica* are useful for nausea. Take up to 12 doses every 2 hours until the symptoms settle.

DIARRHOEA

Herbal remedies Geranium, peppermint and chamomile infusions are effective if taken as 45–60 ml/3–4 tbsp of tea three times a day.

Acupressure Use firm pressure four thumb widths above the inside of the ankle just behind the shin bone.

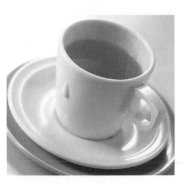

△ Chamomile-containing herbal teas are excellent for soothing anxiety.

Reflexology Apply pressure to the point for the small intestine (which is located between the arch and the heel of the foot) and then the large intestine points on either side.

Homeopathy *Arsenicum album* is the recommended remedy for diarrhoea.

CONSTIPATION

Aromatherapy Gently massage a diluted mixture of rosemary, marjoram and chamomile into the area around the navel.

Herbal remedies Dandelion leaves are a gentle laxative.

Acupressure Place a finger four thumb widths up from the back of the wrist crease. Bend the arm and press the opposite thumb into the outer edge of the elbow crease for a minute, then repeat on the other arm.

Reflexology Use the large intestine pressure point (see picture for exact location). Press firmly and then massage for 10 minutes.

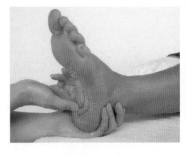

△ A reflexologist is able to massage the large intestine pressure point (the relevant area is drawn on the foot in this photograph) in order to relieve constipation.

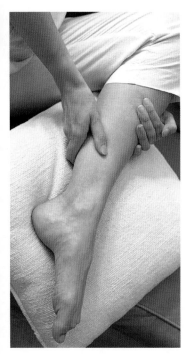

△ Massage cramp with a blend of basil and marjoram diluted in almond oil.

CRAMP

This is when a muscle goes into a painful spasm and feels rock-hard. It occurs most often after exercise, when you are dehydrated, and also often strikes in the middle of the night. Initial measures should involve using the muscle by walking around or stretching and massaging it, and drinking plenty of water every day, at least 2 litres (3 ½ pints).
Aromatherapy Massage with basil and marjoram diluted in almond oil.
Herbal remedies Ginkgo infusion helps ease intractable cramp.
Acupressure Press into the bottom of the calf muscle for 5 minutes.
Homeopathy *Caprum metallicum* tablets may help to ease a cramp-like ache.

▷ Irritability and anxiety are often relieved by massage. Massage is straightforward to learn and easy to do to yourself.

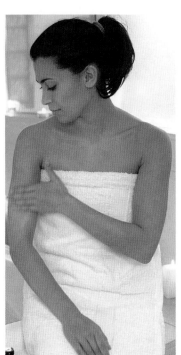

HEADACHE

Stress and tension, which are commonly associated with the trauma of injuries and accidents, may manifest themselves in different ways. One of the most common is headache. The casualty may complain of tightness in the muscles at the back of the scalp and neck.
Aromatherapy Diluted lavender oil rubbed into the temples is wonderful for a tension headache. Inhaling eucalyptus is also very effective for sinus headaches.
Herbal remedies Feverfew may help with a migrainous headache, but should not be taken in pregnancy.
Acupressure Apply pressure to a point between the eyebrows at the bridge of the nose, and on either side of the neck at the base of the back of the skull.
Reflexology Press a thumb firmly to the base of the big toe for 10–20 seconds.
Homeopathy *Kali bichromicum* 6c is good for sinus headache, and *Bryonia* can help a general headache.

△ Try relieving stress headaches by applying gentle pressure to the area around the temples.

SHOCK

Aromatherapy Neroli and lavender oils are known for their relaxing and calming properties.
Herbal remedies Chamomile and lemon balm combine well to make a tea to calm and soothe agitation, and encourage peaceful rest and sleep.
Homeopathy *Arnica* tablets are effective after a bad fall for bruising and shock. Aconite may also be helpful for treating the symptoms of shock.

SOOTHING STRESS AND TENSION

Once any injuries have been treated by a medical practitioner, massage with soothing oils and relaxation exercises can be helpful for easing the stress and tension associated with any accident.

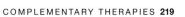

Using complementary therapies 2

SEE ALSO

➤ Refer to index for all other references to these conditions throughout book

Some relatively minor injuries can be treated effectively with one or other of the complementary therapies. There are often a number of options, from which you may choose the one you prefer. For example, to treat bruises you can use *Arnica*, lavender oil or rosemary oil; sunburn can be treated with lavender oil, *Hypericum* (St John's wort), aloe vera or *Calendula*. "Rescue Remedy" combines five of the Bach flower remedies and can be bought as a tincture or a cream – it is useful for reducing the effects of trauma or shock.

There are all kinds of scenarios that respond well to complementary treatments, either used alone or in tandem with conventional first aid treatment. Complementary means exactly that – these treatments are not necessarily an alternative to a more traditional medical approach, and the two approaches should complement each other.

BITES AND STINGS

Aromatherapy Add a few drops of lavender or tea tree oil to a little iced water and apply it to the area. Soak a flannel in the water and

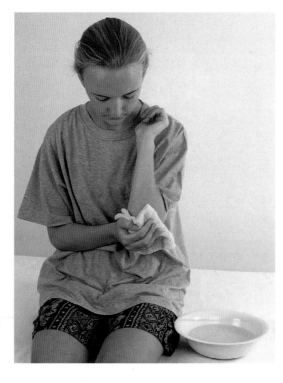

▷ For soothing sore bites and stings, wring a cloth out in iced water or an iced herbal infusion and hold it over the affected area.

place that on the sting, or use cotton wool and apply some of the water every 10 minutes until the pain subsides.

Herbal remedies Fresh onion on an insect bite may take the pain out of the area. Useful herbs for making into an infusion and applying to a burn or sting are chamomile, elderflower or red clover (the latter is also a proven natural alternative to hormone replacement therapy). Fresh leaves of lemon balm, plantain and yellow dock applied to the damaged skin may be soothing and speed up pain relief.

BRUISES

Bruising happens because the blood vessels beneath the skin break and the blood escapes. This is usually after a traumatic event, and it is painful. However, certain people may bruise virtually without injury, perhaps if they are on anticoagulant treatment such as warfarin or have problems with their blood-clotting abilities. This last group of people should always seek medical help.

Aromatherapy Lavender oil made up as a cold compress is very good at reducing swelling and bruising after injury. Diluted rosemary oil massaged into the tissues is also soothing and may speed up healing.

Homeopathy Use *Arnica* on unbroken skin in ointment form or as a bath lotion; the latter is very soothing when suffering from general aching – after an unaccustomed horse ride or aerobics class, for example.

BURNS

Before you do anything to any type of burn you should cool it down. If the burn is bigger than the palm of the victim's hand, they must get medical advice.

Aromatherapy Lavender essential oil is good for numbing the pain of a burn, which can be excruciating. It promotes healing and reduces scarring. Use neat on small areas, on sterile gauze or lint for larger areas.

Herbal remedies Fresh gel from the aloe vera plant is very effective – simply snap off part of a leaf and apply the plant gel directly.

SPRAINS AND STRAINS

Aromatherapy/herbal remedies It can be useful to add some lavender oil or chamomile to water and store them in a

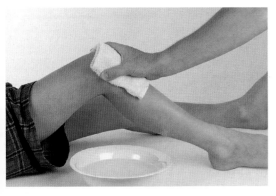

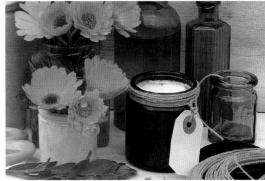

△ Lay the casualty flat to apply a cold compress to sprains and strains.

△ *Calendula* (pot marigold) remedies are ideal for healing cuts and grazes.

bottle in the fridge so that you have something at hand for soothing sprains and strains. A comfrey or marigold leaf infusion applied ice-cold is also good. Comfrey ointment is effective when applied for a few days after a strain has occurred, or to aching muscles.

Homeopathy Homeopathic remedies include *Arnica*, *Rhus tox.* and *Ruta grav.*

SUNBURN

Aromatherapy For widespread sunburn, add some drops of diluted lavender oil to a lukewarm bath. Lavender oil can also be applied directly to the skin, especially if the sunburn is severe. The blood-red oil of St John's wort or aloe vera juice are highly soothing, cooling and healing.

Homeopathy Homeopathic options include *Cantharis* and *Urtica urens*, especially if the pain of the sunburn is intense and persistent. *Hypericum* or *Calendula* cream is also good.

NOSEBLEED

Aromatherapy A pad of cotton wool soaked in cold water with a few drops of lemon oil added is good at slowing down a nosebleed when placed across the bridge of the nose.

Herbal remedies Cotton wool soaked in an infusion of yarrow and then squeezed at the end of the nose for a few minutes may prove effective in stopping a nosebleed.

CUTS AND GRAZES

Aromatherapy Lavender and tea tree can be used neat on small cuts and scratches, added to a bowl of water for cleaning the wound, or used on a dressing applied over the injury. These oils have a disinfectant effect so may well reduce the chances of infection settling into the wound.

Herbal remedies Witch hazel can be used directly on small wounds or on a dressing, as can tinctures of marigold or myrrh. Comfrey is also a powerful tissue-healer.

Homeopathy A homeopathic compress of *Hypericum* (St Johns wort) or *Calendula* can be used direct on dressings, or in ointment form once the skin has healed over.

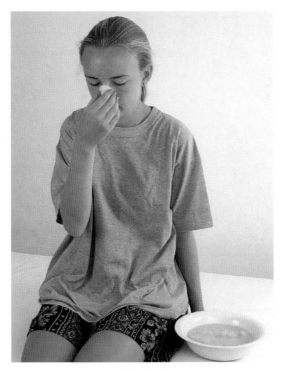

◁ To stop nosebleeds, try applying a pad of cotton wool soaked in a cooled yarrow infusion over the soft part of the nose.

SKILLS CHECKLIST FOR
COMPLEMENTARY
THERAPIES

KEY POINTS

- The remedies described in this chapter are intended to be complementary or additional rather than alternatives ☐

- Always seek qualified medical assistance initially ☐

SKILLS LEARNED

- How to treat minor injuries with natural, complementary treatments ☐

- Recognizing that complementary treatments may be effective in the aftermath of injury, trauma or accident, for treating anxiety, insomnia, depression and stress ☐

- Recognizing that complementary treatments can have side-effects just as conventional medical treatments do ☐

15

KEEPING SAFE

Safety in the home, safety in the garden and safety on the road are supremely important considerations in the prevention of accidents. The great majority of accidents are preventable. This chapter looks at the hazards to be encountered both in the home, especially in the kitchen and the bathroom, and outside it. Being aware and taking sensible precautions will help you to minimize the chances of an accident befalling either you or a member of your family. When accidents do occur, coping with them quickly and effectively can do much to mitigate the effects and prevent further injury.

CONTENTS

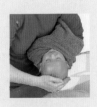

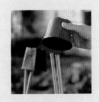

Keeping yourself safe

Most people do not give enough thought to their own safety when they spot someone in danger and in need of assistance. However, you must do everything you can to protect yourself while helping a casualty. Taking time to survey the scene and think through your actions is essential. You should not, for example, rush in to rescue someone from a burning building. Without the necessary training, you are likely to become a casualty yourself and may hinder a rescue operation. It is wiser to wait for the professionals.

The first rule of first aid is not to put yourself in any danger. You may make matters worse if you jump into the scene without first standing back and assessing the situation. You should be aware of your limitations and training. For example, even a strong swimmer should be wary of diving into the water to help someone struggling. You should always consider safer ways to help first, such as throwing in a rope and life ring or an inflatable ball. Rescue attempts often end in a double tragedy that could have been avoided had more time been taken to survey the scene. Always take a few moments to look for danger – there may be flammable chemicals, electric cables or other hazards present.

CARE WITH BODY FLUIDS

Helping a casualty may involve coming into contact with body fluids. There has never been a recorded case of anyone catching HIV or hepatitis from mouth-to-mouth, but this should not lead to complacency.

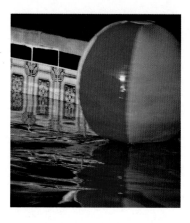

△ Throw an inflatable ball or rope to someone who is having difficulties in deep water rather than jumping in yourself.

Generally, HIV needs contact with fresh blood or semen to be dangerous. It is a relatively fragile virus that does not survive outside the body for long. Hepatitis B, on the other hand, can still be active in dried blood, even when it is several days old. It is also possible to contract tuberculosis (TB) and meningitis from body fluids.

To protect yourself, use a mouth shield when giving mouth-to-mouth, or place a handkerchief across the casualty's mouth. This gives you some protection while still allowing air to pass into their lungs.

AGGRESSIVENESS

You should never underestimate how violent a person might be, particularly if they appear to be drunk or on drugs. If in any doubt about your own safety, wait for the emergency services to arrive and keep away, especially if you suspect that the person might be carrying a weapon.

Sick people may become aggressive for many reasons, including low blood sugar as a result of diabetes or lack of oxygen. If you are worried about getting hurt, it is best to leave them until someone from the emergency services arrives and is able to give them appropriate treatment.

AVOIDING INFECTION FROM BLOOD AND OTHER BODY FLUIDS

The best way to guard against infection is to avoid the casualty's body fluids altogether. However, if that is not possible, there are several ways to minimize the risk.

➤ Wear disposable gloves and wash your hands after contact with blood or other body fluids.

➤ Protect any wounds on your own body from infection by using plasters or bandages to cover them.

➤ Wear plastic goggles or plastic glasses to protect your eyes from splashes.

➤ If body fluids come into contact with your mouth, eyes or nose, wash the area thoroughly for 10 minutes under briskly running water.

➤ If you receive an injury that comes into contact with body fluids, see a doctor. It is possible to detect infection with hepatitis B early on, and to reduce the risk of contracting the disease.

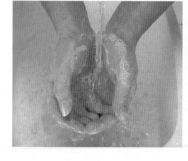

△ Wash your hands thoroughly under running water if you come into contact with body fluids such as blood or semen.

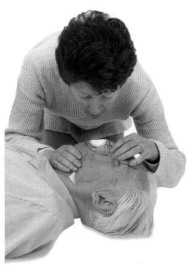

△ Use a mouth shield if you are giving mouth-to-mouth resuscitation. If you do not have one placing a handkerchief over the casualty's mouth gives some protection.

▷ Be wary of approaching anyone who is drunk or aggressive. You do not know whether they may lash out or if they have a weapon.

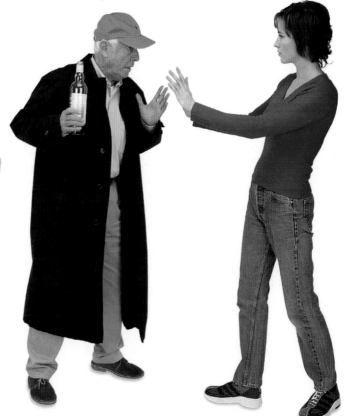

PSYCHOLOGICAL STRESS

It can be exhilarating and rewarding to help someone who is injured or in danger, but it can also be upsetting and disturbing however psychologically strong you are.

You may have witnessed scenes that you find difficult to get out of your mind, even weeks, months or years after the event. You may have disturbing dreams that disrupt your sleep even when you thought you had forgotten the incident. Talking to other people about the event or speaking to a trained counsellor may help you come to terms with the trauma.

Life-threatening emergencies can be frightening affairs, and if death is involved you may feel guilty that you did not do enough to help. You should accept that you may need support to help you to get back to normal.

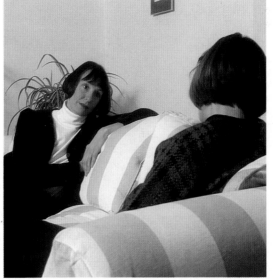

◁ Following a serious accident, bystanders, helpers and paramedics risk developing post-traumatic stress disorder. If you feel agitated or you are sleeping badly after witnessing a trauma, ask your doctor to refer you to a trained counsellor for help.

Safety on the road

SEE ALSO
➤ What is first aid?, p16
➤ Cardiac compressions, p36
➤ Full resuscitation sequence, p38

The most common site for people to have a road accident is within two miles of their own home – perhaps because of fatigue or because drivers exercise less care when on their home turf. Other common causes of road accidents include inexperience and carelessness by young and newly qualified drivers, being distracted by children in the back and driving while under the influence of alcohol. The best way to avoid accidents is to drive not only safely but also watchfully, so that you can compensate for the mistakes of others on the road.

Roads around the world are becoming increasingly busy. Although there are stringent laws governing road safety in many countries, most of the accidents are caused by human error – 95 per cent are somebody's fault, rather than simply an unlucky twist of fate. Perhaps surprisingly, most road traffic accidents happen in daylight; less surprisingly, these often occur in the rush hours: 7–9 a.m. and 3–7 p.m.

WHY ACCIDENTS HAPPEN

Alcohol is a big factor in many accidents. It affects multiple aspects of driving ability – decision-making, self-criticism, balance, coordination, touch, sight, hearing and judgement to name a few. It is best not to drink at all if you are planning on driving rather than trying to stick to a general "safe limit" that may not be safe for a particular individual at all.

Inexperienced and young drivers, especially men, often drive without enough thought for road safety or their responsibility as drivers. This is why those under 20 years old have to pay large amounts for their car insurance – and can then be a hazard on the road.

Older drivers can be a danger to themselves and others if their eyesight and reaction speeds are failing, particularly if they do not have any insight into the problem. Lack of concentration caused by

WARNING
You should never use mobile phones when driving – neither hand-held nor hands-free models.

chatting to others in the car, turning to reprimand children or talking on a cellphone can also cause an accident.

Tiredness is a major killer. Its incidence is probably underestimated because no one can know the exact details of what has gone on before a fatal car crash. Planning regular breaks, being aware of times when you are likely to feel drowsy (for example, just after lunch or between

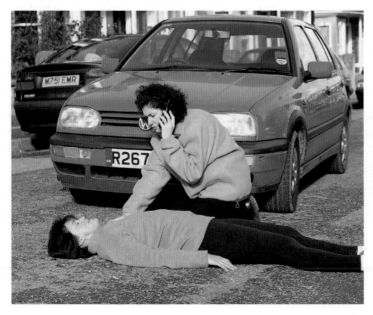

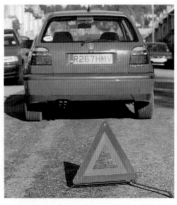

△ Always carry a warning triangle in your car. Place this near the stationary vehicle to warn approaching drivers of an accident.

◁ Make sure that the casualty is in a safe place – move them if necessary – then call the emergency services for help.

the hours of 2 a.m. and 6 a.m.) and stopping for a nap or a coffee if tiredness hits can all help to prevent a tragedy.

Motorways are particularly hazardous because the monotony of driving on long, straight roads and the lack of gear changing can cause the driver to feel tired or be inattentive. But fatigue and lack of concentration can also cause accidents on urban and suburban roads just as easily. Most road accidents occur within two miles of the driver's own home.

WHAT TO DO IN A CAR ACCIDENT

If you witness a road accident, be aware that stopping could jeopardize your own safety. Check all your mirrors before pulling up at the scene. Stay calm and ensure that your car is visible and that the accident scene is protected from oncoming traffic. Switch on your hazard lights as soon as you have stopped.

If the accident has happened on a bend, try to warn approaching drivers by using a hazard warning triangle or asking another driver to flag the cars down. Watch out for broken glass and metal. Make sure that your handbrake is on and that your car is safe to leave.

On motorways, the speed that vehicles travel at may well make stopping to help too hazardous. If this is the case, drive on and use a telephone to summon help.

TO REDUCE THE RISK OF FIRE

Turn off the damaged car's engine and, if possible, disconnect the car battery. Stop people from smoking at the scene, and cover any fuel spillage with soil or sand.

WARNING

Motorcyclists are 24 times more likely to be killed or injured for every kilometre or mile travelled compared with car drivers. This is partly because they are often inexperienced, young drivers, and partly because they are in a more physically vulnerable situation.

FIRST AID FOR ROAD TRAFFIC CASUALTIES

People are often trapped in cars after accidents. This should not stop you from initiating first-aid measures. You can still protect and open the airway on a casualty in the upright position.

Make the area safe. Move people to safety if possible. But do not move anyone who is injured unless they are in further danger.

Telephone the emergency services with precise details of your location.

Stop heavy bleeding.

Instigate CPR if needed.

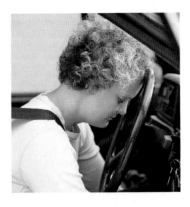

△ A casualty slumped forward in the driver's seat should be moved so their airway is opened, even if spinal injury is a possibility.

▽ To clear the airway of a casualty who is still in the car, tilt their jaw slightly upwards and remove any blood or vomit. Then use the resuscitation techniques.

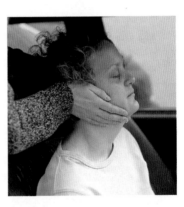

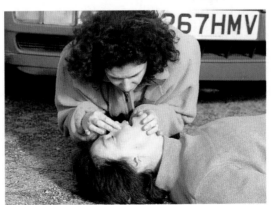

◁ When dealing with any roadside casualty, assume that there may be a neck/spinal injury and handle with great care. Wherever possible, treat the casualty in the position found.

Safety in the home

One in three of all accidents happen in our own homes, the place where we feel safest and at our most comfortable. Our houses are filled with hazards – from faulty electrical appliances to ill-fitting carpets or sticking-out nails in the floorboards. Even a hot pan of soup can cause a serious injury. Most of these accidents are preventable, so making our homes safe must be a prime consideration. The majority of home accidents involve children. So, if you have children or if children may visit your house, home safety is all the more important.

Most of us love our homes, and we feel secure and safe when we are in them. However, although we may feel protected from the dangers of the outside world, our home environments are actually filled with potential hazards.

Domestic accidents are what keep the country's accident and emergency departments busy. On average, more people are killed every week in domestic accidents than die in road traffic accidents. A lot of these accidents are due to a combination of carelessness, ignorance and human frailty – and most of them are preventable.

HOME HAZARDS

Almost anything has the potential to be a hazard. For example, accidents suffered by elderly people are most commonly a result of them putting their slippers on to the wrong feet, and then attempting to walk in them. Trousers are another unsuspected hazard, especially in the elderly and less physically able. Simply sitting down before attempting to put on a pair of trousers cuts down the chance of an accident. Naked feet are also vulnerable – stepping on broken glass or dropping something on your foot can cause a nasty injury.

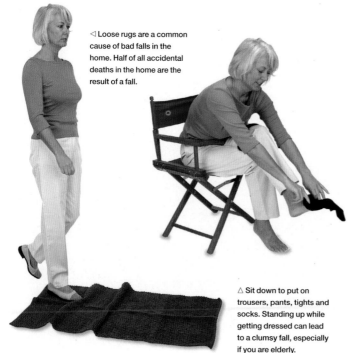

◁ Loose rugs are a common cause of bad falls in the home. Half of all accidental deaths in the home are the result of a fall.

△ Sit down to put on trousers, pants, tights and socks. Standing up while getting dressed can lead to a clumsy fall, especially if you are elderly.

AVOIDING ACCIDENTS

Most accidents can be prevented by taking a few simple precautions.

➤ Don't leave toys lying around.
➤ Don't leave plastic bags within easy reach of children.
➤ Don't smoke in bed.
➤ Don't leave shoes in people's way.
➤ Don't leave flexes trailing or hanging.
➤ Don't allow pets to play on the stairs.
➤ Don't ever put a mat at the top or bottom of stairs.
➤ Don't place anything on a table with an overhanging cloth if you have children.
➤ Don't hang a mirror or toys over a fire.
➤ Don't put plants on the television – it is hazardous when you water them.
➤ Repair or throw away rickety ladders.

A TIDY HOME

Messy houses are without a doubt more dangerous than immaculate ones. Falls – the number one killer in the home – are much more likely to occur if the floor is covered with clutter. Glossy magazines strewn across a sitting room floor can be as slippery as a sheet of ice, and a bean bag in a hallway is difficult not to trip over. Children's toys left scattered across the floor are another major source of accidents.

Keeping a house clear of hazards is obviously a good idea, but this can be difficult when you are busy. The best policy

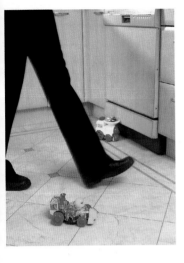

◁ Never leave toys or shoes lying around on the floor because they are a common cause of falls.

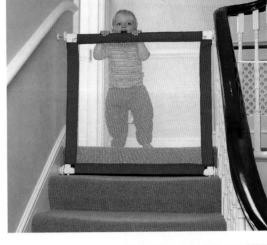

▷ Protect toddlers from falling down stairs by fitting gates at the top and bottom of each flight.

is to have a place for everything and to make sure that all walkways are kept as free of clutter as possible.

SAFE STAIRWAYS

It is particularly important to keep the stairs absolutely clear. Leaving objects on the stairs to be taken up (or down) later on, when you get around to it, is a major hazard. A vacuum cleaner left at the top of the stairs while you are dusting a room, for example, is easily tripped over.

Stair carpets wear out quickly and may develop lethal holes or tags. Repair any damage as soon as possible. Fitting stair gates helps to protect children from falls. These gates need to be at the top and bottom of the stairs.

PREVENTING FIRE HAZARDS

Cracked plugs, loose flexes, old wiring, furniture placed too close to the fire and unguarded fires are all common factors in house fires. Fire is one of the most serious hazards in the home, and yet one of the most preventable. Smoke alarms cut deaths from fires by 60–80 per cent, but even people who install smoke detectors often fail to maintain them by ensuring the batteries they contain are in working order.

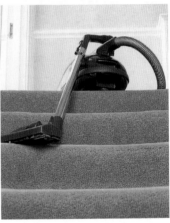

△ Always keep the stairs free of appliances, cables, toys and pets to reduce the chance of an accidental fall.

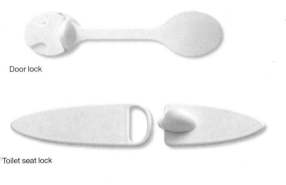

Door lock

Toilet seat lock

△ Child-safety gadgets such as these are a worthwhile investment for your home. Other items include covers for electrical sockets.

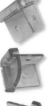

Table corner protectors

CAUSES OF ACCIDENTS IN THE HOME

➤ Falls – 50 per cent.

➤ Accidental poisoning from taking medicines – 20 per cent.

➤ Fires – 10 per cent.

➤ Other, miscellaneous causes, including DIY – 20 per cent.

Safety in the kitchen

SEE ALSO
➤ Safety in the home,
   p228
➤ Dealing with fire,
   p236
➤ Avoiding electrical
   accidents, p237

Hundreds of thousands of accidents occur in kitchens every year. This is not surprising since many of us spend a lot of time in the kitchen, where we come into contact with many potential hazards from sharp knives to hot surfaces and electrical appliances. The kitchen is also a place where we use both water and electricity, which must be kept separate. As well as making the kitchen as safe as possible, you should keep a fire extinguisher, a fire blanket and a sturdy pair of oven gloves always within sight, in case an accident does occur.

A few simple precautions taken when planning and designing a kitchen will prevent a lot of the problems that occur in this part of the house. In addition, laying down some basic kitchen rules may serve a useful purpose in protecting you and other house-dwellers from avoidable accidents.

CLEAR UP CLUTTER

It is impossible to stop children bringing toys into the kitchen, but having to dodge dolls, small metal cars or a farmyard on your way to the sink is an obvious and avoidable hazard. Take special care to clear toys from the floor.

Likewise, keep counters and tabletops clear of appliances unless they are in daily use. Even then, it may be much safer to put them away.

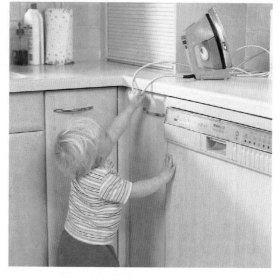

◁ Ensure that flexes and cables are kept to the back of kitchen worktops to prevent a child from pulling down a heavy appliance.

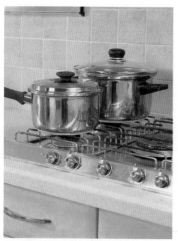

△ Use the back burners in preference to the front ones and turn handles away from the edge.

GUARD AGAINST BURNS

- Toddlers are at a perfect height for grabbing and yanking things off kitchen surfaces. If what they reach for is attached to a kettle or an iron, they could be badly hurt. Put irons away when you have finished with them, and never leave an iron unattended on the ironing board.
- Buy appliances with coiled flexes since these are neater and more difficult to catch hold of by accident. Don't choose appliances with long flexes.
- Remember that tablecloths have dangling edges that are very tempting to small children wandering past.
- Use mugs for hot drinks. As civilized as it is to drink out of cups and saucers, they are much more likely to be tipped over than mugs.

- Don't try to drink your coffee or tea with a small child in your lap; they may wriggle and cause you to spill it.
- Make a habit of always using the back rings on the hob, and of turning the handles of pots and pans away from the edge of the cooker. Cooker guards are not a great idea – they can get very hot, they make it awkward to cook and lift pans off the hob, and they don't stop a child from poking their fingers through and burning them on the gas flame.
- Oven doors can get very hot. The time around opening the oven door and getting the food out can be an especially dangerous one. Your attention may be on ensuring that you get the food on to the kitchen surface in one piece, and not on the small child heading for the oven.

- Burning oil is one of the biggest hazards in a kitchen. If you deep-fat fry a lot, you should seriously consider buying an electric fryer.
- Putting a shelf above your cooker is never a good idea. As you stretch over the cooker to reach it, you may burn yourself. If the shelf is made of wood or contains flammable objects, it will also increase your chances of setting the kitchen on fire.
- Leaving the gas on and unlit for more than 10 to 15 seconds can result in a fireball, which will burn you and whoever is beside or near you. If you can smell gas, but cannot see anything left on that is causing it, get out of the house immediately and call the emergency number for your local gas authority. They are available 24 hours a day.

PREVENT SKIDS AND FALLS
- Try to wash floors in the evenings when everyone is settled and out of the kitchen.
- Keep drawers and doors closed when not in use – when open, they are an obstacle.
- Baby chairs that screw on to kitchen tables are dangerous. Avoid them.
- Always wipe up immediately any grease and food spills, and wipe the patch with a dry cloth afterwards.
- Keep the floor clear of obstacles.

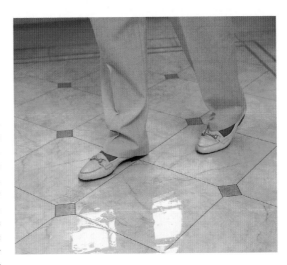

◁ A wet floor can be as slippery as an ice rink – and a fall could put out someone's back for weeks.

MINIMIZE HAZARDS
- Most people store their bleach, cleaning fluids and dishwasher powder under the sink. Although they are fiddly to fit, cupboard locks prevent a child gaining access to these harmful substances.
- Never leave wiring exposed; if wiring starts to fray, stop using the appliance until it is repaired. Every plug socket should be at least 1 m (3 ft) from any water supply, so that there is no chance of someone having one hand on an electric source and the other in water.

- Lacerations from careless chopping account for a lot of kitchen injuries. Keep knives sharp as blunt ones are more likely to slip. Use a proper chopping board and cut with all your fingers above the blade of the knife.
- Beware of searching for broken glass in a sink full of water. Let the water drain out and then clear up the glass.
- Do not use broken crockery and glasses; throw them away.
- Store plastic bags, knives and matches out of sight and reach of children.

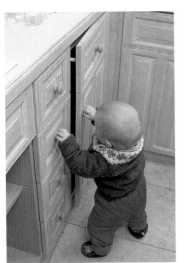

◁ Fit all low-level cupboards and drawers with childproof catches to stop an inquisitive toddler from pulling out heavy objects.

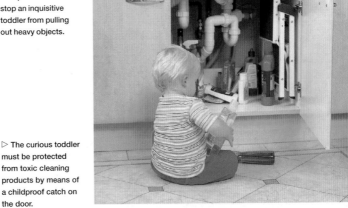

▷ The curious toddler must be protected from toxic cleaning products by means of a childproof catch on the door.

Safety in the bathroom

SEE ALSO

➤ Dealing with shock, p72

➤ Safety in the home, p228

➤ Avoiding electrical accidents, p237

Some 90 per cent of accidents in the home that involve electricity happen in the bathroom. The chief hazards here are the combination of water and electricity, water itself and medicines left within reach of young children. Getting in or out of the bath is another hazard. It is a common cause of falls, particularly among elderly people, but these can be minimized by choosing a bath with side grips and placing a non-slip mat on the base. Children love bathtime but need to be supervised – leaving them alone in the bath could have fatal results.

The two big dangers that come together in the bathroom are water and electricity. Together they form a lethal combination that, if not treated with the greatest care, may lead to tragedy. Water alone is a particular hazard to children, making careful supervision during bathtime essential. Electrical equipment – unless designed to be used in a bathroom – should be avoided at all cost. You should not, for example, take a mains-operated sound system into the bathroom.

All medicines should be kept in a medicine cabinet – this is particularly important if children live in the house or are likely to come to visit. The cabinet should be safely screwed to a wall, well out of the reach of children.

BABIES AND YOUNG CHILDREN

Bathing babies and children up to the age of 5 years should always be supervised by an adult. Young babies should always be bathed in a baby bath or on a specially shaped foam insert for a normal bath. For toddlers and older children, make sure you do not overfill the bath and avoid using slippery bath foams.

It is essential that you test the temperature of the water before the baby or child is immersed. For a baby, use your elbow – the water should feel just warm.

TEENAGERS

Favourite teenage pursuits usually include soaking in the bath for several hours at a time, and bathing by candlelight and while

> **SAFETY IN THE BATHROOM**
>
> ➤ Turn down the hot water thermostat to 54°C (130°F).
>
> ➤ Make sure that all bathroom lights have pulley switches; do not use wall-mounted switches.
>
> ➤ Have a non-slip floor. Avoid using rugs and mats in the bathroom.

listening to music. Make sure they know the dangers of dragging a sound system into the bathroom using an extension lead. Water is a great conductor of electricity, so electric shocks in the bath are usually fatal.

Teenagers should also be made aware that falling asleep in the bath and bathing after they have consumed alcohol or illegal drugs is potentially very dangerous.

OLDER PEOPLE

Fatigue, reduced mobility and lapses in concentration or memory can lead to the elderly having accidents in the bathroom. They may run a bath that is too hot and scald themselves. They may slip and have a nasty fall. They may fall asleep in the bath making drowning a real possibility.

Make sure that the bathroom of an elderly person is as safe as possible. You should install a bath with hand grips in the sides and place a non-slip mat in the bath, to reduce the risk of a fall when getting in and out of the bath. Elderly people should wear a call alarm to enable them to raise the emergency services in the event of an accident.

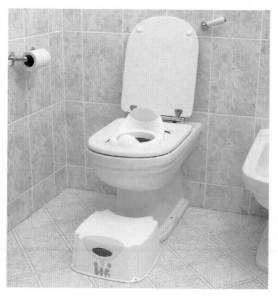

▷ The bathroom should be kept completely clear of obstacles. Invest in special lavatory stools and seats for infants and toddlers so that they can learn to use the toilet without any danger of accidents.

BATHING A BABY

Until your baby starts to demand the right to sit up and play, this is the way to hold them safely in the bath so that they cannot slip or roll over. Always remember to check that the water is not too hot before you begin bathing.

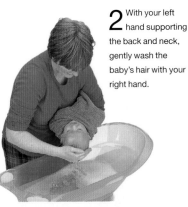

1 Hold the baby cradled in your left arm (right arm if left-handed).

2 With your left hand supporting the back and neck, gently wash the baby's hair with your right hand.

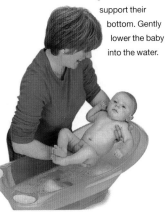

3 Hold high up under the baby's left arm and use your right hand to support their bottom. Gently lower the baby into the water.

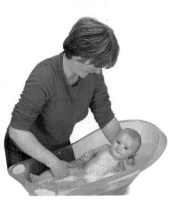

4 Use your right hand to wash, while continuing to keep a firm grip of the baby with your left hand.

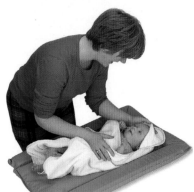

5 Once you've finished bathing the baby, wrap their head and body in a towel and dry thoroughly.

TIPS FOR BATHING BABIES

➤ Never leave a baby (or child) unattended in the bath.

➤ Be wary of leaving bath duty to someone who is not familiar with bathing children. Drowning accidents happen most often when the bathing is carried out by someone who does not realize the dangers.

➤ Even if the baby is in a baby bath seat, do not leave them unattended.

➤ Ignore a ringing telephone or doorbell – or get your child out of the bath before you answer it.

TIPS FOR BATHING CHILDREN

➤ Always run the cold water into the bath before the hot. This avoids any risk of the child scalding themselves if they get into the water unaided.

➤ Never leave a step or chair near or next to the bath. Toddlers are fearless, and if they see a toy floating invitingly on the surface of the water they will reach for it.

➤ Don't ask an older child to watch your toddler in the bath. They are unlikely to exercise the same care as an adult.

➤ Don't give children baths in shifts if it means leaving in the bath water with no adult in attendance. Empty the bath while you put small children to bed, and refill it for the older children later.

➤ Be aware that a razor looks like a toothbrush to a toddler, so they might try to use it like one. Keep all sharp objects out of their way.

➤ Bathroom doors should be impossible for a child to lock. The easiest way to achieve this is to place the lock high up out of small children's reach.

Safety in the garden

SEE ALSO
➤ Drowning: what to do, p64
➤ BURNS AND SCALDS, p177
➤ Avoiding electrical accidents, p237

The garden can be an oasis of calm in a busy life. However, ponds, bonfires, barbecues, and even plants can all present hazards, particularly if children are around. To ensure your garden is a safe haven for everyone, you'll need to take a few sensible precautions. Choose water features that are child-friendly, fence off a swimming pool, and make sure that paths are easy to negotiate. Check that children and pets are out of the way before you start to mow, and store garden tools and implements in a locked shed together with all garden chemicals.

A little forward planning and common sense will go a long way towards preventing accidents in the garden. Many accidents happen when a child or elderly person is visiting a garden that has not been made safe for them. Small children, including those from neighbouring houses, often go wandering. Your elegant ornamental pond with its shimmering goldfish may be a fatal attraction for them.

CARE WITH CHEMICALS

Lock away garden chemicals in a dark, dry and cool place, out of reach of children and animals. Follow the instructions for use exactly and do not decant chemicals into other bottles; keep them in their original containers so you know what they are. Minimize chemicals in the garden: for example, rather than using slug pellets, use environmentally-friendly methods such as dishes of beer sunk into the soil.

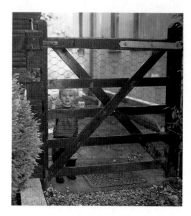

◁ Do not underestimate the climbing abilities of a toddler; this type of gate has been designed to keep out horses not children.

Covering the water with wire netting can give a false sense of security since they could still fall in if they landed on top of it. Placing a sturdy cover over the pond is the safest option. If you really want a water feature but have children, install one in which the water cascades out of a container to drain into a bed of stones rather than into a pool of water. All swimming pools should be fenced off.

WATER SAFETY

Garden ponds are a major hazard for children. They have interesting things floating on the surface that invite curious children to lean over and grab at them. They are also usually placed at ground level, so are easy for a toddler to fall into.

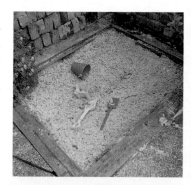

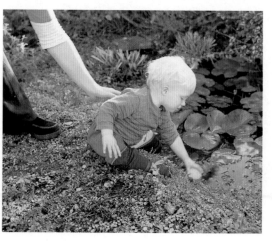

▷▽ A pond can be converted into a sandpit to provide children with an extra play area. When not in use, a sturdy cover will help to keep the sand clean.

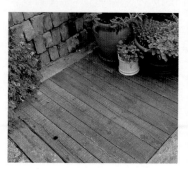

◁ Children are curious to explore their environment through taste and touch. A pond is particularly inviting – but is a potentially fatal hazard.

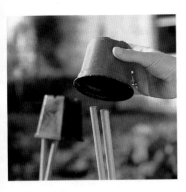

△ Place plastic containers or flowerpots on top of your garden canes, to protect your eyes when you are bending down near them.

ELECTRICITY IN THE GARDEN

- All electric garden tools should be plugged into residual current circuit breakers, so that the current switches off instantly if there is an accident.
- When using electric tools, keep the cable over your shoulder and well away from lawnmower blades and hedge trimmers.
- Keep children out of the garden when you are mowing the lawn or using anything electrical in the garden.
- Water conducts electricity, so great care should be taken when using the two together in a water feature. Many of the pumps available for water features are completely sealed and will automatically switch off if the system fails in any way.
- Exterior lights are designed to be used safely in the garden. If you are unsure, get an electrician to install or check them.

USING LADDERS SAFELY

Accidents on ladders are common but almost entirely avoidable. Make sure that all the rungs are safe before climbing up a ladder. Do not place it so that you have to lean over or stretch up to do the job – move the ladder or use a taller one if necessary. When pruning trees, use two ladders with a plank between them. If you are using a ladder up against the side of the house, ask someone to stand at the bottom to secure it; or if it is a long job, put up scaffolding.

MAKING YOUR GARDEN SAFE

- ➤ Steps should be well lit. They should have a handrail if elderly people are to use them.

- ➤ Moss gathers on patios and can be slippery. Wash surfaces with diluted bleach to get rid of it.

- ➤ Nylon line trimmers throw up stones and other potentially dangerous things, including irritants from plant sap. Wear goggles, long-sleeved shirts and trousers when using them.

- ➤ Get into the habit of wearing heavy boots and thick gloves when you are working in the garden.

- ➤ To stop canes from poking your eyes, place film canisters, plastic bottles or flowerpots over the top of them.

- ➤ Keep all garden tools tidy and store them in a locked shed. Lock away petrol, kerosene and chemicals.

- ➤ Ensure that a clothesline is not positioned at children's neck level.

CHILDREN AND PLANTS

Few children die from eating poisonous garden plants. However, they can become ill with stomachache and diarrhoea. It is best to discourage young children from eating any flowers, fruit or foliage, rather than teach them which ones to avoid.

Certain toxic plants are best kept out of the garden altogether since they are very poisonous in small amounts. These include laburnum, foxgloves, monkshood, woody nightshade and deadly nightshade. Others, such as yew, could be fenced off. Cut back trailing plants, such as thorny brambles and roses, if they could catch a child across their face.

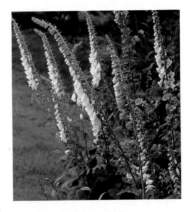

△ Foxgloves are poisonous and have no place in a garden where young children play.

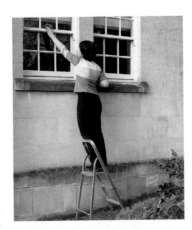

△ The golden rule of DIY safety is to be on top of the job – these steps are too low.

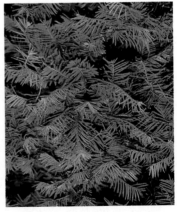

△ Yew is a common toxic plant. To protect children, fence off dangerous plants and trees.

Dealing with fire

SEE ALSO
➤ Tackling fume inhalation, p62
➤ BURNS AND SCALDS, p177
➤ Avoiding electrical accidents, p237

Fires in buildings produce invisible toxic fumes that kill in a few minutes. It is the suffocating effect of these as much as the flames that kill. No one should enter a burning building unless they are trained to do so. Oxygen feeds the flames, and if a door is opened into a burning room, the effect will be a massive explosion. Even a small amount of smoke should be a warning to keep out. Fire may be hidden behind walls, under floors and above ceilings. The most useful thing an untrained witness to a fire can do is to call the local fire department.

An untrained person is easily able to put out small fires, such as one in a chip pan (see Warning box) or in a wastepaper basket. However, once fire starts to spread, expert help is needed and the best thing you can do is to get away from the flames.

FIRE IN A BUILDING
• Try to stay calm, and if you are at work or in a public building follow the evacuation protocol. Walk to the nearest fire exit quickly and calmly. Do not go back for a bag, coat or any other possessions.
• Don't use elevators. Some have heat-activated panels that prevent them stopping at the fire floor, but if the electricity fails you may be trapped in the elevator. The elevator shaft can act like a chimney, sucking up flames and fumes.
• If you find yourself in smoke, stay close to the floor. If possible, cover your mouth and nose with a damp cloth or towel.

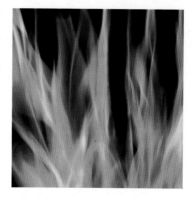

△ Fire is unpredictable and you should not underestimate how quickly it can spread.

• Close doors on the fire as you leave the building, thus starving it of oxygen.
• Never open a door that feels hot or has hot door handles – this suggests that there is a fire raging behind.
• If you cannot find an escape route, find a fire-free room with a window, shut the door, open the window and shout for help. Keep close to the floor.
• Don't turn on a light even if it is dark, since this may cause an explosion.
• Breathing in toxic fumes quickly leads to disorientation and confusion. If you have to enter a smoky area keep to the walls to guide you in and out.
• Remember that children may hide away from fumes in places such as wardrobes and cupboards.

What to do when clothing is on fire
Remember to STOP, DROP and ROLL. STOP the victim from running around.

WARNING
Deep-frying pans are a very common cause of fires in the kitchen. Never put water anywhere near a burning oil pan. Water will feed the flames and cause a massive flare-up. Cover the flames with a pan lid or blanket to deprive them of the oxygen they need.

This fans the flames. DROP them to the ground. Having them lie horizontally stops the flames rising to their face. ROLL them on the ground to put out the flames, ideally after wrapping them in non-flammable material such as that of curtains or a winter coat.

Once the flames are extinguished, you should assess the victim's airway, breathing and circulation. Start resuscitating if necessary. Carry out first aid on burns.

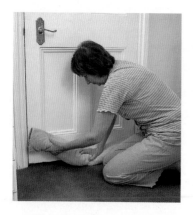

△ Blocking a door helps to keep fumes out of the room you are in and may deprive a fire of oxygen.

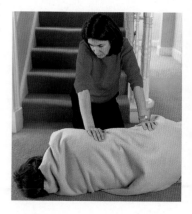

△ Stop, drop and roll someone whose clothing is on fire. Place them in the recovery position.

Avoiding electrical accidents

SEE ALSO
- Safety in the home, p228
- Safety in the kitchen, p230
- Safety in the bathroom, p232

The danger of electricity is that it surrounds us in our everyday lives, and it is easy to become complacent about it. The fraying plug on the iron, the bare wires on the vacuum flex, and the gaping plug sockets left uncovered with a toddler in the house are all electric shocks waiting to happen. Electricity harms because it can cause the heart to beat irregularly and then stop; the muscles, nerves and blood vessels to fry and the skin to burn. One-third of all victims of electrical accidents are children, and 20 per cent of these children die as a result.

One of the main causes of electric shock is contact with faulty electrical appliances or exposed wiring. Children poking sharp objects into sockets or chewing on electrical cords are other hazards, as is flashing from high-voltage power lines.

LIGHTNING INJURIES

The severity of an injury due to lightning depends on several factors:
- How long the victim is in contact with the electric current – the longer the contact, the greater the damage.
- The type of current – Alternating Current (AC) is used in mains electricity and power cables, because it allows greater amounts of electricity to be sent down the power lines. It is more likely to cause cardiac arrest at lower voltages than Direct Current (DC), which is what batteries produce. AC may also cause muscle spasms, with the result

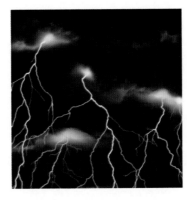

△ Keep away from metal, from cars, from trees, and from power cables during a lightning strike.

that the victim cannot let go of the electrical source.
- The size of the current – overhead power cables and lightning are more damaging than mains electricity and batteries.

ELECTRICAL ACCIDENTS

If you touch someone who is still in contact with a live circuit, they may electrocute you. Make sure that the power source is turned off at the fuse box, or unplugged at the socket. Simply turning off the appliance will not work.

If you cannot turn off the power at source or unplug the appliance, try to separate the victim from the power using a non-conducting object, such as a wooden or plastic broom handle or chair or a rubber doormat. Try to do this while standing on something dry and non-conducting such as a pile of dry newspapers, a telephone directory or a board.

If the source is a high-voltage current from a power line, be aware that the currents can jump a considerable distance. Do not approach the casualty until the power lines are off. Once they are free of the current, check if the casualty is breathing. If not, begin CPR.

Treating the casualty

Once you have excluded any further danger to yourself, approach the victim and assess them. If you are alone, call the emergency services now. Otherwise get someone else to do it for you.

Open the casualty's airway, being aware that if they have fallen or been thrown, they may have cervical spine damage. Avoid moving the head and neck, particularly if they are unconscious. If they are not breathing, begin to do mouth-to-mouth. Start to give cardiac compressions if they are not trying to breathe or move.

Be alert to other injuries if they have been thrown, and splint if necessary. If they have obvious burns, remove any clothing and rinse the burn under cool, running water. Apply a sterile dressing.

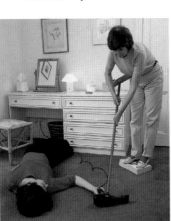

△ Separate a casualty from the source of electricity using a wooden or plastic object.

PREVENTING ACCIDENTS

- Cover sockets with childproof guards.
- Never use electrical appliances when you are wet, or if there is any water on crucial parts of the appliances.
- Teach children about electrical dangers.
- Never place a socket less than 1 m (3 ft) away from a water source.

Safe home for infants

SEE ALSO
➤ Safety in the kitchen, p230
➤ Safety in the bathroom, p232
➤ Safety in the garden, p234

When safety-proofing your home for a new baby, be at your most paranoid and suspicious. Accidents happen in seconds, and most of them are preventable. It helps if you crawl around at your baby's level, seeing what looks interesting, what dangles enticingly, and what might be eaten, opened, poked or climbed. But remember that children grow fast, and their safety needs change just as quickly. In trying to make your home safe, you must be prepared to keep re-evaluating the potential hazards in the light of your child's development.

There is a wide range of dangers for babies and young children in the home, and they will vary depending on the child's age. For example, an 18-month-old may have neither the interest nor the dexterity to do any damage with your lighter, whereas a 2-year-old could burn the house down. Don't forget that an older child could potentially harm a baby, and their age and sense of mischief should be taken into account. Another possible hazard is a grandparent or person who is not tuned into children – they may keep medication where a child can reach it or forget to empty the bath.

CHILDHOOD ACCIDENTS

Accidents involving children happen more often when there are more than two adults in the house, probably because the carers are distracted by their guests. Try to get a child used to a playpen at a young age, so that you can use this to keep them safe when your attention is elsewhere.

Protection from falls and crushing

• Avoid using baby walkers – the baby may walk over steps, off landings or into burning fireplaces.
• Use stair gates at the top and bottom of stairs. For older children, make sure all stairs have handrails and are well lit.
• Keep beds, cupboards and toy boxes away from windows, and make sure all windows have locks on them.
• Use seating appropriate to the child's age and strap them in at all times.
• Make sure that bookshelves and other pieces of furniture are screwed to the wall in case your infant tries to climb up them.
• Place safety catches on toy boxes or the lid may crush their fingers.

COT SAFETY
Make sure that your baby's cot is a safe place for them to sleep.

➤ The cot bars should be no more than 7cm (2⅜in) apart.

➤ The top railing should be at least 65cm (26in) higher than the lowest level of the mattress support.

➤ The mattress should be the correct size for the cot, with no gaps.

➤ Do not place the cot next to a radiator or in a draughty place.

➤ Avoid any soft, squashy articles such as pillows or duvets.

Avoiding poisoning and choking
• Lock up all potential poisons and do not take medicines in front of children.
• Remember that some plants are toxic.
• Avoid toys with buttons or removable bits, or breakable toys.

Preventing burns and drowning
• Put away hairdryers, irons, and toasters.
• Use the back burners on your hob and turn handles to the back.
• Cover all electric outlets.
• Cover hot pipes and radiators.
• Use a fixed fireguard in front of the fire.
• Do not leave the bathwater unattended or leave a child alone in the bath.
• Cover fish-tanks with a fixed top.

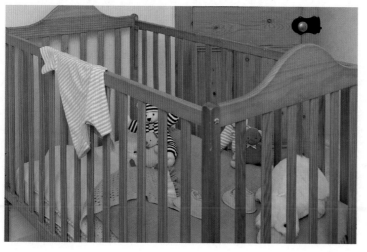

◁ Choose a good cot with a well-fitting mattress and high sides.

Avoiding cot death

SEE ALSO
➤ Resuscitating a baby or child, p50
➤ Recognizing childhood illness, p114

Most cot deaths occur quickly and while the baby is asleep, with no outward signs of suffering. Any death of a child is a tragedy for the parents, but cot deaths can be particularly traumatic because they are unexpected and sudden and may initially be treated as suspicious by the police. Cot deaths are most likely to occur in babies aged between 1 and 4 months. Nobody knows exactly why they happen, but there are certain risk factors that make them more likely. Protecting your baby from these reduces the chance of cot death.

There are many theories about why cot death occurs, but the causes are still unknown. Some of the known risk factors, such as smoking around the baby, can be avoided; and others, such as prematurity and poverty, cannot. Cot death is known to be more common in the winter months and in male babies.

REDUCING THE RISK

- Do not smoke while pregnant or if you have a baby. It is also advisable to discourage anyone living in your home from smoking, too. The risk of cot death is higher in families where a smoker lives.
- It is also best to prevent visitors smoking in the house, and avoid taking the baby into smoky areas.
- Place the baby on their back to sleep. Babies lose heat from their faces and if they lie prone they may overheat. They are no more likely to choke if they sleep on their backs.

- Do not overheat the baby. Try to keep the bedroom at about 16–20°C (60–68°F). Avoid heaters, hot-water bottles, placing the baby in direct sunshine to sleep and electric blankets. If the baby's stomach feels hot to touch or they are sweating, take off the blankets. If they have a fever, take off blankets.
- Never put a baby to bed with a hat on, as they lose a lot of heat through their heads.
- Never sleep on a sofa with the baby. Avoid sleeping in the same bed with a baby if you smoke, have drunk alcohol, are excessively tired or have taken sedatives.
- Do not use duvets until a baby is over 1 year old.

BREATHING MONITORS

Some parents buy breathing monitors for their babies. These have not been shown to prevent cot death, but they do create anxiety as they are prone to false alarms and may go off several times in a night.

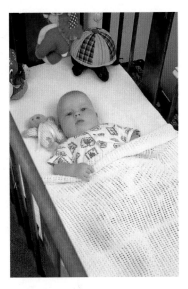
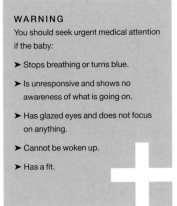

△ Make sure that your baby does not get overheated when asleep; don't use too many blankets, keep the room cool and do not cover their head.

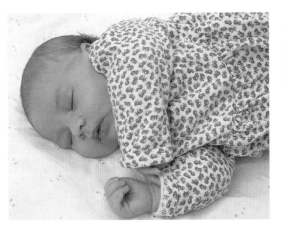

◁ A baby should initially be placed on their back to sleep, but it is quite normal for them to move on to their side as they nap.

WARNING

You should seek urgent medical attention if the baby:

➤ Stops breathing or turns blue.

➤ Is unresponsive and shows no awareness of what is going on.

➤ Has glazed eyes and does not focus on anything.

➤ Cannot be woken up.

➤ Has a fit.

SKILLS CHECKLIST FOR
KEEPING SAFE

KEY POINTS

- Most road accidents occur within two miles of the driver's own home ☐

- Keep your stairway clear ☐

- The kitchen is the most hazardous area of the home ☐

- Never leave a young child unattended in the bath – even for a moment ☐

SKILLS LEARNED

- Making your kitchen a safe place to be ☐

- How to bathe babies and children ☐

- Using common sense to make your garden a less hazardous place ☐

- Putting out a deep-fat fire ☐

- STOP, DROP and ROLL to put out burning clothing ☐

- Making your home safe for babies and young children ☐

16

OUTDOOR SAFETY

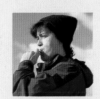

Outdoor pursuits offer a wide variety of hazards for which the sensible person must be fully prepared and properly informed. Appropriate clothing, footwear and equipment, together with a basic first-aid kit, are essential to enjoy your chosen sport or activity without unnecessary risk. Always be on the alert for changing environmental conditions (such as weather and tides) and for warning notices by seas, rivers and lakes. When travelling, be as informed as possible about your surroundings and about issues such as the safety of local drinking water and where to contact a doctor who speaks your language.

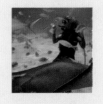

CONTENTS

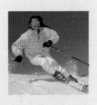

Safety in sport

SEE ALSO

➤ What is first aid?, p16

➤ Managing heat and cold disorders, p110

➤ Assembling a first-aid kit, p202

The thrills of outdoor sports are great, but sometimes the risks can be even greater. Being aware of potential risks is vital and taking appropriate actions to avoid accidents in the first place is a much better approach than just learning how to deal with an emergency. Safety is the key word, and this doesn't take away all the fun. So, if you're undertaking an outdoor sport in a new location, be prepared – even find out where the nearest hospital is. On the subject of having fun, it goes without saying that alcohol and sporting pursuits never mix.

Adventure sports have never been as popular or as accessible as they are today, each new one a little more dangerous and thrilling than the last – whitewater rafting, bungee jumping and abseiling down mountains are all possible, even for the novice. But all such activities have strict safety guidelines and provisions to ensure your safety at all times.

Even though some outdoor sports require a certain level of training, it is surprising that many people embark on outdoor pursuits, such as mountain or hill climbing, with little or no training and little or no thought to safety issues at all. It's a good idea when setting out on an outdoor activity to be prepared for the worst-case scenario – in that way, you'll be alert to potential hazards and be able to avoid them, if possible, and if not, then be best placed to deal with them.

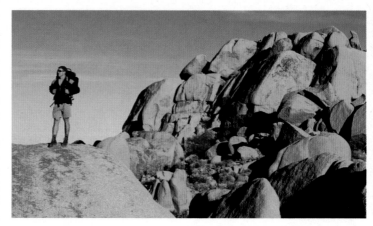

HIDDEN PERILS

It is not always amateurs that come to grief, but inexperience and ignorance of a sport's risks and dangers inevitably increase the chances of mishaps and accidents. Most problems can be traced back to poor training, a lack of fitness or poorly maintained equipment. While a certain amount of risk adds to the enjoyment and attraction of some sports, prevention of accidents through awareness of the safety aspects is the best course of action when considering engaging in any outdoor pursuit. Initial training is a good way to find out about risks, and practising with experienced people reinforces this.

△ Weather can change without warning so be prepared with waterproofs and extra layers.

UNPREDICTABLE WEATHER

All outdoor pursuits have one thing in common – exposure to the elements. Weather in cities and towns is often a minor irritation that happens high above the rooftops, but in isolated situations a sudden and unexpected change in the weather can make the difference between

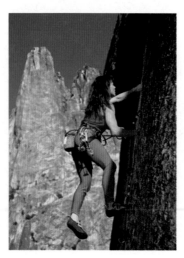

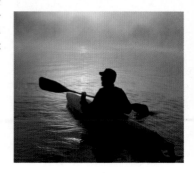

◁ Never climb alone. Climbing as part of a team means that a rescue and first aid can be easily organized if necessary.

▷ Weather at sea is notoriously changeable. Be sure to carry flares, a cellphone and warm clothing and always wear a life jacket.

life and death if you are unprepared. Certain areas of the world are renowned for their sudden and unpredictable changes in weather, but it's a good idea to be prepared for the worst wherever you are and whatever you are doing.

PEER PRESSURE

Although it is certainly safer to perform many outdoor sports in a group, there is sometimes a herd mentality at work in group activities, particularly when there is a physical challenge such as climbing up a mountain. It's easy to be spurred on by the group to do things that you know are unwise and possibly beyond your level of skill and stamina. In such circumstances, try to hold on to your common sense and resist the urge to undertake a challenge to be "part of the group". You'll probably know instinctively if an activity is one step beyond your capabilities or confidence.

It is also worth remembering that many people view extreme sports as the ultimate challenge, a way of proving something to themselves and others. They may not be willing or able to accept their limitations until it is too late and they are in trouble.

FIRST AID – BACK TO BASICS

All of the principles of first aid are as applicable out in the wilds of a windswept mountain as they are in a domestic or workplace setting. The main difference is that the victim may be isolated and a long way from any rescue centre or hospital, and may have to wait some time for treatment in the case of illness or accidental injury.

Keeping a clear head (and making sensible, safe decisions) is just as important as knowing the correct first-aid approach for a particular condition. Applying the perfect leg splint, for example, is a useless skill if you then abandon the casualty with no or little protection against the elements and/or equipment to continue to call for help while you go for assistance.

Try to remember that first aid is often about knowing what not to do, just as much as it is about knowing what to do.

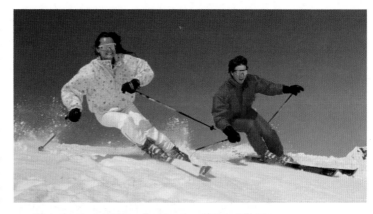

△ Skiing off-piste is the ultimate challenge, but carry a bleeper or cellphone in case of snow drifts or avalanches.

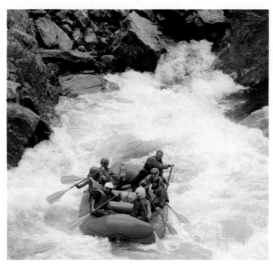

◁ Check that adventure sports organizers are qualified and experienced before you set out on an activity with them.

A BASIC SURVIVAL FIRST-AID KIT

Whatever your choice of outdoor activity, always carry a basic first-aid kit with you. A suitable kit need not be heavy or widely comprehensive but should contain the following items:

➤ A few plasters in various sizes.

➤ Sterile dressings in various sizes.

➤ A couple of triangular bandages.

➤ A lightweight foil survival blanket, cellphone, whistle and torch are other advisable items.

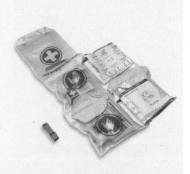

△ A basic first-aid kit is an essential part of any outdoor-based pursuit.

Safety in land sports

Mountaineering, walking, trekking and cycling all have their hazards as well as presenting exciting and tremendous challenges. As well as being alert to potential dangers of the activity itself, remember to be aware of the possibility of changes in your environment and the havoc these can wreak – sunburn, heat stroke and frostbite, to name a few. Always carry maps of the area you're exploring and make sure you're well equipped regarding footwear and clothing. Also, tell someone where you're going and never go alone – there's safety in numbers.

Like many people, you probably love to escape civilization once in a while. Putting on a pair of walking boots or getting on a bike are two of the most accessible and popular leisure activities. What's more, they are also fantastic ways of getting fit.

But any outdoor activity comes with its own hazards and it's a good idea to know what these are so that you can avoid them or, in the worst cases, have some idea what first aid you might need to give.

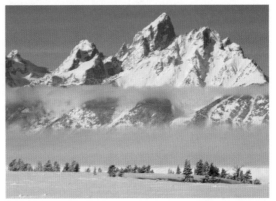

◁ Weather in mountainous regions is unpredictable, so be aware that loss of visibility and drops in temperature can be amazingly sudden.

CYCLING IN SAFETY

Almost 75 per cent of cyclists killed in accidents die from injuries to the head. So no wonder safety pundits recommend that all cyclists – whether in cities or the countryside – wear a cycle helmet. Such safety helmets reduce the chances of death from a head injury by 80 per cent.

On the roads, most cycling accidents happen at junctions, but cycle-related injuries don't just happen on roads. With the ever-increasing popularity of mountain biking, a growing number of accidents take place on hills and mountains well away from traffic. As with other pursuits, it is important not to push yourself too far too soon on rough terrain, and to always cycle as part of a group. Make sure at least one person has a first-aid kit and a cellphone. Many mountain bikers carry water reservoir rucksacks on their back. Having plenty of water is vital to avoid dehydration – a condition that could lead to dizziness, fatigue and ultimately to an accident while cycling.

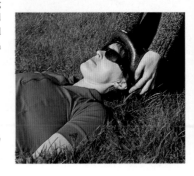

△ Do not move the casualty if you suspect a neck or spine injury. Call for help immediately on your cellphone.

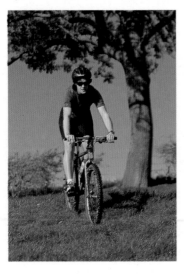

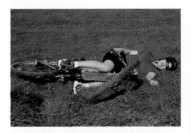

◁ Always wear a well-fitting helmet and appropriate footwear for safety's sake. And a padded pair of shorts will cushion your ride.

▷ Reassure the casualty and try to obtain some information about the accident so that you can give this to the emergency services.

Common causes of biking accidents are:
- Wet surfaces, leading to loss of control (wet bike brakes).
- Travelling too fast downhill or around corners.
- Mechanical bike failure.
- Hitting an animal or pedestrian.

HAZARDS WHEN WALKING

Most of the following hazards are avoidable by being aware and taking adequate precautions before you set out on a trek.

Blisters

Some people are prone to getting blisters, but commonly they develop in those with ill-fitting boots and in those who don't undertake such walking very often. Make sure your boots are comfortable, you wear natural-fibre socks and that your boots are not too loose nor too tight. If you do get a blister, stick a plaster over the area; never pop it as it could become infected.

Heat exhaustion

To avoid heat exhaustion, make an early start when hiking so that most of the walk is done in the cool of the morning.

WHAT TO TAKE WALKING

Even a short day walk in the hills may lead to problems if weather conditions deteriorate or if there is an accident. It is best to take the following equipment:

➤ Waterproof clothing.

➤ Strong footwear.

➤ Spare dry inner clothing – in the summer one other warm article will do.

➤ Map and compass.

➤ Whistle.

➤ Torch.

➤ First-aid kit.

➤ Reserve food and drink.

➤ Sunglasses.

➤ Pocket knife and matches.

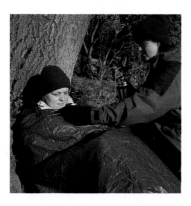

△ Prevent a casualty with hypothermia from losing more heat and rewarm them slowly.

Hypothermia

Walking in cold conditions requires a serious approach to the risks of such extreme low temperatures. If a person appears confused, quiet or is stumbling a lot, they could have hypothermia. In such instances, get them into some shelter and wrap them in spare clothes, sleeping bags or anything warm and dry. Then, give them something warm to drink, avoiding caffeine- and alcohol-containing drinks.

Soft-tissue injuries

Sprains and strains are common injuries and are difficult to prevent. As anywhere, the basic RICE (rest, ice, compression, elevation) first-aid techniques apply.

Sunburn

Always wear at least 15SPF sunscreen, and sunblock on the lips and eye area. Remember to reapply every few hours.

MOUNTAINEERING SAFETY

Mountains should be treated with great respect. Demanding climbing combined with unpredictable weather can mean accidents are more likely. Any mountain rescue can be difficult, especially when changing weather causes a loss of visibility and plummeting temperatures.

In cases of serious injury or in severe cold, use a cellphone to alert the mountain

SIGNS AND SYMPTOMS OF MOUNTAIN SICKNESS

This is one of the most serious problems that can hit anyone above 2,400 m (8,000 ft). It is usually caused by ascending a mountain too fast and is due to reduced atmospheric pressure and oxygen levels at high altitudes – it can be fatal if urgent action is not taken. Early symptoms include increasing fatigue, breathlessness that is unrelieved by rest, headache and vomiting.

If the person continues to climb, they may develop:

➤ Confusion, unsteadiness and lassitude.

➤ Pulmonary oedema, in which the lungs fill with fluid.

➤ Cerebral oedema, in which the brain swells.

The golden rule is that if the mild symptoms do not settle after a day of rest and plentiful fluids or if they worsen, the person must descend at least 300 m (1,000 ft) until they recover.

rescue team; or send one or two people from your party to get help. If you have to leave an injured person, protect them from the elements, leave them a flashlight and whistle, mark the site and note local landmarks. Learn the international distress signal: six successive whistle blasts or light flashes, repeated after a 1-minute pause.

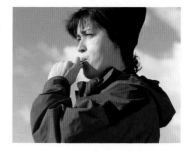

▽ Acknowledge a distress signal by blasting three times, repeating after 1 minute.

Safety in water sports

SEE ALSO

➤ Understanding
resuscitation, p30

➤ Drowning: what to
do, p64

➤ Managing heat and
cold disorders,
p110

Splashing about at the seaside, zooming about on jet-skis or windsurfers or skimming the waves in a motorboat are just a few of the ways we enjoy the water. Like other sports, all water sports come with their own hazards and a watery environment poses its own unique risks too. To be safe in the water, you must be a proficient swimmer and be aware of the power of the sea and the dangers of animals and plants that live beneath the water's surface. Also, bear in mind that many water-related accidents happen when people have been drinking.

Both salty and fresh water areas provide chances for recreational activities. Like any outdoor pursuit, water sports should be treated with great respect. It is vital to be aware at the outset of the possible hazards involved – many people underestimate water-related dangers.

Bodies lose heat more quickly in the water than on land, even in warm tropical waters, so it's advisable to wear a wet suit for sports such as scuba diving or windsurfing. A full wet suit, or what's called a dry suit, with head and hand gear is required during the colder months.

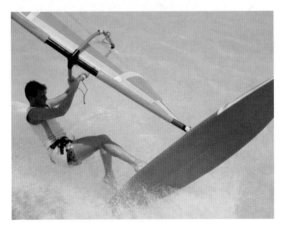

◁ Windsurfers should beware of spring tides and rip tides pushing them far out of their depth.

WEATHER AND THE WATER

Water skiing on all but the calmest waters is ill-advised, but sailing in high winds and choppy seas is what experienced sailors thrive on (although it is not advisable for a novice). Always check the weather forecast to ensure that it suits your plans and that you are prepared. Sunglasses are vital in most water sports as the water increases the sun's glare which can burn the eyes' cornea, causing temporary or even permanent damage. Don't forget that you can still get sunburn even when you are in the water so it is vital to wear waterproof sunscreen lotion and replenish it regularly.

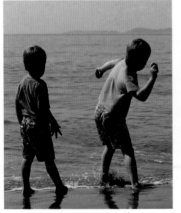

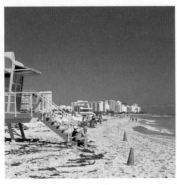

◁ Children should always be supervised when near the water's edge.

SWIMMING SAFELY IN THE SEA

Some beaches are patrolled by lifeguards and are safer than others. These beaches are usually marked by flags and sealed by joined floats to keep watercraft out of the area. If conditions are dangerous, the lifeguards will fly a warning flag. It's good practice to check the colour of the flag flying before setting off for the water. Know what the different flags mean.

• Green flag – It's safe to swim.
• Red/yellow flag – Lifeguards are on patrol and you should bathe only in the area between the flags.
• Red flag – Dangerous to bathe. You should not enter the water.
• Black/white check flag – Area is zoned for surfboards and it is not safe for swimmers.
• Blue/white flag – Divers in the area.

◁ If you have young children it is a good idea to choose a beach that is patrolled by lifeguards.

Any non-swimming child, or child under 12, should be supervised near the water's edge, especially if wading or swimming. Keep clear of rocks when swimming and keep an eye out for animals in the water such as sea urchins and jellyfish. In tropical waters, avoid swimming near the beautiful but dangerously sharp coral.

TIDES AND RIP TIDES

A large part of the sea's danger lies in the tides. Sands seemingly miles away from the shore can be covered by an incoming tide in seconds. Rip tides are narrow bands of current that create a powerful force in the water, often pulling swimmers or surfers out to sea. Swimming against these forces is pointless; it rapidly leads to exhaustion and the risk of drowning. The simplest way to safety is to work out the direction the rip tide is taking you and swim at right angles (90°) to this for about 10–20 m (33–64 ft), and then swim towards the shore.

SCUBA DIVING

Anyone taking part in scuba diving has to undergo rigorous training in the use of equipment, signalling between divers and how diving affects the body. Even so, accidents can happen, such as near drowning, decompression ("the bends") and ruptured eardrum and/or lung.

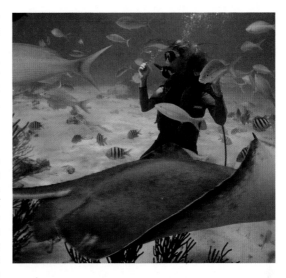

◁ The world beneath the ocean's surface can be exciting to explore, but you should be aware of potential dangers. For example, if coral grazes the skin it can lead to infection.

HAZARDS IN FRESH WATER

Most water-related accidents involve swimming in strong currents or cold water. Ponds, rivers, lakes and reservoirs can be extremely cold and pose a serious threat to life from drowning and hypothermia.

Deep rivers and lakes often have dangerous debris hidden beneath the surface. Pollution can cause skin reactions and infections such as Weil's disease. Getting in and out of the water can be tricky, and slimy banks with reeds and grasses can be hazardous.

▽ Diseases like bilharzia are carried by blood flukes like these. People can become infected by bathing or swimming in contaminated water.

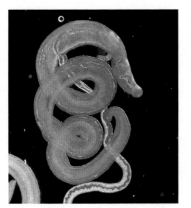

▽ Avoid fast-flowing water and be aware that sharp branches and other hazards may be hidden in deep water.

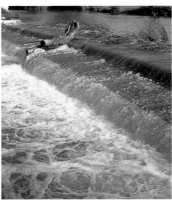

MAKING A WATER RESCUE

Giving first aid while in the water is extremely difficult, so unless you have proper training get the casualty to dry land before resuscitating them.

Avoid getting into the water: use a branch to pull them in or throw a float.

Once out of the water, protect them from the wind and lay them on their back.

Open their airway and check breathing. Be prepared to start resuscitation.

Remove any wet clothing and wrap in warm blankets to avoid hypothermia.

Safety in snow sports

SEE ALSO

➤ Managing heat and cold disorders, p110

➤ Handling lower-leg injuries, p168

➤ Managing sprains and strains, p172

Having a good attitude towards safety will mean that snow sports are enjoyable rather than dangerous. Your first considerations should be clothing and footwear. Make sure you've got enough warm layers on and a waterproof jacket. A hat will keep you cosy as a huge amount of heat is normally lost through your head. Gloves are a must, as are ski goggles or sunglasses. Boots need a good grip and should be roomy enough for thick, warm socks. Once properly kitted out, you can concentrate on having fun in the snow.

People who live where there is rarely much snow sometimes seem to go slightly mad when the first snowflakes fall. They seize any item they can sit on – plastic bags, trays or plastic crates – and hurl themselves down the nearest snow-covered hillside. It's not surprising that many injuries occur in this way, from a bruised back and ribs to fractured ankles and limbs.

With the increasing popularity of snow sport holidays, such injuries are becoming more common as people spend only a week a year on the slopes and underestimate the level of fitness and skill required.

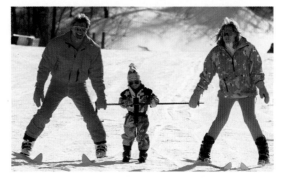

◁ Help your child to learn properly on lower slopes before taking them on steeper slopes.

AVOID INJURIES ON THE SLOPES

• Ski in control. Some people seem to delight in skiing or snowboarding on slopes beyond their level, but they risk injuring others as well as themselves.

• Train beforehand. Snowboarding and skiing are arduous sports. Make sure you build stamina, strengthen leg muscles and improve flexibility before you go.

• Use properly maintained equipment. Wearing someone else's ski boots and an old pair of skis is just asking for trouble.

• Stop as soon as you feel tired or cold, because this is when injuries happen.

If you fall while skiing, try to keep your knees flexed and do not try to get up until you have stopped moving or sliding. Ski patrols regularly check the slopes and are trained in first aid. To warn others that you are injured, get someone to plant your skis in an X pattern just uphill from where you're lying. Stay calm until help arrives.

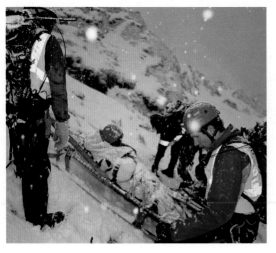

◁ This mountain rescue team have wrapped the casualty in a waterproof covering to protect him from the cold. The team paramedic assesses the injuries before they transport the casualty down the mountain.

SIGNS AND SYMPTOMS OF FROSTBITE

➤ The affected area of skin goes white and is painful – the sensation is similar to pins and needles.

➤ Sensation is gradually lost and the skin feels numb. The colour changes from white to blotchy.

➤ The skin and underlying tissue start to feel hard and stiff.

➤ The affected skin turns blue.

If the skin tissue colour then changes from blue to black that means that gangrene has set in.

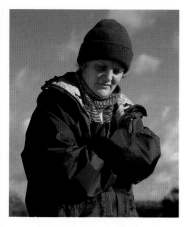

◁ If you suspect you have frost-bitten fingers, warm your hands under your armpits.

DEALING WITH FROSTBITE

In temperatures below freezing, the body diverts blood to the vital organs and away from the ears, nose, hands and feet. If tissues freeze, the condition is known as frostbite. Freezing temperatures or cold and windy conditions can cause frostbite, which often occurs with hypothermia.

If you suspect someone has frostbite, it is essential that you try to warm them up slowly and arrange to get them to hospital.

- Initially, get them out of the cold, replace any wet clothes and warm their hands by placing in your hands or lap or under their armpits, after removing rings and any other constricting objects.
- Once in the warm, put the frostbitten part in a sink or bowl of warm (never hot) water and dry it without rubbing.
- Elevate the affected limbs and support them to reduce any tissue swelling.
- Arrange transport to hospital.

COMMON INJURIES

Propelling yourself at high speed down the rough terrain of a mountainside is bound to entail the risk of falling. Most injuries on the slopes are sprains and strains, and so you should follow the RICE (rest, ice, compression, elevation) first-aid guidelines.

Knee injury

There are several ligaments in the knee. The one that is most commonly damaged in skiing is the anterior cruciate ligament.

If a skier straightens their leg at the knee, often while still in motion, and a ski edge catches their knee twists nastily. The knee does not always swell, but it is extremely painful and may give way suddenly.

Skier's thumb

If the thumb becomes jammed by the ski poles in a fall, a small ligament in the lower part of the thumb (the ulnar collateral ligament) may become sprained or even completely ruptured.

Snowboarder's wrist

Injuries to the wrist and bones in the hand are common in snowboarding where people use their hand to steady themselves and land on it outstretched.

SNOW BLINDNESS

The sun reflects off the snow, thus doubling its harmful effects. Without sunglasses or ski goggles, the sun may burn the layer of cells covering the eyeball (the cornea). This causes temporary blindness and great pain. As a first-aider, cover their eyes and get them to medical help.

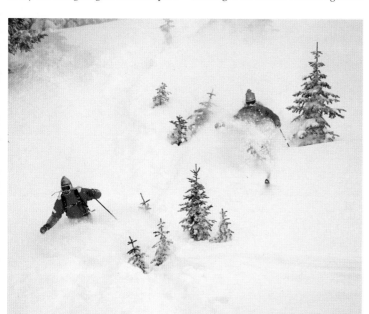

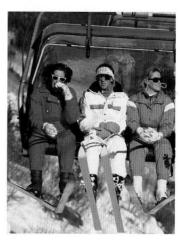

△ Ensure that your skis are always lifted well off the ground when you are travelling back up the mountain.

◁ Only ski off-piste if you are very experienced and have checked conditions before leaving.

Travelling safely

Whether you are going to France or Fiji, it pays to prepare for the trip. As airfares become cheaper, people travel to more and more exotic destinations. With far-flung places come new and sometimes deadly hazards. But, by following a few simple guidelines, you can ensure that your trip will be as safe as possible. Even the journey can be hazardous – so stretch your legs, drink plenty of water and avoid alcohol. And don't forget to take out travel insurance; if you do have an accident abroad it is vital for prompt medical assistance.

If you are heading somewhere off your usual beaten track, it's advisable to visit your doctor or practice nurse for travel advice at least six weeks before going away. You may need to have certain immunizations or start a course of antimalarial tablets in advance of your departure date.

DO YOU NEED ANY JABS?

Immunization offers protection against particular diseases. Some immunizations, such as that against yellow fever, are mandatory, and a certificate dated with the time and place of immunization is an entry requirement for some countries.

Even if you're heading for places such as North America, Europe, Australia or New Zealand, you need to be up-to-date on tetanus and polio (though no other immunizations are required at the time of writing). Common conditions to be immunized against include hepatitis A and typhoid. Which immunizations are needed for which countries varies over time, so always check in plenty of time.

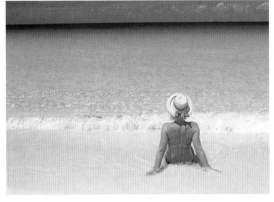

◁ The sun's rays are intensified as they are reflected off the water. Protect yourself by wearing a wide-brimmed hat, sunscreen and sunglasses.

TRAVELLER'S DIARRHOEA

This common condition usually strikes in the first two weeks of a visit; most often it's due to bacteria or viruses in the food and/or local water. Follow these simple prevention tips and you will stand a good chance of avoiding the problem:

• Wash hands before you eat anything.

• Wash all fruit, vegetables and salad leaves in purified water, or peel if possible.

• Avoid eating undercooked shellfish, meat and fish.

• Buy bottled water or purify local water using iodine, puritabs or a water-purifying pump.

• Avoid uncooked foods or cold drinks that may have been in contact with local water (and therefore possibly loaded with germs) – drinks with ice cubes, ice cream, salads, fresh fruit and vegetables.

• Use bottled water (check the seal is intact) to rinse your teeth after brushing and for any washing of fruit or vegetables that you prepare yourself.

PROTECTING YOURSELF AGAINST MALARIA

Certain areas of the world put the traveller at risk of catching malaria through mosquito bites. The actual tablets that protect against malaria vary with the country being visited. Check with your doctor or nurse which tablets you need to take; they can be bought from any pharmacist and the course should be started a few weeks before you depart for your trip.

Follow these simple guidelines for a malaria-free trip:

➤ Keep arms and legs fully covered after dusk and when trekking through forested areas.

➤ Use an insecticide (ideally one containing the chemical DEET) to keep mosquitoes away at night; they come in coils, mats and vaporized forms.

➤ If you're staying in jungle areas, take an insecticide-impregnated mosquito net with you. (Staying in an air-conditioned hotel room cuts down on exposure to mosquitoes.)

➤ Bear in mind that mosquitoes are most common in country areas, near water and that they are more active at night.

➤ Apply mosquito-repellent cream for added protection – day or night.

What to do if you have diarrhoea

The main concern when suffering from diarrhoea is to prevent dehydration, so drink plenty of fluids. Oral rehydration salts are an excellent remedy for dehydration. These can be bought from a chemist – ready-made in individual sachets – before your trip, and then made up as and when needed. If you don't have any such salts, you can easily make some from water, salt and sugar. Use 1 level tsp of salt and 8 level tsp of sugar and add these to 1 litre (1¾ pints) of boiled, purified or bottled water.

For each loose motion passed give a quarter of a mug to babies (but seek medical help as soon as possible), half a mug to small children, a mug to older children and two mugs to adults, plus plenty of bottled or boiled water.

If you need to travel or don't have time for the rehydration salts to work, then you could take one of the following medicines:
• An antidiarrhoeal drug called loperamide will help to "dry up" the diarrhoea.
• An antibiotic called ciprofloxacin taken after the first loose stool will cut the duration of uncomplicated watery diarrhoea down to one day.

In any case, if you are suffering from a high fever, there is blood in your stools, or the diarrhoea persists for more than four days, then it is advisable to seek medical help as soon as you can.

▽ Drink plenty of fluids; rehydration fluids are best for relief from diarrhoea.

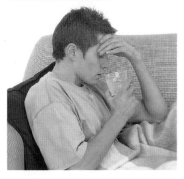

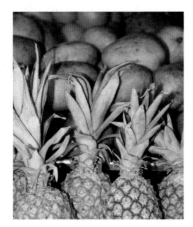

△ If you buy fruit from a stall make sure that you peel it or wash it with bottled water.

THE RISK OF BLOOD CLOTS

Reduce the risk of clots on long-haul flights by following these tips:
• Drink plenty of non-alcoholic fluid.
• Wear elasticated stockings to thigh level.
• Walk up and down the aisle for a few minutes at least once every two hours.
• Be aware that pregnancy, recent operations, obesity and the contraceptive pill can all increase the risk.
• Take aspirin (a 75–150mg tablet) on the day of the flight (or clopidogrel if allergic).

PRACTISE SAFE SEX

Many sexually transmitted infections are contracted on holidays or trips abroad. The best form of protection against diseases such as hepatitis B, HIV and gonorrhoea are condoms, although they cannot protect against all of them 100 per cent. Take plenty of condoms with you if you think you're going to be sexually active while away; in some countries, condoms are not as reliably made or are not as easy to buy.

DEALING WITH TRAVEL SICKNESS

Some people are prone to motion or travel sickness regardless of the mode of travel, but boats are particular culprits. If you suffer regularly from motion sickness, there are drugs to prevent it. Acupressure bands (also suitable for children), may help to quell nausea. Try these tips, too:
• Keeping your eyes on the horizon or on a fixed point.
• Keeping your head still by lying down or leaning upright against a pillar or wall.
• Staying in the fresh air, rather than cooped up indoors.
• Sitting in the front passenger seat of a car rather than the rear seat.

GETTING THROUGH JET LAG

When flying across time zones, your natural body clock can find it difficult to readjust to the local time. This jet lag is a common problem. Symptoms of jet lag include: tiredness, difficulty concentrating, loss of appetite and constipation. It can take several days to adjust and it's a good idea not to do too much initially. Try to fit in with local times but rest when you need to.

USEFUL MEDICINES FOR A TRAVEL FIRST-AID KIT

The following suggestions for travel medicines are given only as a guide. If travelling to a remote area, it is wise to discuss malaria treatment and antibiotics for traveller's diarrhoea with your doctor before you leave.

➤ Antihistamines are useful for insect bites and itchy rashes. They are also useful in travel sickness.

➤ Hydrocortisone cream (1%) can be bought over the counter in many pharmacies – it is good for allergic skin rashes, insect bites and sunburn.

➤ Antifungal creams are good for itchy rashes (which are often due to a fungus) in hot sweaty places, such as between the toes or in the armpits.

➤ Antidiarrhoeal tablets to help prevent and control diarrhoea.

➤ Painkillers – such as paracetamol or ibuprofen – always come in handy for quelling headaches and toothache or for bringing down a fever.

SKILLS CHECKLIST FOR
OUTDOOR SAFETY

KEY POINTS

- Prevention is far preferable to cure, especially in outdoor activities when it may take considerable time to obtain assistance ☐

- Don't be tempted to push yourself beyond your abilities ☐

- Always supervise children in hazardous situations ☐

- Always carry a basic first-aid kit and a cellphone ☐

- Get as much information as possible before you set out ☐

- Move about regularly when flying in a plane ☐

SKILLS LEARNED

- How to have fun while minimizing risk ☐

- Recognizing the value of researching your sport or activity and location ☐

- Checking out your equipment, first-aid kit and maps ☐

- Obtaining in advance specific medicines for various medical complaints ☐

- How to avoid a bout of diarrhoea – the most common travellers' complaint ☐

GENERAL RULES FOR DEALING WITH
MEDICAL EMERGENCIES

Many people panic when faced with a medical emergency because they think that they cannot help unless they can immediately bring to mind complex specific rules for dealing with each particular situation. In fact, there are just a few basic guidelines that are extremely useful in most scenarios. These are simple to remember and are summarized here because it is so easy to lose sight of the general ground rules:

- If people have serious injuries or you are in any doubt at all about the extent of the injuries, call the emergency services without delay

- Don't waste any time trying to work out what to do yourself before getting professional help

- Stay as calm as you can

- Keep reassuring the patient – and others around you

- Ensure that neither you nor the injured person are in danger

- If there are bystanders, make good use of them – to go and call for help while you stay and reassure the patient, for example

- Assess the injured person as well as you are able, and try to follow these basic first-aid steps:
  Unconsciousness: If the person is unconscious and there is no sign of life, call the emergency services. Only if you have the skills, give mouth-to-mouth resuscitation until help arrives
  Burns: Cool with water for at least 10 minutes, cover with a non-adhesive dressing (cling film is excellent), and keep the patient warm while you wait for help to arrive
  Bleeding: Stem heavy blood loss by applying firm pressure to the wound with a clean, dry dressing and raise the affected area above the heart. In general, you should lay the person down and loosen their clothes but keep them warm
  Broken bones: Avoid any movement as far as possible

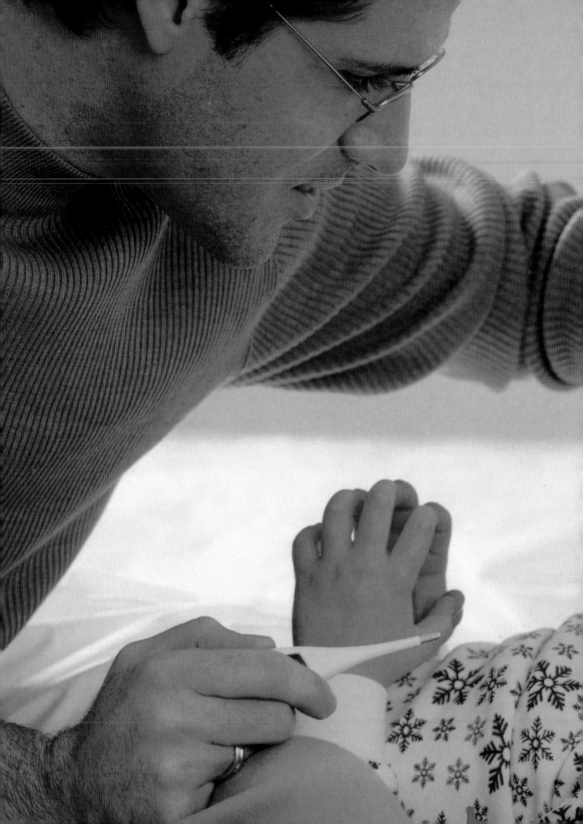

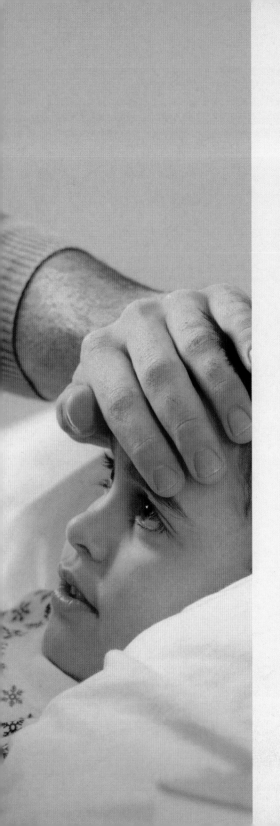

FAMILY HEALTH GUIDE

This section of the book will help all the family diagnose a vast range of ailments – from the common cold to chronic fatigue syndrome. Most of the chapters are organized around systems of the body, such as the digestive system, and begin with a thorough explanation of how those organs function within the body. Other chapters deal with vital issues such as maintaining a healthy lifestyle and caring for children or the elderly. Throughout, special feature boxes provide handy symptom summaries and point you towards related articles in other chapters.

How to use the family health chapters

Clearly written text, special feature boxes, carefully selected photographs and detailed, annotated artworks combine to make this invaluable health guide both accessible and easy to use.

The guide begins with a general Healthy Living chapter that introduces you to all kinds of strategies for keeping yourself and your family fit and healthy. The chapters that follow are conveniently organized around each of the major systems of the body, from the heart and circulation to the blood and the immune system. The chapters begin with an introduction to that bodily system, which gives a valuable background context to what follows. The chapter then goes on to deal with the various conditions that commonly affect that particular part of the body.

Within an entry for a specific condition, you will find other features that help you to gain a concise and clear understanding of the main issues involved. These features are outlined below.

See Also boxes
These cross-references point the way to other entries or features in the family health section that may provide useful extra information.

Specialist photographs
Hundreds of full-colour photographs help you to recognize problems and to see specific conditions and processes under the microscope.

Entry text
Each entry explains the most important issues in a clear, informed and non-technical way, offering readers the most up-to-date facts.

Signs and Symptoms boxes
These blue boxes let you see the main symptoms of a condition at one quick glance, without having to hunt through the main text.

Full-colour artworks
Specially commissioned, fully annotated artworks are featured throughout, giving vital additional information.

Information boxes
Beige-coloured boxes are there to provide all kinds of fascinating information, from prevention tips to related conditions.

HEALTHY LIVING

It is important to think carefully about lifestyle choices and their effect on your health. And it is never too late to take stock and discover how healthy (or unhealthy) your lifestyle really is. You can influence many areas of your life – and therefore health – whether in terms of dealing with stress more effectively, eating a more balanced diet, including more exercise in your daily routine or checking your alcohol consumption. A completely new lifestyle is not always necessary because small changes can be highly beneficial and gradual healthy choices are more likely to become an integral part of your life and so help you live more healthily for longer.

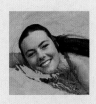

A healthy lifestyle

SEE ALSO

➤ Learn to manage
stress, p260

➤ Exercise for life, p266

➤ Routine health
checks, p272

Your health is something that you can influence – for better or for worse – through the lifestyle choices you make every day. People today are generally much better informed than their parents' generation and the expectations of what medicine can do is also higher. It is possible to make small changes to the way you live which will lead to a healthier and longer life. Simple, realistic changes are by far the best – drastic measures usually prove difficult to sustain and tend to be followed for only a short time. Healthy choices are those that you make for life.

In the 21st century more people are living for longer – in fact, most of the world's population is living 20 years longer than their parents. What's the secret? Today, we have access to better food, sanitation and healthcare services.

CHANCE AND CHOICE FACTORS

Having a healthy lifestyle comes down to two factors – chance and choice. The chance factors are those you cannot change, such as your genetic make-up, which may protect you from or predispose you to illness throughout your life. But, if you find out

▽ Being self-aware means that you will notice abnormal symptoms earlier and so can alert your doctor to possible problems.

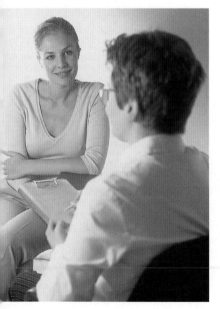

▷ Spending time doing things you enjoy can be invaluable to both your physical and your mental health. Gardening can be an active pursuit while giving your mind something to focus on during any stressful times.

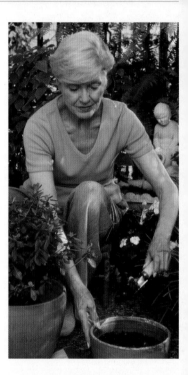

that you are more likely to develop a condition, you can take positive steps to help you prevent the situation from arising. The choice factors are being aware of the foods you eat, whether you drink alcohol (and to what extent), whether you smoke, how much exercise you take and how you deal with day-to-day stress.

IT'S ALL IN THE BALANCE

As with most things in life, having a healthy lifestyle is all about a balanced approach. Occasional overindulgence won't, on the whole, damage your health irreparably but your body will need time to recover afterwards and some tender loving care.

Making changes to your life, say from having a cooked breakfast every morning to eating a bowl of yoghurt and muesli, can be a positive healthy choice but it's unlikely to be sustained if you just switch in one go. Start off with a change that you are more likely to sustain, such as switching half of your breakfasts to the more healthy option and then perhaps eventually just keep fried breakfasts for a weekend treat.

The same goes for exercise. It is a matter of deciding which activities you enjoy and which will fit in to your daily routine. The key is to increase the amount of exercise you do gradually. Whether it's a brisk 20-minute walk in the fresh air or a session at the gym, both will be beneficial to your heart, muscles, bones and lungs.

SELF-AWARENESS
Your doctor relies on information provided by you to diagnose a problem. So, make an effort to note what is normal for you on a regular basis – this could relate to functions such as eyesight and bowel movements, or the appearance of the skin, breasts and testicles for example. This means that you are much more likely to notice something out of the ordinary, which means you can mention it to your doctor at an earlier stage so that it can be treated more effectively.

START THEM OFF YOUNG

Healthy habits are best started in childhood because most bad habits are picked up then, too. If you have children, then one of the most effective ways to influence them is to lead by example – it won't do any harm to have a few hours in front of the television if it is balanced by something more active earlier or later in the day. But bad habits can soon become part of your child's normal life and changing these habits will become much more difficult later on.

Education on health-damaging habits, such as smoking, can also begin at a very early age and probably has the best effect when your children can see plainly that you yourself, for example, don't smoke.

Positive health influences can take many different forms, from promoting a healthy diet to making an effort to organize family-group activities on a regular basis. Bike rides or walks to the woods, for example, that allow you to spend time together as a family, will set a pattern for later in life.

▽ Involving children from an early age in fun and energetic activities can help to set the pattern for a healthy and active adult life.

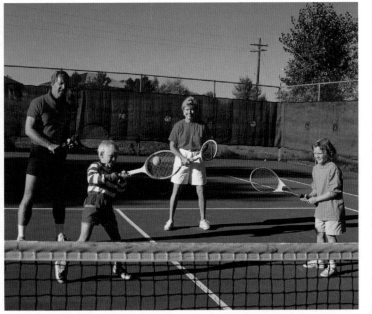

POSITIVE THINKING

Keeping our lives happy and harmonious can very often be difficult and studies have shown that positive thinking can help us to deal more effectively with everyday stress as well as having a beneficial effect on our emotional health. Research has also demonstrated that a person's emotional wellbeing plays an important part in his or her physical health. It can be enormously beneficial, psychologically and physically, to make an effort to integrate positive thinking into every aspect of your life. You will reap the health rewards if you follow a few basic guidelines:

- Consider that it is often much easier to be negative and critical so make an effort to be positive and encouraging to yourself and to others.
- Keep crises in perspective and if possible try to see them simply as problems that you can solve.
- Focus on the good things in your life.
- When faced with a situation that you find stressful, try calming strategies such as taking deep breaths or visualizing tranquil scenes or images.

HEALTH SCREENING

Your doctor now has access to an ever-increasing array of sophisticated screening checks that can often detect potential diseases and conditions many years before they become apparent. By picking up such problems at an early stage, doctors hope that medical interventions will prevent disease progression or at least lead to more successful treatments.

▽ High blood pressure usually has no obvious symptoms so routine checks are vital to detect this condition.

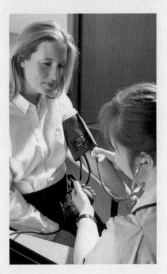

INFORMATION IS POWER

Health information has never before been so comprehensive and accessible, although some sources are not especially accurate or reliable. If your doctor suspects a particular condition, find out all you can about it by searching the Internet or by visiting your local library; there are plenty of patient groups and foundations for particular conditions, so you are very likely to find the facts you need. The more information you have the easier it will be to make decisions with your doctor about your healthcare. You will feel more confident and better able to ask questions, too.

Learn to manage stress

Our lives seem to become increasingly stressful. We work harder than ever and our personal lives have become more complex. Family and community support systems are often not so readily available. So, stress is a major factor in most people's lives. Some stress may be beneficial: many people need a certain level of stress to perform at their best. It is when stress becomes excessive and unmanageable, with no apparent resolution, that problems start to arise. This is why it is very important to be able to recognize stress and know how to manage it.

SIGNS AND SYMPTOMS

Psychological symptoms of stress include:

➤ Mood fluctuations.

➤ Depression.

➤ Anxiety.

➤ Difficulty sleeping.

➤ Poor mental performance – difficulty concentrating and forgetfulness.

➤ Relationship problems.

Physical symptoms of stress include:

➤ Stomach acidity.

➤ Changing bowel habit, alternating bouts of diarrhoea and constipation.

➤ Breathing problems.

➤ Asthma.

➤ Palpitations.

➤ Migraines.

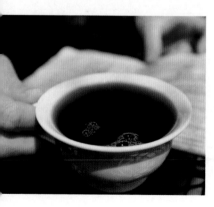

It is usually possible to recognize when levels of stress become unmanageably high. Stress tends to manifest itself in either psychological or physical symptoms, but sometimes as both.

HOW TO DEAL WITH STRESS

As soon as you begin to feel that things are getting on top of you and your health is starting to suffer, try any or all of these approaches, first to identify, and then to deal with, stress in your everyday life.

• Work at identifying sources of stress in your life and consider whether or not you can make any changes that will leave you in greater overall control.

• Learn to manage your time better. Many people's stress is due to an overwhelming workload. To make work more manageable, write a list of goals for the day and list them in order of priority. Ticking off tasks as you complete them gives you a sense of achievement.

• Breathe deeply. A very effective and easy way to relieve stress is to focus on your breathing and make your breaths progressively deeper.

• A number of illicit drugs worsen feelings of stress and anxiety, including crack, cocaine and ecstasy.

• Look after your health. Eat healthily and drink alcohol and caffeine in moderation. By maintaining good overall health you reduce your tendency to illness and increase your ability to cope with whatever life throws at you.

◁ Caffeine-containing drinks, such as coffee and hot chocolate, are useful stimulants but can also contribute to anxiety and insomnia.

• Try to avoid substances that might increase anxiety. A few cups of strong black coffee may wake you up in the morning but caffeine can increase levels of anxiety, especially in people already suffering from the effects of stress.

• Get into the exercise habit. Regular exercise helps to mobilize and utilize excessive amounts of adrenaline (caused by stress) and so helps to calm you down.

• Try to include some positive relaxation techniques on a daily basis. There is a range of alternative therapies that are all effective methods of relaxing and so reducing anxiety levels. These include yoga, massage, shiatsu, aromatherapy, reflexology and acupuncture.

WHAT IS YOUR STRESS SCORE?

Many life events can be a major source of stress; even when an event is a wholly desirable one, such as a wedding or house move. Read through the following stress "ratings" to see how they are linked to various major and minor life events. This will help you to focus on the factors that may be causing stress in your life and to establish if you can make any changes to alleviate the problem.

• Very high stress – Death of a spouse; divorce or marital separation; loss of job; house move; personal injury or illness.

• High stress – Retirement; pregnancy; change of job; death of close friend; serious family illness.

• Moderate stress – Large debts such as mortgage; trouble with parents-in-law; spouse starting or stopping work; trouble with boss; legal proceedings over debt.

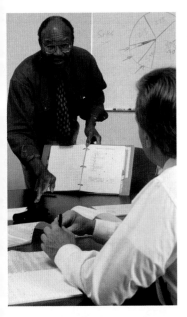

feel that you cannot allow time for the luxury of a good night's sleep. But studies have shown that long-term sleep deprivation will eventually predispose a person to a range of physical and psychological problems.

PROBLEMS SLEEPING

If you are having difficulty sleeping or feel that you have poor-quality sleep, it may well be helpful to discuss the situation with your doctor. If you have already tried some of the self-help suggestions then it may be that you need a mild hypnotic drug to help you to re-establish a sleep pattern.

Overtiredness is a leading cause of reduced productivity at work as well as being a major cause of road accidents. Insomnia may also be a manifestation of anxiety and/or depression, both of which require specific treatment.

△ You will tackle challenges at work much more effectively if you have seven to eight hours of good-quality sleep every night. Arriving at work feeling refreshed means higher energy levels to handle stress.

▽ Try to make a relaxation session part of your daily routine. Even if you have only 10 or 15 minutes to spare each day, you will benefit greatly from the calming influence of any relaxation technique.

SELF-HELP FOR A GOOD NIGHT'S SLEEP

If you have problems sleeping or feel that you don't get enough sleep, try out the following suggestions.

➤ Don't eat heavy meals late at night.

➤ Avoid caffeine-containing drinks late at night – remember that traditional bedtime drinks such as cocoa and hot chocolate contain caffeine.

➤ Don't drink too much alcohol.

➤ Tire yourself out physically by exercising during the day: physical activity has a calming effect on both mind and body. But, avoid exercising too late in the evening as it tends to be stimulating and keep you awake rather than promoting sleep.

➤ Practise meditation, yoga and/or relaxation exercises in the evening to create a relaxing mood, and a relaxing routine leading up to bedtime.

• Low stress – Change in work conditions; change in schools; change in eating habits; small mortgage or debts; Christmas or other family holidays.

GET A GOOD NIGHT'S SLEEP

We spend approximately one-third of our lives asleep but many of the elements of this fundamental biological process – exactly why we sleep and how our bodies know when to sleep – still elude sleep science researchers.

An adequate period of sleep is necessary to allow the body and mind to rest properly and what is adequate will vary from person to person. Making sure that you have enough sleep is vital in terms of stress management so it is perhaps surprising then that many people do not allow themselves adequate periods of sleep.

An increasingly complex lifestyle that means you are continually struggling to deal with competing demands may lead you to

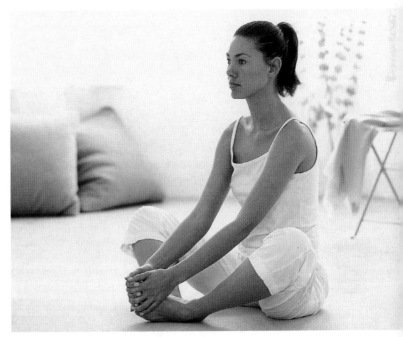

Eat healthily

It may be a cliché to say "you are what you eat" but it is true. Your body requires a healthy combination of different foods and fluids in order to function properly and maintain good health. Balance is a key word in dietary matters. A healthy balanced diet comprises the three basic food types – protein, carbohydrate and fat – in the right proportions for optimum physical health. The foods your body needs will depend on how active your life is: if you have a demanding manual job your energy needs are higher than someone who works at a desk.

Eating patterns and diets vary around the world and studies have shown that this often bears a direct relation to the prevalence of certain diseases.

DIETS AROUND THE WORLD

The traditional British and American diets are often high in cholesterol and rich in calories. Such diets lead to an increase in obesity and heart disease. In contrast, a traditional Mediterranean diet, rich in fibre, olive oil, garlic, red wine and fish, lowers cholesterol and fat consumption. As a result, fewer people from Greece and Italy, for example, suffer from conditions such as obesity and heart disease.

The Japanese have always had a low incidence of heart disease because of the high quantities of fish that they eat. They also have low levels of colorectal cancer because their diet is generally high in fibre. These patterns are changing, however, because more Japanese people are adopting Western patterns of eating, and that includes higher fat consumption.

DIET-RELATED PROBLEMS

A range of digestive tract problems such as haemorrhoids, diverticular disease and constipation are related to the lack of fibre in Western diets.

Levels of obesity in the developed world are also increasing. Researchers believe this rise to be linked both to high levels of fat consumption and to diets that are increasingly rich in sugars.

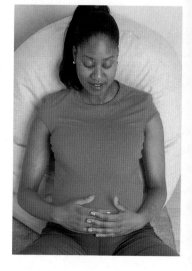

△ At certain times of life, such as during pregnancy, your body's demand for particular nutrients increases. Talk to your doctor about this to make sure you don't miss out.

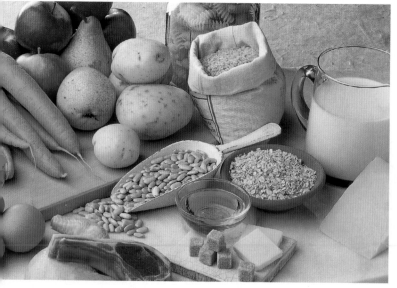

◁ It is important that you eat a variety of foods from the main food groups in order to provide your body with the balance of nutrients it needs to stay healthy.

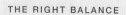

THE RIGHT BALANCE

Try to ensure that you eat the correct combination of different food types every day. Current recommendations state that you should aim for:

➤ At least 40 per cent carbohydrate.

➤ About 30 per cent protein.

➤ No more than 30 per cent fat.

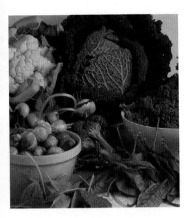

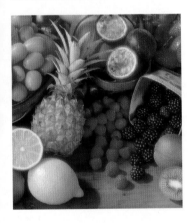

△ ▽ Fresh fruit and vegetables are a good source of carbohydrate (in the form of fibre), vitamins, minerals and natural sugars. To stay healthy aim for five portions of fruit and vegetables each day – this can include juices, dried fruit and tinned produce.

NOT JUST A COFFEE ISSUE

Caffeine is found in coffee, tea, hot chocolate, cocoa and a range of cola drinks, as well as in chocolate bars. Caffeine stimulates the brain and as a result is widely used to energize us in the morning and to help us stay awake at night if necessary. Too much caffeine, however, can irritate the digestive system and lead to a fast heart rate and raised blood pressure. Caffeine may also heighten feelings of anxiety and can be disruptive to sleep patterns.

WHAT IS A HEALTHY DIET?

A healthy diet needs to balance the consumption of the three basic nutrients – carbohydrate, protein and fat – and the micronutrients of minerals and vitamins. The healthiest diet relies heavily on sources of carbohydrate and protein and less on fat.

SOURCES OF CARBOHYDRATE

Carbohydrates – sugars and starches – are found abundantly in bread, potatoes, rice, cereals and pasta, most of which also provide rich sources of fibre. Wholegrain and unprocessed foods such as wholemeal pasta, brown rice and brown bread provide the healthiest carbohydrate sources but normal pasta, white rice and white bread also contain carbohydrate.

SOURCES OF PROTEIN

Meat and fish provide a rich source of protein and readily available energy. Furthermore, white meat from chicken and turkey contains a much lower proportion of fat than red meats such as beef and lamb. Eggs, fruits, nuts, beans, peas and lentils are sources of protein, and are particularly important foods for people following vegetarian and vegan diets.

SOURCES OF FAT

Fats are an important source of energy and supply the basic building blocks for your body's cells as well as helping you absorb certain vitamins. But the balance is important because too much fat, especially too much saturated fat, can lead to various health problems.

Try to choose most of your fat intake from the healthier unsaturated fats. These fats are believed to provide some protection against heart disease whereas saturated fats promote the clogging up of arteries in the body (atherosclerosis).

High levels of saturated fat are found in red meat, butter, some cheeses, some ice-creams and many biscuits, cakes and chocolate bars. Milk and dairy products can be high in fat but do supply rich sources of vitamins and minerals.

DEGREES OF SATURATION

The fats or oils you choose when cooking count in your fat consumption. Choose those from the unsaturated fats wherever possible to keep your intake of saturated fats to a minimum.

➤ Polyunsaturated fats:

Safflower oil.

Sunflower oil.

Corn oil.

➤ Monounsaturated fats:

Peanut oil.

Olive oil.

➤ Saturated fats:

Butter.

Coconut oil.

VITAMINS AND MINERALS

These micronutrients are found in abundance in fresh fruit and vegetables, nuts, beans, wholegrains, meat and fish. Most people can obtain enough vitamins and minerals from their diet and don't need to take daily supplements. (Although if you prefer to take a multivitamin then make sure it's a balanced one.) However, at certain times, such as during pregnancy or when breastfeeding, a person needs a higher supply of micronutrients, as do those with certain illnesses, such as the digestive condition coeliac disease.

▽ Choose your cooking oils wisely to increase the healthiness of a meal.

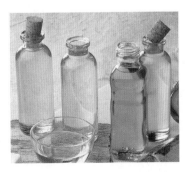

Weight control

SEE ALSO

➤ Heart disease, p282
➤ Obesity, p296
➤ Diabetes, p314
➤ Stroke, p328
➤ Osteoarthritis, p360

A healthy weight is one where you are not too thin (light) or too fat (heavy) for your height. Being overweight or obese puts your health at risk, but so does being underweight. A healthy weight is one that you can maintain throughout life; fluctuating weight levels push up your risk of disease. Since the 1950s, increasing affluence, poor eating habits and more sedentary lifestyles have meant that obesity has become much more common in developed countries. Obesity affects both men and women, and recently is increasingly apparent among children.

Healthcare professionals use a particular method of working out whether a person is a healthy weight for his or her height. This method is known as the body mass index or BMI. The values differ for men and women but the calculation is exactly the same.

WORK OUT YOUR BMI

BMI = your weight in kilograms divided by (your height in metres) squared. (To convert your weight from pounds to kilograms multiply by 0.4536; to convert your height from feet to metres multiply by 0.3048.)

For example, Nikki weighs 65 kg and is 1.64 metres tall, so her BMI is
$65 \div (1.64)^2 = 24.17$

A healthy weight/height balance should give a BMI of between 18.5 and 25. If your BMI is under 18.5 then you are underweight. If your BMI is over 25 then you are overweight and if it exceeds 30 you are obese. However, some people feel more comfortable at a higher weight while others feel healthier carrying less weight around.

ARE YOU A HEALTHY WEIGHT?

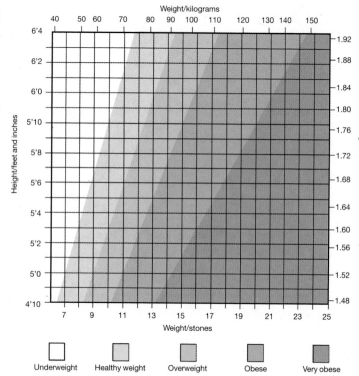

△ This chart shows at a glance whether your weight is healthy or unhealthy for your height. How does your weight score?

Underweight | Healthy weight | Overweight | Obese | Very obese

WEIGHTY ISSUES

Being overweight puts you at risk; obese people are more likely to suffer from:

➤ Heart disease.

➤ Stroke.

➤ Diabetes.

➤ Musculoskeletal problems, such as osteoarthritis.

WHAT ABOUT BODY FAT?

Sometimes the BMI reading alone is misleading and you may have to undergo a body fat measurement and waist–height ratio before your doctor decides if your weight is putting your health at risk.

Doctors also use waist size as another useful measurement of obesity and health risk. So whether you're an "apple" or a "pear" shape affects your heart's health. Fat around the waist indicates an increased risk of heart problems. A waist measurement of more than 89 cm (35 in) in women and 102 cm (40 in) in men indicates such a risk.

Although obesity is usually obvious, weightlifters or body builders, for example, have high BMIs but may well have a low proportion of body fat, which means that the risk of cardiovascular problems is low.

BURN CALORIES THROUGH EXERCISE

Exercise helps to use up calories and promote a higher level of health. If you are not used to exercising, simply taking a long, brisk walk two or three times a week will provide some benefit. But if you are able and motivated to exercise at a higher and more strenuous level, activities such as running, cycling and swimming are more effective at helping you to shed those unwanted pounds.

LOSING WEIGHT

If you have decided that you are overweight and wish to lose weight there are a number of important factors to consider:
• There are no short-term solutions.
• A short, sharp, shock diet is invariably followed by a gradual return to previous weight levels.
• Rapid weight loss is unhealthy.

It is probably a good idea to start out by assessing your diet and identifying high-fat and high-sugar foods that you eat. Try to calculate how many calories, on average, you usually consume; bear in mind that alcohol is high in calories – how often do you drink alcohol? If you do not eat much fat, you need to reduce your overall calorie intake or to increase your energy expenditure or both.

The recommended daily intake of

▽ Your waist measurement can help your doctor to work out whether your weight is unhealthy for your height.

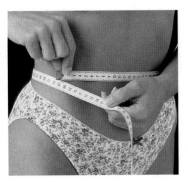

calories is 2000 for women and 2500 for men but if you are unsure and want to discuss your requirements further visit your doctor or dietitian for advice.

APPORTIONING YOUR CALORIES

To achieve a steady, healthy weight loss, you should aim to reduce your daily intake of calories by about 600. For most women, this means a daily intake of between 1200 and 1500 kcal while the figure for men stands at about 1750–1950 kcal.

So that you never go hungry, try to spread your allowance throughout the day. Eating smaller meals more frequently will help to maintain steady blood sugar levels and make you less likely to feel the urge to binge on unhealthy foods.

MAKE A PLAN AND STICK TO IT

Follow this advice for a successful weight-loss programme.
• Set realistic and achievable goals.
• Alter your diet with a view to maintaining any changes for life.
• Reduce your consumption of high-calorie foods, such as fried foods, red meats, cakes, chocolates and sweets, cheese and dairy products.
• Cut down your consumption of alcohol and fizzy drinks.
• Choose low-calorie foods such as fruits, vegetables and lean meats.
• Drink 1.5 litres (2½ pints) of water a day;

▽ If you are on a weight-loss diet check the scales once a week. Checking every day shows a negligible change and can be discouraging.

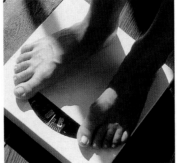

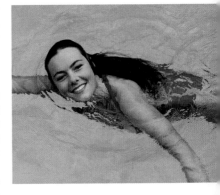

△ Swimming at least 20 lengths at your local pool can raise your metabolism, burn extra calories and help you to lose weight.

a good fluid balance improves health in general and assists the metabolic changes necessary to lose weight.

FIGHT MIDDLE-AGE SPREAD

Putting on weight as you get older is not inevitable. Although your body's metabolic rate slows down with age, the effect is modest. The best way to prevent weight gain during life is to remain physically active. Most people's middle-age spread is the result of becoming more sedentary but eating more or less as they did when they were active. This excess energy intake is stored in the body as fat.

HOW TO DIET EFFECTIVELY

➤ Avoid quick fixes.

➤ Do not undertake punitive short-term diets, as they are less likely to result in long-term weight loss.

➤ Only ever use slimming pills under the direct supervision of your doctor. Most slimming pills are amphetamines that suppress appetite but will also increase blood pressure and heart rate, cause insomnia and increase levels of anxiety.

Exercise for life

Most people are aware that regular activity is a vital part of a healthy lifestyle. However, that doesn't make it any easier to find the energy and time for exercise in our busy lives. However, there are plenty of options for improving health besides a strenuous session at the gym and simply deciding to walk to work can have significant health benefits. Studies have shown that increasing levels of physical activity on a day-to-day basis is the key to long-term health. So, take a new look at how you can build activities into your life every day.

The amount of exercise that people take during their lives has dropped significantly over the past 50 years or so. An increasingly mechanized, automated and computerized world has reduced the amount of walking and heavy work that most of us need to do. There is therefore a greater potential role for regular physical activity, which should ideally be encouraged from a young age.

HEALTH BENEFITS OF EXERCISE

It's never too late to become more active. Just look at the many health benefits:

• Cardiovascular – Exercise that speeds up

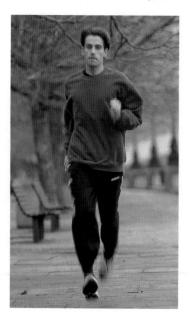

▽ Within four weeks of starting regular aerobic exercise, your heart and lungs will not need to work as hard so you will feel more energized.

GET THE GO-AHEAD FROM YOUR DOCTOR

If you haven't exercised for some time or are starting a new sporting pursuit then it is a good idea to visit your doctor. He or she can give advice on exercise intensity, assess your current fitness level and discuss the implication of any conditions you may have. In this way, you and your doctor can agree a safe but effective plan of action for exercising regularly.

the rate of the heart and is taken for at least 30 minutes, three or more times per week, is an effective way of promoting cardiovascular health. Such exercise – known as aerobic exercise – strengthens the heart muscle so that it becomes more efficient at pumping blood around the body. As a result your heart rate (or pulse) slows down, showing that you are becoming fitter. Regular cardiovascular workouts also improve circulation, lower blood pressure and reduce blood cholesterol levels.

• Respiratory – People with lung conditions such as asthma and chronic obstructive lung disease often find that doing exercise that makes them slightly out of breath helps to improve their lung capacity and breathing patterns.

• Musculoskeletal – Regular exercise will help to keep muscles, tendons and ligaments strong and supple, reducing the tendency to problems such as lower back pain, particularly later in life. Building strong muscles requires working against a resistance, which is often provided by weights. Strength-building exercises also serve to stabilize joints and reduce the effects of diseases such as rheumatoid arthritis. Weight-bearing exercises, such as walking, dancing or skipping, can build strong bones and help to counteract the natural tendency of the bones to thin with age – a condition known as osteoporosis.

• Psychological – People who are active or exercise regularly enjoy a strong feel-good factor. Exercise also helps to relieve stress, channel aggression, lift depression and promote good sleep.

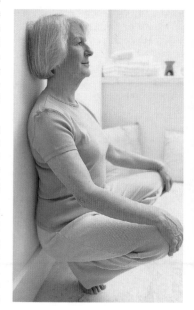

▽ Take time at the end of a workout to relax and stretch muscles. Cooling your body down in this way helps you to stay injury-free.

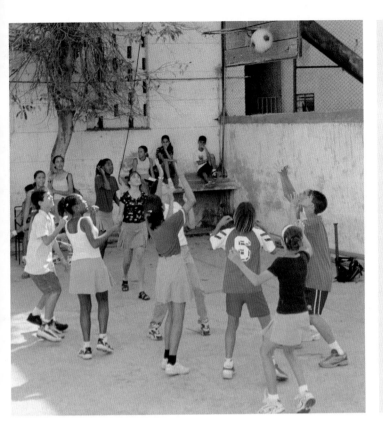

ADD UP YOUR ACTIVITIES

Experts agree that we should aim for 30 minutes of moderate activity five times a week. You can add up everyday activities – even cleaning and DIY – to see if you are meeting your quota. Aim for a weekly total of 2000 kcal for optimum health.

Activity	kcal/min
Dusting	3
Walking at 3km/h (2 mph)	3
Cycling at 9.5 km/h (6 mph)	4
Light DIY (decorating)	4
Light gardening	4
Mopping	4
Walking at 6.5 km/h (4 mph)	4
Vacuuming	4
Moderate DIY (carpentry)	6
Dusting and polishing	6
Scrubbing floors	6
Cycling at 16 km/h (10 mph)	7
Heavy DIY (e.g. mixing cement)	8
Heavy gardening	8
Cycling at 19 km/h (12 mph)	9

To work out how many calories you have burned, add up the minutes you spend doing each activity and multiply it by the value given in the table.

△ Taking part in team sports and games from an early age will help to develop physical and social skills that will be beneficial in adult life.

• Social – Many people enjoy playing as part of a team or in competitions. Such team activity expands your circle of friends and encourages feelings of mutual respect and shared responsibility while learning new skills.

WHICH ACTIVITY TO CHOOSE

This, of course, is a wholly personal choice. Some people naturally gravitate towards strenuous activities and thrive, while others never feel the need or desire to undertake such vigorous exercise.

The most important point to bear in mind is to choose an activity that you enjoy and is fun. Try to make time for regular periods of exercise (about three to five times a week). If you are not the gym-going type or running does not appeal to you, what about taking long walks, dancing or yoga?

As with all exercise and activity, it is important to have the proper equipment and any special training beforehand.

FITNESS PLANNING

When planning a structured exercise programme consider the following:

➤ Frequency – How often can you exercise?

➤ Intensity – How energetic do you want to be?

➤ Time – How long can you put aside for each exercise session?

➤ Type – What sort of activities do you enjoy doing?

WARM UP AND COOL DOWN

It can be easy to overexert yourself or pull a muscle when you start exercising so make sure that any bouts of activity are preceded by ten minutes or so of gentle "warm-up" exercises and stretches. Marching on the spot or cycling can raise your heart rate and the temperature of your muscles. Such aerobic activity should always be followed by some "cool-down" stretching exercises for the muscles and joints.

Never stop exercising so suddenly that you go straight from intense levels of activity to a complete standstill. Gradually step down the level of effort you put in towards the end of your session and then spend approximately 15 minutes stretching all the muscles you have worked. As well as improving your flexibility, such stretching will help reduce any stiffness in your muscles the next day.

Smoking and your health

In the Western world, almost 20 per cent of deaths are related to smoking. But despite such statistics, people continue to smoke and put their health at risk, mainly because they become addicted to the effects of nicotine in tobacco. This addiction puts the smoker in a vicious cycle or feeding his or her cravings. To be able to give up this disease-inducing habit, you must be motivated to do so and have a lot of willpower. Your doctor can discuss other strategies that can help you quit – it could well be the best health decision you ever make.

SMOKING HEALTH RISKS

There is overwhelming evidence to prove that smoking causes or is a contributory factor for a range of diseases, such as:

➤ Asthma.

➤ Bladder cancer.

➤ Chronic obstructive lung disease.

➤ Colorectal cancer.

➤ Excessive ageing of the skin.

➤ Heart disease.

➤ Lung cancer.

➤ Oesophageal cancer.

➤ Peptic ulcers.

➤ Stomach cancer.

➤ Stroke.

➤ Throat cancer.

Scientific studies have shown that smoking has various and wide-ranging effects (almost all harmful) on your body. There is also evidence that passive smoking increases the risk of disease.

SMOKE DAMAGE

• Cardiovascular system – Smoking encourages the development of atheroma, or fatty plaques, inside arteries around your body. Such furring up of arteries greatly increases the risk of heart attack and stroke. Smoking raises blood pressure and, by stimulating adrenaline production, it can cause disturbances to heart rhythms (arrhythmias). Smokers are more likely to develop clots in a blood vessel (thrombosis), which could prove fatal if part of the clot breaks off and travels to the lungs or the brain. Anyone who has smoking-induced lung disease will go on to develop smoking-related heart disease.

• Respiratory system – Toxic substances in cigarette smoke directly damage the protective linings of both the upper and the lower respiratory tracts. This makes it much easier for germs to invade and cause a respiratory tract infection, and it also increases the chances of developing asthma. Long-term smokers risk destroying their lungs, a condition known as chronic obstructive pulmonary disease. Smoking is the direct cause of 80 per cent of all cases of lung cancer.

• Digestive system – Nicotine acts on the digestive system in various ways via the bloodstream and by targeting the nerves supplying the digestive tract. Smoking promotes cancers of the oesophagus, stomach and colon/rectum. It also causes inflammation of the stomach and ulceration of its lining.

• Urinary system – Carcinogenic (cancer-causing) chemicals from inhaled tobacco smoke travel from the lungs in the bloodstream and promote cancer in other organs such as the bladder.

• Ears, nose and throat – The hundreds of harmful chemicals in tobacco smoke contribute to most cases of throat and laryngeal cancer.

• Skin – Smoking prematurely ages skin because, among other adverse effects, it is known to block blood vessels and limits the oxygen the skin needs to stay healthy.

• Pregnancy – Smoking is dangerous during pregnancy because the baby will be much smaller and its chances of survival are decreased. Children with parents who are smokers are more likely to suffer from asthma.

▽ As a smoker inhales, nicotine transfers from the tobacco onto tiny droplets of tar, which then travel deep into the lungs.

▽ This microscopic view of tissue taken from the lungs of a heavy smoker shows tar deposits clearly as black areas.

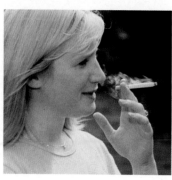

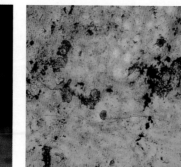

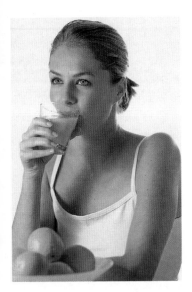

△ Orange juice accelerates the loss of nicotine from your body, which can help you fight your addiction more quickly.

GIVE UP FOR LIFE

Whatever your circumstances, giving up smoking increases both the quality and the quantity of your life. See how your body recovers from smoking's effects:

➤ After 20 minutes – Your circulation starts to improve.

➤ After 8 hours – Your blood can carry more oxygen as half of the carbon monoxide and nicotine have now been eliminated from the blood.

➤ After 24 hours – Your red blood cells are now fully loaded with oxygen as all carbon monoxide is now gone.

➤ After 2 days – All the nicotine has now been removed from your body.

➤ After 2 weeks – Your heart rate and blood pressure return to normal.

➤ After 5 years – Your risk of a heart attack is half that of a smoker.

➤ After 10–15 years – Your risk of lung cancer is half that of a smoker.

PLAN TO GIVE UP

Once you have decided that you want to stop smoking, make a plan and tell people that you are going to stop and ask for their support. Try some of the following tips on quitting smoking for good.

- Make a list of all the health benefits of giving up and stick it to the fridge or in another prominent place.
- Keep low-calorie snacks to hand to snack on when you get the urge to smoke.
- Start your day off with a glass of freshly squeezed orange juice. Not only does it taste great, it also speeds removal of nicotine from your body.
- Make a note of how much money you save each week by not smoking and then work out how much money you will save over the next year.
- Cut down on caffeine. Some research shows that caffeine can make nicotine cravings worse so reduce the amount of tea or coffee you drink.
- Avoid bars and alcohol for a while. Many people want a cigarette when they have a drink and so the association between the two is often strong.
- Use your willpower to avoid giving in to temptation. Having a few puffs on a cigarette will just weaken your resolve so do not be tempted. If you do succumb, do not despair – many ex-smokers were successful only on their second or third time around.

ADVICE FROM YOUR DOCTOR

From time to time your motivation and willpower will need an extra boost so ask your doctor to provide you with details of any reputable, specialist clinics or self-help groups that are available in your area. It is often useful to talk to other people about what they have found helpful.

One of the most effective strategies against nicotine addiction is to adopt a three-pronged attack:

- Nicotine substitution – Whether as patches or chewing gum, using nicotine substitution therapy for a few months may help to break the ritual habit of smoking while at the same time gradually reducing the body's dependence on this powerful chemical.
- Medication – Drugs are now available to help to reduce nicotine dependency. These drugs need to be taken under medical supervision over a period of several months and so far have shown encouraging results.
- Complementary treatments – Some therapies, such as acupuncture and hypnotherapy, help people stop smoking. Many therapists offer a money-back guarantee if you start smoking again. Be sure to visit qualified professionals.

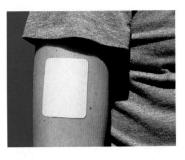

△ Nicotine patches deliver a continuous low dose of nicotine to the body. Some people find these helpful in the battle against smoking.

▽ Acupuncture – the placing of fine needles in specific "meridians" of the body – has helped many people to give up smoking.

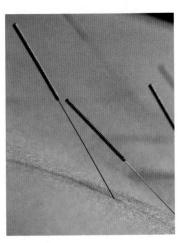

Sensible drinking

Alcohol is enjoyed by people around the world at all kinds of celebration and social occasion. It has a relaxing effect and complements the taste of many foods, but it can also cause considerable physical and psychological ill-health. A moderate intake of alcohol may protect against heart disease, but excessive binge drinking or sustained high intakes of alcohol can damage the liver irreparably and reduces life expectancy. Alcohol abuse and dependency can also cause or lead to serious physical, psychological and social problems.

When you drink alcohol, a small amount is absorbed in the stomach but the majority slips into your bloodstream via the small intestine. From here it goes to the liver, whose role it is to detoxify the blood and break down most of the alcohol. Excess alcohol then travels around the body, affecting different organs in various ways.

SHORT-TERM EFFECTS

Initially, alcohol depresses your central nervous system, leading to feelings of well-being and confidence and impaired judgement and thought processes. Your skin becomes redder as alcohol causes blood vessels in the skin to dilate. Alcohol also has a diuretic effect and so increases urine production, leaving you dehydrated.

▽ Drinking with friends can help you to relax after a day at work, but it is always a good idea to stay within your limits.

Heavier drinking may result in further effects on the nervous system, which include slurred speech, memory loss, lack of coordination and control of your body's movements, and aggressive and antisocial behaviour patterns.

IN THE LONG TERM

When alcohol is drunk in excess over long periods, there are a number of detrimental side-effects and social consequences. The physical effects are:
• Liver damage.
• Heart muscle damage.
• Impotence.
• Reduced fertility.
• Brain damage.
• Increased risk of cancers of the mouth, throat and oesophagus.
• Pancreatitis, a condition where the pancreas becomes inflamed.

WHY SOME PEOPLE CAN'T TOLERATE ALCOHOL

Some people seem to be quite incapable of metabolizing alcohol and for such people alcohol can be a very dangerous substance. Even very small amounts of alcohol result in rapid drunkenness and may precipitate collapse. This problem arises when enzyme systems within the digestive system are incapable of breaking down and detoxifying alcohol. Such enzyme deficiencies are more common among Asian populations.

As well as damaging your physical health, alcoholism has far-reaching psychosocial consequences, including:
• Loss of employment.
• Family and marital breakdown.
• Loss of friends.

BENEFITS OF DRINKING

Moderate alcohol consumption appears to have beneficial effects on the circulation and research has shown that it may even have protective effects on your heart. Scientists are studying different alcoholic drinks for their beneficial properties and it is believed that red wine might offer significant cardioprotective benefits.

WHAT'S IN AN ALCOHOL UNIT?

If you are planning to drive or operate machinery then any alcoholic drink, no matter how small, will affect your ability. Alcohol intake is measured in units. Current recommendations state that men should not drink more than 3–4 units a day

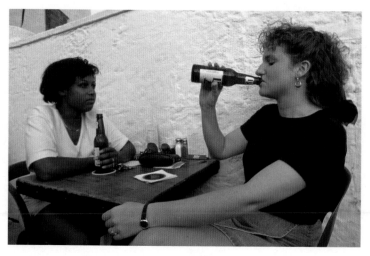

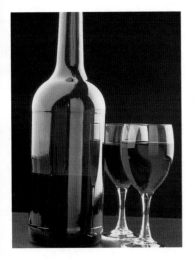

△ It is a good idea to be aware of the number of units you are drinking. For example, a small glass of wine counts as roughly one unit.

while for women the level is a maximum of 2–3 units. These recommendations were changed from weekly limits because there was a danger that people thought they could save up a week's worth of units and drink them all at the weekend.

One unit of alcohol is drunk in:
• Half a pint of beer (250 ml /8 fl oz).
• A small glass of wine (125 ml /4 fl oz).
• One measure of spirits (25 ml /⁴/₅ fl oz).

Beers, wine and spirits have very different strengths in terms of alcoholic content. Normal-strength beer, for example, may be 4 per cent alcohol whereas whisky is about 40 per cent; wine varies from 9 to 14 per cent (red wine is generally stronger than white wine).

ARE YOU DRINKING TOO MUCH ALCOHOL?

If you regularly drink more than the recommended safe limit of alcohol you could be putting your health at risk. Answer yes or no to the questions below (and be honest) to see if your drinking is affecting your lifestyle and whether it could soon become a habit that is controlling you.

1 Have you ever thought you should cut down on your drinking?
2 Have other people ever annoyed you by criticizing your drinking habits?
3 Have you ever felt guilty about your drinking?
4 Have you ever had an "eye opener" drink first thing in the morning?

If you said "yes" to two or more of the questions above, your drinking habits may be becoming problematic. Think about how you could reduce your alcohol consumption and perhaps make an appointment to visit your doctor for professional health advice.

WHEN DRINKING BECOMES A PROBLEM

Any of the following may indicate a potential problem with alcohol:
• Regular episodes of excessive consumption.
• Not being able to stop drinking once you have started.
• Days off work because of hangovers.
• Drinking in the morning.
• Not being able to remember what happened the previous night.
• Friends commenting on your drinking.
• Injury to yourself or someone else as a result of drinking alcohol.

WHERE TO GET HELP

Always consider consulting your doctor, who can help you assess the severity of your situation and consider appropriate strategies for dealing with the problem. Most countries have a range of specialist services available that can provide information, support and counselling. There are also centres that specialize in alcohol detoxification and rehabilitation. Certain drug treatments can also help people to stop drinking as well as reducing cravings for alcohol after stopping.

▽ Group therapy sessions at Alcoholics Anonymous have helped enormous numbers of people kick their addiction to alcohol.

METABOLIZING ALCOHOL

The rate at which alcohol is metabolized by the liver varies between individuals. It also depends on a person's weight, build, whether they are male or female and how regularly they drink alcohol (regular drinkers can metabolize it more quickly). On average, it takes 1 hour to eliminate 1 unit of alcohol from the body. But if you're having a heavy drinking session then your body can only deal with 1 unit per hour and so it takes a lot longer to metabolize the many units you've drunk during the evening. After a particularly drunken night out, you may still be intoxicated the next morning.

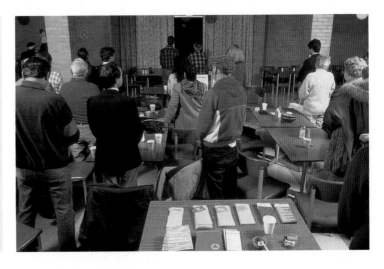

Routine health checks

There are a number of relatively simple interventions that can pick up potential medical problems before any symptoms or complications have developed. These are usually very simple tests that can be done or organized by your doctor. The number of these screening tests is gradually increasing. Many developed countries have national screening programmes for various types of cancer – breast cancer, cervical cancer, prostate cancer and colorectal cancer – while other vital checks monitor your hearing, sight, teeth, blood pressure and blood cholesterol.

Doctors now have a whole armoury of screening tests at their disposal to optimize their patients' health and to pick up any health problems as early as possible.

BLOOD PRESSURE MONITORING

Blood pressure rises gradually with age and this small increase is normal. Some people are more likely to develop high blood pressure as it may run in their family. High blood pressure increases the risk of several serious conditions but has no symptoms, which is why doctors often check your blood pressure as a matter of course. It is

▽ In one test in the haematology laboratory blood is placed in a tiny tube in a centrifuge machine and spun at high speeds to separate the blood cells from the blood plasma.

important that high blood pressure is picked up because most of the complications of this condition can be prevented by taking appropriate measures. This may involve lifestyle changes and/or taking regular medication.

It is recommended that you have your blood pressure checked on a regular basis, and ideally it should be checked by your doctor at least every two to three years from the age of 40 onwards.

BLOOD CHOLESTEROL TESTING

High levels of cholesterol have been linked to an increased risk of cardiovascular disease in general. A blood test measures cholesterol and other blood fats – what doctors refer to as your "lipid profile".

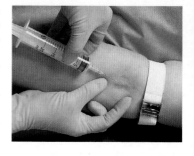

△ A sample of blood is taken from a vein in the arm. Several different tests can be carried out on one sample of blood.

Research has established healthy and "at risk" levels of blood cholesterol, but your age, blood pressure and whether or not you smoke must be taken into account. These levels are measured in millimoles per litre:
• More than 6.5 mmol/l means higher risk.
• Between 5.4 and 6.5 mmol/l means moderate risk.
• Less than 5.4 mmol/l means lower risk.

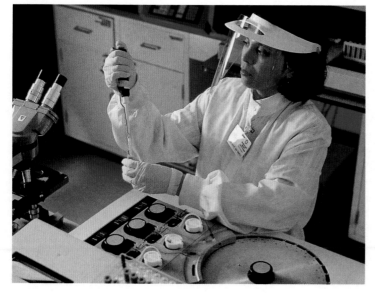

DENTAL CHECK-UPS
Regular trips to the dentist can help him or her spot the signs of gum disease early and give appropriate treatment. There may be some work needed, depending on how well you look after your teeth, to keep your oral hygiene to optimum standards. The gums are indicators of more general disease and your dentist may pick up early warning signs. Frequency of check-ups varies from dentist to dentist, but most recommend a six-monthly or annual check.

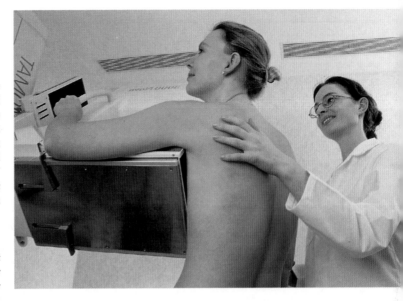

▷ Routine mammography screenings for breast cancer target older women, but many younger women also choose to be screened.

MAMMOGRAPHY

A mammogram is a simple X-ray of the breast to check for cancerous and precancerous tissue and hopefully catch the disease early on. It is routinely available in many developed countries for women between the ages of 50 and 65 and should be carried out every three to five years.

If your family has a history of breast cancer then routine screening from a much earlier age is very important.

CERVICAL SMEAR TESTS

A regular screening programme means that a cervical smear test can pick up on any cellular changes in the cervix so that further tests can be made and, if neccessary, treatment can begin before the development of cervical cancer.

A cervical smear test is a simple procedure that can take place at your doctor's surgery. The test will sometimes be done by your doctor but more often by the practice nurse. During an internal examination, a speculum is inserted in order to check the cervix. A spatula or small brush is then swept around the cervix to obtain a small sample of cervical cells. These samples are placed on a microscope slide and sent away to a hospital laboratory for analysis.

It is recommended that all women who are, or have been, sexually active have a smear test at least every three years.

PROSTATE TESTS

As a man ages, his prostate gland enlarges. In some men this is accompanied by cancerous changes. A blood test for prostate-specific antigen levels provides a non-specific indicator for prostate gland disease and the possibility of prostate cancer. This test is being increasingly used in men over the age of 50. It is hoped that this test will be done at regular and planned intervals in the future.

HEARING TESTS

Hearing becomes less acute with age. Over half of all people over the age of 70 have some degree of hearing loss, which is exacerbated when trying to hear above a background noise or music. Significant hearing loss may result in depression and loss of confidence.

It is not easy to monitor because it happens so gradually, but if you feel that you can't hear sounds well or clearly or if people have mentioned that you're not hearing what they say, ask your doctor to arrange a formal hearing test to see whether or not a hearing aid would correct the hearing deficiency.

EYESIGHT TESTS

It is normal for vision to diminish with age and this can often be corrected by an appropriate lens prescription for near and/or distant vision. As well as assessing your vision, ophthalmic practitioners can examine the eyes for evidence of cataracts and glaucoma, both of which become more common with age and which can be treated. Other diseases, such as diabetes or high blood pressure, can also be picked up because they affect your eyesight and your optician may refer you to your doctor for further tests. It is a good idea to have a routine eye check once a year, even if you don't wear glasses, because you don't always notice deterioration in your eyesight.

DIABETES

Your doctor can carry out a quick test to check a sample of your urine for signs of diabetes. Where there is a strong family history of diabetes, tests may be carried out on a frequent basis.

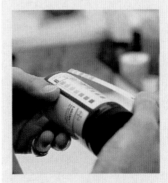

△ This simple dipstick test, to test urine for the presence of sugars, is over in under a minute or so.

Travel health and safety

Now that air travel is relatively inexpensive, more of us are travelling to exotic places. Whatever the destination, it is vital to know what precautions to take when travelling abroad – even for a two-week holiday. On the journey itself it is advisable to drink plenty of water, stretch your legs and avoid alcohol – to reduce the risk of deep vein thrombosis. Travel insurance comes high up the list of travel essentials, along with adequate planning in terms of prevention – via immunizations, malaria tablets and supplies of medicines.

PLANNING AHEAD

If you have a medical problem that requires attention from time to time, make sure you check out what medical facilities will be available at your destination. If you have a complex medical problem, visit your doctor or specialist so that they can write a medical summary for you to take with you.

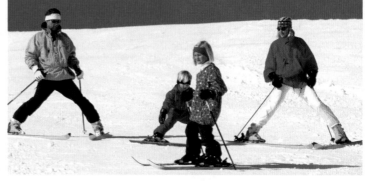

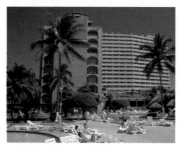

△ Even a short sun-and-sea package holiday will need some health preparation.

▽ Make sure you have sunscreen (minimum SPF15), and apply it often. Also remember that water intensifies the burning effects of the sun.

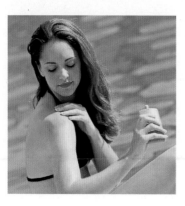

ESSENTIAL COVER

It is essential to take out suitable travel insurance before any holiday. It is also a good idea to make sure that your insurance cover is appropriate to the activities that you intend to undertake on your holiday. So, bear this in mind if your holiday involves high-risk activities such as skiing, diving or hang-gliding.

STOCK UP ON MEDICINES

If you have to take medicines on a daily basis, make sure that you have more than enough to take away with you. It is a good idea to carry medication, stored in its original containers, in your hand luggage in case your suitcases go missing en route.

ARE YOU UP TO DATE?

A minimum of six weeks before you go on holiday, you should visit your doctor or practice nurse for advice on which immunizations are recommended or essential for your intended destination. It is also advisable to find out whether you need

△ If you are going on a holiday that involves high-risk activities such as skiing, make sure that you have suitable medical cover.

to take antimalarial tablets and if you do which of the many types available provide the right protection for your destination.

SAFE SEX

Many sexually transmitted infections are contracted on holidays or trips abroad. The best method of protection against such infections is using a condom. Be prepared and take a plentiful supply with you as they may not be quite so easy to come by once you are overseas.

AVOID STOMACH UPSETS

If there are any doubts about the safety of local water, drink bottled water and also use it for brushing your teeth and rinsing your mouth. In places where the water is unsafe it is a good idea to have drinks without ice and avoid foods that may have been washed in local water, such as salads, raw vegetables, shellfish and unpeeled fresh fruit.

2

THE HEART AND CIRCULATION

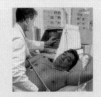

Your heart's beat is one of the most evocative sounds, symbolizing life itself. How you look after this amazing organ has great bearing on its health specifically and your health in general. Millions of people in the developed world suffer with disorders of the heart and circulation, many of which can be deadly. Because atherosclerosis and heart disease along with stroke are such major killers in the Western world, much medical research has already been done. Awareness of the major cardiovascular conditions, along with their symptoms, diagnosis, treatment and any preventative information, could help minimize your risk of such disorders.

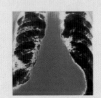

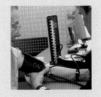

CONTENTS

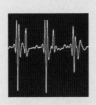

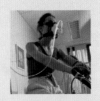

The cardiovascular system

Your heart and circulation are also known as the cardiovascular system (cardio means heart, vascular means blood vessels), and have developed to fulfil your body's constant need for oxygen and other nutrients dissolved in the blood. The driving force at the centre of this system is the heart, a powerful but simple pump. Every heartbeat pumps blood rich with oxygen and nutrients to every part of your body through a complex network of "pipes" – these are the blood vessels that carry the blood, and which make up the body's circulation system.

Your heart beats an amazing 100,000 times a day and has a pacemaker called the sinoatrial node, which sits in the right atrium. Electrical signals are generated from here and spread first to the atria, causing them to contract and push blood into the ventricles. After a short delay, which allows the ventricles to fill, the signals pass through the ventricles, which contract and pump blood out to the body and the lungs. Sometimes this pacemaker malfunctions and the heart beats more slowly or much faster than it should. In such cases, an artificial pacemaker can be installed to regulate its rate and rhythm.

MOVING BLOOD FORWARDS

To keep blood flowing in the right direction, there is a series of one-way valves. The mitral valve sits between the left atrium and ventricle, and the tricuspid valve sits where the right atrium and ventricle meet; these valves prevent backflow into the atria when the ventricles contract. Another pair of valves separate the ventricle from the arteries they pump into; these prevent blood flowing back into the heart when the ventricles relax. The aortic valve lies between the left ventricle and the aorta (the body's largest artery), and the pulmonary valve sits between the right ventricle and pulmonary artery.

When a doctor listens to your heart, he or she hears the familiar "lubb-dupp" sound; this sound is the snapping shut of the two pairs of valves. If the valves don't open or close properly, the blood can flow turbulently – like water down rapids – and cause extra sounds, known as a murmur.

THE HEART

▽ The heart is divided into a right and left side, and each side is divided further into an upper chamber (atrium) and a lower chamber (ventricle). The atria act as pre-filling chambers for the ventricles, which are the main pumping chambers. The left side pumps blood around the whole body so it is bigger and more powerful than the right side, which pumps blood around the shorter circuit to the lungs.

NOTE: Blue = deoxygenated (oxygen-depleted) blood; its oxygen has been used up by the body's cells. Red = oxygenated (oxygen-rich) blood. Blood vessels supplying the heart make sure that deoxygenated blood from the body is taken to and from the lungs to pick up oxygen and that oxygenated blood is pumped out to the body.

When the heart muscle contracts it is called systole (systolic pressure), and when the heart relaxes between contractions it is called diastole (diastolic pressure).

The difference in size between the two halves gives the heart its characteristic shape. Contrary to popular belief, the heart does not lie in the left side of the chest. It sits in the middle but the larger left side spreads to the left.

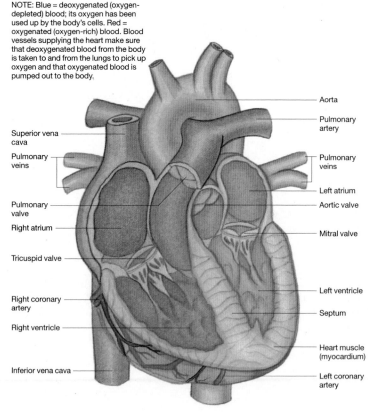

- Aorta
- Pulmonary artery
- Superior vena cava
- Pulmonary veins
- Pulmonary valve
- Right atrium
- Tricuspid valve
- Right coronary artery
- Right ventricle
- Inferior vena cava
- Pulmonary veins
- Left atrium
- Aortic valve
- Mitral valve
- Left ventricle
- Septum
- Heart muscle (myocardium)
- Left coronary artery

THE HEART AND CIRCULATION SYSTEM

▷ Mirroring the two sides of the heart, the circulation is made up of two separate systems – one supplying the body (systemic circulation) and one supplying the lungs (pulmonary circulation). The systemic circulation exits the heart from the left side and carries the blood to all parts of the body and returns to the right side of the heart. The pulmonary circuit carries blood from the right side of the heart to the lungs and then returns it to the left side, ready to be pumped around the body.

THE CIRCULATION SYSTEM

A journey around the body's circulation system begins in the heart's left ventricle. This contracting chamber forces a surge of blood into the aorta that passes through a network of ever-smaller arteries and capillaries. Blood then passes into bigger and bigger vessels until these form the vena cavae veins, which dump blood into the right atrium. From here, it passes into the right ventricle and is pumped into the pulmonary trunk and on to the lungs' capillaries. Here, oxygen dissolves into the blood and carbon dioxide is removed. Oxygen-rich blood travels through the pulmonary veins, into the left atrium and on to the left ventricle, ready to start the journey again.

THE BLOOD VESSEL "FAMILY"

There are five types of blood vessel – artery, arteriole, capillary, venule and vein. Arteries and arterioles carry blood away from the heart to the capillaries, which nourish the tissues, while venules and veins deliver blood back to the heart. The blood pressure in arteries is high and, because their walls are muscular and elastic, they pulse with the pressure wave of each heartbeat. By the time blood reaches the veins, blood pressure is very low. Veins have valves that snap shut to stop backflow and keep the blood flowing in the right direction as it travels back to the heart. If the leg valves deform and become blocked, they appear as purple "cords" of varicose veins.

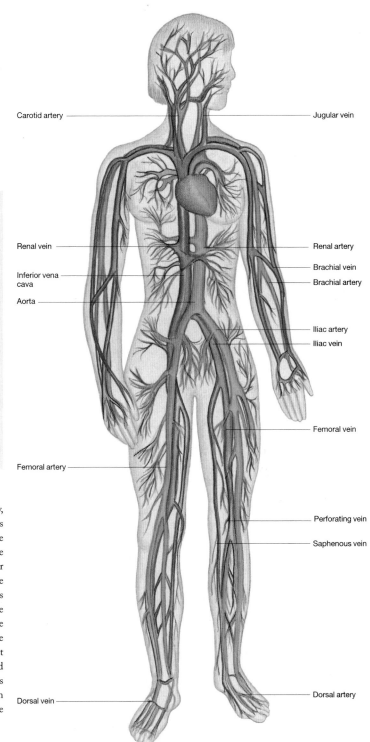

Carotid artery

Renal vein

Inferior vena cava

Aorta

Femoral artery

Dorsal vein

Jugular vein

Renal artery

Brachial vein

Brachial artery

Iliac artery

Iliac vein

Femoral vein

Perforating vein

Saphenous vein

Dorsal artery

High blood pressure

Persistently high blood pressure, also known as hypertension, can damage arteries and body organs, including the kidneys and the heart itself. This insidious disease is a major factor for heart disease, heart attacks and strokes. In fact, high blood pressure increases the risk of stroke six times and the risk of a heart attack threefold. Health education and screening programmes aid the early detection of high blood pressure and, together with improved treatments, have helped to significantly reduce the incidence of strokes and heart attacks.

Persistently high blood pressure is a common problem and it is important to treat it when it occurs because it significantly increases the risk of a stroke.

There are times when everyone's blood pressure is high. Your blood pressure fluctuates throughout the day, being lowest during sleep then rising on getting up, and reaching its higher value sometime mid-morning. On top of your normal values are times of stress, nervousness, excitement and physical activity – all of which raise your blood pressure.

Although people's blood pressure has a range of values that are acceptable, doctors will consider 120/80 mmHg as a "normal" reading. The first number of the reading relates to the blood pressure when the heart muscle contracts – systole – and the second number relates to pressure during its relaxation phase – diastole.

SIGNS AND SYMPTOMS

The difficulty with high blood pressure (hypertension) is that it usually occurs without any obvious symptoms. So, it is advisable to have regular health checks and to have your blood pressure checked at least every 4 to 5 years.

WHAT COUNTS AS HIGH BLOOD PRESSURE?

Most doctors agree that blood pressure is high if the reading is more than 150/95 mmHg (or 130/80 mmHg in people with diabetes). However, as blood pressure varies, it is important to take at least three consecutive high readings before a diagnosis can be made.

For some people, the very act of going to see a doctor or nurse makes their blood pressure shoot up – a phenomena known as "white coat hypertension". To obtain an accurate blood pressure reading, these patients may wear a small machine, that takes readings over a 24-hour period.

DIFFERENT TYPES OF HIGH BLOOD PRESSURE

There are three basic types of high blood pressure or hypertension:

1 Essential or primary hypertension – Nine out of ten people with high blood pressure have this type and the exact cause is unknown, although it involves many risk factors.

2 Secondary hypertension – About 10 per cent of people have high blood pressure due to another disease, such as kidney disease, rare endocrine disorders or heart valve problems, or in rare cases it is due to interactions with a drug.

MEASURING BLOOD PRESSURE

Doctors usually use a device called a sphygmomanometer to measure blood pressure, although some doctors now have electronic machines instead. This device has an inflatable cuff linked to a column of mercury or sprung dial. The blood pressure values are given in millimetres of mercury (written as mmHg for short).

A blood pressure reading is shown as two numbers, for example, 140/90 mmHg. The first number on the reading is the systolic pressure – the pressure when the heart contracts and when the pressure is at its highest. The second number is the diastolic pressure and corresponds to the

resting and therefore the lower pressure between the heartbeats.

The cuff is placed around the upper arm over the main artery – the brachial artery – and inflated to block the blood flow. The doctor places a stethoscope just below the cuff on the inside of the elbow. As the cuff is gradually deflated, blood rushes through the artery and this turbulent flow can be heard via the stethoscope (or microphone in electronic devices). The doctor can monitor the changes in the sounds and identify the point at which the blood is flowing smoothly (through the unsquashed brachial artery), this is the diastolic pressure.

▽ Routine blood pressure tests are vital for at-risk groups such as the elderly because hypertension may show no symptoms.

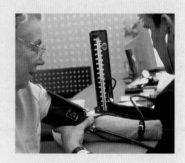

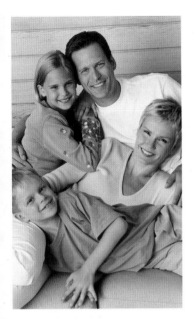

△ High blood pressure can run in families, so if this is the case in your family make an appointment for a check with your doctor.

3 Malignant hypertension – In this rare type, blood pressure can soar to dangerous levels, requiring urgent hospital treatment.

KNOW THE RISK FACTORS

High blood pressure can run in families, but doctors have identified other factors that can put you at risk of high blood pressure; some are similar to those for heart disease.
• Increasing age (as you get older, your arteries become stiffer and push your blood pressure up).
• Being overweight.
• Excessive alcohol consumption.
• Smoking.
• High-salt diet.

DIAGNOSING HIGH BLOOD PRESSURE

If your doctor measures your blood pressure and it is consistently high, they will also want to do a few extra tests. Tests include using a dipstick to check a sample of urine for the presence of protein (which would

indicate kidney damage) or glucose (which would indicate diabetes) as well as taking a blood sample to send to a laboratory to assess your kidneys' function. Your doctor may also examine the back of your eye using an ophthalmoscope as high blood pressure can cause damage to the light-sensitive layer of the retina. Other tests can be done to check for any underlying disorder and include a chest X-ray and electrocardiogram (ECG).

TREATMENT OPTIONS

The first line of treatment is not medication. Your doctor will recommend lifestyle changes to reduce high blood pressure. These changes include losing weight if overweight, reducing alcohol intake, cutting down salt consumption, taking regular exercise and, most importantly, giving up smoking.

Some doctors advocate biofeedback training. In biofeedback, you learn how to enter a relaxed state at will. Specialized equipment feeds back information about your heart rate, muscle tension and stress levels. You receive a continuous stream of this information as you practise certain relaxation techniques. In time, you learn to control your body's responses and help to reduce your high blood pressure.

If such measures fail, the next line of attack is drug therapy, which is a lifelong strategy. There are many antihypertensive drugs available; the common groups are:
• Thiazide diuretics.
• Beta-blockers.
• ACE inhibitors.
• Calcium antagonists.
• Alpha-blockers.

Many doctors use a thiazide or beta-blocker as first-line treatment; although ACE inhibitors work better for people with diabetes. Many antihypertensive drugs can cause side-effects, making people reluctant

▷ If the heart works against high pressure over a long period of time, the heart muscle becomes thicker – indicated in red on this coloured chest X-ray image.

HIGH BLOOD PRESSURE DURING PREGNANCY

Pregnant women will have their blood pressure checked at regular intervals during their pregnancy as high blood pressure can indicate one of two serious conditions – pre-eclampsia and eclampsia. These conditions occur in about 5–10 per cent of pregnancies and in severe case can be life-threatening for both the mother-to-be and her developing baby. Left untreated, pre-eclampsia and eclampsia can cause seizures and result in coma. Pre-eclampsia and eclampsia are probably caused by a placental problem.

to continue taking their medicine. It is important to bear in mind that the benefits of treatment include significantly reducing the risk of a heart attack or stroke. This is particularly pertinent for people with diabetes, who are more susceptible to the effects of high blood pressure.

It is quite usual to have to take two or more drugs. Furthermore, you may have to try several combinations until you find the one that works for you.

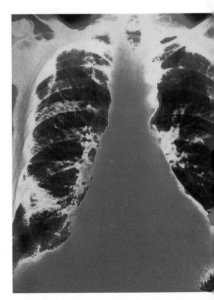

Atherosclerosis

Atherosclerosis is the furring up of arteries by the formation of fatty plaques called atheroma. Such narrowing of the arteries restricts blood flow and oxygen supply to the body's tissues. Atherosclerosis can affect arteries in any part of the body, the most serious, being when it blocks up the heart arteries or those that supply the brain. There are often no symptoms – the first sign could be a heart attack. It is vital, therefore, that you recognize the risk factors and do all you can to minimize your risk of atherosclerosis and any associated conditions.

The word "atherosclerosis" comes from Greek – *athere* meaning porridge and *skleros* meaning hardening. This word derivation conjures up an image of exactly what happens as atherosclerosis develops.

The plaques that form and fur up arteries are made of atheroma – this is a mixture of cholesterol, dead muscle cells, fibrous tissue, clumps of platelets and sometimes calcium.

NO ARTERY IS SAFE

Atherosclerosis can silt up arteries in any part of the body and may affect:

• The heart, causing heart disease (the coronary vessels are easily blocked).
• The brain, causing a stroke.
• The legs, causing poor circulation (see box on peripheral vascular disease) or even gangrene.
• The intestine, causing parts to die.

PERIPHERAL VASCULAR DISEASE

If the fatty deposits of atherosclerosis form in arteries taking blood to the legs, most commonly in the arteries of the pelvis and the artery just above the knee, they will cause the leg muscles to become cramped and painful with exertion. This pain usually occurs in the calf muscle and subsides with rest. Doctors refer to this condition as intermittent claudication. As the blockage gets worse, the exercise needed to produce the pain gets less until pain may be present even at rest. In this situation the leg barely has enough blood to survive and, if left untreated, gangrene will develop, possibly requiring an amputation.

As with all effects of atherosclerosis, you can help to prevent such a condition developing by giving up smoking and exercising regularly. The exercise will prevent the claudication from worsening and in many cases will improve it. If the condition is very severe, surgeons can bypass the blocked vessel using a patient's own vein or an artificial artery.

RECOGNIZE THE RISK

There are a number of well-recognized risk factors for atherosclerosis, and of these many can be changed for the better. Making changes to these risk factors where possible saves lives.

These factors fall into two categories: those you can change and those you cannot. Because some of these risk factors are unchangeable, it is all the more important that you reduce those that you do have the power to change.

HOW ATHEROSCLEROSIS DEVELOPS

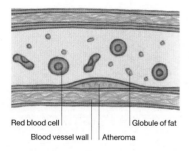

Red blood cell | Globule of fat
Blood vessel wall | Atheroma

1 The underlying process of atherosclerosis can start even before you are born. A tiny deposit, or plaque, mainly of fats – called an atheroma – develops on the inside of a blood vessel wall.

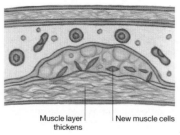

Muscle layer | New muscle cells
thickens

2 Over years this plaque grows, furring up the artery and reducing the blood flow. If the flow of blood in the arteries in the legs is reduced, for example, it can cause pain on walking, known as claudication.

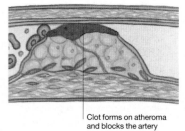

Clot forms on atheroma
and blocks the artery

3 As the plaque grows it can split and rupture. If this happens, the body forms a clot on the plaque. This clot and plaque can permanently block the blood vessel, starving the tissue of vital oxygen.

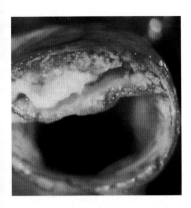

△ This magnified view of a slice through an artery shows a thick deposit of atheroma caused by atherosclerosis.

CHANCE FACTORS

The non-modifiable risk factors include:

- Age – The older you are, the greater the risk of developing this condition.
- Ethnicity – Studies have shown that some ethnic groups are more likely to suffer from atherosclerosis.

ANEURYSMS

Another result of atherosclerosis is a weakening of the blood vessel wall caused by the fatty deposits. A weak spot in the wall can balloon and form an aneurysm. Aneurysms most commonly affect the aorta, especially as it passes through the abdomen. As an aneurysm gets larger it becomes increasingly likely to burst, which can cause sudden and massive blood loss and is usually fatal.

Aortic aneurysms are usually detected by chance when a doctor examines your abdomen or an investigation is done for another reason. If they are detected they can be repaired surgically. This is a major operation, but has a very good success rate. Sometimes an aneurysm may leak before it bursts, resulting in severe sudden back pain that radiates to the thighs. In this case, surgeons can try to repair the aneurysm before it bursts and prevent future ruptures.

- Genetic inheritance – Heredity plays a part in the health of the cardiovascular system and atherosclerosis often runs in families. The inherited condition hyperlipidaemia, which causes high levels of fat in the blood, also increases the risk of atherosclerosis.
- Gender – Men are more likely to suffer from atherosclerosis because it seems that the production of oestrogen protects women against the development of atheroma but it is not clear if this protection continues after menopause for those taking hormone replacement therapy. The risks even out once women stop producing oestrogen.
- Diabetes – People with diabetes are at high risk of developing atherosclerosis because it can be associated with high cholesterol levels. In diabetes, the fatty plaques form much faster. Well-controlled glucose levels lessen the risk but it is especially important to control other factors, such as high blood pressure and high blood cholesterol levels.

CHOICE FACTORS

Factors you can influence for the better include the following:

- Smoking – Cigarette smoking promotes atheroma formation within the arteries.
- High blood pressure – Hypertension increases your risk of atherosclerosis.
- High blood cholesterol levels – Recent studies have shown that high levels of cholesterol in the blood increase the risk of atherosclerosis.
- Obesity – Being overweight or obese is linked both to poor cardiovascular health in general and to a higher risk of atherosclerosis.
- Inactivity – Regular physical exercise lowers the risk of atherosclerosis.

It would be a mistake to think you are too young to worry about atherosclerosis because it can be present for years before it causes symptoms. The first signs can start in adolescence – or even in childhood – so the earlier you make changes the better.

ASPIRIN – A WONDER HEART DRUG

The humble aspirin in small doses is the most useful drug doctors have for treating heart disease. It thins the blood, thereby preventing clots forming on fatty plaques, and also slows the growth of the plaques themselves. In cases of heart disease, angina or after a heart attack, doctors will prescribe a daily dose of aspirin (75 mg, one quarter-strength aspirin tablet).

PREVENTING ATHEROSCLEROSIS

Your doctor will discuss your risk factors and recommend lifestyle changes you can make. You may have a cholesterol test, where a sample of your blood is analysed in a laboratory. Your doctor will check your "lipid profile" for values of HDL and LDL cholesterol (high- and low-density lipoproteins). HDLs give some protection against arterial disease but LDLs do not.

Cholesterol levels can be kept low by eating plenty of fresh fruit and vegetables and cutting down on animal fats, such as full-fat milk, cheese, eggs and red meat. However, someone with high cholesterol levels will probably take cholesterol-lowering drugs as well as eating a low-fat diet. Recent studies have shown that these drugs improve the long-term risk of developing heart disease.

▽ Regular activity from an early age can help prevent the development of tiny plaques of atheroma within the arteries.

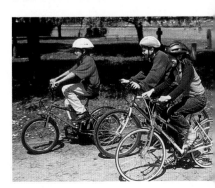

Heart disease

Heart disease is inextricably linked with atherosclerosis and the two are responsible for the biggest cause of death in the Western world. When atherosclerosis furs up the heart's arteries it is known as coronary artery disease or heart disease. As with atherosclerosis, it is vital to know if any risk factors for heart disease apply to you and then take steps to minimize these. Heart disease may develop insidiously and the first symptom could be a heart attack. It is never too early to start looking after your heart and visiting your doctor for a check-up if necessary.

When one or both of the heart's coronary arteries is blocked by deposits of atheroma, the tissue beyond the blockage no longer receives a blood supply and so the heart muscle dies due to oxygen starvation.

KNOW THE RISK FACTORS

There are well-recognized risk factors for heart disease and these mirror those for atherosclerosis. In order to assess your risk factors, your doctor will probably ask you questions about your state of health, diet, exercise habits and smoking as well as checking your blood pressure.

SIGNS AND SYMPTOMS

In the early stages of heart disease there may be no symptoms. In later stages, the first symptom is usually chest pain (angina) on physical exertion or a heart attack. Some people develop arrhythmias (see box) and suffer from associated palpitations and dizziness.

Some risk factors you can change and some you cannot. So it is vital to reduce any choice factors that apply to you.

CHANCE FACTORS

The non-modifiable risk factors include the following:
- Genetic inheritance – Heart disease often runs in families and is more common in people from northern Europe.
- Gender – Statistically women under 65 are less likely to suffer heart disease than men under 65; oestrogen offers women protection until menopause but then the risk rises to equal that of men.
- Ethnicity – Some ethnic groups have been shown to be at higher risk of suffering from heart disease.

HEART ARRHYTHMIAS

You may have felt at times that your heart is pounding, thumping or racing, especially when you are feeling anxious. Such palpitations can be explained by the fact that you have suddenly become aware of the beating of your heart (something you may not normally notice). However, such abnormal heart rhythms – also known as arrhythmias – can occur due to clogging of the heart's arteries by heart disease.

- Atrial fibrillation – In this common abnormal rhythm, the atria of the heart fail to contract properly, causing the heart to beat irregularly and sometimes to beat incredibly fast. The person may become short of breath and faint. It can be controlled or corrected with drugs. A small electric current (defibrillation) may be passed through the heart to restore normal atrial rhythm.

- Ventricular fibrillation/tachycardia – If the heart's ventricles enter one of these rhythms the heart stops and the person collapses and loses consciousness. No blood flows to the brain and death can occur quickly. Cardiopulmonary resuscitation (CPR, or mouth-to-mouth) keeps blood flowing to the brain and allows time for medical or paramedical staff to attempt to restart the heart.

- Bradycardia – In this condition the heart beats abnormally slowly, causing a person to feel very unwell, short of breath and faint. It can occur as a side-effect of certain heart drugs but may also result from a heart disorder. If this condition persists, a person may have to undergo surgery to have a temporary or permanent artificial pacemaker fitted which will restore a normal rhythm to the heartbeat.

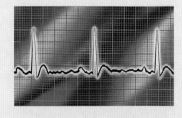

△ This electrocardiogram (ECG) shows the electrical activity in a normal heart.

▽ This ECG shows abnormal activity within the heart's electrical system, in this case causing a fast heartbeat (tachycardia).

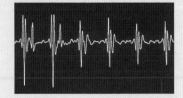

HEART MURMURS

When blood flows through the heart it usually does so silently and smoothly. Sometimes the blood may become turbulent – like water rushing down river rapids. This turbulent flow causes a heart murmur. The commonest murmur is a flow murmur. It is completely normal and shows that a healthy heart is beating vigorously enough to cause turbulent blood flow. The exact nature of a murmur is best confirmed using the diagnostic technique of ultrasound scanning of the heart – known as echocardiography.

In children, abnormal murmurs are most often due to "holes in the heart". In most cases this causes no problems, but the condition can be corrected surgically if necessary.

In adults, an abnormal murmur may be the result of a heart attack or it can be due to a heart valve that was damaged by rheumatic fever as a child. Most adult murmurs need no treatment apart from antibiotic protection during any invasive procedure, such as operations or dental extractions. Artificial or pig heart valves can be used to replace severely damaged valves.

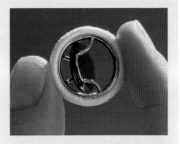

△ Surgeons can replace faulty valves that may cause a murmur with artificial ones.

- Age – In general, heart disease is more common with increasing age.
- Diabetes – People with diabetes are at high risk of developing heart disease and stroke. Well-controlled glucose levels lessen the risk but it is especially important to control other risk factors.

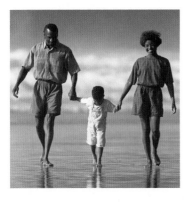

△ Studies have shown that African-Americans are more at risk from heart disease. Take care of your heart to ensure that it is as healthy as it can be and visit your doctor regularly.

CHOICE FACTORS

If the following factors apply to you it is important to remember that you have the power to change them.

- Smoking – Between 30 and 40 per cent of deaths from coronary artery disease can be attributed to smoking. The more you smoke, the higher the risk – there is

▷ This coloured angiogram shows a blockage in one of the heart's coronary arteries. Such a blockage could cause a heart attack.

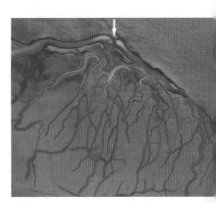

no safe level. Even one cigarette a day increases the risk of heart disease. After quitting the level of risk decreases rapidly, although it can take up to 20 years to dwindle to that of a non-smoker.
- High blood pressure – Hypertension increases your risk of heart disease threefold. If you manage your high blood pressure, your risk is reduced, although it is still higher than someone with normal blood pressure.
- High cholesterol levels – Doctors now know that there is a direct link between high levels of cholesterol in the blood and the risk of heart disease.
- Obesity – Being overweight is linked to poor heart health and the risk of heart disease can be easily three times more than a person of healthy weight.
- Inactivity – Regular physical exercise can dramatically reduce the risk of developing heart disease.

TREATING HEART DISEASE

The treatment options for heart disease are covered on the next pages when we look at the commonest symptom of heart disease – angina. Symptoms can be controlled with drugs but in severe cases or after a heart attack surgery may be the only option.

HEART INFECTIONS

Infections of the heart, particularly of the heart valves (rheumatic fever and endocarditis) used to be quite common, but occur less and less in the developed world. Pericarditis, an inflammation of the tough fibrous sac around the heart (the pericardium), is quite common and may be due to infection by viruses, bacteria or fungi. Symptoms include crushing pain in the centre of the chest and shortness of breath. Fortunately this condition is most often caused by a virus and will settle, leaving no long-term damage. Occasionally fluid may build up around the heart, which can interfere with its beating and so doctors will operate to drain this in order to restore normal heart function.

Angina

Angina is chest pain that originates in the heart muscle itself. The blood vessels taking blood to the heart – the coronary arteries – can become partially blocked with the fatty plaques caused by atherosclerosis (in this case also known as heart disease). There may be enough blood for the heart at rest, but during activity – when the heartbeat can increase from 75 to 190 beats per minute – the muscle cannot get enough blood and it "hurts". This is reflected by the fact that angina is brought on by exercise but subsides when activity is stopped and the person rests.

SIGNS AND SYMPTOMS

Angina can be mild or severe. The pain, which is heavy or crushing, is typically in the centre of the chest and can radiate up the neck and down the arms, most commonly the left arm. You may also feel short of breath and sweaty.

Angina is not easy to diagnose from physical symptoms, particularly as the symptoms of other conditions, such as indigestion, are similar.

HOW IS IT DIAGNOSED?

Testing usually begins with an exercise electrocardiogram (ECG) – where you walk on a treadmill (or cycle on an exercise bike) while hooked up to a machine that records the heart's electrical activity. The level of exercise is slowly increased until the patient feels pain and the electrocardiogram pattern changes.

Further tests include a coronary angiogram, in which you lie flat on a table and a doctor inserts a fine tube into your heart via an artery in your groin. A special dye is injected into the arteries and X-ray pictures are taken. Any narrowed arteries are clearly visible on the X-ray images.

TREATMENT OPTIONS

Angina usually responds well to drug treatment. The most common drugs used in treating angina are the following:

- Nitrates – These drugs come as fast-acting sprays or tablets that go under the tongue and ease the pain during an angina attack. Daily long-acting tablets reduce the need for the sprays.
- Beta-blockers – These tablets reduce the workload of the heart, prevent pain and slow the gradual worsening of angina.
- Calcium antagonists – These drugs ease the heart's workload to help prevent pain.

A standard treatment is a low, daily dose of aspirin to prevent more atheroma from building up within the heart's arteries.

LIFESTYLE ISSUES

Once angina is diagnosed, your doctor will assess your risk factors for heart disease and probably suggest lifestyle changes, such as quitting smoking or a low-fat diet.

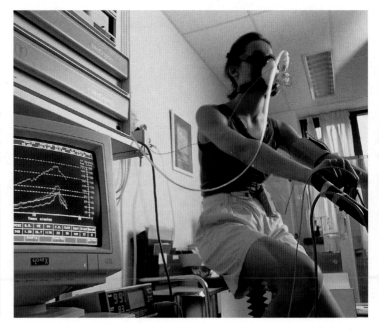

▽ During an exercise ECG electrodes attached to the chest relay information about the heart's electrical activity while a cuff on the arm monitors blood pressure.

UNSTABLE ANGINA

Angina gets worse over time and less and less activity will provoke the pain. If your angina suddenly worsens or you are experiencing pain at rest, it could be due to a blocked coronary artery causing a heart attack. If this happens, you should see a doctor urgently.

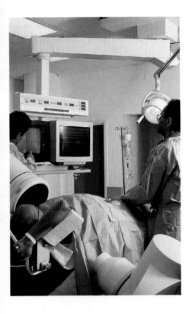

◁ This surgeon is carrying out an angioplasty. A balloon catheter is inserted into the patient's groin and advanced slowly up an artery into the heart. Once in the partially blocked coronary artery, the balloon is inflated and deflated to widen the artery and increase blood flow.

MEDICAL INTERVENTIONS TO TREAT BLOCKED ARTERIES

There are two levels of intervention for reinstating blood supply to the heart muscle once a coronary artery has become blocked or narrowed by plaques of atheroma. The intervention chosen will depend on how badly the arteries are narrowed. As with any operation, these carry certain risks.

1 Angioplasty – During this procedure for narrowed but not completely blocked arteries, a fine hollow tube (catheter) is inserted into your heart and a tiny balloon at the catheter's tip is inflated and deflated a few times to squash the plaque and widen the artery. Such a procedure is carried out on an outpatient basis and is performed using local anaesthetic

2 Bypass surgery – If coronary arteries are very narrow or completely blocked, a new route for the blood supply is made using what is known as a bypass graft. Surgeons have two options for the bypass graft – they either use an artery that already lies within your chest or they remove a piece of a vein from your leg. Sometimes a person may have two, three or four blockages to bypass. In these cases the procedure would be called a double, triple or quadruple bypass. Bypass surgery is done under general anaesthetic and takes between three and five hours. It is now one of the most frequently performed surgical procedures.

BYPASS SURGERY OPTIONS FOR BLOCKED CORONARY ARTERIES

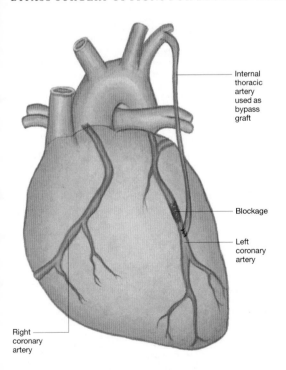

Internal thoracic artery used as bypass graft

Blockage

Left coronary artery

Right coronary artery

△ In the first option, heart surgeons detach an artery – the internal thoracic artery – from the chest wall and re-attach it beyond the blockage to reinstate the heart muscle's continuous blood supply.

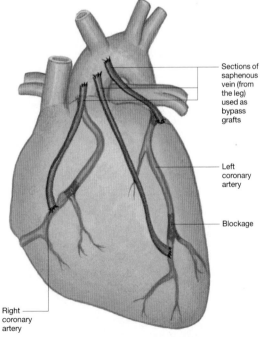

Sections of saphenous vein (from the leg) used as bypass grafts

Left coronary artery

Blockage

Right coronary artery

△ Alternatively, pieces of a vein in the inside of the leg – the saphenous vein – are removed and cut into sections, which can then be used to re-route the blood supply around any number of blockages.

Heart attack

SEE ALSO

➤ High blood pressure, p278
➤ Heart disease, p282
➤ Angina, p284
➤ Diabetes, p314

A heart attack, or myocardial infarction, occurs when a blood vessel has become blocked. When a part of the heart muscle loses its blood supply in this way it can suffer irreversible damage and die. Having a heart attack can be a very frightening experience but a large proportion of heart attack sufferers return to normal life after a recovery period. A heart attack can also damage the heart's pacemaker and cause arrhythmias. Studies have shown that one in four heart attacks goes unnoticed – these "silent" heart attacks only become apparent on ECGs.

SIGNS AND SYMPTOMS

The pain of a heart attack is similar to angina but may be more severe. It also lasts longer than angina pain, is not eased by rest and is not relieved by nitrate sprays or tablets. Symptoms include shortness of breath, sweating, nausea and dizziness. An angina sufferer who has chest pain for more than 20 or 30 minutes may be having a heart attack and should seek urgent medical help.

The key to a good outcome in treating a heart attack is speed in clearing the blockage in the artery so that there is less likely to be permanent damage to the heart.

ACTION AT THE HOSPITAL

• On arrival, an ECG test or blood tests confirm a diagnosis instantly.

▽ Speed is key to the successful treatment of a heart attack. Ambulance paramedics can start treatment on the way to hospital.

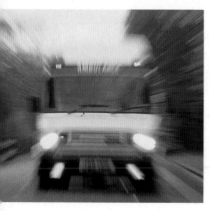

• The first treatment is aspirin, which will be given by the ambulance crew or your doctor to prevent further clot formation.
• Oxygen given via a mask will also help limit the damage.
• Morphine or another strong opiate may be given to lessen the pain.
• Doctors will try to dissolve the clot causing the blockage using drugs or may have to perform an angioplasty.

TYPICAL REHABILITATION SCHEDULE

DAY 1
Sit up and walk around the bed. Perform breathing exercises in bed.

DAYS 2 AND 3
Get up without help and take short walks to the bathroom.

DAYS 4 AND 5
Walk with the cardiac physiotherapist along hospital corridors.

DAYS 6 AND 7
Continue walking further each time; go home Day 7 if have not before.

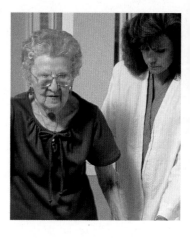

△ A rehabilitation schedule means that, with expert help, a patient can make as fast a recovery as possible after a heart attack.

LIFE AFTER A HEART ATTACK

The first step to recovery is to build up the heart again to cope with everyday life. So, during your week's hospital stay you won't just rest in bed, you will start special exercises, usually with a physiotherapist or cardiac nurse. Risk factors for heart disease have to be identified and changes made to prevent future heart attacks.

Many people recover completely from a heart attack, and it is largely due to a structured rehabilitation programme. Positive thinking also plays an important part in the recovery. It is easy to become depressed after such a life-threatening event – many people fear another attack and that can be enormously stressful. Studies have shown that a positive attitude speeds up the recovery process and return to a normal life.

Heart failure

SEE ALSO
- Heart disease, p282
- Obesity, p296
- Diseases of the thyroid gland, p316
- Anaemia, p450

Heart failure does not mean that the heart has stopped working; it indicates that it has become less efficient at pumping blood around the body and so cannot meet the body's constant demand for oxygen-rich blood. This condition tends to be most common in those over the age of 80 and is afflicting increasing numbers of people in developed countries every year. The degree to which someone is affected by their heart failure varies: some individuals have no symptoms at all while others may be severely disabled by the restricted mobility it confers.

The heart has two sides and either side or both can be affected by heart failure. In left heart failure, the left ventricle is unable to pump oxygen-rich blood out to the body and so fluid accumulates in the lungs, known as pulmonary oedema. Right-side heart failure causes fluid to build up in the body tissues – the legs, ankles and feet being the most obvious places. Initially, only one side may be affected but in time both sides usually fail.

CAUSES OF HEART FAILURE

Any disorder that affects the heart's ability to pump blood effectively can cause heart failure. About 70–80 per cent of cases are due to damaged heart muscle from heart

▽ Ultrasound scanning of the heart, known as echocardiography, is used to assess the heart's structure and function.

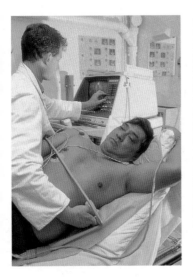

disease and/or a heart attack. High blood pressure is another common cause: a heart that has pumped against high pressure for years on end suffers from the strain put on the muscle tissue. Other conditions that can also lead to heart failure are leaking or stiff heart valves, and, rarely, anaemia, extreme obesity and hyperthyroidism.

MAKING LIFESTYLE CHANGES

Once a diagnosis of heart failure has been made, your doctor will talk to you about how making simple changes to your everyday life can also help your condition. You should avoid strenuous exercise, although gentle exercise can actually help your condition. Smoking should definitely be given up and being overweight puts unnecessary strain on your heart. Avoiding salty foods is also a good idea.

SIGNS AND SYMPTOMS

Many people suffer heart failure without any symptoms whatsoever, especially in the early stages of the disease. When symptoms do eventually become apparent, they may include:

- Muscle weakness and fatigue.
- Loss of appetite.
- Cold hands and feet.
- Swollen ankles.
- Breathing difficulties (typically in left-sided heart failure) such as shortness of breath, which often becomes worse when lying flat and on exertion.

HOW IS IT DIAGNOSED?

Your doctor may make a diagnosis after asking you about your symptoms and an examination. He or she may want to carry out a few confirmatory tests, such as:

- ECG – This test assesses the electrical activity within the heart.
- Chest X-ray – This imaging technique checks the size of the heart and whether there is fluid on the lungs.
- Echocardiography – This investigation looks at the heart's internal structure and function.

TREATMENT OPTIONS

Although heart failure is a progressive disease, current drug treatments are powerful and have been shown to improve the length and quality of life for people suffering from the condition. Heart failure cannot be cured but it can be controlled, and your doctor may prescribe the following drugs as part of a long-term treatment:

- Diuretics – These drugs eliminate excess fluids via the kidneys. This reduces the amount of blood to be pumped and decreases the strain on the heart.
- ACE inhibitors – These drugs work by widening the blood vessels, thereby reducing the workload of the heart.

Drug therapy is usually successful at treating symptoms and improving quality of life. Unfortunately, heart failure is a progressive disease and so tends to become more severe over time.

Thrombosis and embolism

SEE ALSO

➤ Exercise for life, p266

➤ Travel health and safety, p274

➤ Obesity, p296

➤ The roles of blood and lymph, p448

In thrombosis, a blood clot (or thrombus) forms in a blood vessel and blocks the blood flow. Occasionally clots form spontaneously, most commonly in the veins of the legs. Clots below the knee are very common and don't usually cause problems; if the clot sits above the knee, the affected leg can become hot, swollen and painful, indicating a deep vein thrombosis. If a fragment of clot – called an embolus – breaks off, it travels through the heart and circulation until it becomes stuck in a blood vessel. An embolus lodged in the lung is potentially fatal.

Blood clotting is a vital survival mechanism, but when the blood clots for no reason it can be very dangerous. A clot can form in any artery or vein in the body, but most commonly in the veins in the legs, due to a lack of movement of the blood flow. If such a clot forms in a deep vein, in the leg or in an artery, it can be serious and needs prompt medical diagnosis and treatment.

If a clot, or a clot fragment, blocks an artery, blood cannot reach the tissues. If a blockage occurs in an artery supplying the brain, lungs or heart, it could be fatal.

KNOW THE RISK FACTORS

Many factors increase the chance of developing a deep vein thrombosis:

• Family history.
• Obesity.
• Smoking.
• Immobility, such as sitting for long periods during a long journey or while recovering from surgery.
• Dehydration.
• Drugs, such as the contraceptive pill.
• Surgical procedures.

SIGNS AND SYMPTOMS OF THROMBOSIS AND DVT

The symptoms of thrombosis depend on the location of the clot. Symptoms of a deep vein thrombosis include:

➤ Pain in the legs, even at rest.

➤ Enlarged veins beneath the skin.

➤ The area becomes hot, swollen and red.

MINIMIZING THE RISK OF DEEP VEIN THROMBOSIS

If you are going on a long journey (by car, train, bus or plane), take a few simple steps to avoid a DVT.

➤ Wear special support socks just before and during the journey.

➤ Get up and stretch your legs every now and then.

➤ Drink plenty of water and avoid drinking alcohol.

➤ Point and flex your toes, to help return the blood in your legs to your heart.

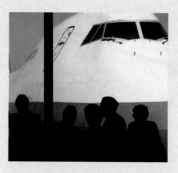

△ Long-distance travel increases the risk of a DVT developing so take note of the precautionary measures to minimize the risk.

HOW CLOTS ARE DIAGNOSED

Your doctor may suspect you have a clot in a deep vein after taking your medical history and after examining you. To confirm any clinical suspicions, the doctor may then arrange for you to have an ultrasound or Doppler ultrasound scan of the affected area. This imaging technique enables doctors to assess the blood flow and to establish if the vessel is blocked and, if so, how badly.

If the test results show the signs of a possible pulmonary embolism, then an urgent hospital appointment for a specialized test called a ventilation-perfusion scan will be arranged. Doctors will probably take a blood sample to check the levels of blood gases – oxygen and carbon dioxide – which will give them more information on your condition and confirm how the treatment should proceed.

▽ This back view clearly shows redness and swelling in the lower half of the left leg – caused by clotting in a vein deep within the leg muscle.

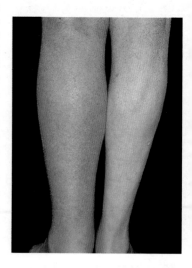

DISSOLVING CLOTS

If you are at high risk of thrombosis, such as after surgery, you'll be given special support stockings to improve the circulation in your legs. Furthermore, doctors may administer a blood-thinning (anticoagulant) drug to prevent clots from forming and those that already exist from enlarging.

If a clot has already developed, doctors will want to thin the blood with bigger doses of anticoagulants – initially this is done by injection (heparin) and afterwards by mouth (warfarin). A clot in a deep vein may need such anticoagulant treatment for six weeks or so, whereas a pulmonary embolism would be treated for at least three months. Some people are prone to clots in their deep leg veins and so have to take anticoagulant drugs for life.

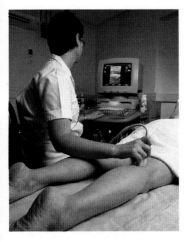

△ This patient is undergoing a Doppler scan, which is used to check for evidence of deep vein thrombosis.

SIGNS AND SYMPTOMS OF A PULMONARY EMBOLISM

The symptoms depend on how many clots or fragments are lodged within the lungs. If a major lung artery is blocked, a massive pulmonary embolism can cause sudden death without any warning.

Single or small clots may produce some of the following symptoms:

➤ Sharp chest pain.

➤ Shortness of breath.

➤ Feeling faint.

➤ Coughing up blood.

➤ Racing heartbeat or palpitations.

Raynaud's disease and phenomenon

SEE ALSO
➤ Autoimmune diseases, p459

Having painfully cold hands on a frosty winter's day, if you are not wearing gloves, is a perfectly normal response. Your body is conserving heat by taking blood away from the skin. However, in those suffering from Raynaud's disease this response sends the arteries into spasm.

Raynaud's disease is most commonly seen in young women. It usually affects the fingers and toes but can affect the ears, nose and lips. Some diseases, such as systemic sclerosis, and certain drugs can cause symptoms that appear identical to those of Raynaud's disease but in these cases it is referred to as Raynaud's phenomenon.

▽ This Raynaud's sufferer has abnormal blood flow due to arterial spasms.

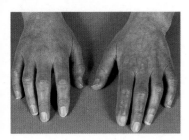

SIGNS AND SYMPTOMS

Usually both hands or feet are affected, and attacks may last minutes or hours. The changes follow a certain pattern:

➤ The small blood vessels go into spasm, reduce the blood flow and cause a dramatic colour change. The skin may turn white or dark purple.

➤ There may also be a "pins and needles" sensation.

➤ As the skin begins to warm up, the affected area changes to blue as the blood starts to flow more normally again. Finally the skin becomes red as the arteries open up once more. This red phase can be very painful.

TREATMENT OPTIONS

One of the most effective treatments is keeping the hands and feet as warm as possible, and mild cases can be remedied by wearing extra-thick gloves and socks in cold weather. Smoking constricts the arteries and worsens the symptoms of Raynaud's disease so giving up smoking will also be helpful.

During an attack, exercises that stimulate circulation may speed up recovery.

In severe cases, your doctor can prescribe calcium channel blockers. These drugs promote the relaxation of the muscle in the artery wall, which goes into spasm in Raynaud's disease, and so keeps the arteries open and blood flowing to the area.

Varicose veins

SEE ALSO
➤ Weight control, p264
➤ Exercise for life, p266
➤ The cardiovascular system, p276

Varicose veins are a very common problem that often runs in families. They occur when the small superficial veins in the skin of the legs become distorted and dilated, and appear on the surface as lumpy, purple cords. Faulty valves in superficial or deep veins mean that blood can flow backwards, from deep to superficial, and overfill the small veins. Some people mistakenly believe varicose veins are due to jobs which involve a lot of standing, such as hairdressing or working in a shop. Standing will aggravate an existing problem but not actually cause it.

Women are more susceptible to varicose veins than men, and being overweight increases the pressure on the superficial veins, which can lead to varicose veins.

SIGNS AND SYMPTOMS
Varicose veins can ache, occasionally bleed and most seriously lead to ulcers around the ankle, which can be very difficult to treat. For some reason varicose veins can cause the skin at the ankle to change, causing, first, an itchy rash and, second, a brown pigmentation that can easily break down into an ulcer.

SIMPLE SELF-HELP MEASURES
If you have varicose veins, the following suggestions may help you feel more comfortable:
• Avoid standing for long periods of time.
• Exercise or walk about during the day to keep the blood flowing in your legs.
• Put your feet up when you can.
• Wear elasticated support stockings if your doctor has recommended these.
• Lose some weight if you are overweight.

TREATMENT OPTIONS
Although varicose veins can be unsightly and painful, surgery is most commonly carried out if there is thought to be a danger of leg ulcers developing. However, some people have varicose veins removed for cosmetic reasons.

There are four basic treatment options:
1 People with mildly problematic varicose veins may find that wearing support stockings is helpful.
2 Painful veins may subside after injection with a sclerosing agent, a substance that shrivels up the vein and closes it off.
3 Tying off the superficial veins so that no blood flows into them (see below).
4 The last option is to remove the vein completely. Two small incisions are made at the top and bottom of the vein, and the surgeon literally strips the vein out.

TYING OFF VARICOSE VEINS

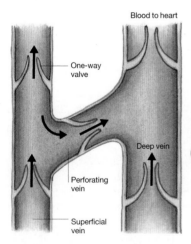

△ In healthy veins there are one-way valves to make sure that the blood flows in the right direction – from superficial to deep veins and then to the heart.

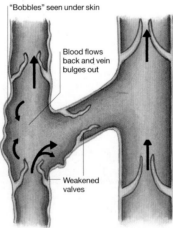

△ A weak valve in a superficial vein, or in a vein connecting superficial to deep veins, allows blood to flow back and overfill the superficial vein, causing the vein to bulge.

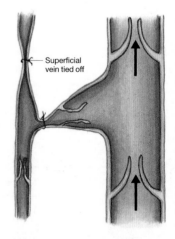

△ Tying off problem veins is an effective technique to prevent blood from flowing into them. The blood flow is diverted via the deep vein on its trip back to the heart.

3

THE DIGESTIVE SYSTEM

The digestive system is the body's power source. It breaks down food so that sugars, fats, proteins, vitamins, minerals and water can be absorbed into the blood, and used to provide energy for growth and repair. Anything the body cannot use is expelled as faeces. Fibre in food is not used by the body for fuel but is essential to the passage of faeces – and may help to protect against disease. Keeping to a healthy weight, following a balanced diet and eating regularly helps to keep the digestive system functioning.

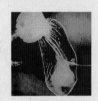

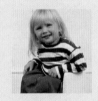

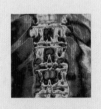

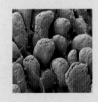

The process of digestion

Your digestive system comprises the digestive tract and the accessory organs of the liver, pancreas and gallbladder. The digestive tract is a tube about 8 metres (26 feet) long. It is divided into various sections, each with a specialized function. The aim of the system is to provide your body with energy and the raw materials for growth and repair, and to get rid of any waste. To work efficiently, your body needs sugars, fats and proteins. Special proteins called enzymes help break down the foods you eat into simple components for your body to use.

The process of digestion starts in the mouth. Here the teeth work with the muscular tongue and with saliva to cut, crush and mix food to a mush, ready to be swallowed. The chewing and grinding increases the surface area of the food so that a special enzyme found in saliva can start to break down the food's sugars. Once a ball of food is swallowed it travels down the throat into the oesophagus; to prevent food entering the respiratory system via the other "tube" in the throat (the trachea), a small flap called the epiglottis closes over it.

ON THE WAY TO THE STOMACH
Food travels down the length of the oesphagus to the stomach by a process of muscular contraction and relaxation called peristalsis. You are unaware of this, as with other movements within the digestive tract. At the end of the oesophagus, a ring of

▽ Projections called villi cover the small intestine's surface. Nutrients are absorbed into the bloodstream through capillaries in the villi.

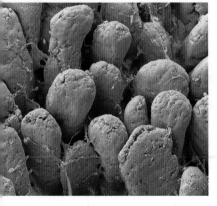

muscle (sphincter) opens to allow food into the stomach. The food changes very little as it passes through the oesophagus.

AN ACTIVE ENVIRONMENT
The stomach's many muscle layers twist and turn to grind, churn and mix the food with a germ-killing acid and a host of enzymes that have various functions. The stomach is a J-shaped muscular bag that acts like a water system header tank – it stores food after a meal and then allows it bit by bit into the next part of the digestive tract, the small intestine. Another ring of muscle called the pyloric sphincter controls how much food squirts into the duodenum, the first part of the small intestine.

HOW FOOD IS ABSORBED
Part of the way along the duodenum, substances from the gallbladder (in the form of bile to help fat digestion) and the pancreas (enzymes and an alkaline substance to neutralize the stomach's acid) are released. They are then mixed with the mush that was once food. Digestion continues within the small intestine but its main function is one of absorption – about 80 per cent of food molecules are absorbed through the walls of the small intestine. These walls are covered in tiny, finger-like projections called villi, which increase the surface area available for the absorption of food molecules into the bloodstream.

GUT FLORA
Your body houses trillions of bacteria and a huge proportion of these live in your large intestine – your gut flora. These "friendly" bacteria feed off the material that passes through and in return they produce a range of vitamins, help to break down bile pigments and keep harmful bacteria at bay by competing with them for food.

IN THE LARGE INTESTINE
The large intestine has three parts: the caecum, colon and rectum. This is where water, vitamins and minerals are absorbed from our food, through the large intestine's walls. Food material is also gradually compacted in the large intestine, a process that starts at the caecum.

The dehydrated food remains finally finish their journey through the colon at the rectum, where they are stored (now known as faeces), ready for excretion. Strong anus sphincters control when the faeces are excreted.

THE FIBRE FACTOR
Your diet comprises three food types – carbohydrates, fats and proteins. An important sub-type of carbohydrate is fibre, which has a major effect on the health of your digestive tract. Fibre exists as water-insoluble fibre (found mainly in cereals, fruit, vegetables and pulses) and water-soluble fibre (found in oats, bran, beans and pulses). Insoluble fibre absorbs water on its passage through the large intestine, making larger, softer faeces; it also reduces the transit time in the colon, which it is thought may help to prevent cancer of the colon. Soluble fibre, on the other hand, forms the main food for your gut flora.

THE DIGESTIVE ORGANS

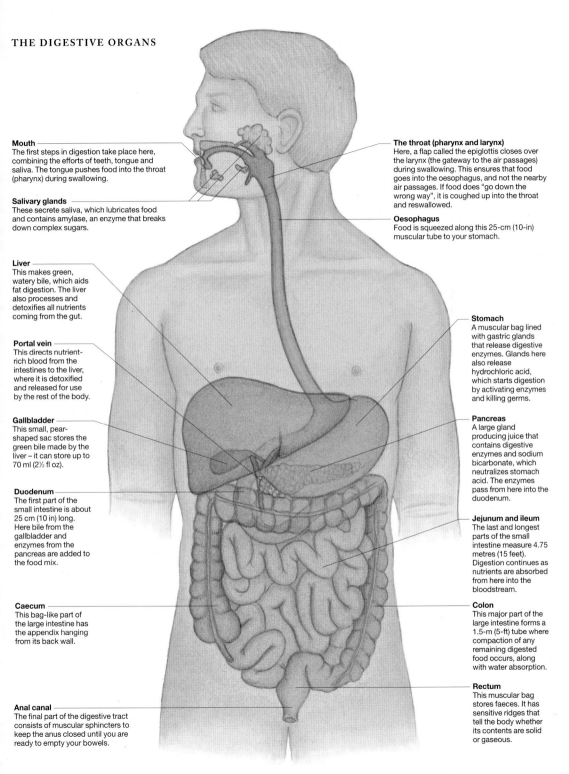

Mouth
The first steps in digestion take place here, combining the efforts of teeth, tongue and saliva. The tongue pushes food into the throat (pharynx) during swallowing.

Salivary glands
These secrete saliva, which lubricates food and contains amylase, an enzyme that breaks down complex sugars.

Liver
This makes green, watery bile, which aids fat digestion. The liver also processes and detoxifies all nutrients coming from the gut.

Portal vein
This directs nutrient-rich blood from the intestines to the liver, where it is detoxified and released for use by the rest of the body.

Gallbladder
This small, pear-shaped sac stores the green bile made by the liver – it can store up to 70 ml (2½ fl oz).

Duodenum
The first part of the small intestine is about 25 cm (10 in) long. Here bile from the gallbladder and enzymes from the pancreas are added to the food mix.

Caecum
This bag-like part of the large intestine has the appendix hanging from its back wall.

Anal canal
The final part of the digestive tract consists of muscular sphincters to keep the anus closed until you are ready to empty your bowels.

The throat (pharynx and larynx)
Here, a flap called the epiglottis closes over the larynx (the gateway to the air passages) during swallowing. This ensures that food goes into the oesophagus, and not the nearby air passages. If food does "go down the wrong way", it is coughed up into the throat and reswallowed.

Oesophagus
Food is squeezed along this 25-cm (10-in) muscular tube to your stomach.

Stomach
A muscular bag lined with gastric glands that release digestive enzymes. Glands here also release hydrochloric acid, which starts digestion by activating enzymes and killing germs.

Pancreas
A large gland producing juice that contains digestive enzymes and sodium bicarbonate, which neutralizes stomach acid. The enzymes pass from here into the duodenum.

Jejunum and ileum
The last and longest parts of the small intestine measure 4.75 metres (15 feet). Digestion continues as nutrients are absorbed from here into the bloodstream.

Colon
This major part of the large intestine forms a 1.5-m (5-ft) tube where compaction of any remaining digested food occurs, along with water absorption.

Rectum
This muscular bag stores faeces. It has sensitive ridges that tell the body whether its contents are solid or gaseous.

Digestive disorders

Your bowel habit is probably the best indicator of how well your digestive system is functioning. And when it comes to your bowel habit, you are unique. Everyone's digestive system functions slightly differently – so "normal" can be seen as anything from bowel movements three times a day to just three times a week. The most important aspect of monitoring your digestive health is that you are aware of what is normal for you. That way, you will be able to spot anything out of the ordinary and bring it to the attention of your doctor if necessary.

The digestive system copes very well with a wide range of substances – but it can react violently if you take in contaminated food or drink, poisons, some drugs or other irritants. Some digestive symptoms, such as vomiting and diarrhoea, can be the body's straightforward and relatively brief response to a harmful substance – enabling it to expel the substance as quickly as possible. Others, such as constipation or bloating, may be the result of eating the wrong things over a longer period of time – causing the digestive system to work less efficiently. Minor symptoms such as indigestion can

often be a result of the person eating in the wrong way – for example, when they are in a hurry or stressed or when they are sitting in an awkward position that impedes the digestive process.

Although most digestive symptoms are the result of a short-term problem, they can also indicate several serious disorders that need prompt medical treatment. A pain in the abdomen, for example, could be the result of cancer, or a less serious but still uncomfortable condition such as peptic ulcers, or of a temporary complaint such as a mild attack of gastroenteritis.

It is often difficult to determine the cause of a digestive symptom – peptic ulcers and stomach cancer cause pain in the same area of the abdomen, for example. Because of this it is important to see a doctor for a proper investigation if a symptom continues for longer than a few days – or if it is particularly violent.

DIGESTIVE SYMPTOMS

Most people experience bouts of vomiting, diarrhoea, abdominal pain, constipation, flatulence and bloating from time to time. These episodes are usually few and far between and often settle within a day or so. Only if these symptoms are severe or if they persist should you be concerned and visit your doctor. These are some of the commonest digestive symptoms – and how you should act if you notice them.

- Blood – Whether it is in vomit or in the stools, the presence of blood is never normal. There may be a simple reason for the blood – such as haemorrhoids (piles) or an anal fissure (tear) – but it could

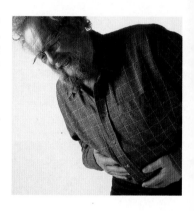

△ Abdominal pain is very common. Often the cause is a minor problem that passes quickly, but regular or very severe pain should be investigated by a doctor.

also indicate a more serious problem. It is therefore essential that you see your doctor for a diagnosis.

- Abdominal pain – Abdominal pain can be the result of a wide range of conditions – from over-eating and menstruation to serious disorders. If you suffer regularly from pain in your abdomen or if the pain changes, consult your doctor.
- Constipation or diarrhoea – Everyone suffers from occasional bouts of these. However, if your bowel habit changes suddenly and remains changed, it could indicate a serious condition and you should visit your doctor without delay.
- Vomiting – Vomiting is a common symptom of many diseases related to digestion, but it also occurs in other disorders. Bouts of vomiting can cause dehydration, so it is important that you drink plenty of fluids. If vomiting persists

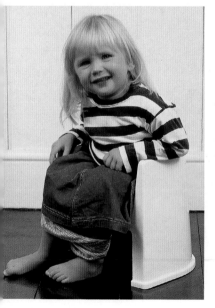

▽ Young children are unembarrassed about going to the toilet, but as we grow older we find it difficult even to discuss our bowel habits.

or if there is blood in your vomit, contact your doctor.

- Tenesmus – This word describes the feeling that you have not completely emptied your bowel after defecation. It can be a sign of serious disease, so it is wise to see your doctor.
- Weight loss – Any unexplained weight loss needs further medical investigation.
- Loss of appetite – Appetite tends to decrease naturally with age, but a sudden loss of appetite can be a sign of certain diseases and needs evaluation by a doctor.
- Bloating and flatulence – These are common symptoms which can produce discomfort and even pain. However, they rarely indicate serious disease.

INVESTIGATING DISORDERS

After asking you a series of questions about your state of health and your specific symptoms, your doctor may perform an

DON'T BE SHY

Many people are embarrassed when they have to discuss any digestive problems. They may either delay going to their doctor or feel unable to tell the whole story when they are there. Never feel embarrassed when talking about anything with doctors – they are used to dealing with such information and it is very important that your doctor has all the information you can give on your symptoms to be able to make an accurate diagnosis.

Your doctor will probably ask the following questions.

➤ How often do you empty your bowels? (A normal range is anything from three times a day to three times a week.)

➤ Is the stool loose and watery, hard and pellet-like, pale or foul smelling?

➤ Is there any blood or mucus in the stool? Is there fresh blood on the toilet tissue after wiping?

▷ X-rays such as this, taken after the patient was given a barium enema, clearly reveal any abnormalities in the small intestine.

examination of your rectum and will use a gloved finger to do so. This should not hurt but it will probably feel undignified and uncomfortable. However, it is important that the doctor is able to carry out a complete examination. Serious digestive diseases are best treated as quickly as possible so it is vital that you are honest with your doctor about any symptoms you are suffering even if you feel embarrassed about discussing them.

FURTHER TESTS

If your doctor feels that further investigation is required, you may be referred to a hospital for any or all of the following tests:

- Contrast X-rays – X-rays of the digestive tract can be very useful in detecting disease, especially if they are combined with a contrast dye or other medium that shows up white on an X-ray image. Barium sulphate is often used for this purpose. It may be mixed with water and drunk (called a barium meal) or injected into the rectum (a barium enema), before a series of X-rays are then taken. The barium makes it possible to see an outline of the inside of the digestive tract on the X-ray that enables a doctor to identify any potential problems.
- Endoscopy – This investigation involves looking inside your digestive tract via a flexible telescopic instrument. A flexible endoscope, which may be passed through the mouth or through the anus and rectum, makes it possible for a specialist to examine almost all sections of the digestive tract. Small instruments can be fed down into special channels within the endoscope to take samples of tissue (biopsies) or even to treat some conditions without surgery.
- Ultrasound scanning – Solid organs of the digestive system such as the liver are usually investigated using the non-invasive method of ultrasound.

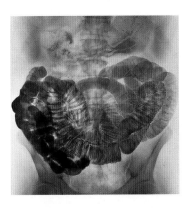

PROCEDURE FOR AN ENDOSCOPY OF THE UPPER DIGESTIVE TRACT

You may be given an intravenous sedative or anaesthetic before the procedure. A local anaesthetic may be sprayed on the back of the mouth, and a mouth guard will be used to protect your lips and teeth.

A flexible tube with a small camera at its tip is inserted through the mouth, oesophagus and into the stomach and duodenum. A steering control enables the specialist to guide the endoscope.

Images from the endoscope camera appear on a screen, allowing the specialist to see any ulcers or other abnormalities.

The specialist may take small samples of abnormal tissue (a biopsy) using a tiny surgical instrument attached to the endoscope. The biopsy is then sent to a laboratory for analysis.

Obesity

Obesity is a condition in which there is excess accumulation of fat. Obesity is growing more common in the developed world, due to modern habits of eating unhealthy "junk" foods and an increasingly sedentary lifestyle. It is not necessarily that obese people eat more than the average person, but that they all eat more than their bodies actually need. However, people do tend to put on weight as they get older, due to metabolic changes. Rarely, obesity is due to an underactive thyroid gland, Cushing's syndrome or to corticosteroid drugs.

Being very overweight puts your health at risk – obese people are at high risk of dying prematurely due to heart disease, diabetes and stroke, and are also more likely to suffer back pain and other complaints because of the extra strain placed on their bodies. However, being moderately overweight will not usually have an adverse effect on your health – especially if you eat a balanced diet and exercise regularly.

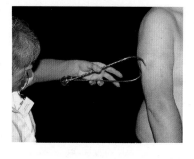

△ Weight-management clinics use various methods to determine the amount of body fat. This specialist is measuring fat with calipers.

Health education programmes aimed at children and adults seek to prevent obesity by emphasizing the importance of a healthy, balanced diet and active lifestyle.

DEFINING OBESITY

Healthcare professionals use the body mass index (BMI) to measure whether or not someone is a healthy weight for their height. The BMI uses a simple calculation (body weight in kilograms divided by height in metres squared). A person is described as obese if their BMI is above 30 if they are male and above 28 if they are female. The BMI serves as a guide only and your doctor will take many other factors into consideration. Waist size, for example, is often significant because extra weight around the waist is linked to cardiac risk.

TREATING OBESITY

The only sure way to lose weight is to eat less and exercise more. Losing weight gradually, and slowly increasing the amount of exercise that you do, is the healthiest and most effective way to reach and maintain a healthy weight. There are also medical options for treating obesity, including drug therapy and, as a last resort, surgery.

• Drugs – A number of drugs have been tried out for obesity with limited success and often with serious side-effects. New drugs, which block the absorption of fat or act on the brain to reduce the appetite, have become available. However, drugs can only do so much, and even people taking obesity drugs need to have, and maintain, willpower.

• Surgery – This is an extreme solution and is used only for the very obese when all diets have failed. The two commonest procedures are wiring the jaws so that only liquid food can be taken, and an operation called a gastroplasty, in which most of the stomach is stapled shut so that only smaller meals can be eaten.

▽ This X-ray shows a hiatus hernia, where part of the stomach protrudes through the diaphragm. Obesity puts extra pressure on the stomach, increasing the risk of a hernia.

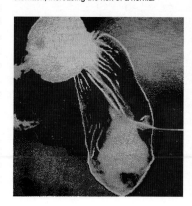

COMPLICATIONS OF OBESITY

Obesity can result in the development of many different complaints and more serious diseases including:

➤ Arthritis of the hips and knees.

➤ Back pain.

➤ Breathlessness.

➤ Gallstones.

➤ Heart disease.

➤ Hiatus hernia.

➤ High blood pressure.

➤ High cholesterol levels.

➤ Menstrual problems.

➤ Post-operative problems, such as chest infection or deep vein thrombosis.

➤ Stroke.

➤ Type II diabetes.

➤ Varicose veins.

Oesophagitis

SEE ALSO
➤ Eat healthily, p262
➤ Smoking and your
  health, p268
➤ Endoscopy, p295

Food travels through the mouth and throat to the stomach via a thin, muscular tube called the oesophagus. Food then travels into the stomach in a one-way system in order that the stomach acid does not flow back in to the oesophagus. A number of conditions, however, can cause acid to flow back, or reflux, into the oesophagus, causing the lining to become inflamed and painful. The condition can usually be brought under control by avoiding provoking factors such as fatty foods or alcohol and by taking antacids or other drugs.

FACTORS THAT MAY PROVOKE OESOPHAGITIS

The reflux of acid into the oesophagus can be a result of:

➤ Eating too many fatty foods, chocolate, coffee and alcohol.

➤ Eating large meals.

➤ Smoking.

➤ Pregnancy or obesity.

➤ A hiatus hernia, in which part of the stomach forces through the diaphragm and affects the valve that prevents acid from flowing backwards.

The swelling and inflammation of the lining of the oesophagus causes chest pain, known as heartburn or dyspepsia, which is made worse by lying down or bending forward. Other factors, such as eating spicy foods or drinking hot liquids or alcohol, can also aggravate the burning sensation. In severe cases, the oesophagus may bleed.

WHAT MIGHT YOUR DOCTOR DO?

Your doctor may suspect oesophagitis from your symptoms. Contrast X-rays or an endoscopy may be carried out if it is not a straightforward case.

The first line of treatment is to avoid or reduce the provoking factors. Acid suppressants are usually the first line of defence and various drugs can be used to reduce stomach acid secretion. In severe cases, surgeons can form a new valve at the top of the stomach to prevent reflux.

FURTHER COMPLICATIONS

In rare instances, severe inflammation causes a narrowing, or stricture, in the oesophagus. If continually exposed to acid, the oesophageal lining can transform itself to resemble that of the stomach. This is known as Barrett's oesophagus and is a precancerous condition. Regular monitoring and lifelong drug treatment is needed in order to suppress the production of acid.

Cancer of the oesophagus

SEE ALSO
➤ Endoscopy, p295

This is the eighth most common cancer in the world. There is a particularly high incidence in Iran, which may be due to the widespread use of stoneground flour and the silicates it contains. The main risk factors in developed countries are smoking and a high alcohol consumption.

One of the main symptoms of oesophageal cancer is difficulty swallowing, which occurs first with solids and eventually even fluids cause pain. The pain is usually only apparent once the cancer has spread.

WHAT MIGHT YOUR DOCTOR DO?

After a history and examination, your doctor may refer you for an endoscopy or contrast X-ray to diagnose the cancer. The only cure is to remove the cancer surgically.

Unfortunately this form of cancer is fast-growing and it is often diagnosed when surgery is no longer an option. Chemotherapy and radiotherapy can be given to slow the disease's development, and other treatments focus on keeping the oesophagus open so that the person can continue to eat and drink.

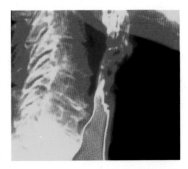

▷ Contrast X-rays are useful diagnostic tools, and allow doctors to see abnormalities such as tumours or ulcers in the oesophagus.

Peptic ulcers

SEE ALSO
➤ Learn to manage stress, p260
➤ Smoking and your health, p268
➤ Stomach cancer, p300
➤ Osteoarthritis, p360

Stomach acid is hydrochloric acid, one of the strongest acids that exists. Its function is to destroy anything unpleasant that may be ingested with food and drink and to activate one of the main stomach digestive enzymes. Despite the mucus coating of the stomach and duodenum, their linings can come under attack from this powerful acid. An ulcer is an area of tissue that has been damaged by acid. Peptic ulcers occur in the duodenum (duodenal ulcers) and the stomach (gastric ulcers). Fortunately, treatment is successful in 90 per cent of cases.

Duodenal ulcers are three times more common than gastric ulcers and the 20 to 45 age group are most likely to be affected. On the other hand, people with gastric ulcers are likely to be over 50.

SIGNS OF PEPTIC ULCERS

Many people affected by ulcers do not have any symptoms – or they may experience only minor discomfort that they put down to indigestion. However, ulcers can cause severe pain in the upper abdomen. With duodenal ulcers, the pain worsens when the stomach is empty – it may be relieved by eating but recurs later. Gastric ulcer pain is usually made worse by eating. The pain caused by either type of ulcer is similar to the pain that occurs as a result of stomach cancer, so prompt investigation is essential.

WHY PEPTIC ULCERS OCCUR

The vast majority of peptic ulcers are caused by infection with *Helicobacter pylori* bacteria. People living in unhygienic living

SIGNS AND SYMPTOMS
➤ The main symptom of peptic ulcers is pain in the upper abdomen. Sometimes the pain is so severe it wakes sufferers at night.

➤ Nausea and vomiting.

➤ Loss of appetite and weight loss.

conditions are particularly at risk from this infection. Other causes include:
• The long-term use of aspirin or non-steroidal anti-inflammatory drugs.
• Excessive alcohol or, possibly, caffeine consumption.
• Smoking.

Stress is a contributory factor, for those suffering from dyspepsia, because it increases acid production. There may be a genetic factor since there often seems to be a family history of the condition.

WHAT MIGHT YOUR DOCTOR DO?

Your doctor may suspect ulcers from your symptoms, but will probably refer you to a hospital for tests. The tests may include a blood test, to establish if there are antibodies against the bacteria in your blood. Your doctor may also recommend an endoscopy where biopsy samples of the ulcer can be taken. These biopsies can be tested in a laboratory, both for the presence of *H. pylori* and to rule out the possibility of stomach cancer. If an endoscopy is not appropriate a urea breath test can be done to confirm the presence of *H. pylori*.

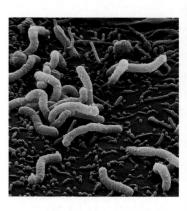

△ *Helicobacter pylori* bacteria, shown here on a human gastric cell, are the commonest cause of stomach ulcers and can also cause gastritis. The infection can be cleared with a simple course of antibiotics.

A NEW DISCOVERY

Doctors used to think that ulcers were caused primarily by stress. However, a revolution in understanding ulcers happened in the 1980s when researchers discovered that a tiny, innocent-looking bacterium, often seen on biopsies of stomach ulcers, was in fact the culprit. The precise mechanism of how *H. pylori* does this is still unclear but it seems to interfere with the mucus layer, making it more vulnerable to attack by the stomach's acid. *H. pylori* plays a role in the development of stomach cancer.

H. pylori can now be detected with blood and/or breath tests. It is also detected by a quick test done on samples of ulcerated tissue taken during an upper digestive tract endoscopy.

AREAS AFFECTED BY PEPTIC ULCERS

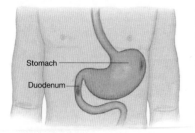

Stomach

Duodenum

△ Peptic ulcers are most likely to develop in the duodenum – the first section of the small intestine – but can also occur in the stomach.

GASTRITIS

This inflammation of the stomach lining demonstrates similar symptoms to ulcers, and can be easily treated by taking antacids for the pain and implementing preventive measures such as reducing alcohol intake and giving up smoking. Gastritis can develop suddenly (acute gastritis) or develop gradually over many months or years (chronic gastritis). The acute form is commonly caused by excessive alcohol consumption or taking anti-inflammatory drugs, such as aspirin.

Chronic gastritis may cause no symptoms other than a vague feeling of ill health. However, it can result in significant damage to the stomach lining, causing bleeding and ulceration. It is also a risk factor for stomach cancer. In the past, the causes of long-term gastritis were not known and so there was no effective treatment available. Now that *H. pylori* has been identified as a major cause of the disease, a course of antibiotics usually clears it up. Chronic gastritis is sometimes caused by sustained, excessive alcohol consumption or smoking.

▽ The classic duodenal ulcer sufferer has long been seen as a 20–45-year-old man with a highly stressful job. However, although stress, along with alcohol and smoking, can exacerbate duodenal ulcers, recent studies show that bacteria may be the main cause.

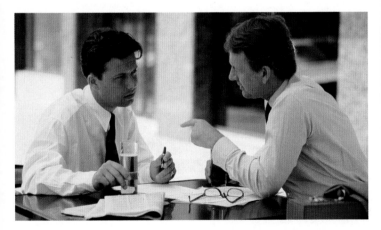

▷ This surgeon is studying screen images of a digestive tract he is exploring with an endoscope. He is able to guide the endoscope to explore any area he wishes to examine.

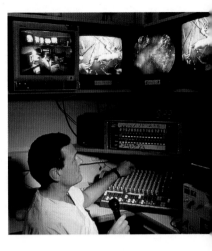

TREATMENT OPTIONS

Treatment of ulcers is more straightforward now that we know that *H. pylori* is often the cause. *H. pylori* eradication relies on the administration of two antibiotics and a PPI (proton pump inhibitor) for seven days, with six weeks' worth of acid-suppressing drugs to help heal the affected areas. If *H. pylori* is present, 90 per cent of ulcers can be healed with one course of treatment. A second course of treatment usually settles the majority of the remaining ulcers.

Those ulcers caused by aspirin or non-steroidal anti-inflammatory drugs usually settle if the drug is stopped. However, in cases of osteoarthritis, for example, such anti-inflammatories are essential. In these cases, your doctor will prescribe a drug to be taken with the anti-inflammatory to protect your stomach and duodenum from ulceration. Recently, Cox 2 inhibitors have been used as an alternative to anti-inflammatories because they have minimal gastrointestinal side effects.

To prevent ulcers from recurring, your doctor may advise you to make long-term lifestyle changes, such as reducing high levels of stress at work, giving up smoking or drinking less alcohol, as appropriate.

COMPLICATIONS OF PEPTIC ULCERS

Surgery was commonly used to remove ulcers before *H. pylori* was found to be the main cause. Today, surgery is used to treat complications of peptic ulcers.

➤ Haemorrhage – Duodenal ulcers tend to occur directly over a large blood vessel and can damage it, causing copious bleeding. This bleeding can usually be stopped with injections via an endoscope, but some cases still need a surgeon to tie off the vessel to halt the bleeding.

➤ Perforation – A hole in the stomach can form at the site of a peptic ulcer and the stomach contents can spill into the abdominal cavity, causing a life-threatening inflammation called peritonitis. It may be necessary for a surgeon to sew up the cavity; this is followed by ulcer drug therapy.

➤ Pyloric stenosis – Peptic ulcers can lead to scarring and narrowing (stenosis) of the exit valve from the stomach (the pyloric sphincter). A bad stenosis stops most food leaving the stomach and results in copious vomiting. Most patients need surgery to repair the pylorus.

Stomach cancer

SEE ALSO

➤ Eat healthily, p262

➤ Smoking and your health, p268

➤ Sensible drinking, p270

➤ Peptic ulcers, p298

Stomach cancer is the second most common cancer worldwide, after lung cancer. It is particularly common in Japan and China, probably due to dietary factors. Unfortunately, the incidence of this cancerous tumour of the stomach lining is increasing in the Western world. Stomach cancer tends to spread rapidly, so treatment is often focused on slowing the disease's progression rather than curing it. In Japan, where there is extensive screening, the disease is diagnosed at an earlier stage and about 90 per cent of those affected are cured.

KNOW THE RISKS

There are several risk factors for stomach cancer. Chronic gastritis (inflammation of the stomach lining) caused by long-term infection by *Helicobacter pylori* is the main factor. Other risk factors include:

➤ Smoking.

➤ A diet that is low in fibre.

➤ Diets rich in salty, pickled and smoked foods.

➤ High alcohol consumption.

Diets that are high in fibre promote general digestive health, and can help to reduce the risk of stomach cancer. Peptic ulcers are not a risk factor for stomach cancer, but it can often be difficult for doctors to distinguish between a peptic ulcer and early stomach cancer.

Stomach cancer usually develops in the lining of the stomach, but may spread rapidly to other sites in the body. Most of those affected are over the age of 50, and men are twice as likely to develop the disease as women.

WHAT MIGHT YOUR DOCTOR DO?

After listening to your symptoms, your doctor may examine you to check for evidence of a mass in the upper abdomen. Your doctor may then refer you to hospital for an endoscopy, in which the stomach will be examined through a thin viewing instrument. Biopsy specimens will be taken during an endoscopy, and then sent for analysis. You may also be sent for a contrast X-ray, which clearly shows the structure of the stomach and any abnormalities.

The stomach is a large "bag" so there is plenty of room for a cancer to grow before it causes any symptoms. Once symptoms start they are usually only mild and are not distinctive – they include abdominal pain, nausea and weight loss. Because of this, stomach cancer is often not diagnosed until the cancer has already spread to other parts of the body.

If diagnosed early in its development, it is usually possible to remove the tumour surgically – this is the procedure in about 20 per cent of cases. The surgery involves the partial or complete removal of the stomach, and removal of the surrounding lymph nodes to which the cancer can spread. Surgery may also be performed to relieve symptoms where the cancer has spread to other areas of the body. Patients are usually given a course of chemotherapy and radiotherapy to control the growth of the tumour and to delay the development of the disease. Strong pain relief may also be necessary.

SIGNS AND SYMPTOMS

➤ Upper abdominal pain, which is indistinguishable from that caused by a peptic ulcer.

➤ Pain in the stomach after eating.

➤ Nausea and vomiting.

➤ Loss of appetite.

➤ Weight loss.

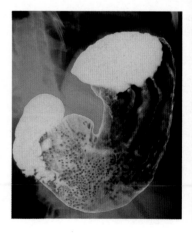

▽ A contrast X-ray shows up the structure of the stomach and can reveal the presence of a tumour – this image shows a healthy stomach.

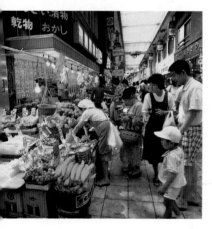

◁ Dietary habits may explain the high levels of stomach cancer in China and Japan – specifically raw fish and smoked, salty and pickled foods.

Pancreatitis

SEE ALSO
➤ Sensible drinking,
  p270
➤ Disorders of the liver,
  p302
➤ Diabetes, p314

Inflammation of the pancreas is an uncommon disorder which may occur suddenly (acute pancreatitis) or develop over a long period of time (chronic pancreatitis). Once it has become inflamed, the pancreas releases its digestive enzymes into the abdominal cavity, rather than into the small intestine. These powerful chemicals then start to digest nearby tissues, causing severe pain, fever and vomiting. The condition can be fatal – in the very worst cases, one in five patients dies – but most people recover with time and treatment.

Acute pancreatitis may be caused by gallstones, alcohol abuse, certain drugs (such as diuretic drugs) and, rarely, viruses. In most cases no obvious cause can be found. The progressive loss of function seen in chronic inflammation of the pancreas is usually a consequence of the long-term abuse of alcohol.

WHAT MIGHT YOUR DOCTOR DO?

Your doctor may suspect pancreatitis from hearing your symptoms and may take a sample of blood for testing. Occasionally, as needed, you will be referred for an abdominal ultrasound or a CT scan. Blood tests to determine blood sugar levels may be carried out.

Treatment focuses on relieving pain and other symptoms. You may need to be treated in hospital and given intravenous fluids and antibiotics to fight infections. Once the acute attack has settled, the underlying cause can be treated. For example, if a gallstone was the cause, you will usually need to have your gallbladder removed, and you may have to abstain from drinking alcohol.

Repeated attacks can seriously damage the pancreas, which ultimately affects both its digestive functions (leading to poor digestion of food) and its hormonal functions (resulting in diabetes). You may need to take enzyme supplements, and will require insulin treatment if diabetes occurs.

SIGNS AND SYMPTOMS
➤ Severe pain in the upper abdomen, which is often more severe when the patient moves.

➤ Fever.

➤ Nausea and vomiting.

➤ Bruised appearance of the skin of the abdomen.

In cases of acute pancreatitis, symptoms appear suddenly and may be severe. Symptoms of chronic pancreatitis develop gradually. In many cases people only notice their symptoms in the later stages of the disease.

Cancer of the pancreas

SEE ALSO
➤ Eat healthily, p262

Pancreatic cancer is a rare cancer that often produces no symptoms until it is well advanced. Doctors do not know the exact cause but it has been linked with diet, particularly diets high in fatty foods and low in fibre. Smoking may also be a contributory factor.

If your doctor suspects pancreatic cancer, from taking a medical history and an abdominal examination, he or she will refer you for a CT scan to check if there is a tumour. Pancreatic cancer spreads rapidly. Surgery to remove the whole tumour is rarely possible and other treatments tend not to be successful.

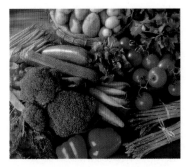

▷ A high-fibre diet that is rich in fruits and vegetables helps to protect against the risk of many cancers, including pancreatic cancer.

SIGNS AND SYMPTOMS
➤ Abdominal pain.

➤ Weight loss.

➤ Yellowing of the skin and the whites of the eyes (jaundice), which is caused by the fact that a cancer in the pancreas can block the bile duct and the flow of bile.

Disorders of the liver

SEE ALSO
➤ The process of
  digestion, p292
➤ Pancreatitis, p301
➤ Sexually transmitted
  infections, p411
➤ Anaemia, p450

The liver is an amazing organ that performs a wide variety of biochemical functions. It is the body's chemical factory and it has a great ability to heal itself when damaged. The liver must be severely damaged before its function is affected but when it does fail, there are serious and life-threatening consequences. This organ responds to most damage in the same way: initially there are signs of jaundice, then the liver becomes inflamed (a condition known as hepatitis) and, if the damage persists, scar tissue forms in the liver (cirrhosis).

WHAT DOES THE LIVER DO?

The liver has a range of vital biochemical functions which include:

➤ Producing blood proteins and controlling blood sugar levels.

➤ Regulating the transport of fat around the body.

➤ Manufacturing bile.

➤ Removing hormones, drugs and toxins from the blood.

➤ Playing a part in the immune system.

HEPATITIS

Hepatitis, or inflammation of the liver, is usually caused by bacteria, viruses and parasites. Hepatitis viruses A, B, C, D and E – are often responsible. These viruses have features in common but vary in the ways they are spread and in their long-term effects. Hepatitis A is the most common cause of hepatitis, followed by hepatitis B.

• Hepatitis A – This is often an epidemic that is spread by mouth, usually by eating contaminated food. The virus causes fever, jaundice, abdominal discomfort and tiredness, which subside over a period of three to six weeks. Long-term effects are rare and no treatment is needed. A vaccine is available for those going to affected areas.

• Hepatitis B – This virus causes a more serious infection and it is transmitted via contaminated blood or needles and by sexual intercourse, particularly among homosexual men. Symptoms may be similar to hepatitis A but many cases show no symptoms. Most people recover, but a few die from acute liver failure. The disease can persist and the patient can become a carrier and infect other people.

• Hepatitis C, and particularly D and E viruses are rarer causes of hepatitis.

THE STRUCTURE OF THE LIVER

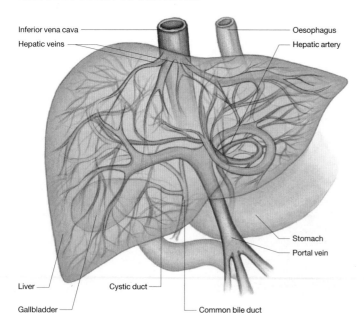

Inferior vena cava
Hepatic veins
Oesophagus
Hepatic artery
Stomach
Portal vein
Liver
Cystic duct
Gallbladder
Common bile duct

◁ The liver acts as a detoxification unit. Blood is sent from the aorta for cleansing via the hepatic artery. It is released into the hepatic veins, which drain into a central vein (inferior vena cava). The liver receives nutrient-rich blood from the small intestine (via the portal vein). The liver also makes bile, which is stored in the gallbladder. When needed for digestion bile is sent via the cystic and common bile ducts to the duodenum.

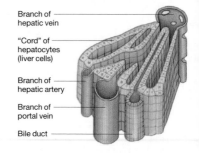

Branch of hepatic vein

"Cord" of hepatocytes (liver cells)

Branch of hepatic artery

Branch of portal vein

Bile duct

△ A section of the liver, served by a branch of the portal vein, hepatic artery and bile duct.

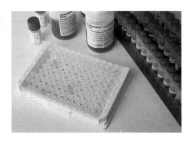

△ In this test for hepatitis C, blood has been added to substances produced by the virus. Infected blood contains antibodies that react with these viral substances – an enzyme has been added so that the sample turns yellow if such a reaction occurs. This test is positive.

A blood test will confirm which type of hepatitis virus is present, and specific antiviral agents are then given to treat the different forms. There are excellent vaccines available for hepatitis A and B that are used both to prevent infection if a person is exposed to the virus and to give lifelong protection to at-risk groups, such as healthcare workers.

ALCOHOLIC LIVER DISEASE

The commonest cause of long-term liver disease in the developed world is excessive alcohol consumption. Excess alcohol can cause permanent damage to body organs.

The liver rapidly removes alcohol from the bloodstream, but if there is too much alcohol the liver cells can become damaged and die. Excess alcohol leads to hepatitis at first, followed by scarring or cirrhosis and

eventually to liver failure and death. This process can take many years, even in very heavy drinkers, and if the alcohol abuse stops the liver can recover to some extent. Damage is more likely to occur in those people who drink to excess on a regular basis rather than occasional binge drinkers. It is also more common in men.

A doctor can diagnose alcoholic liver disease based on a person's medical history and liver function blood tests. The only treatment is to abstain from alcohol.

GALLSTONES

Bile is produced in the liver and then stored and made more concentrated in the gallbladder. The gallbladder contracts in response to a fatty meal and releases bile to break up fats during digestion. Bile pigments give faeces their brown colour.

Stones formed from cholesterol and bile can develop in the gallbladder. Up to 20 per cent of the population have gallstones, which most commonly affect those over 40. Often a person will have more than one stone at a time.

In most cases, gallstones cause few problems, but in severe cases they can block the exit of the gallbladder or the bile duct (a tube that carries bile to the small intestine) and stop the flow of bile. Bile can cause the gallbladder to become inflamed and infected – a condition known as

CAUSES OF JAUNDICE

In jaundice, there are high levels of bilirubin (the breakdown product of red blood cells), and this is what causes the skin and whites of the eyes to turn yellow. High bilirubin levels can be due to a number of factors:

➤ Excessive red blood cell destruction, such as in haemolytic anaemia.

➤ Liver damage, such as cirrhosis.

➤ Bile duct obstruction, such as from gallstones or pancreatic cancer.

▽ Damage to the liver can lead to jaundice, where the whites of the eyes turn yellow.

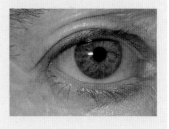

cholecystitis – which causes pain under the ribs on the right-hand side, particularly after a fatty meal.

If a gallstone is forced into the bile duct, it can cause great spasms of pain. A blocked duct may also cause pancreatitis (inflammation of the pancreas). If the stone blocks the flow of bile it can cause jaundice. The stools may also become very pale and hard to flush away, due to undigested fat.

If gallstones start causing problems and the gallbladder stops working properly, the removal of the gallbladder and its stones is the only treatment. A gallbladder cannot recover once it stops functioning correctly, and you can manage without one. Removal of the gallbladder, a procedure known as cholecystectomy, is usually carried out via keyhole techniques and involves only a short stay in hospital. The bile duct usually expands after the operation to form a new storage area for bile.

PARACETAMOL OVERDOSE

Many drugs may adversely affect the liver, but one of the most dangerous is paracetamol. Even a small overdose of as little as 15 paracetomol tablets can be fatal. There is an antidote, but it must be administered within eight hours of the overdose to be most effective. If treatment fails, liver failure can occur, leading to coma and death.

▽ Many gallstones are very small and cause no symptoms, but some are as large as golfballs. This stone is about 2 cm (¾ in) in diameter.

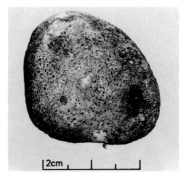

|2cm

Coeliac disease

SEE ALSO

➤ The process of digestion, p292

➤ Diabetes, p314

People with coeliac disease have an allergy to a protein found in gluten. Gluten is present in wheat, rye, barley and oats and their products. In those affected, the lining of the small intestine becomes inflamed and flattened as the finger-like projections (villi) responsible for absorbing nutrients are destroyed. Exactly how the damage is caused is not known, but the only real solution is to avoid gluten by following a strict diet. Most people find that their symptoms improve rapidly and may disappear altogether if they continue with a gluten-free diet.

SIGNS AND SYMPTOMS

➤ Abdominal bloating.

➤ Weight loss.

➤ Loose, foul-smelling stools.

➤ Sometimes, a skin rash.

➤ In children, normal growth patterns are affected.

It may be difficult for a doctor to diagnose the disease because the symptoms are vague.

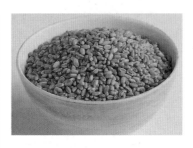

The symptoms of coeliac disease can often be vague and similar to other conditions and so doctors often find it difficult to diagnose the disorder.

◁ Wheat is one of the main foodstuffs to avoid on a gluten-free diet, but other cereals such as oats, corn, rice and millet contain gluten too.

WHAT MIGHT YOUR DOCTOR DO?

Your doctor can confirm a diagnosis by taking a sample of blood and sending it for tests, and by taking a biopsy sample from the jejunum (the middle section of the small intestine) for investigation.

If coeliac disease remains untreated, a range of related conditions can develop and there is also thought to be a higher risk of diabetes and cancer.

Appendicitis

SEE ALSO

➤ The process of digestion, p292

The appendix is a thin sac at the end of the first part of the large intestine, the caecum. In appendicitis, it becomes inflamed and infected. If it is left untreated, it could burst and can be life-threatening. The cause is not always obvious, but it can result from a blockage.

If your doctor suspects appendicitis, you will be referred immediately for hospital treatment. The appendix is removed in an operation called an appendicectomy, which can be performed by keyhole surgery.

There are a range of other conditions that have symptoms similar to those of early appendicitis. To avoid the risk of unnecessary surgery, most surgeons will often observe the patient for a few hours. If the signs and symptoms worsen, then the appendix is swiftly removed. If the patient remains stable or improves, an operation is not thought to be necessary.

POSITION OF THE APPENDIX

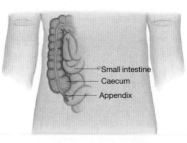

Small intestine
Caecum
Appendix

△ The actual function of the appendix is not clear. In rabbits it is used to store bacteria to digest cellulose, but in humans it is redundant.

SIGNS AND SYMPTOMS

➤ Nausea and vomiting.

➤ Diarrhoea.

➤ A mild fever.

➤ Loss of appetite.

➤ Initially, the pain will be around the navel area.

➤ Later, tenderness will develop on the right-hand side of the abdomen.

Irritable bowel syndrome

SEE ALSO
➤ Eat healthily, p262
➤ Digestive disorders, p294
➤ Endoscopy, p295

Irritable bowel syndrome, or IBS, is a common and poorly understood condition. It is twice as likely to affect women as men, and usually develops between the ages of 20 and 30. It has been given different names, including spastic colon, over the years and is probably the result of abnormal functioning of the large intestine. The large intestine regularly contracts along its length to empty itself during defecation. If this contraction occurs at other times in an uncoordinated manner, it may cause abdominal pain and other symptoms of IBS.

SIGNS AND SYMPTOMS
➤ Colicky abdominal pain, which is often eased by defecation.

➤ Abdominal bloating, also eased by defecation.

➤ Alternating hard and very soft motions.

➤ Flatulence.

Irritable bowel syndrome symptoms tend to come and go and will usually persist for many years.

The symptoms of IBS are often made much worse by stress or depression. There is also evidence that if you suffered from abdominal pain as a child you are more likely to develop IBS in adulthood.

INVESTIGATING IBS
Unfortunately, there is no definitive test for diagnosing IBS and any investigations tend to be aimed at ruling out other more serious conditions that share similar symptoms. The number of tests you are given will depend on your symptoms and your age. The tests may range from simple blood tests to a comprehensive examination of the large intestine with the help of contrast X-rays and endoscopy.

TREATMENT OPTIONS
Many people with IBS respond well if they are put on to high-fibre diets that include plenty of wholemeal bread, cereals and vegetables. Other treatments include antispasmodic drugs to reduce the spasm of the large intestine. Psychological treatment may also help some people. In the most severe cases, the debilitating symptoms of IBS can cause depression and may be treated with appropriate antidepressant medicines.

Diverticular disease

SEE ALSO
➤ Colonscopy, p307

In diverticular disease, diverticula (small, blind-ended sacs or pouches) form at the side of the large intestine. These develop when part of the intestinal wall bulges outwards through a weakened area. This condition affects one-third of people in the West by the time they are 50.

SIGNS AND SYMPTOMS
➤ Bright red blood from the rectum.

➤ Bouts of diarrhoea and constipation.

➤ Pain on the left-hand side of the abdomen, which is relieved by a bowel movement.

➤ If the diverticula become inflamed – diverticulitis – there will be severe pain and tenderness in the lower abdomen.

Diverticula are associated with a low-fibre diet. Most diverticula cause no problems and three-quarters of those with the condition do not realize that they have it. Occasionally the diverticula become blocked and infected – a condition known as diverticulitis. If they perforate or burst, they lead to a severe form of peritonitis.

DIAGNOSING DIVERTICULAR DISEASE
The diagnosis may be obvious from the symptoms but is often confirmed by a barium enema. Your doctor may also refer you for a colonoscopy, in which the colon is examined by means of a flexible tube with a camera attached. CT or ultrasound scanning are also sometimes used.

TREATMENT OPTIONS
A high-fibre diet can minimize the symptoms. Antispasmodic drugs may be prescribed to relieve abdominal pain. Most attacks of diverticulitis settle with antibiotics and a fluid-only diet to rest the intestines. But if you have more than three or four attacks in a year, surgery to remove a section of intestine may be necessary.

Colorectal cancer

SEE ALSO

➤ Eat healthily, p262

➤ The process of digestion, p292

➤ Digestive disorders, p294

Doctors do not know why the colon and rectum are affected so much by cancer – colorectal cancer is one of the most common tumours in the developed world. It rarely affects people under the age of 40, but the incidence increases with age and most people with this condition are over 60. Most large intestinal cancers occur in the very end of the colon (the sigmoid colon) or in the rectum, which is why a rectal examination is so important. Although they can run in families, 90 per cent of colorectal cancers occur in people without a strong family history.

Medical researchers have identified a number of risk factors in connection with colorectal cancers, which include:

• Diet – Diets high in animal fat and low in fibre increase the risk of colorectal cancer. The disease is rare in countries where a high-fibre diet is the norm.

• Ulcerative colitis – People affected by this inflammatory bowel disease have an increased risk of colorectal cancer.

• Familial polyposis coli – This inherited

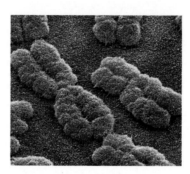

◁ Human chromosones hold the key to one in ten cases of colorectal cancers. Tests may soon be available to pinpoint those at risk.

condition causes the formation of fleshy growths called polyps in the large intestine. These polyps tend to become cancerous and people with this condition have regular examinations by endoscopy to check their intestinal health.

• Genetics – The genetic changes in DNA that lead to colorectal cancer are now well understood. For tissue to transform from normal to cancerous, a chain of events has to occur. Some links in the chain are inherited, making members of some families more prone to colorectal cancer. Tests are being developed to pick up these genetic changes and find out who is most at risk. Aspirin and other anti-inflammatory drugs may offer some protection from colorectal cancer.

THE STRUCTURE OF THE COLON

▽ The colon is a tube that absorbs water from food remains and compacts faeces. It divides into four parts: ascending (moving up the right of the abdomen), transverse (crossing to the left), descending (moving down the body) and the sigmoid colon (which meets the rectum). Doctors can examine the colon with tubes called sigmoidoscopes and colonoscopes.

WHEN TO SEE YOUR DOCTOR
If you notice a sudden and persistent change in your bowel habit, blood or mucus in the stools and/or regular abdominal pain,

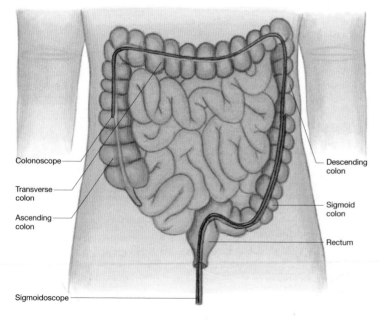

Colonoscope

Transverse colon

Ascending colon

Sigmoidoscope

Descending colon

Sigmoid colon

Rectum

SIGNS AND SYMPTOMS

➤ Abdominal pain.

➤ Change of bowel habit.

➤ Passage of blood or slime with the stool.

➤ Loss of appetite.

➤ Rectal discomfort or a feeling of fullness after defecation.

you should make an appointment to see your doctor. Another symptom is the feeling that the rectum has not emptied properly after defecation.

Like many cancers, colorectal cancer is curable if it is diagnosed early enough, so prompt investigation of any symptoms is very important.

INVESTIGATING COLORECTAL CANCER

Colorectal cancer can be picked up before any symptoms appear by screening. If you visit your doctor with symptoms, you will probably have an abdominal examination where your doctor will examine your rectum using a gloved finger. You will be asked for a stool sample, which will be tested for the presence of blood.

Your doctor is likely to refer you to a hospital for a series of tests such as a sigmoidoscopy (which involves a flexible tube being passed through the rectum to allow examination of the sigmoid colon) together with a contrast X-ray, or a colonoscopy (which involves a flexible endoscope being passed around the entire length of the colon). In both of these cases, the whole of the large intestine can be examined for evidence of tumours.

During an endoscopy, a biopsy sample of tissue can be taken and tested in a

▽ This coloured contrast X-ray shows a cancer in the colon, highlighted in red.

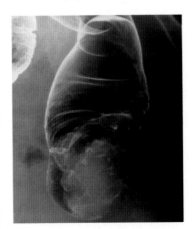

SCREENING FOR COLORECTAL CANCER

Colorectal cancer can be picked up early using specific screening tests. Testing for blood in the faeces (known as a faecal occult blood test) is now done routinely (over the age of 50) in the United States and Australia. The opinion of doctors is divided over this test because it has a high false-positive rate – that is, blood in the faeces is very often an indication of a non-cancerous condition. It is therefore recommended that people with a strong family history or other known risk factors for the disease undergo regular colonoscopy to survey the large intestine from an earlier age.

laboratory for signs of cancer. If cancer is confirmed, a CT scan will usually be performed to check how far the cancer extends and whether it has already spread to other parts of the body.

PROCEDURE FOR A COLONOSCOPY

The day before the procedure, you will be given laxatives to empty the bowels. A sedative or anaesthetic may also be given intravenously just before the procedure.

⬇

The colonoscope, a narrow, flexible tube with a camera attached to its tip, is then inserted into the rectum and guided around the colon.

⬇

Images from the camera are displayed on a monitor, allowing a specialist to guide the instrument to see any areas of abnormality. A biopsy sample may be taken for further investigation.

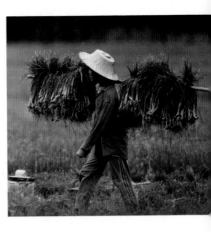

△ In many Asian countries, people live closer to the land and eat high-fibre diets that help protect against colorectal cancer.

TREATMENT OPTIONS

If colorectal cancer occurs, the only chance of a cure is to remove the entire tumour at an early stage. The affected area of the large intestine is removed (a procedure known as a colectomy) and the two free ends joined together. In most cases, surgeons rejoin the two ends of the bowel but sometimes the bowel may be brought up to the abdominal wall to create a temporary opening through which faeces can pass – this is known as a colostomy. Not all colostomies are permanent – some may be done as a temporary measure before the bowel is rejoined in a second operation.

If the cancer is limited to the intestinal wall, more than 90 per cent of people remain free from cancer five years after treatment. If the cancer has spread to the lymph nodes, especially to those within the liver, the survival rate is much lower.

In recent years chemotherapy has prolonged life in advanced cases, but surgery is still the best option. The sooner the operation is carried out, the better the chance of survival. Studies have shown that the biggest time delay in treating colorectal cancer is the time the person spends wondering whether or not to visit the doctor. If you have suspicious symptoms do not delay – see your doctor at once.

Crohn's disease

Crohn's disease is a type of inflammatory bowel disease that causes swelling through the whole thickness of the wall of the digestive tract. Over time, this wall becomes thickened and scarred, and a narrowing may form. Crohn's disease can affect any part of the digestive tract from mouth to anus, although it often affects the last part of the small intestine (ileum) and the large intestine (colon). The cause is unknown, although it tends to run in families and smokers are three times more likely than non-smokers to develop the disease.

SIGNS AND SYMPTOMS

➤ Abdominal pain.

➤ Diarrhoea, sometimes with blood.

➤ Fever.

➤ Generally feeling unwell.

➤ Weight loss.

Crohn's disease occurs worldwide but it is more common in the West, where it particularly affects those of Jewish origin. It usually occurs in people between the ages of 15 and 40 and affects both men and women equally. There is no actual cure for the disease, which produces episodic attacks of symptoms with periods of remission in between. However, symptoms can usually be brought under control with drugs.

WHAT MIGHT YOUR DOCTOR DO?

If you visit your doctor with the typical symptoms of Crohn's disease, he or she will check your mouth for ulcers and feel your abdomen, although these may show nothing out of the ordinary. Your doctor may take a sample of blood to do a full blood count, to show the level of inflammation and to check levels of iron, folic acid and vitamin B_{12}. You may also have to supply a stool sample.

You are likely to be referred to hospital for further tests including a colonoscopy, in which a flexible tube is passed through the anus and rectum and used to inspect the length of the colon. Biopsy samples of tissue may be taken. A contrast X-ray may also be performed.

MANAGING CROHN'S DISEASE

If your attacks are relatively mild, you may be treated with standard antidiarrhoeal drugs such as loperamide or codeine. Anti-inflammatory steroid drugs (given as tablets or enemas) and immunosuppressant drugs are the mainstay of treatment. Severe attacks often require hospitalization.

Elemental diets, which contain simple, easily digested nutrients and so serve to rest the digestive tract, may be recommended. Following this type of diet for six weeks can settle an attack of Crohn's; unfortunately, such diets are expensive and unpalatable.

Between 70 and 80 per cent of people with Crohn's disease need surgery, either to remove an affected area not responding to drugs or to remove a narrowing that is causing a blockage. Because many operations may be needed during a person's lifetime, surgery is kept to the absolute minimum to preserve as much of the digestive tract as possible.

Fortunately, attacks of Crohn's disease usually settle down and most people do not need to take any drugs between attacks and can lead normal lives. About ten per cent of people with Crohn's disease will develop other associated disorders. These include a form of arthritis known as ankylosing spondylitis, kidney stones, gallstones, conjunctivitis and skin rashes such as *erythema nodosum*.

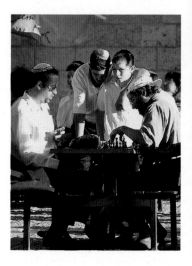

△ Studies show that people of Jewish origin are particularly susceptible to Crohn's disease, but the cause of the condition remains unknown.

▽ Contrast X-rays are an effective way of highlighting any abnormalities in the digestive tract, and are helpful in the diagnosis of Crohn's disease.

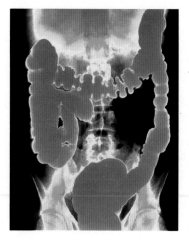

Ulcerative colitis

This type of inflammatory bowel disease affects only the large intestine – that is, the colon and the rectum. The disease often starts in the rectum and then spreads into the colon. The cause is unknown, but ulcerative colitis results in inflammation of the lining of the large intestine, which then breaks down or ulcerates, and bleeds. Ulcerative colitis usually starts between the ages of 20 and 40, and is more likely to affect women than men. As with Crohn's disease, ulcerative colitis tends to occur in distinct attacks with symptom-free periods.

SIGNS AND SYMPTOMS
- Diarrhoea with blood and mucus in the stools.
- Abdominal pain.
- Fatigue.

As in Crohn's disease, severe cases of ulcerative colitis can also affect:

- The skin – producing a rash such as *erythema nodosum*.
- The eyes – causing conjunctivitis.
- The liver – causing fatty deposits.
- The kidney – causing kidney stones.
- The gallbladder – causing gallstones.
- The joints – causing types of arthritis such as ankylosing spondylitis.

Most people with ulcerative colitis take a drug called 5-ASA to minimize the number of attacks and induce remission. Immunosuppressants are sometimes needed. In severe cases, steroids may be given. If drug therapy fails, affected areas of the colon can be removed. In some cases, the whole colon will be removed so that the intestine ends at the ileum (the final part of the small intestine). The surgeon then redirects the ileum into an artificial opening in the abdomen. A bag is attached to this opening, so the bowel contents can be drained.

Surgeons now try to form a new storage pouch from the ileum and connect this to the end of the rectum. This means patients go to the toilet as normal, although motions are looser. However, this does leave a small part of the colon behind, which may be affected by ulcerative colitis in the future.

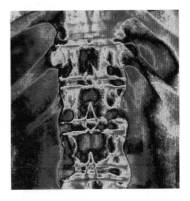

△ This X-ray shows a spine in which the vertebrae have fused together. This is the result of ankylosing spondylitis, which is an inflammatory arthritic condition that can be associated with ulcerative colitis.

COMPLICATIONS
Both Crohn's disease and ulcerative colitis may lead to serious complications.

- Perforation – A hole can form in the wall of the digestive tract so the contents of the bowel leak out, causing peritonitis, an inflammation of the abdominal cavity lining.

- Toxic dilatation – The large intestine can expand, like a balloon, and then burst. If the ballooning fails to settle, the affected area must be removed. Toxic dilatation is most likely to occur in ulcerative colitis.

- Colorectal cancer – Ulcerative colitis increases the risk significantly and so those affected are monitored closely.

HOW A COLECTOMY IS CARRIED OUT

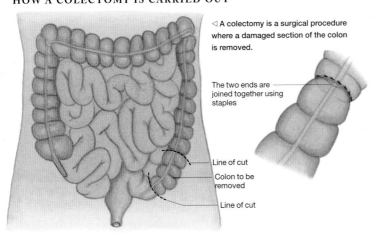

◁ A colectomy is a surgical procedure where a damaged section of the colon is removed.

The two ends are joined together using staples

Line of cut

Colon to be removed

Line of cut

Anorectal disorders

SEE ALSO
➤ Eat healthily, p262
➤ The process of digestion, p292

Many people suffer from an anorectal disorder at some point in their lives. Piles are a particularly common problem – up to 50 per cent of us will suffer from them. Fortunately, disorders that occur around the anus tend not to be serious and are easily treated. Fresh blood in the stool or on the toilet tissue after wiping is almost always due to piles or one of the other conditions below. However, it can be a sign of more serious disorders, so it is extremely important to visit your doctor promptly for a diagnosis if you notice bleeding.

HAEMORRHOIDS

Haemorrhoids or piles are very common. They are due to swollen veins in the anus and rectum, and occasionally these veins can be forced out of the anus. Straining to pass hard stools – often the result of a low-fibre diet – can be the cause. Piles are the most common reason for rectal bleeding.

Piles do not usually hurt, but if a blood clot forms in them they can be extremely painful. Most cases of piles disappear if you eat a high-fibre diet and use soothing anal ointments. Larger more troublesome piles can be destroyed by cutting off their blood supply at the base of the pile with injections and elastic bands.

ANAL ABSCESSES

Mucus-secreting glands around the anus can become infected, and a painful abscess (collection of pus) may form. Anal sex increases the risk of these abscesses.

Antibiotics often fail to cure the infection and many abscesses have to be drained of pus surgically, which is done under a general anaesthetic.

FISTULA

Sometimes an infected anal gland can burst on to the skin and into the anal canal to form an abnormal passage between the inside of the anus and the skin. Unfortunately these passages, known as fistulas, often fail to heal and have to be surgically removed.

ANAL FISSURE

It is quite common for the lining of the anus to tear, such as during the passage of hard faeces. Such tears usually heal. If they are very large, however, they can be pulled apart by the anal sphincter muscle and fail to heal, causing persistent anal bleeding and pain on defecation.

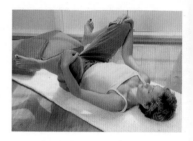

△ Doing pelvic yoga exercises is believed to help protect against anorectal disorders and may be helpful for easing an existing complaint.

A nitrate cream is applied to relax the sphincter muscle and allow the fissure to heal. If this fails an operation is performed to gently weaken the sphincter muscle without affecting control of defecation.

PILONIDAL SINUS

The hair follicles in the cleft between your buttocks can become infected and break down to form an abscess. These abscesses (pilonidal sinuses) do not heal and need to be removed surgically.

UNEXPLAINED ITCHING

Pruritus ani is anal itching that has no obvious cause but which can be related to poor hygiene, piles or threadworm infestation. The itching makes you want to scratch, which in turn makes the itching worse. Most cases settle if the anus is kept clean and dry, and by avoiding touching the skin. After washing, the anus should be blotted dry (or dried with a hairdryer), not wiped.

REMOVING LARGE HAEMORRHOIDS

▽ The treatment of large haemorrhoids is a straightforward procedure. The doctor passes a short tube (a proctoscope) into the rectum, then grasps the haemorrhoid using forceps. A rubber band is attached to the base of the haemorrhoid, which eventually drops off.

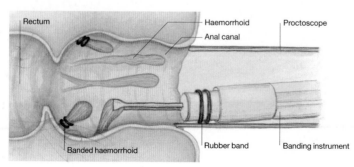

Rectum · Haemorrhoid · Anal canal · Proctoscope

Banded haemorrhoid · Rubber band · Banding instrument

THE HORMONE SYSTEM

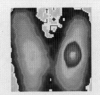

A whole family of hormones is responsible for maintaining constancy within your body's biochemical world. The word "hormone" derives from the Greek term meaning to impel or set in motion. All hormones are essentially chemical messengers that travel in the bloodstream to produce a bodily reaction, either specifically or generally. Occasionally, the glands which manufacture the hormones – known as endocrine glands – are affected by disease or malfunction in some way. Because hormones play such an important role in the functioning of every part of your body there is a wide range of potential endocrinological problems.

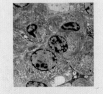

CONTENTS

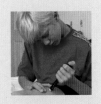

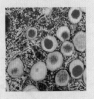

The endocrine glands

SEE ALSO

► The cardiovascular system, p276
► Diabetes, p314
► Diseases of the thyroid gland, p316

Hormones are manufactured by a number of endocrine glands found in different parts of the body. These specialized glands produce and secrete essential hormones which then travel through the bloodstream to their specific site, or sites, of action. For example the adrenal glands produce adrenaline, which affects the heart, brain, blood vessels, muscles, intestines and breathing. The major hormone-producing glands in the body are the pituitary, thyroid, parathyroid and adrenal glands, and the pancreas, ovaries and testes.

Many of the body's hormone-producing glands are controlled by the pituitary – a vital endocrine gland found just beneath the brain. Also called the "master gland", the pituitary produces stimulating factors that prompt other glands to release their hormones into the bloodstream. Disease of the pituitary can have widespread health effects.

A FINE BALANCE

The endocrine system is a complex web of finely tuned mechanisms. The diagram below shows just one aspect of this system – the control of blood sugar by the

▽ Negative feedback. To maintain correct hormone levels in the blood, the release of most hormones is controlled by a process called the negative feedback loop. This diagram shows how one loop controls our blood glucose levels.

hormone insulin – in action. In general, things go wrong when these delicate mechanisms are disrupted in some way and the endocrine glands produce either too much (hyper-) or too little (hypo-) of a particular hormone. The most common cause of hormonal disorders is a non-cancerous growth called an adenoma. An adenoma can either block hormone production or it can overstimulate the gland so that it produces far too much.

GLUCAGON AND GLYCOGEN

Any excess glucose in the bloodstream is converted into glycogen so that it can be stored. The hormone glucagon breaks down the stores of glycogen into glucose so that it can be released as needed into the bloodstream.

DIAGNOSING PROBLEMS

Doctors analyse the levels of hormone in a person's bloodstream to compare it with normal values. Such tests also help to monitor hormone or drug therapy. Doctors also use imaging techniques, such as ultrasounds or CT scans, to check endocrine glands for signs of an adenoma.

TREATMENT OPTIONS

The most common endocrine disorders are diabetes mellitus (sugar diabetes) and an underactive thyroid (hypothyroidism). Other disorders are uncommon, and can be treated using one of the following options:
1 Replace or supplement the hormone.
2 Use drugs to block the action of excess amounts of hormone.
3 Remove the offending adenoma surgically or through radiotherapy.

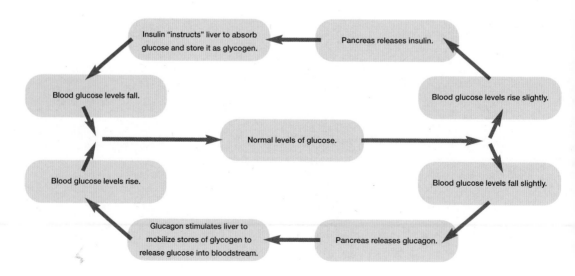

Insulin "instructs" liver to absorb glucose and store it as glycogen.

Pancreas releases insulin.

Blood glucose levels fall.

Blood glucose levels rise slightly.

Normal levels of glucose.

Blood glucose levels rise.

Blood glucose levels fall slightly.

Glucagon stimulates liver to mobilize stores of glycogen to release glucose into bloodstream.

Pancreas releases glucagon.

THE MAJOR ENDOCRINE GLANDS

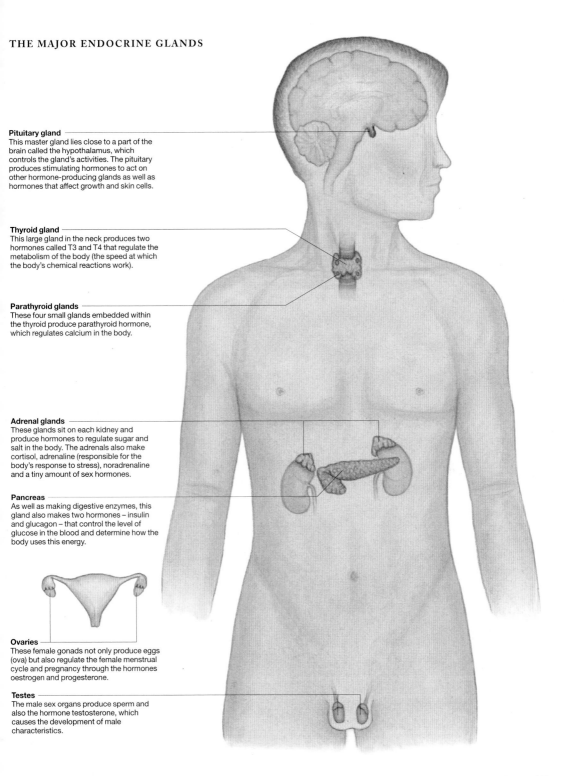

Pituitary gland
This master gland lies close to a part of the brain called the hypothalamus, which controls the gland's activities. The pituitary produces stimulating hormones to act on other hormone-producing glands as well as hormones that affect growth and skin cells.

Thyroid gland
This large gland in the neck produces two hormones called T3 and T4 that regulate the metabolism of the body (the speed at which the body's chemical reactions work).

Parathyroid glands
These four small glands embedded within the thyroid produce parathyroid hormone, which regulates calcium in the body.

Adrenal glands
These glands sit on each kidney and produce hormones to regulate sugar and salt in the body. The adrenals also make cortisol, adrenaline (responsible for the body's response to stress), noradrenaline and a tiny amount of sex hormones.

Pancreas
As well as making digestive enzymes, this gland also makes two hormones – insulin and glucagon – that control the level of glucose in the blood and determine how the body uses this energy.

Ovaries
These female gonads not only produce eggs (ova) but also regulate the female menstrual cycle and pregnancy through the hormones oestrogen and progesterone.

Testes
The male sex organs produce sperm and also the hormone testosterone, which causes the development of male characteristics.

Diabetes

Many people will know diabetes mellitus by its more common name, sugar diabetes. Diabetes results in chronically raised levels of blood sugar because of either a lack of the hormone insulin or of a resistance to it. It is a very common disease affecting 30 million people worldwide and is increasingly widespread in nations of the developed world. In the past, the outlook was fairly bleak for those with diabetes but now, with improved insulin formulations and other drugs to control its complications, people with diabetes have relatively normal and healthy lives.

The hormone insulin is manufactured by specialized cells in tiny areas of the pancreas called the islets of Langerhans. Insulin makes it possible for every cell in the body to access the sugar glucose from the bloodstream as well as influencing the way in which the liver stores any temporary excesses. All sugars will eventually be converted to glucose, which is one of the body's main fuels.

TYPES OF DIABETES

There are two types of diabetes, known simply as type I and type II.

• Type I – In this form of diabetes the pancreas stops producing insulin or produces only small amounts. This condition usually starts in children and young adults, and mainly affects Europeans and North Americans. Approximately 1 person in 20 has type I diabetes. They will usually be very thin

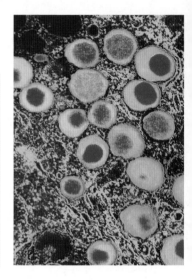

▷ This shows hormone-secreting cells in the islet of Langerhans area of the pancreas. The red circles are hormones (insulin or glucagon) ready to be released into the bloodstream.

SIGNS AND SYMPTOMS

The main symptoms of both type I and type II diabetes are listed below. Type I symptoms tend to develop faster.

➤ Thirst and a dry mouth.

➤ Excessive urination.

➤ Lethargy.

➤ Blurred vision.

➤ Poor-quality sleep because of the need for frequent trips to the toilet.

and will probably first visit their doctor with symptoms of passing a lot of urine (polyuria), thirst and weight loss.

• Type II – This form of diabetes occurs when the pancreas manufactures normal or even increased amounts of insulin but

COMPLICATIONS OF DIABETES

If you have diabetes, you will probably already be aware of its complications. Your doctor will ensure that you have check-ups for signs of these on a regular basis. People who manage their blood sugar levels efficiently will reduce the risk of complications but there are a number of other risk factors:

➤ Vascular disease – Diabetes accelerates the furring up of arteries (atherosclerosis), which makes people with the condition more likely to develop life-threatening complications such as angina, heart

attacks, strokes and gangrene of the foot. It is important to control or minimize any risk factors for atherosclerosis, including high blood pressure, high blood cholesterol levels and smoking.

➤ The nerves – Diabetes damages the small blood vessels supplying nerves. This can lead to a loss of feeling, especially in the feet. The skin of the feet can become damaged without the person knowing it and large ulcers, which do not heal well, can result.

➤ The eyes – Diabetic eye disease (retinopathy) is very common and all people

with diabetes should ensure that they have regular eye checks.

➤ The kidneys – The kidney's small vessels can become damaged, reducing the kidneys' ability to function. This damage shows up as protein in the urine, which can be detected with a simple dipstick test.

➤ Infections – People with diabetes, even those who control their blood sugar levels carefully, are prone to infections. The skin, kidneys, bladder and lungs are particularly vulnerable to infection.

DIABETES IN PREGNANCY

Some pregnant women develop a temporary diabetic condition called gestational diabetes. It is treated with insulin to safeguard the mother's and the baby's health and usually disappears once the child is born. However, half of the women who have gestational diabetes develop diabetes later in life.

the body becomes insensitive or resistant to its actions. Type II is the more common form of diabetes and tends to affect older people of all racial groups. It is sometimes referred to as adult-onset diabetes. (However, doctors are now detecting this type of diabetes in children in developed countries.) In contrast to type I, patients will tend to be overweight but other symptoms are the same in that they will urinate a lot and feel thirsty. Other than that, most patients will complain only of general feelings of tiredness and lethargy.

▽ Many people with type II diabetes can control their blood sugar levels by following a healthy diet and taking regular exercise.

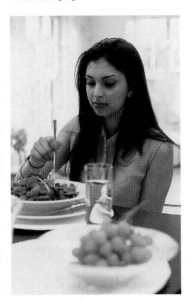

HOW IS IT DIAGNOSED?

First your doctor will want to ask about your symptoms and perhaps perform a physical examination. Usually, you will be asked to supply a urine sample, which can be tested with a simple dipstick while you wait in the doctor's surgery.

After testing a sample of urine for the presence of glucose, your doctor may also take a blood sample. This sample is sent to a laboratory to check its glucose levels. Normally, doctors would want two consecutive measurements to confirm a diagnosis. Such tests are also used to monitor and adjust ongoing treatments.

TREATMENT OPTIONS

All types of treatment aim to maintain glucose levels within a normal range, without too many swings (high or low). Lifelong dietary modification is always essential and may be combined, if necessary, with insulin injections or drug therapy.

- Diet – A good diabetic diet is no different from that considered healthy for everyone. It should be high in fruit and vegetables, low in fat and include complex carbohydrates (such as pasta, rice and bread). Complex carbohydrates release a steady stream of glucose (as do unrefined sugars found in fruit and vegetables) rather than the short-lived surges of glucose from refined sugars (found in sweets and biscuits). Some people with type II diabetes can control their blood glucose levels with diet alone.
- Drug therapy – There are many different types of tablets and they are designed to increase the amount of insulin produced or increase the person's sensitivity to insulin. People with type II diabetes may have to take one or more types of tablets.
- Insulin injections – All people with type I diabetes need regular insulin injections. Some people with type II diabetes also need insulin. Those injecting insulin usually take a long-acting form once or twice a day and a short-acting insulin at meal times. If someone injects too much insulin accidentally, it results in an

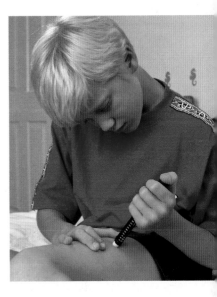

△ Children over a certain age are usually taught to inject insulin themselves. Most diabetics use insulin pens like this one, rather than a syringe.

extremely low blood sugar level, also known as hypoglycaemia. In this state, they become tired, sweaty and confused and may even fall unconscious. To reverse the hypoglycaemia, glucose is given urgently as a sweet, a drink or as an infusion into a vein.

DIABETIC KETOACIDOSIS

This diabetic emergency affects only people with type I diabetes. It is caused by a lack of insulin. The most common cause is patients reducing or omitting their insulin because they are not eating due to nausea and vomiting. Insulin treatment should never be stopped.

The lack of insulin means the body cannot use the glucose in the blood. The glucose passes out with lots of water (as urine) making patients extremely dehydrated. Without glucose, the body has to use other fuels, such as fat, but this can lead to a build-up of toxic substances called ketones that can prove fatal. Ketoacidosis is treated with intravenous fluids and an insulin infusion.

Diseases of the thyroid gland

SEE ALSO

➤ The endocrine glands, p312

➤ Pituitary gland disorders, p320

➤ Bipolar affective disorder, p348

The thyroid gland sits at the front of the neck surrounding the windpipe (trachea). The thyroid hormones regulate the metabolic rate of many tissues. Diseases may cause the thyroid to under- or overproduce the two thyroid hormones called T3 and T4. The thyroid hormones are released into the bloodstream in response to a regulating hormone from the pituitary gland called thyroid-stimulating hormone (TSH). Thyroid disorders are common and often develop gradually. They may lie undetected for months or even years.

HYPOTHYROIDISM

This underactivity of the thyroid gland causes levels of T3 and T4 to be low, while TSH levels remain high.

WHAT CAUSES AN UNDERACTIVE THYROID GLAND?

There are many causes of hypothyroidism.

• Atrophic (autoimmune) hypothyroidism – This is the commonest cause in which the body's own immune system attacks and destroys the thyroid gland. Women are more commonly affected than men.

• Hashimoto's thyroiditis – An auto-immune disease where attacking antibodies cause the thyroid to become enlarged and tender.

• Iodine deficiency – This is common in mountainous areas with little iodine in the water or diet; the thyroid enlarges to form a goitre (see goitres box, opposite).

• Pituitary disease – An underactive pituitary gland will not produce enough

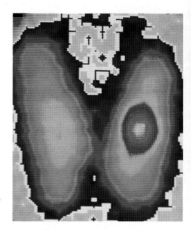

▷ This radionuclide scan of a thyroid shows a non-cancerous adenoma in the right-hand portion of the gland, seen as red and white.

TSH to stimulate the thyroid gland and so in turn causes hypothyroidism.

• Thyroid cancer – Rarely, a cancerous growth destroys the gland.

TREATMENT OPTIONS

Treatment replaces the thyroid hormones T3 and T4 with thyroxine tablets. A low dose is given at first and is then increased until the blood tests show normal levels of thyroid function. Determining the optimal dose is vital for successful treatment. Thyroxine has to be taken for life.

THYROID FUNCTION TESTS

To assess thyroid function, doctors take a sample of your blood and send it to a laboratory for detailed analysis. Such tests measure the levels of:

• The thyroid hormones T3 and T4.
• The pituitary hormone TSH.

These test results should enable your doctor to make a diagnosis or if necessary to advise other investigations, such as a radionuclide scan.

THE STRUCTURE OF THE THYROID GLAND

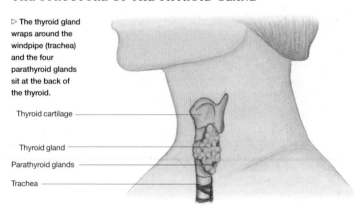

▷ The thyroid gland wraps around the windpipe (trachea) and the four parathyroid glands sit at the back of the thyroid.

Thyroid cartilage ———

Thyroid gland ———

Parathyroid glands ———

Trachea ———

SIGNS AND SYMPTOMS OF HYPOTHYROIDISM

Hypothyroidism has various symptoms, many of which are "general". Typical symptoms are tiredness, intolerance of the cold, feeling depressed and gaining weight despite having no appetite.

You may have dry, thin hair, a slow pulse and a swelling in your neck. These are only a few of the features of this disease and doctors often do thyroid function blood tests when they are not sure of the diagnosis.

INVESTIGATING A LUMP IN THE THYROID

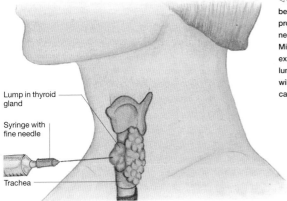

◁ Cells and fluid can be removed in a procedure called fine-needle aspiration. Microscopic examination of the lump in the thyroid will reveal if it is cancerous or not.

Lump in thyroid gland

Syringe with fine needle

Trachea

HYPERTHYROIDISM

An overactive thyroid is quite common and is again more often seen in women. The commonest cause is Grave's disease – an autoimmune disease in which attacking antibodies stimulate the thyroid to release T3 and T4 so their levels in the blood rise.

Rarely, a non-cancerous tumour (adenoma) or thyroid growth produces too much thyroid hormone. Rarer still, a non-cancerous pituitary tumour produces excess TSH, making the thyroid over-secrete.

TREATMENT OPTIONS

Once the cause has been investigated there are three possible options for the treatment of an overactive thyroid gland:

1 Anti-thyroid drugs that block the formation of thyroid hormones.
2 Radioactive iodine to reduce the amount of thyroid hormone produced (this is a sensitive treatment and can easily result in hypothyroidism).
3 Surgery to remove part of the thyroid gland is only an option if drugs fail or produce too many side-effects, or if the patient has a large goitre. It is not always successful and is considered the last resort.

THYROID CANCER

Cancers of the thyroid are rare and thyroid cancer has one of the highest treatment success rates. Treatments vary depending on the growth rate and nature of the cancer.

GOITRE (THYROID ENLARGEMENT)

Many diseases can cause goitre and some have already been mentioned, such as Grave's disease, Hashimoto's thyroiditis, iodine deficiency and thyroid cancer. The commonest type is multinodular goitre. This generally harmless condition is caused by the overgrowth of part of the thyroid gland. Goitre can also be a side-effect of lithium, a drug prescribed for people with bipolar affective disorder.

Goitres may produce low, normal or high levels of thyroid hormones, so doctors will often use a standard thyroid function blood test to measure the hormone levels. An ultrasound scan and fine-needle aspiration of the thyroid gland itself will determine the cause of the swelling and whether it is cancerous.

Surgery to remove the goitre is sometimes performed if the goitre is large and unsightly and, in rare cases, when it compresses the windpipe.

▽ The enlarged thyroid gland or goitre in this woman's neck is clearly visible. Most goitres are painless.

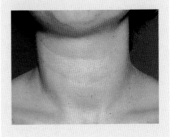

SIGNS AND SYMPTOMS OF HYPERTHYROIDISM
Typical symptoms include:

➤ Feeling restless.

➤ Loss of weight despite having an increased appetite.

➤ Low tolerance of heat.

Other symptoms could include experiencing tremors, having a fast pulse and a neck swelling. In Grave's disease one of the symptoms is staring eyes, known as exophthalmos.

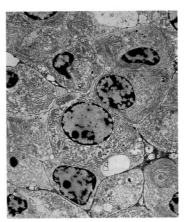

TREATMENT OPTIONS

Usually surgery to remove part or all of the thyroid gland is carried out. This procedure is called a thyroidectomy. If the thyroid gland is removed, and this usually offers the best chance of a cure, a patient will need lifelong thyroxine hormone replacement.

◁ This coloured photomicrograph shows cells taken from a cancerous thyroid. The rapidly-dividing cancer cells have abnormally large nuclei (seen in green).

Adrenal gland disorders

SEE ALSO

➤ High blood pressure,
   p278
➤ The endocrine
   glands, p312
➤ Autoimmune
   diseases, p459

The two adrenal glands sit on fatty pads above the kidneys and consist of two parts – an outer cortex and an inner medulla. The adrenal cortex produces corticosteroid hormones (cortisol and aldosterone) that are involved in regulating sugar, salt and blood pressure; the medulla produces adrenaline and noradrenaline. Diseases occur if there is an insufficient level of a hormone (hypoadrenalism) or if any is present in excess (hyperadrenalism). A non-cancerous adenoma is often the cause of adrenal disorders, which on the whole are rare diseases.

THE STRUCTURE OF AN ADRENAL GLAND

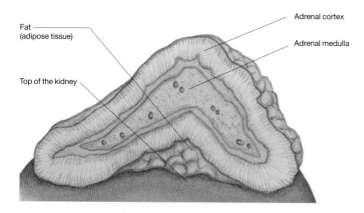

Fat
(adipose tissue)

Top of the kidney

Adrenal cortex

Adrenal medulla

△ Located on top of your kidneys, your adrenal glands consist of two parts, each with its own definite functions.

SIGNS AND SYMPTOMS OF ADDISON'S SYNDROME

Symptoms tend to develop slowly and are often just a feeling of ill-health. Other symptoms you may experience include:

➤ Fatigue and weakness.

➤ Loss of appetite.

➤ Fever.

➤ Weight loss.

➤ Skin pigmentation – dark patches of skin on creases of palms, elbows and knees.

Your doctor may also discover you have low blood pressure (hypotension).

ADDISON'S SYNDROME

This is caused by an underactive adrenal gland (hypoadrenalism) and can be due to autoimmune conditions where the body produces antibodies that destroy the adrenal cortex. Rarer causes include HIV and AIDS, tuberculosis and hypopituitarism (underactive pituitary gland). Corticosteroid hormone production can be suppressed in someone taking long-term steroid therapy or who has undergone surgery.

Whatever the cause, the production of corticosteroid hormones in the cortex falls, upsetting the body's chemistry with dangerous consequences. Addison's syndrome is twice as common in women as in men and appears to run in families.

HOW IS IT TREATED?

Synthetic corticosteroids are often prescribed to substitute natural hormones. Occasionally patients have a severe shortage of salt and sugar in their urine and are dehydrated. Their blood pressure is very low and they fall unconscious. This "Addisonian crisis" can be fatal without rapid fluid and steroid replacement. People with Addison's syndrome should always carry a Medic-Alert bracelet, which gives details of their disease if they are found unconscious.

People who have been taking steroid drugs long term for other diseases can also have an Addisonian crisis if they stop their medication suddenly. It is always advisable to step down your dosage of steroids gradually. It is also recommended that you discuss any change in your medication with your doctor first.

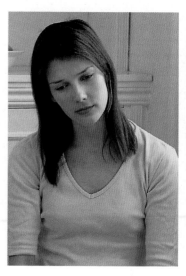

▽ Addison's syndrome is twice as common in women as in men and very often the only symptom may be a vague feeling of ill-health.

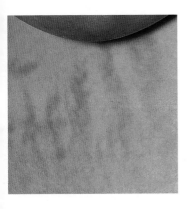

△ Excess levels of corticosteroid hormones in the blood (Cushing's syndrome) can cause streaky marks on the skin, seen here under the breast.

CUSHING'S SYNDROME

In stark contrast to its actions in Addison's syndrome, in Cushing's syndrome the adrenal cortex produces excessive corticosteroid hormones, causing a different upset in the body's chemistry. Cushing's syndrome is more common in women than in men and may be accompanied by depression and other psychological problems.

WHAT CAUSES IT?

It can be caused by an adrenal tumour or by excessive stimulation by adrenocorticotropic hormone (ACTH) from the pituitary gland; ACTH stimulates the adrenals to release their hormones. However, the most common cause is long-term steroid drug therapy. Steroid drugs mimic the action of the body's own adrenal hormones and so, when combined with natural levels, cause dramatically high corticosteroid levels in the body's circulation.

HOW IS CUSHING'S SYNDROME TREATED?

It is vital that Cushing's syndrome is treated as it could be fatal. If the condition is due to steroid drug therapy, your doctor will reassess your dosage or, if possible, discontinue treatment. If a tumour is the cause, your doctor can arrange for the affected gland to be removed surgically.

PHAEOCHROMOCYTOMA

The hormone adrenaline and its counterpart noradrenaline are produced within the adrenal medulla. Adrenaline and noradrenaline increase the heart beat and blood pressure in reaction to times of stress, exertion or fear. Phaeochromocytoma is a rare condition and it is caused by a non-cancerous tumour that secretes far too much adrenaline and noradrenaline, and consequently your body behaves as if under constant state of agitation resulting in a variety of distressing symptoms.

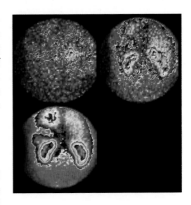

△ This coloured scan shows a tumour of the adrenal gland. The scans are made by injecting the patient with a radioactive "tracer" which shows up any abnormalities.

SIGNS AND SYMPTOMS OF CUSHING'S SYNDROME

People with Cushing's syndrome (or those taking long-term steroids) may develop the following symptoms:

➤ Tiredness.

➤ Excessive facial hair.

➤ The face becomes rounder.

➤ Skin becomes thin and bruises easily.

➤ Tendency to become overweight.

➤ Streaky marks (striae) may develop on the skin.

➤ High blood pressure.

SIGNS AND SYMPTOMS OF PHAEOCHROMOCYTOMA

Physical exercise or heightened emotion can trigger the tumour to release hormones into the bloodstream and also produce typical symptoms such as:

➤ Palpitations.

➤ Nausea and vomiting.

➤ Intense anxiety.

➤ Headache.

➤ Pallid skin.

➤ Profuse sweating.

➤ High blood pressure.

HYPERALDOSTERONISM (CONN'S SYNDROME)

The adrenal cortex produces the hormone aldosterone, which is involved in the regulation of salt balance and blood pressure. Overproduction of this hormone (known as hyperaldosteronism) results in an accumulation of salt within the body and a loss of the mineral potassium in urine.

Conn's syndrome is often caused by an adenoma in the cortex area of the adrenal gland. Signs and symptoms of hyperaldosteronism include:

➤ Muscle weakness and cramps.

➤ Frequent passage of large volumes of urine.

➤ Thirst.

➤ High blood pressure.

Treatment options include drugs to block the actions of the excessive hormone or removal of a tumour that may be prompting oversecretion.

TREATMENT OPTIONS

First, your doctor will treat you to normalize your blood pressure and then look at removing the offending tumour. Surgery is usually successful and people normally make a full recovery.

Pituitary gland disorders

SEE ALSO

➤ The endocrine glands, p312

➤ Cushing's syndrome, p319

➤ Meningitis, p332

The pituitary gland – often referred to as the "master gland" – sits at the base of the brain. It produces many hormones – both releasing factors to stimulate other organs to secrete their hormones and hormones that directly affect the body. Most pituitary disorders are the result of non-cancerous tumours (adenomas) that change the amounts of hormones that the gland produces. Adenomas that secrete growth hormone, adrenocorticotropic hormone (ACTH, for short) and prolactin are the most commonly encountered.

HYPOPITUITARISM

An underactive pituitary gland can affect one or many of the hormones that the pituitary produces. It can be caused by:
• A non-cancerous tumour.
• Infections such as meningitis.
• Trauma, for example a skull fracture.
• Surgery.

The pituitary hormone most likely to be affected by hypopituitarism is the growth hormone, which controls growth rates.

Doctors suspect growth hormone deficiency in a child who fails to grow at the normal rate. A synthetic growth hormone injection can restore normal growth patterns.

PROLACTINOMA

This pituitary tumour causes oversecretion of the hormone prolactin. Prolactin promotes breast development and lactation (milk production in women) and it also helps regulate sexual function. If overproduced, it can cause menstrual disturbance in women and reduced fertility in both sexes.

TREATMENT OF PITUITARY GLAND PROBLEMS

➤ Replacement of hormone deficiencies.

➤ Reduction of excess hormones, by surgically removing part of the gland or by using drugs to block the formation or effects of the hormone involved.

➤ Removal of the tumour, surgically, with radiotherapy or with drugs that shrink the pituitary gland tumour.

Treatment can lead to hypopituitarism, necessitating lifelong hormone therapy.

PITUITARY HORMONES AND FACTORS

➤ Luteinizing hormone (LH) and follicle-stimulating hormone (FSH) – Affect male and female sex organs.

➤ Melanocyte-stimulating factor (MSH) – Affects skin pigmentation.

➤ Adrenocorticotropic hormone (ACTH) – Affects the adrenal glands/body's general metabolism.

➤ Thyroid-stimulating hormone (TSH) – Also affects body's metabolism.

➤ Oxytocin – Affects milk release and uterine contractions.

➤ Antidiuretic hormone (ADH) – Affects kidney function.

➤ Growth hormone – Affects cell division, and bone and cartilage development.

➤ Prolactin – Affects female breast development.

THE STRUCTURE OF THE PITUITARY GLAND

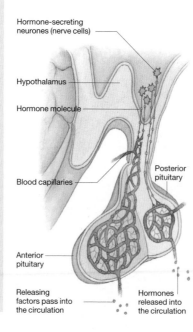

Hormone-secreting neurones (nerve cells)

Hypothalamus

Hormone molecule

Blood capillaries

Posterior pituitary

Anterior pituitary

Releasing factors pass into the circulation

Hormones released into the circulation

ACROMEGALY/GIGANTISM

In children, the overproduction of growth hormone is gigantism, in adults it is called acromegaly. This overproduction from a pituitary tumour causes body parts – usually the tongue, face, hands and feet – to enlarge. The changes happen slowly and may not be obvious. If doctors suspect acromegaly, they may ask for old photographs to compare with your current appearance. People with gigantism can grow more than 2 metres (7 feet) tall.

Other physical changes can include increased growth of coarse body hair, deepening of the voice and excessive sweating. Other symptoms may include headaches and defects of vision as the pituitary tumour presses on the optic nerve.

◁ The pituitary gland has two lobes (anterior and posterior). It hangs from the hypothalamus by a stalk of nerve fibres and a blood vessel network. Releasing factors exit the anterior lobe and the posterior lobe deals with hormones.

5

THE NERVOUS SYSTEM

The nervous system includes the brain, and the central and peripheral nervous systems. It controls all our body's functions, from vital life support mechanisms, such as breathing, to the ability to sense and react to stimuli. The brain is the control centre that regulates physical functions and makes us conscious and able to feel emotions. Yet, like all our body systems, the nervous system is prey to disorders, from interruption to its blood supply to life-threatening infections. The brain is also prone to subtle chemical change that can cause emotional disturbance and psychological illness.

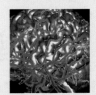

CONTENTS

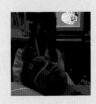

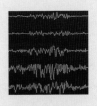

The brain and nerve network

SEE ALSO
➤ Stroke, p328
➤ Multiple sclerosis, p336
➤ Depression, p346
➤ The musculoskeletal system, p354

The brain is the control centre of your body, and other parts of your body play an important role in supporting your brain by feeding it with oxygen and nutrients, for example, and by supplying it with information. The brain functions via billions of interconnected nerve cells and various information-signalling chemicals called neurotransmitters. A fine chemical balance exists in terms of the levels of neurotransmitters in the brain and any shift in balance can cause unusual psychological functions such as mood swings or depression.

Your nervous system can be seen as comprising two parts:
- The central nervous system – The brain and spinal cord.
- The peripheral nervous system – All other nerves throughout the body.

THE BASIC BUILDING BLOCK

The brain is composed of about 100 billion nerve cells, or neurones. Everything you see, feel, think and do depends on their ability to communicate with one another.

Neurones function in different ways:
- Motor neurones – Cause muscles to contract when instructed to by the brain.
- Sensory neurones – Carry sensory information, such as pain or touch, from the body to the brain.
- Interneurones – Connect neurones to each other.

FAST-TRACKING SIGNALS

Your nerves are made up of bundles of nerve cells, or neurones, which pass information between specific sites in the body and the brain and spinal cord. This information travels as electrical messages along the length of a neurone's axon, and via outgrowths called dendrites. The messages pass from one neurone to another across a gap called a synapse, and are taken across in the form of chemical "neurotransmitters". Doctors are able to measure the electrical activity in the brain by using an electroencephalogram (EEG).

To speed the transmission of nerve impulses, some axons are insulated by a fatty white substance called myelin. In some diseases, such as multiple sclerosis, this myelin insulation is destroyed or damaged, which stops nerve signals getting through.

PROTECTION AND SUPPORT

As your brain and spinal cord perform absolutely vital, finely tuned functions, they have to be well-protected and supported against possible physical injury and infection. The bones of the skull and the vertebrae do a good job of protecting the brain and spinal cord from physical damage. The brain and spinal cord are also enveloped by three protective membranes, called the meninges, and are bathed by a nourishing and lubricating fluid known as cerebrospinal fluid. Both the membranes and fluid act to cushion movements within the head and spine. However, infectious micro-organisms can invade the nervous system. This may lead to inflammation of the membranes – meningitis – and clouding of the cerebrospinal fluid, which can be detected by taking a sample via a procedure called a lumbar puncture.

THE STRUCTURE OF THE BRAIN

▽ The brain is divided into two cerebral hemispheres – the left and right hemispheres – which are linked by a network of nerve fibres. This nerve network is called the corpus callosum. Each hemisphere is in turn divided into four areas known as cerebral lobes.

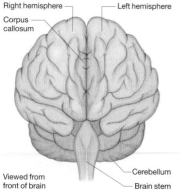

Right hemisphere
Corpus callosum
Left hemisphere
Cerebellum
Brain stem
Viewed from front of brain

Frontal lobe
This area of the brain deals with planning, forethought and other intellectual functions.

Temporal lobe
This area at the side of the brain deals with information on smell and hearing as well as making sense of language.

Viewed from side

Parietal lobe
This area deals with information on sensation from the entire body.

Occipital lobe
This lobe is concerned with vision.

Cerebellum

Brain stem

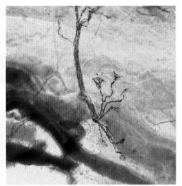

△ This picture shows a nerve–muscle connection – the synapses between a motor neurone axon and the muscle fibres that it controls (the muscle appears as pale bands).

BASIC BRAIN DIVISIONS

The human brain has three divisions:

- Cerebrum – Made up of left- and right-hand cerebral hemispheres.
- Brainstem – Connects the cerebral hemispheres to the spinal cord; it controls the automatic functions of the body, such as heart rate and breathing.
- Cerebellum – This large, flat, tree-shaped area at the back of the brainstem controls and regulates movement.

ANATOMY OF A NEURONE

▽ Neurones of all types consist of a cell body, a long "tail" called an axon and branching projections called dendrites.

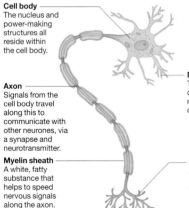

Cell body
The nucleus and power-making structures all reside within the cell body.

Axon
Signals from the cell body travel along this to communicate with other neurones, via a synapse and neurotransmitter.

Myelin sheath
A white, fatty substance that helps to speed nervous signals along the axon.

Dendrite
These projections seek out other neurones to make contact and collect information.

Synaptic knob
At the end of each axon branch is a knob that sends signals across a tiny gap (a synapse) to the next neurone.

THE CENTRAL NERVOUS SYSTEM

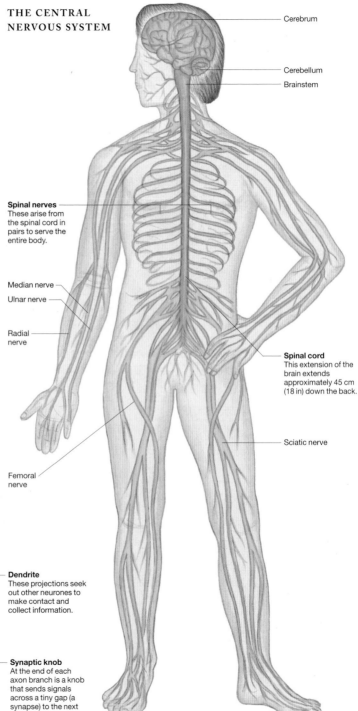

Cerebrum

Cerebellum

Brainstem

Spinal nerves
These arise from the spinal cord in pairs to serve the entire body.

Median nerve

Ulnar nerve

Radial nerve

Spinal cord
This extension of the brain extends approximately 45 cm (18 in) down the back.

Sciatic nerve

Femoral nerve

Headaches and migraine

SEE ALSO
➤ Learn to manage stress, p260
➤ Meningitis, p332
➤ Migraines in children, p478

The majority of people have the occasional headache but this usually disappears spontaneously within a few hours. In some people, though, headaches can persist for longer and cause great distress. The pain itself may focus on the back of the head, the forehead and behind the eyes, and the quality of the pain varies from dull and continuous to sudden and sharp. However, it is rare for a headache to have a life-threatening cause. Most headaches are not serious in nature, although they can be hard to explain and treat.

Doctors tend to talk about four different types of headache:
• Tension headache.
• Analgesic headache.
• Cluster headache.
• Migraine.

A headache may also accompany a feverish illness such as influenza and is an all-too-familiar symptom of the common cold and of sinusitis. Excessive consumption of alcohol can also lead to a headache the following morning.

There are some more serious, but much rarer, causes of headache. These include a brain tumour (benign or malignant), which can be the cause of recurrent headaches, or inflammation of the arteries in the brain, which causes a sudden throbbing pain in one or both temples. Other serious but rare conditions associated with headache include meningitis and subarachnoid haemorrhage.

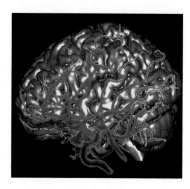

△ Widening and subsequent narrowing of the blood vessels in the brain is a probable cause of the pain of migraine headaches.

It is recommended that you consult your doctor as soon as possible if you experience any of the additional symptoms listed in the box on recognizing serious headaches.

TENSION HEADACHE
This is by far the most common form of headache. Such headaches can be moderately or severely painful. Doctors believe the pain to be due to spasm in the muscles of the scalp and neck. The headache usually feels like tightness across the forehead, often spreading back into the neck. Slight nausea is a common accompanying symptom, although vomiting is not. Usually these headaches last only a few hours but sometimes they can persist. This type of headache generally affects more women than men.

Many factors can trigger tension headaches, including stress, noise, fumes, problems with eyesight and depression. Tension headaches can often result from bad posture and from long periods staring at a computer screen. These headaches respond well to relaxation techniques and over-the-counter painkillers. Tension headaches often improve if you perform some vigorous exercise.

If you suffer from recurrent headaches, your doctor will want to know about the severity and frequency of your symptoms, so it is often useful to keep a note of these. In some cases a CT scan may be carried out in order to discover the underlying cause of recurrent or persistent headaches.

ANALGESIC HEADACHE
It may seem unlikely but painkillers can actually cause a headache. Studies have shown that regular long-term use of painkillers for a headache can in turn lead

∇ Most tension headaches are quickly relieved by over-the-counter painkillers. However, medical advice is needed if headaches recur.

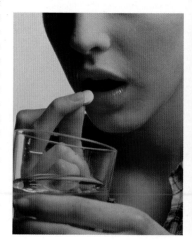

RECOGNIZING A SERIOUS HEADACHE
Seek medical advice without delay if you suffer any of the following symptoms:

➤ A severe headache that develops quickly and suddenly.

➤ A headache that gets worse and worse despite painkillers.

➤ Vomiting after the onset of headache.

➤ Significant numbness and weakness of the limbs.

➤ Blurred vision wiith eye pain.

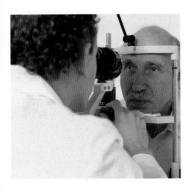

△ Some eye conditions can lead to headaches. An eye examination may be needed in certain cases of persistent or recurrent headaches.

to a pain that is similar to a tension headache. For sufferers there is a temptation to use ever-stronger painkillers, but this will only make the problem worse. This type of headache can be avoided by using painkillers as sparingly as possible. However, if you have a headache that is not relieved by taking simple painkillers, you should always consult your doctor, who will investigate the cause.

CLUSTER HEADACHE

This unusual condition is poorly understood. Sufferers, most commonly men, are often woken in the middle of the night with excruciating pain through one eye. Such attacks generally last 15 to 30 minutes. The headaches tend to follow a pattern and they may occur between one and four times a day.

The pain is exceedingly resistant to painkillers and antimigraine drugs, although lithium, a drug that is also used to treat certain psychiatric disorders, may help prevent attacks and inhaling oxygen may stop an attack. Smoking and drinking alcohol can increase the risk of a cluster headache occurring.

MIGRAINE

This severe form of headache can be extremely debilitating. Millions of people worldwide experience migraines each year. Susceptible individuals usually have their

TYPES OF MIGRAINE
Doctors describe migraine as being either classical or common.

➤ In classical migraine the headache usually affects one side of the head. Many people get a warning – or aura – before the headache starts that usually consists of seeing flashing lights, stars or zigzag lines. About 20 per cent of migraines are classical.

➤ In common migraine, the only symptom may be a one-sided headache.

first migraine before the age of 30 but children as young as three may suffer from this condition. It is rare to experience a first migraine after the age of 40 and the frequency and severity of attacks usually diminishes with age.

Migraine-sufferers usually have other symptoms, such as disturbance to vision, as well as a headache. The cause of the condition is not apparent but it is probably due to the dilation of certain blood vessels in the brain. Just before the symptoms start, small arteries in the brain become narrower, thereby reducing blood flow. For reasons that are not clear, as the headache begins, these small arteries become wider again.

SIGNS AND SYMPTOMS OF A MIGRAINE
As the headache develops there may also be some of the following symptoms:

➤ Vomiting.

➤ Aversion to bright light (photophobia).

➤ Feeling irritable.

Once the migraine has passed, the person will often just want to sleep. It is unusual for a migraine to last for more than 24 hours, although some people suffer recurrent migraines with a day or so gap between them.

POSSIBLE CAUSES
Certain factors seem to trigger a migraine attack in some people, including:

• Stress.
• Foodstuffs such as chocolate, coffee and cheese.
• Red wine.
• Missed meals.
• The contraceptive pill.
• Menstruation.
• Sexual intercourse.

A high percentage of migraine sufferers will have other family members who also suffer from them.

TREATMENT OPTIONS
The priority in the prevention of migraine attacks is to avoid any known precipitating factors. It may help to keep a diary of what you have eaten and other possible factors to help you determine what the cause may be. In many cases, a simple dietary change is all that is needed to prevent a recurrence.

As a migraine begins, painkillers or antimigraine drugs, which act on the brain's blood vessels, can help. Your doctor can recommend antiemetics to quell nausea and/or vomiting, or prescribe drugs that prevent attacks as a long-term treatment.

▽ A variety of relaxation techniques can be effective in cases of tension headaches. Scalp massage is often of benefit.

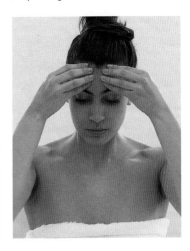

Fatigue

Each day, large numbers of people visit their doctor complaining of tiredness. Yet many come away from consultations feeling that they have had no satisfactory explanation for the way they feel. Fatigue is such a generalized symptom that it is not easy for anyone except the sufferer to assess it, plus it also depends on comparisons with previous energy levels. Fatigue can be caused by a range of conditions, from lack of oxygen in the blood to depression. If there are no other accompanying physical symptoms, then the cause can be very hard to pin down.

COMMON CAUSES OF FATIGUE

➤ Anaemia.

➤ Hypothyroidism.

➤ Diabetes.

➤ Sleep disorders.

➤ Depression.

The first step in a diagnosis is for your doctor to take your medical history in order to find out if there are any other symptoms that may explain your fatigue. If there are symptoms, a physical examination may be carried out to help identify possible causes. Your doctor may then take a sample of blood and send it for laboratory testing. Testing will include:

• A full blood count to check for anaemia.

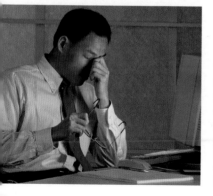

▽ Fatigue may result from long hours in a stressful job or from physical factors such as poor ventilation or glaring computer screens.

• Thyroid function tests to look for an underactive thyroid gland.
• Sugar levels to look for diabetes.

These blood tests are normal in more than 90 per cent of people.

LOOKING FOR CAUSES

Your doctor may not find a physical cause for your lack of energy and may consider whether depression could be to blame. If neither of these seem to be the culprit, then the underlying cause is likely to be stress – probably the main cause of fatigue in the Western world today.

LOOKING AT YOUR LIFESTYLE

Most people live hectic lives, having to cope with demands and strains our bodies were not designed for. Once physical disease and psychological health problems have been excluded, most people feel better if made to recognize that their fatigue may simply arise from the pace of modern life and if they are given some simple, sensible advice to follow. Many of us "burn the candle at both ends" trying to meet the demands of a busy work schedule and home or social life. This may mean you are getting too little sleep, which can lead to a build-up of fatigue. You may be skipping meals or eating too much junk food, thereby missing out on essential nutrients. You should also consider if your alcohol consumption is too high – a major cause of fatigue. Importantly, lack of physical exercise can lead to lethargy and sluggishness. Regular exercise, particularly outdoors, can have a remarkable effect in boosting energy levels.

CHRONIC FATIGUE SYNDROME

Also known medically as myalgic encephalomyelitis (ME), chronic fatigue syndrome is a controversial subject and the symptoms are often vague and non-specific. For this reason the condition is often misdiagnosed. The main symptoms, which may last for about six months, are:

➤ Fatigue and poor quality sleep.

➤ Poor concentration and memory.

➤ Fever.

➤ Aching muscles.

The condition may occur in the aftermath of infection by certain viruses. In other cases it seems to develop in response to severe emotional stress. But in many cases there is no obvious triggering infection or life event. However, many doctors are not convinced that this is a physical illness, preferring a psychiatric or psychological explanation for the symptoms.

Studies have shown that chronic fatigue syndrome occurs most often in women between the ages of 25 and 45, but it is possible for those of either sex or of any age group to be affected.

The treatment for this condition is mainly supportive and psychological, although a programme of graded exercise can be beneficial for many sufferers. Depression is common in people with chronic fatigue syndrome and in such cases antidepressant drugs can be very helpful.

Head injury

SEE ALSO
➤ The brain and nerve network, p322
➤ Epilepsy, p330
➤ The musculoskeletal system, p354

Minor bumps and bangs to the head are extremely common and in most cases leave no long-term ill-effects – the skull is a very resilient structure. As for more serious head injuries, the principal cause of these is road traffic accidents. Many developed countries have made it compulsory for motorcycle riders and drivers to wear helmets and seatbelts respectively. These preventive measures have resulted in significant reductions in the number of road accident-related head injuries. Helmets for cyclists and horse riders also help to minimize injuries.

SIGNS AND SYMPTOMS OF A SERIOUS HEAD INJURY

Look out for any of the following symptoms, which may appear up to 24 hours after the injury:

➤ Vomiting.

➤ Blurred vision.

➤ Loss of memory, especially of events after the injury.

➤ Drowsiness and/or confusion.

➤ Headache that gets progressively worse despite taking painkillers.

If you have injured your head and have any of the symptoms listed in the above box on serious head injury, visit your doctor immediately or go to the nearest accident and emergency department.

TYPES OF INJURY

The brain can be injured by:
- Shearing and rotation, which means that the brain's nerve cells are battered and bruised inside the skull. This is the commonest form of brain injury.
- Direct nerve damage caused by penetrating injuries.
- Swelling of the brain as a result of inflammation.
- Lack of oxygen to the brain while the patient is unconscious.
- Raised intracranial pressure, which can occur if the pressure within the skull rises. This may be caused by an expanding blood clot from a torn blood vessel, for example. As a result the brain is forced out of the bottom of the skull, causing severe damage.

INVESTIGATING HEAD INJURIES

Doctors may examine you physically and ask about the incident and any symptoms. They may X-ray your skull to look for fractures, although this will reveal little about any underlying brain damage.

Most minor head injury patients are allowed home if someone can keep an eye on them. Serious problems can develop in the first 24 hours and so monitoring is vital.

TREATMENT OPTIONS

If the head injury is severe, the patient may be kept in hospital for observation. In such cases, a brain scan may be done to look for brain damage.

In severe head injuries, the patient may remain unconscious for a long time. In a

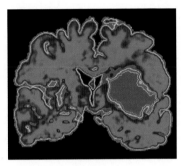

△ A computer-enhanced scan of the brain shows bleeding within the brain (red area). This may be caused by a serious head injury.

few cases the problem lies with an expanding blood clot or haematoma, which needs to be removed by a neurosurgeon.

The key treatment is to assist a person's breathing so that the brain gets plenty of oxygen and nutrients. Drugs may be given to prevent the brain swelling. Recovery from a severe brain injury may take weeks or months and the degree of recovery is variable and not easy to predict early on.

▽ When taking part in any activity with a risk of head injury it is advisable to wear a helmet to prevent serious damage if an accident occurs.

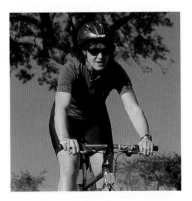

POSSIBLE COMPLICATIONS AFTER A HEAD INJURY

The commonest complication is post-head injury syndrome – consisting of headache, nausea and tiredness – which can occur even after very minor head injuries. In most cases this settles with a few weeks' rest. More serious possible long-term consequences can include epilepsy, loss of higher brain function, personality changes and hydrocephalus (water on the brain).

Stroke

SEE ALSO

➤ Exercise for life, p266

➤ Atherosclerosis, p280

➤ Thrombosis and embolism, p288

➤ The brain and nerve network, p322

Brain damage caused by an interruption in the brain's blood supply – and therefore its oxygen supply – is a common cause of death in many developed countries and a major cause of long-term disability. Stroke is more common in those over 70 and the risk of stroke increases with age. It can occur with little or no warning and have devastating effects, depending on which part of the brain is affected. With the help of staff in specialized rehabilitation units, stroke victims often make a full recovery, although about a third may be left with some form of disability.

Strokes, also known as cerebrovascular accidents (CVAs), can be caused by several different types of disruption to the blood supply to the brain. The main types of stroke are:

• Cerebral infarction – This is the commonest form of stroke and occurs when a blood vessel in the brain becomes blocked – either by a clot formed within the blood vessel (thrombus) or by a clot that has formed elsewhere in the body and has travelled to the brain (embolus). The area of the brain supplied by that blood vessel dies and the functions that were provided by that area are affected. The main underlying cause of this type

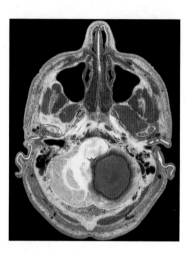

△ The red colouring in this scan of the brain indicates the area affected by a cerebral haemorrhage in the cerebellum.

of stroke is atherosclerosis – where fatty plaques (atheroma) form on the lining of blood vessels, which encourages the formation of blood clots in the brain and elsewhere. Less common causes of cerebral infarction include disorders such as sickle-cell disease, in which the blood tends to form clots too easily, and disorders of heart rhythm or heart valves.

• Cerebral haemorrhage – In this form of stroke a blood vessel in the brain bursts and as a result blood leaks out and causes damage to the surrounding brain tissue. This can occur as a result of an underlying weakness of the blood vessels in the brain, and is perhaps exacerbated by high blood pressure, or if the blood-clotting process is impaired – for example by drug treatment.

MINI-STROKES

Also known by doctors as transient ischaemic attacks (TIAs), mini-strokes are short-lived versions of a stroke that may last from a few seconds to an hour. Symptoms are often similar to those of a stroke but they disappear over 24 hours. They are caused by lack of oxygen to the brain due to temporary blockage of a blood vessel. Sudden visual loss in one eye and bouts of confusion, that usually pass in a few hours, are characteristic of such mini-strokes.

After a series of mini-strokes, doctors often perform a Doppler ultrasound scan of the carotid arteries in the neck to see if they are furred up with atheroma. Treatment options include aspirin, surgical removal of the plaques or balloon angioplasty to widen the arteries narrowed by atheroma.

SIGNS AND SYMPTOMS

➤ Loss of consciousness.

➤ Weakness or inability to move on one side of the body.

➤ Blurred or fuzzy vision or loss of vision in one eye.

➤ Numbness on one side of the body.

➤ Loss of control of fine movements and tremor.

➤ Speech difficulties.

➤ Difficulties maintaining balance and vertigo.

RISK FACTORS FOR STROKE

There are several adjustments that you can make to your lifestyle in order to reduce your risk of atherosclerosis and stroke. These are some of the risk factors that can be controlled by you:

• High blood pressure – This increases the risk of atherosclerosis by putting strain on the blood vessels in the brain.

• Smoking – As well as the many other risks associated with it, smoking leads to narrowing of the blood vessels and encourages the formation of blood clots.

• High blood cholesterol levels – This condition, which may be the result of an inherited tendency or a high fat diet, can lead to atherosclerosis.

• High alcohol intake – Although drinking small amounts of alcohol may be beneficial for the circulation, studies have shown that regular high alcohol consumption increases the risk of stroke.

- Inactive lifestyle – Taking regular exercise reduces the formation of atherosclerosis and helps to maintain healthy blood pressure.
- Diabetes – This condition carries an increased risk of atherosclerosis. So it is important that a diabetic's blood pressure is monitored very carefully.
- Obesity – There is a strong correlation between being severely overweight and circulatory problems of all kinds.

AREAS OFTEN AFFECTED BY STROKE

In theory, any brain function could be affected by a stroke but certain areas of the brain are more at risk. These areas include:
- Motor strip – This region is concerned with muscle control and damage to this area on one side of the brain results in weakness and/or paralysis on the opposite side of the body.
- Broca's and Wernicke's areas – These areas of the left side of the brain are principally concerned with speech. People affected by strokes in these areas have difficulty understanding speech or find it difficult to find the right words.
- Brainstem – In this area, which controls vital functions such as breathing, the nerve fibres are tightly packed as they pass into the spinal cord and even very small strokes can cause life-threatening damage. Victims of strokes in this part of the brain rarely survive in the long term.

▽ Fast foods and convenience dishes are often very high in fat. Controlling your fat intake is an important way of reducing your risk of stroke.

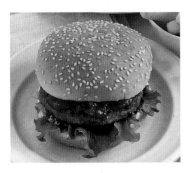

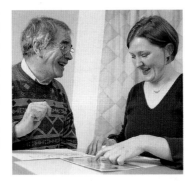

△ Special therapists can help those recovering from the effects of a stroke. Activities and games are used to rebuild speech, cooordination and thought processes.

DIAGNOSING A STROKE

There are rarely any warning signs of a stroke, although someone who has experienced repeated transient ischaemic attacks or mini-strokes is at increased risk. Anyone displaying symptoms of a stroke requires immediate medical attention. A doctor may be able to diagnose the condition from the obvious physical symptoms or after making a detailed physical examination to find out whether any functions are not working as normal and by taking a medical history. The precise site of the stroke can be confirmed by a CT or MRI brain scan.

TREATMENT OPTIONS

If a cerebral infarction is picked up early the main aim of treatment will be to try to minimize damage and reduce the long-term ill effects. Specific treatment to reverse the stroke may not always be possible, although drugs to reduce blood pressure or to combat inflammation may be administered.

Long-term treatment following a cerebral infarction may include regular low doses of aspirin to prevent further clots forming. Once the victim's condition has stabilized following a stroke, the focus of treatment is likely to be rehabilitation and returning the patient to as near normal life as possible.

STROKE REHABILITATION

The brain has an amazing capacity to "rewire" itself and bypass damaged areas so that most people who have had strokes recover some of the lost function, although to what extent is variable and unpredictable.

Rehabilitation following a stroke starts soon afterwards with physiotherapy to get your body moving again. It is important to regain mobility as quickly as possible because there is a greater the chance that surviving nerve cells can remodel themselves to acquire lost functions. Specialist interventions may also include hydrotherapy and speech therapy.

Once an individual is ready to leave hospital, an occupational therapist will help to implement any adaptations that may be needed in the home, such as grab rails or a stair lift, in order that as much independence can be retained as possible. If necessary, speech therapists and physiotherapists continue to visit the patient after discharge from hospital to pursue their programme of treatment.

THE LONG-TERM OUTLOOK

Improvements to functions damaged by stroke can continue to happen for as long as six months after the stroke. However, any remaining disability after this time is more likely to last. Some people are severely disabled by stroke and require long-term, full-time nursing care. One person in five dies within a month of a stroke.

▽ Taking regular exercise throughout adult life, and particularly later in life, can make a vital contribution to the health of your blood vessels.

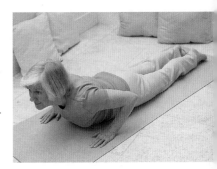

Epilepsy

SEE ALSO

➤ Stroke, p328
➤ Dementia, p338
➤ Febrile convulsions, p479

An epileptic fit or seizure occurs when part or all of the brain's nerve cells create electrical signals in an uncontrolled manner. If you have an isolated seizure this does not necessarily mean that you have epilepsy. Doctors need evidence of recurrences of such seizures on two or more occasions to carry out a proper diagnosis. Epilepsy is a very common condition, affecting 2 per cent of the population in developed countries. Many people with epilepsy lead normal lives, although some activities, such as driving, are prohibited.

Epileptic seizures can be categorized into two types – these are generalized seizures or partial seizures:

- Generalized seizures are the most common and there are two sub-categories – tonic-clonic and absence. A tonic-clonic (or grand mal) generalized seizure may start with a vague sense of foreboding (an "aura"), after which the person suddenly becomes rigid and falls to the ground, often uttering a cry. They may bite their tongue, lose control of their bowel or bladder and start to shake all over. Finally, as the fitting subsides and ends, the person becomes very drowsy. Fits usually occur one at a time; fits that follow on from one another are a dangerous sign and the person needs to go to hospital as soon as possible.

- Absence (or petit mal) generalized seizures are more common in childhood and adolescence. In such cases the child "goes blank", often with the eyes open and staring, for up to 30 seconds.

- Partial seizures are less common. In this case the fit is limited to just one part of the brain. The person may simply look blank or vacant for a few minutes, may experience odd sights or smells, or may have uncontrolled movement of one part of their body.

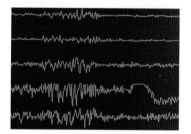

△ Traces produced by an EEG (electroencephalography) show increased electrical activity during an epileptic seizure.

▽ During an EEG electrodes are placed on the scalp. The electrodes monitor and record electrical activity in the brain.

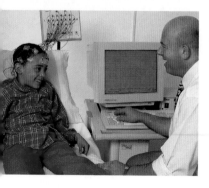

CAUSES OF EPILEPSY

In most people no obvious cause for epilepsy is found, although the condition does tend to run in families. Most epileptics experience their first seizure as children and many outgrow the condition during adolescence. A person who has a first fit in adulthood is unusual and this should be investigated further.

Other causes of seizures include:
- Brain trauma or surgery.
- Brain tumour.
- Drugs and alcohol.
- Alzheimer's disease.
- Stroke.

WHAT TO DO IF SOMEONE HAS AN EPILEPTIC FIT

Seeing someone having a fit can be very frightening. The main thing is not to panic as fits usually only last a short time.

The first priority is to try to prevent the person hurting themself while they are having a fit.

Once the fit is over, place him or her on their side with the uppermost leg bent at the knee to keep him or her from slumping forward – this is known as the recovery position.

Do not try to keep the mouth open during a fit. You will only cause injury and may end up having your fingers bitten.

- High fever – Young children with a fever can have a fit, which is known as a febrile convulsion, but this is a fairly normal response and there is little risk of this developing into epilepsy as an adult.

Some things can trigger a seizure or make it more likely, and these include strobe lighting, excessive stress and lack of sleep.

DIAGNOSIS AND TREATMENT OPTIONS FOR EPILEPSY

Epilepsy can be confirmed with a tracing of the electrical activity of the brain, called an electroencephalogram or EEG. Brain scanning may also be performed to shed light on any physical defects that could be causing the epilepsy, such as a brain tumour.

In the long term there are a wide range of anticonvulsant drugs to control the fits. The correct dosage varies greatly between individuals and it may take a little while for the doctor to find the optimum dose to control fits in each case. Most people with epilepsy have no or very few fits once they are stabilized on medication.

The danger to other road-users means that in many countries people with epilepsy must have had three fit-free years before they can drive again. Commercial drivers, such as lorry drivers and bus drivers, may be prohibited from driving altogether. Anyone who has suffered from epilepsy should seek medical advice before undertaking potentially dangerous sports such as rock climbing or scuba diving.

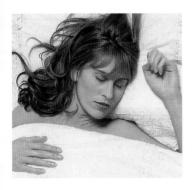

△ Lack of sleep can trigger seizures. Most epileptics benefit from an ordered lifestyle with regular meals and low stress levels.

Brain tumours

SEE ALSO
➤ Lung cancer, p384

Brain tumours can either originate in the brain or spread from a cancer elsewhere, such as the lungs or breast. Tumours can be cancerous or non-cancerous, but because of the restrictions of the skull any such growth may affect brain function. Fortunately, such tumours are rare.

If your doctor suspects a brain tumour from your symptoms and a thorough physical examination, then you will be referred to a neurologist and for brain scanning. In certain cases, additional tests such as

SIGNS AND SYMPTOMS

Symptoms often appear due to compression of part of the brain by the growing tumour; they include:

➤ Headache, usually worse in the morning.

➤ Nausea and vomiting.

➤ Blurred vision.

Symptoms are often specific to the part of the brain affected, including:

➤ Difficulty reading or writing.

➤ Slurred speech.

➤ A change of personality.

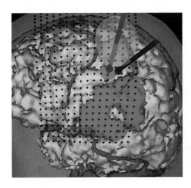

△ The green area in this MRI (magnetic resonance imaging) scan shows a tumour in the motor cortex (blue dotted area) of the brain.

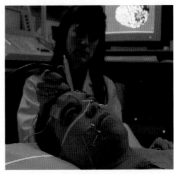

△ A technician prepares a patient for brain surgery by creating a computerized map of the brain, which is then used to guide the surgeon.

cerebral angiography or a brain biopsy (in which a sample of tissue is removed for analysis) are carried out.

Some benign brain tumours may be removed surgically and recovery chances tend to be good. Removing benign tumours may pose operative risks, such as brain damage, as they lie close to vital structures, such as the brain stem. Radiotherapy to shrink the brain tumour may be advised. Depending on its location and spread, a cancerous tumour may be removed surgically. If surgery is not possible, the tumour may respond to radiotherapy, but the outlook in cases of brain tumours that have spread from other organs is poor.

Meningitis

Meningitis is the inflammation of the membranes surrounding the brain (the meninges). It is usually caused by an infection. Viral meningitis is the most common, and less dangerous, form and generally affects young adults. Bacterial meningitis is a more serious condition that mainly affects children. This life-threatening condition often begins with symptoms similar to those of a common cold or flu. However, the child's condition rapidly worsens and the classic symptoms of the disease, described below, develop.

Meningitis is the result of an infection by one of a number of different viruses or bacteria. In rare cases, usually among those with reduced immunity, it may also be caused by a fungal infection. Although treatment depends on the type of infection, all forms of the disease are serious and any suspected case of meningitis warrants immediate medical assessment and possible admission to hospital.

MAKING THE DIAGNOSIS

A doctor will usually make a provisional diagnosis based on observation of the symptoms and an examination of the

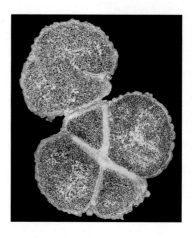

△ *Neisseria meningitidis*, seen here in the process of dividing, is the bacterium that causes meningococcal meningitis.

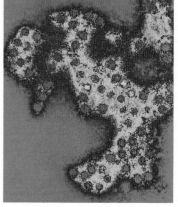

△ The coxsackie virus shown here is a common cause of colds as well as being a frequent cause of viral meningitis.

SIGNS AND SYMPTOMS

If the infection is due to a virus, the symptoms tend to develop gradually. In bacterial meningitis, however, symptoms appear rapidly. Symptoms of meningitis include the following:

➤ Fever.

➤ Headache.

➤ Neck stiffness.

➤ Dislike of bright lights (photophobia).

➤ Sometimes a rash will develop.

In addition, children and babies may be:

➤ Very drowsy and unrousable.

➤ Floppy.

➤ Have a high-pitched cry.

Fitting may occur if treatment is not given as soon as possible.

patient. Further investigations, which may be carried out after treatment has already started, are likely to include a lumbar puncture, in which a sample of cerebrospinal fluid is removed from around the spinal cord in the lower back and examined under the microscope for signs of infection. In some cases a brain scan may be carried out.

TREATMENT OPTIONS

Viral meningitis generally requires no specific treatment beyond analgesics to provide pain relief and reduce fever. Full recovery from the condition takes one to two weeks.

In cases of suspected bacterial meningitis, prompt administration of intravenous antibiotics is essential. Time is vital and minutes can save lives. In some cases, corticosteroids may be given to reduce inflammation. Recovery from the bacterial form of the disease is much slower than from viral meningitis, but recovery times vary from case to case. Even with the best treatment, approximately 15 per cent of patients die from the condition.

WHAT ARE THE LONG-TERM EFFECTS?

Although most people make a full recovery from viral and bacterial meningitis, some people are left with long-term problems following bacterial meningitis. These include hearing loss and impaired memory.

PREVENTING MENINGITIS

Many people are concerned, when there is a case of meningitis locally, that they or their children may be at risk. However, bacterial meningitis is actually quite difficult to catch from another person. You would need to be breathing the same air as the affected person for a number of hours to be even slightly at risk. The spread of infection among such close contacts is usually effectively prevented by the administration of a two-day course of antibiotics.

Children in many developed countries now receive immunization against *Haemophilus influenzae* type B (HIB) bacterium, which is a common cause of meningitis. The meningococcal bacterium has two main strains that cause meningitis in Europe. There is now a vaccine to the C strain and it is part of the standard childhood vaccination programme. A vaccine for the more common B strain is likely to be available shortly.

HOW TO RECOGNIZE A MENINGOCOCCAL RASH

It is possible that meningitis resulting from infection with meningococcal bacteria may also result in an infection in the blood stream. This sometimes leads to a characteristic purpuric rash which looks like a bruise, appears suddenly and spreads quickly. The rash consists of small, blotchy dark-red-purple spots. One of the factors that may help you recognize this rash is that it does not "blanch" (seem to disappear) when it is pressed – typically using the side of a glass tumbler. However, if you have any doubts at all about the nature of a rash, particularly if it is accompanied by any of the other symptoms, consult a doctor, or take your child to hospital, as soon as possible.

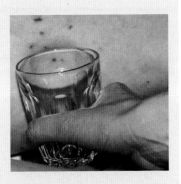

△ The tumbler test is the best way to find out if it is a meningococcal rash. Press the side of a glass over the affected area. If the rash does not disappear when pressed, then you must seek medical advice immediately.

Viral encephalitis

SEE ALSO
▶ Viral infections, p466

This viral infection of the brain tissue itself results in inflammation and raised intracranial (inside the skull) pressure. It is a rare condition that is usually fairly mild in nature and settles rapidly. Viral encephalitis most commonly affects babies and the elderly.

This condition may develop as a complication of another viral illness and is often caused by the same viruses that cause mumps and measles. It may also be caused by the herpes simplex virus. This form of the disease can be life-threatening. In some parts of the world there are more severe forms, such as Japanese encephalitis in South-east Asia, California encephalitis in the US and Ross River fever in Australia.

If your doctor suspects viral encephalitis, immediate hospital admission is necessary. A lumbar puncture to take a sample of cerebrospinal fluid may be necessary. A CT or MRI brain scan may also be carried out. In some cases, an electroencephalogram (EEG) is done.

There is no specific treatment for some forms of viral encephalitis and most patients recover spontaneously. However, acyclovir may be given intravenously in cases of herpes simplex infection. A vaccine exists for preventing Japanese encephalitis.

SIGNS AND SYMPTOMS

Typical symptoms of viral encephalitis include the following:

▶ Fever.

▶ Headache.

▶ Drowsiness.

These symptoms are similar to those of meningitis and a doctor's main concern will be to discount this possibility as quickly as possible.

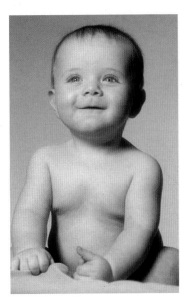

▷ Babies are among those most susceptible to viral encephalitis. Fever and drowsiness are the most common symptoms.

Prolapsed disc and sciatica

SEE ALSO

➤ Exercise for life, p266
➤ The brain and nerve network, p322
➤ Backache, p365

The intervertebral discs sit between the bones of the back (vertebrae). These discs consist of a tough, fibrous ring that holds the bones together and a spongy centre that acts as a shock-absorber. A prolapsed disc, which is also known as a slipped or herniated disc, occurs when the fibrous ring splits and some of the spongy centre is forced out; this in turn presses on the nerves leaving the spine, thereby causing pain. A slipped disc very often leads to a common condition called sciatica – severe nerve pain felt in the buttocks and legs.

SIGNS AND SYMPTOMS OF A PROLAPSED DISC

➤ Pain in the back that radiates down one leg.

➤ Weakness and numbness in a leg.

-PROLAPSED DISC

The symptoms of a slipped disc may appear to develop suddenly but this condition arises from long-term changes in the discs caused largely by poor posture and exercise habits. The normally plump and resilient discs can dry out and become brittle as a result of poor circulation in the spine and strain from long periods spent sitting. The affected discs then become vulnerable to

▽ Doing regular toning and stretching exercises, and working on maintaining good posture, will dramatically decrease the risk of developing sciatica.

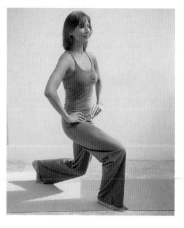

damage, often from relatively minor strains such as bending to pick something up.

To check for a slipped disc, your doctor will consider your medical history and make a thorough examination. A classic sign is that you experience pain when you are lying down and try to lift one leg straight up in the air. A CT or MRI scan of your back can identify the location of the slipped disc.

TREATMENT OPTIONS FOR A PROLAPSED DISC

Most slipped or prolapsed discs will settle after a few weeks of rest and some gentle activity. It is important to keep comfortable and to have adequate pain relief. Many people find that treatment by a physiotherapist is helpful.

If the pain fails to settle or if there is any weakness or numbness, an MRI scan of the back can show how big the prolapse is. It may be necessary to have an operation (microdiscectomy) to remove the affected disc and release the pressure on the nerves.

SCIATICA

This form of pain can be felt anywhere along the course of one of the sciatic nerves that run from the lower back, through the buttocks and down the back of each leg. The pain may be brought on by twisting the back and is made worse when coughing or sneezing. Rarely, there may be weakness and numbness of the leg.

CAUSES OF SCIATICA

In the majority of cases, sciatica is caused by a slipped vertebral disc but other causes can include severe degenerative bone

THE SCIATIC NERVE

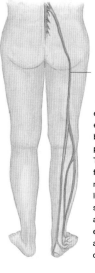

Sciatic nerve

◁ The sciatic nerves extend the length of each leg and end in branching nerve pathways in the foot. The nerves originate from the branching nerve roots in the lower part of the spinal cord. (Note: although occurring in each leg, the nerves are shown in one leg only for simplicity.)

changes to the spine. In rare cases, secondary bone tumours press on spinal nerves and this may affect both legs and the nerves to the bladder and bowel.

TREATMENT OPTIONS

Persistent sciatica should always be assessed by a doctor. If you suffer from sciatica and have difficulty passing urine or opening your bowels, see your doctor immediately or go straight to the hospital. You may need an operation to remove a disc from your spine to prevent paralysis of the legs.

In less severe cases, once a serious underlying condition has been excluded, rest and painkillers are usually the only treatments required.

Spinal injuries

SEE ALSO
➤ The brain and nerve network, p322
➤ Backache, p365

Injuries to the spinal cord are often the result of a major trauma such as a fall or a road traffic accident. If the impact was severe, the spinal cord may be damaged beyond repair. The spine is most likely to be damaged at its most mobile parts, which are the neck and lower back. The consequences of a severe spinal cord injury are profound because all muscle and sensory function is usually lost from the point of the injury downwards. A more common and less severe form of spinal injury is whiplash – also caused mainly by road traffic accidents.

Injuries to the neck vertebrae at the top of the spine are immediately fatal because the nerves supplying the breathing muscles are paralyzed. In damage below the fourth neck vertebra, breathing can continue as the nerves to the diaphragm are unaffected. Injuries to the spinal cord in the neck produce quadriplegia (paralysis of all four limbs) whereas lower back injuries can cause paraplegia (paralysis of the legs).

People with spinal cord injuries are also prone to bladder and chest infections and can develop pressure sores on the heels and buttocks due to immobility and the lack of pain sensation.

WHIPLASH INJURY

This common spinal injury occurs when the neck is quickly and violently bent forwards and/or backwards. It usually occurs after a road traffic accident, particularly one in which there is impact from behind. The effects can be long-lasting and debilitating.

THE SPINAL NERVES

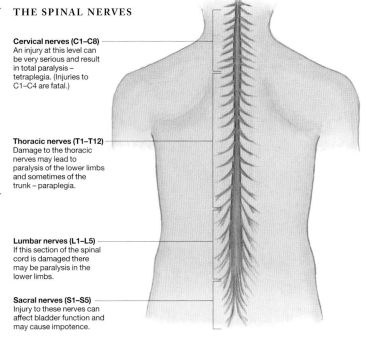

Cervical nerves (C1–C8)
An injury at this level can be very serious and result in total paralysis – tetraplegia. (Injuries to C1–C4 are fatal.)

Thoracic nerves (T1–T12)
Damage to the thoracic nerves may lead to paralysis of the lower limbs and sometimes of the trunk – paraplegia.

Lumbar nerves (L1–L5)
If this section of the spinal cord is damaged there may be paralysis in the lower limbs.

Sacral nerves (S1–S5)
Injury to these nerves can affect bladder function and may cause impotence.

△ The vital spinal nerves enable your body to move and function, so any damage to them can have serious consequences.

SIGNS AND SYMPTOMS OF WHIPLASH INJURY

There may be no pain initially, but neck pain and stiffness start to develop after a few hours. Other symptoms may include:

➤ Headache.

➤ Swelling of affected area.

➤ Shoulder pain.

Seek urgent medical advice if you develop numbness or weakness in your arm or if pain persists or suddenly gets more severe.

It is very often the case that the pain in the neck may not develop until a day or two after the accident.

It is important to seek medical advice if you have been involved in a traffic accident that has affected your neck. Your doctor may refer you to a specialist for an X-ray to assess the extent of any damage.

TREATMENT OPTIONS

Most people with a whiplash injury simply require bed rest, and painkillers to relieve the pain and discomfort. Non steroidal anti-inflammatory drugs such as ibuprofen are most effective. It is advisable that anyone who has had a previous neck problem, or someone whose symptoms do not show any sign of settling after two weeks, should return to their doctor, who may refer them for physiotherapy.

For a long time it was usual practice to issue soft neck collars to whiplash victims however, doctors now know that these tend to stiffen the neck which slows down the healing process, so that it takes much longer for the pain to subside.

Multiple sclerosis

SEE ALSO

➤ The brain and nerve network, p322

➤ The roles of blood and lymph, p448

➤ Autoimmune diseases, p459

Many of the nerve cells in the brain and spinal cord are insulated by sheaths of a fatty substance called myelin, which speeds signals along the nerves. In multiple sclerosis, damage is caused to these myelin sheaths. This is due to abnormal activity of the immune system and the trigger may be infection, but genetic factors may also play a role. This means that the nerve cells cannot function properly. In some cases steroids and the drug beta-interferon can reduce the severity and length of a relapse, but there is no long-term cure for the condition.

SIGNS AND SYMPTOMS

➤ Weakness and/or numbness of limbs.

➤ Loss of coordination.

➤ Urinary frequency, and sometimes incontinence.

➤ Blurred vision.

The symptoms of multiple sclerosis tend to develop in young people over the age of 20. There are two main forms of this disease. The most common is the relapsing-remitting form, in which there are frequent attacks of disabling symptoms with periods of recovery between. Over time, recovery between attacks becomes less complete and there is increasing disability. In the chronic-progressive form, the disabling symptoms advance more slowly and there are no periods of recovery in between.

Doctors may not make a diagnosis until two or more episodes of symptoms have occurred. An MRI brain scan will probably show areas of damage within the brain. If this is unhelpful, taking a sample of the fluid from the spinal cord can aid diagnosis.

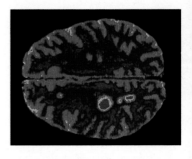

△ This brain scan shows damage, coloured red and yellow, caused by multiple sclerosis. The symptoms vary depending on which nerves have been damaged.

Motor neurone disease

SEE ALSO

➤ The brain and nerve network, p322

This rare progressive disease affects the nerves in the brain and spinal cord that control movement – the motor neurones. Also known as amylotrophic lateral sclerosis, this debilitating disease usually develops after the age of 40. It is more common in men.

SIGNS AND SYMPTOMS

Initially, someone affected by motor neurone disease may not realize anything is wrong. Symptoms develop slowly and insidiously. Over time, a person may start to stumble or notice a weaker grip or increasingly stiff muscles. As the condition progresses, muscles that are involved in swallowing and speech control may be affected. The condition results in severe physical disability but despite this a person's senses and intelligence remain intact.

It may take some time and several visits before your doctor can diagnose motor neurone disease, as the symptoms tend to be general and so could point to a number of different diseases.

You may undergo several investigations before a firm diagnosis is made. These include an MRI scan of the spine and a lumbar puncture (taking a sample of cerebrospinal fluid to check for inflammation). Electromyelography – a test that monitors electrical activity in the muscles – may be performed to show if nerves supplying muscles are damaged.

TREATMENT OPTIONS

As there is no cure for this condition, treatment focuses on relieving any symptoms. Antidepressants may be prescribed and antibiotics may be needed to treat chest infections, to which motor neurone disease sufferers are particularly prone. Physiotherapy to maintain mobility for as long as possible is likely to be offered as well as practical support in dealing with the patient's increasing disability. People with this condition have been known to survive for as long as ten years, but a higher proportion die within three years.

Other neurological problems

SEE ALSO
▶ Diabetes, p314
▶ Diseases of the thyroid, p316
▶ Rheumatoid arthritis, p362
▶ Acupuncture, p493

Many neurological problems are localized and affect only the very limited area of the body served by a particular nerve or nerves. They may be painful and distressing and, in some cases, difficult to treat. Symptoms may result from inflammation of nerves as a result of infection or other factors. In other cases the nerve problem is caused by compression from surrounding tissues. Although none of these conditions is a threat to general health, medical advice is needed to obtain effective treatment, possibly including surgery.

TRIGEMINAL NEURALGIA

The trigeminal nerve transmits sensations from parts of your face to the brain as well as controlling muscles that move your jaw. If this nerve is compressed, inflamed or damaged, sharp shooting pains may be felt in the cheeks, lips or one side of the face.

This condition is common among elderly people and its cause is unknown. Pain occurs in short bursts which then subside. Attacks may be triggered by activities such as washing, being out in a cold wind or eating. If painkillers do not help, your doctor may prescribe an anticonvulsant drug called carbamazepine. In a few cases surgery is required.

BELL'S PALSY

The facial nerve carries taste sensations from the front of the tongue and controls muscles of expression in the face. If this nerve is compressed, inflamed or damaged, it causes paralysis of muscles on one side of the face and loss of taste on the front part of the tongue. Often the eyelid and the corner of the mouth will droop. In some cases, the symptoms appear over the course of 24 hours. It may be caused by a virus and usually settles in a couple of weeks, with no after-effects. A course of steroid drugs may help to resolve the paralysis problem. The front of the eye (cornea) needs to be protected if the eyelids cannot be closed and you may have to use artificial tears.

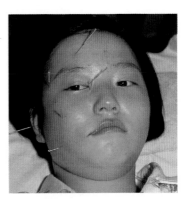

△ Acupuncture, a traditional Chinese therapy, is being used here to treat Bell's palsy, but the symptoms of this condition often disappear without any treatment at all.

THE BRANCHES OF THE TRIGEMINAL NERVE

▷ The trigeminal nerve is the largest in the face and has three main branches – ophthalmic, maxillary and mandibular.

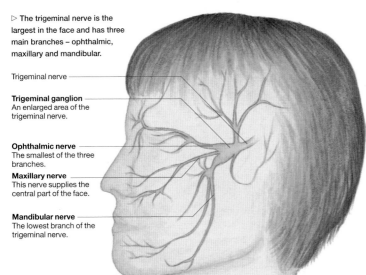

Trigeminal nerve

Trigeminal ganglion
An enlarged area of the trigeminal nerve.

Ophthalmic nerve
The smallest of the three branches.

Maxillary nerve
This nerve supplies the central part of the face.

Mandibular nerve
The lowest branch of the trigeminal nerve.

CARPAL TUNNEL SYNDROME

The carpal tunnel is a narrow space in the bones of the wrist and the median nerve runs through it on its way to the hand. If the median nerve becomes trapped and/or constricted it can cause pain and tingling in the hand and forearm. Carpal tunnel syndrome is a common condition. Typically it causes weakness of the thumb and pins and needles in the index, middle and ring fingers, which may be worse first thing in the morning. In most cases there is no obvious cause, although carpal tunnel syndrome is sometimes related to hypothyroidism, diabetes, pregnancy, obesity and rheumatoid arthritis.

Splints and steroid injections can be helpful, but an operation to relieve the pressure on the nerve may be required in some cases.

Dementia

Dementia is a deterioration in mental ability due to a disorder of the brain. It has a combination of symptoms – memory loss, confusion and intellectual decline. It is common and becoming more so as a larger section of the general population is living longer. In severe cases, it is very disabling and distressing for both patients and their friends and families. Dementia usually affects those over 70, but can occur in younger people. Some disorders, such as depression, behave like dementia but once identified and treated, the dementia symptoms soon disappear.

SIGNS AND SYMPTOMS OF DEMENTIA

The following are typical symptoms of dementia and are all related to the loss of higher brain functions:

➤ Impaired memory, particularly of recent events.

➤ Loss of the ability to think.

➤ Noticeably reduced verbal and conversational skills.

➤ Inability to learn new skills or facts.

➤ Loss of emotional control.

➤ Increasing restlessness and a tendency to wander.

➤ Behavioural difficulties.

➤ Depression and/or anxiety.

There is no single test to identify dementia or its specific cause. If your doctor suspects an underlying condition is causing symptoms of dementia, then he or she will arrange for tests to confirm or exclude the suspected diagnosis.

Your doctor may take a sample of blood to send for laboratory analysis, in order to determine the possibility of a vitamin deficiency. Brain scanning may provide revealing information and rule out the more uncommon causes of dementia. Your doctor may also carry out a detailed questioning session aimed at assessing mental ability.

The commonest causes of dementia are Alzheimer's disease and multi-infarct dementia. Rarely, dementia is caused by Creutzfeldt-Jakob disease, known as CJD. Conditions that can cause symptoms similar to those of dementia include vitamin deficiency or anaemia, and adverse reactions to certain drugs.

TREATMENT OPTIONS

There is no specific treatment for any of the forms of dementia and the symptoms get progressively worse with time. Recently, new drugs have become available that improve the symptoms for a short time, but unfortunately in the long term there is nothing that can be done to halt the progress of the disease.

Treatment is based on caring for the increasingly dependent sufferer and most patients end up requiring full-time supervision and nursing care for the remainder of their life.

It is also vital to care for the needs of those looking after a person with dementia.

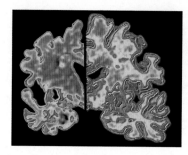

△ A brain affected by Alzheimer's disease (left) is considerably shrunken compared with a normal brain (right).

The impact on carers can be profound, especially if a loved one becomes violent or is unable to remember the carer. No matter how devoted someone is, all carers need plenty of support from medical advisers and social services, and the opportunity to take a break from their responsibilities by taking advantage of respite care.

ALZHEIMER'S DISEASE

This is the most common cause of dementia. This is a progressive degenerative brain condition that causes 70 per cent of the cases of dementia. It results from the loss of nerve cells in the brain, a reduction in neurotransmitter levels and the development of "protein tangles" around the nerve cells. These abnormalities can be detected by a brain scan, which can distinguish Alzheimer's disease from other possible causes of dementia. The underlying cause of the condition is not known, but studies have shown that the tendency to develop Alzheimer's disease may be genetic because it appears to run in families.

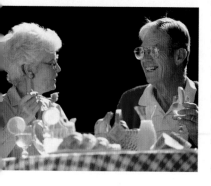

▽ Alzheimer's disease is the most common cause of dementia and it is most likely to develop later in life, specifically in those over 70 years of age.

SIGNS AND SYMPTOMS OF ALZHEIMER'S DISEASE

➤ Limited memory. Short-term memory of a few minutes may be intact, but long-term memory is lost with the most recent events being affected first. Many people with dementia can recall their early lives in great detail, but are unable to remember anything that happened to them on the previous day.

➤ Inability to learn new information or use previously learned information.

➤ Loss of language skills.

➤ Inability to perform complex muscular activity, even though muscle function remains normal.

➤ Inability to recognize objects.

➤ Rapid mood swings.

➤ Personality changes.

➤ Wandering off and getting lost, even in familiar surroundings.

➤ Neglect of personal hygiene.

HOW THE CONDITION PROGRESSES

The symptoms of the disease develop very gradually, and the person will start to become increasingly forgetful and absent-minded. As the disease progresses, among the most distressing symptoms are personality changes and the failure to recognize family and close friends.

Although modern drug treatment can help some symptoms and slow the progress of the disease in certain cases, most Alzheimer's disease sufferers do not survive for longer than ten years following the initial diagnosis.

MULTI-INFARCT DEMENTIA

This condition is also known as vascular dementia. Multi-infarct dementia is the second most common cause of dementia. It occurs as the result of small ischaemic episodes, which mean there is an inadequate supply of blood reaching a part of the body. These episodes result in oxygen deprivation in the surrounding areas of the brain, causing the gradual death of nerve cells and loss of the functions that they control. Like other forms of stroke, the underlying cause is usually atherosclerosis (the furring up and narrowing of arteries), which is usually the result of lifestyle factors such as a high-fat diet, heavy smoking and lack of exercise. High blood pressure is also a very important risk factor.

The precise nature of the symptoms of this dementia depends on the area of the brain that has been affected, but the process of the condition is gradual and there are not usually any neurological symptoms such as weakness or slurred speech.

MAKING THE DIAGNOSIS

This form of dementia can often be diagnosed from the pattern of symptoms, but in most cases a CT or MRI brain scan is usually carried out to confirm the diagnosis and rule out other possible causes of the symptoms of dementia.

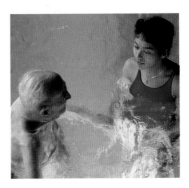

△ Regular gentle exercise such as swimming is particularly important for sufferers from multi-infarct dementia as it can help to reduce the risk of future attacks.

TREATMENT OPTIONS

Brain damage caused by multiple infarcts cannot be repaired. Treatment is therefore focused on the prevention of future episodes and most importantly the risk of a potentially fatal major stroke. Drugs are usually prescribed to reduce blood pressure and regular doses of aspirin may also be taken to reduce the chance of the formation of blood clots.

CREUTZFELDT-JAKOB DISEASE (CJD)

An unusual infectious agent called a prion causes this rare disease. It causes spongy areas to develop in the brain, leading to dementia and ultimately death in around six months. Other symptoms include:

➤ Depression.

➤ Unsteadiness and poor coordination.

➤ Seizures.

➤ Impaired vision.

This disease has a very long incubation period and may occur anything up to 20 years after the initial infection. A new variant of CJD (vCJD) has also developed that tends to affect younger people. Scientists have linked vCJD with eating meat from animals infected with "mad cow disease" – bovine spongiform encephalopathy (BSE).

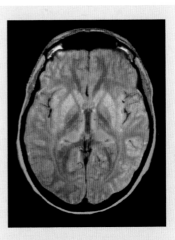

△ This MRI scan shows a section through a CJD-affected brain. The diseased parts of the thalamus (areas of grey matter in the front of the brain) are indicated in green.

Parkinson's disease

SEE ALSO
➤ The brain and nerve network, p322
➤ Dementia, p338
➤ Depression, p346

The symptoms of this common neurological condition, which mainly affects the elderly, are the result of degeneration of nerve cells in a part of the brain that controls movement. The degeneration means that the affected area of the brain no longer produces sufficient dopamine, a chemical neurotransmitter that normally works in balance with another neurotransmitter called acetylcholine, to fine-tune your muscle control. The resulting chemical imbalance in the brain is the cause of the typical symptoms of Parkinson's disease.

SIGNS AND SYMPTOMS OF PARKINSON'S DISEASE

Typical symptoms are:

➤ Tremor of a hand, arm or leg on one side of the body, which may stop as the person attempts a task. Over time both sides may be affected.

➤ Rigidity of the muscles.

➤ Difficulty in initiating movement.

➤ A stooped, shuffling walk.

➤ Expressionless or mask-like face.

➤ Slurred speech.

➤ Depression.

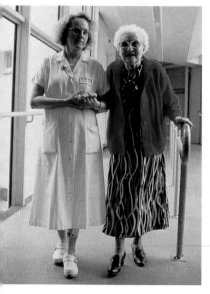

◁ Mobility problems are among the chief symptoms of Parkinson's disease. Plenty of support is needed to maintain an active life.

The underlying cause of the spontaneous degeneration of the nerve cells in the basal ganglia, the part of the brain affected by Parkinson's disease, is unknown. What is known is that susceptibility to the disease appears to run in families and that men are more commonly affected than women. Parkinsonism – which has symptoms similar to those of Parkinson's disease but is due to identifiable factors – can be caused by certain drugs or by head injuries.

HOW THE DISEASE PROGRESSES

In 1817, James Parkinson described this disease as the "shaking palsy", which quite accurately conveys the classic symptoms of this disease – tremor and stiffness. These symptoms develop very gradually. As these movement difficulties grow progressively worse, it can become almost impossible for individuals to perform even the most simple everyday tasks. Many people with Parkinson's disease develop depression and some also develop dementia.

HOW IS IT DIAGNOSED?

Because Parkinson's disease often develops gradually it may take some time for your doctor to diagnose the condition, based on a medical history and physical examination. Long-term observation of muscle activity may be needed to make a definite diagnosis. Blood tests can be carried out to eliminate other conditions. Further tests may include brain scans to establish if the symptoms are caused by a stroke or a brain tumour.

WHERE DAMAGE OCCURS

▽ The area of the brain affected by Parkinson's disease is the basal ganglia. It is this part of the brain that controls smoothness of movement.

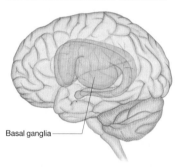

Basal ganglia

Questions will be asked about various factors including exposure to drugs or viruses to establish if it is Parkinsonism.

TREATMENT OPTIONS

Parkinson's disease is usually treated primarily by drugs. The drug most commonly prescribed is levodopa, which is converted to dopamine in the brain and

FUTURE THERAPIES

Some patients undergo brain surgery but this procedure is still experimental. Scientists are currently experimenting with the use of stem cell implants in the treatment of Parkinson's disease. Another possibility for treatment in the future is a pacemaker-type implant that dramatically reduces tremor by stimulating the brain directly. However, none of these therapies are currently used routinely.

restores levels of this neurotransmitter. In excess, this drug can cause unpleasant side effects and the dose is carefully tailored to each patient. In some cases the dose needed to control symptoms is so high that the side effects are unacceptable. In such cases, an alternative drug is prescribed.

Another group of drugs that are sometimes used are anti-cholinergic drugs. These block the effects of acetylcholine, thereby bringing it back into balance with the reduced levels of dopamine. It may take some time to find the right dose of drug for each person and side effects such as dry mouth and impaired vision can create difficulties for some people.

In some cases, most commonly when the disease affects a younger person, surgery

▽ A computer image of a dopamine molecule. Lack of this chemical in the brain is responsible for the symptoms of Parkinson's disease.

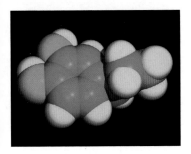

CAUSES OF PARKINSONISM
The symptoms of this condition are very similar to those of Parkinson's disease and can be produced by:

➤ Certain drugs, such as some antipsychotics.

➤ Rare viral infections, such as the strain of flu virus that caused an epidemic in the 1920s.

➤ Abuse of the drug known as MPTP.

➤ Head injury, particularly repeated head injuries such as those sustained by boxers.

BENIGN ESSENTIAL TREMOR
This is a common inherited condition where the tremor usually affects the upper limbs of elderly people. The condition displays symptoms similar to Parkinson's disease but the two are actually not related.

In most cases, treatment may not be needed, although small doses of alcohol or beta-blocker drugs can help reduce the severity of symptoms.

may be considered. The aim of such treatment is to destroy tissue in the area of the brain that governs the tremor. Other more experimental treatments include brain cell transplantation and electrical stimulation of the brain.

SUPPORTIVE MEASURES
Maintenance of mobility is of utmost importance to people with this condition. Parkinson's disease sufferers should try to take as much gentle exercise as possible, including stretching exercises such as yoga, taught by a qualified practitioner. Many people benefit from physiotherapy to help with mobility problems. Rest is also important, as excessive tiredness can make symptoms worse.

As the disease progresses, an individual with Parkinson's disease may also need various physical aids to make everyday tasks achievable. It is important to make clothing, cutlery, chairs, shoes and floors as easy as possible to use. An occupational therapist can advise on adaptations to equipment and to the home that will help to maintain independence. Speech therapy may also be useful. Increasing depression is a common feature of the disease, and in such cases plenty of support from health professionals, as well as family and friends, is very important.

Although Parkinson's disease is debilitating and reduces quality of life, people with the condition can survive for many years following the diagnosis.

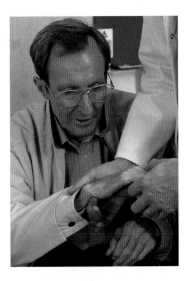

△ A doctor examines the hand of a Parkinson's disease patient. A tremor is one of the classic symptoms of this condition.

HUNTINGTON'S DISEASE
Also known as Huntington's chorea, this rare inherited brain disorder causes jerky, uncontrolled muscle movements and increasing dementia. The disease is caused by the presence of an abnormal gene. The Huntington's disease gene is "dominant", which means that, to be affected, a person has to inherit the defective gene from only one parent. A genetic test, which can be done at any age, can tell you whether you have the abnormal gene.

In those who carry the gene for Huntington's disease, symptoms commonly develop between the ages of 30 and 50. The diagnosis can be confirmed by a CT or MRI scan of the brain, which can detect the type of degeneration that is characteristic of the condition. Drug treatment can ease the spasms and jerks, but the disease gets progressively worse over time, with most patients requiring high levels of care in the later stages. Most sufferers do not survive for more than 10–20 years following the onset of symptoms.

Anxiety

SEE ALSO

➤ Learn to manage
   stress, p260
➤ Diseases of the
   thyroid gland, p316
➤ Phobias, p344
➤ Depression, p346

We all experience feelings of nervousness or apprehension in different situations at different times in our lives and this is a completely normal response – whether it is butterflies in the stomach before a big test or exam or worrying about a job interview. Such feelings often lead us to perform better but if anxiety persists or becomes a common response to everyday situations, it can start to have a detrimental effect on normal life. In such cases, particularly when feelings of anxiety occur without apparent cause, professional advice is needed.

SIGNS AND SYMPTOMS

Common symptoms of anxiety are:

➤ Feelings of general unease and
   agitation.

➤ Inability to relax.

➤ Disturbed sleep.

➤ Episodes of panic.

➤ Feelings of being unable to cope.

A number of factors can contribute to persistent feelings of anxiety but often no underlying cause can be clearly identified. A susceptibility to this condition may be inherited or be brought about by events and experiences in early childhood.

The inherent ability to cope with everyday stress in your life is also influenced by a number of other factors:
• The levels of support available from family and friends.
• Socioeconomic circumstances.
• The number of factors provoking anxiety.
• The intensity of those provoking factors.

Symptoms of anxiety may be felt intermittently when the immediate cause is present (for example when exposed to the object of a phobia) or when the cause is uppermost in a person's mind (reading a bank statement when you have financial problems, say). In other cases there may be almost constant feelings of agitation and fear with no readily discernible cause. In extreme circumstances, when a person cannot cope with overwhelming feelings of anxiety, they may suffer from acute episodes of anxiety known as panic attacks.

Anxiety can result in hyperventilation or overbreathing. This occurs when the stress of a situation causes you to take conscious control of your breathing and you overdo it. The levels of carbon dioxide in the blood fall and your automatic breathing mechanism switches off. The sensation of not being able to breathe is extremely distressing and makes you take deeper breaths. Breathing in and out of your mouth into a paper bag breaks the cycle and normalizes oxygen and carbon dioxide levels in the blood. Hyperventilation is a common feature of panic attacks.

THE CAUSES OF ANXIETY

Common causes of anxiety are:

➤ Relationship problems.

➤ Loss and bereavement.

➤ Health problems.

➤ Financial worries.

➤ Work-related problems.

➤ Unresolved conflicts.

➤ Phobias or obsessive-compulsive
   disorder.

➤ Physical causes, such as
   hyperthyroidism.

Anxiety may also accompany or alternate with depression, or may be part of a more serious psychiatric disorder such as schizophrenia. Often, however, no particular cause can be found.

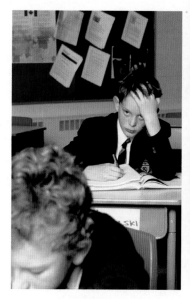

△ The stress of exams and of school life in general can easily lead to anxiety in children and teenagers. It is never too early to learn how to recognize the symptoms and how to deal with what is causing the anxiety effectively.

TREATMENT OPTIONS

The first step in treatment is to consider whether your anxiety may have a root cause in a set of complex physical and/or mental health problems. In the first instance, discussing your situation with your doctor or with a counsellor could help shed some light on the factors that may be important in your case. It is also possible that your doctor may decide to arrange blood tests to rule out the possibility of a physical cause for your symptoms, such as excess production of thyroid hormone.

individual's reactions to anxiety-provoking situations. If a phobia or obsessive-compulsive disorder is at the root of the anxiety, specialist therapy to overcome the underlying psychological problem may be recommended.

LONG-TERM OUTLOOK

In most cases, the earlier a person suffering from anxiety receives treatment, the faster they recover from the condition. Without appropriate treatment the anxiety could become ingrained and develop into a lifelong condition.

SELF-HELP

In addition to specific medical treatment and professional counselling, anxiety-sufferers often find that they benefit from making a variety of lifestyle changes. Scientific studies have shown that increasing the amount of regular physical activity taken helps to burn off excess adrenaline, and also provides a healthy outlet for feelings of restlessness. Studies have also shown that exercise helps to lighten mood and encourage a more positive outlook. Forms of exercise that incorporate relaxation techniques, such as yoga, are particularly effective for dealing with anxiety. In addition, cutting down consumption of stimulants such as caffeine can often dramatically reduce the physical symptoms of anxiety.

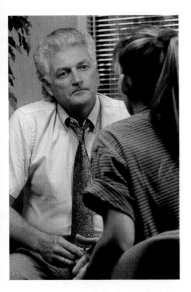

△ Professional counsellors are skilled at helping to discover the root of a problem. Tackling the cause of anxiety is an important part of the treatment for sufferers.

Some patients are reassured when their doctor tells them their symptoms are anxiety-related, as they may have thought that they had developed a serious heart condition, for example. Shortly afterwards, their symptoms may settle and the anxiety is likely to abate.

There are two courses of recognized treatment for anxiety – drug therapy and supportive therapies:
• Drug therapy – The most commonly used anti-anxiety drugs belong to the benzodiazepine family. These drugs can be beneficial in the short term for anxiety and disturbed sleep but the danger is that they are highly addictive and can have counter-productive side effects, so long-term use is not an option. In cases where a patient's anxiety is associated with a depressive illness, antidepressant drugs may be prescribed.
• Supportive therapies – Counselling may allow an affected person to focus on the root causes of his or her anxiety. A psychological approach (cognitive-behavioural therapy) tries to alter the

▽ Studies have shown that it is often beneficial for people who suffer from anxiety to own a pet. Caring for and petting an animal has been shown to have a calming influence.

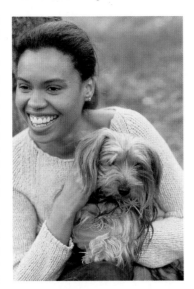

PANIC ATTACKS

Someone with an anxiety disorder may suffer from episodes of severe physical symptoms that result from high levels of adrenaline being released into the bloodstream in response to a fear-provoking situation. (Under normal circumstances, this neurotransmitter is released in order to prepare the body for "fight or flight" when confronted by a threatening situation, by increasing the heart rate and breathing rate and causing blood to be diverted to the muscles from other parts of the body.) Typical symptoms of a panic attack are:

➤ Palpitations.

➤ Tightness and pains in the chest.

➤ Difficult or rapid breathing.

➤ Light-headedness and faintness.

➤ Sweating, trembling and nausea.

➤ Heaviness in the arms.

➤ Tingling in the fingers.

➤ Sense of impending death.

Panic attacks may result from exposure to the object of a phobia or they may be a recurring feature of a generalized anxiety disorder.

A panic attack can be alarming to witness and may be hard to distinguish from a heart attack. Although a panic attack usually passes without any harm to the sufferer, if you are present when someone has such an attack and are unsure whether it is a panic attack or something more serious, it is best to summon medical help without delay.

Phobias

SEE ALSO
➤ Anxiety, p342
➤ Panic attacks, p343

A phobia is an irrational and intense fear that is focused on one specific object, activity or situation. There are many common phobias, such as fear of spiders, flying, or heights. Some people become fearful of leaving their home. Certain phobias are minor and, because they do not have a significant impact on daily life, they require no treatment. In other cases the phobia presents a major obstacle to everyday life, preventing the sufferer from pursuing normal activities, and this is where treatment is essential in order to restore quality of life.

When a phobia develops, an affected person will often go to considerable lengths to avoid a specific object or animal, or a fear-provoking situation such as flying or going to the doctor. Exposure to the provoking factor tends to result in hysteria or a panic attack.

WHAT CAUSES PHOBIAS?

It is often not easy to identify the cause of a phobia. A bad experience in early life may result in phobic symptoms. People who are already anxious are more likely to develop phobias, which may be an expression of an underlying generalized anxiety disorder.

TREATING PHOBIAS

Phobias often respond very well to a gradual process of treatment called desensitization. While being given support by your doctor or therapist, you are exposed in stages of increasing intensity to the provoking object or situation. At first, you will experience anxiety but as the treatment progresses you will gradually learn to overcome these feelings. Simple phobias usually respond very well to such treatment, but more complex phobias may be more difficult to treat in this way and therefore require a range of psychological and/or psychiatric interventions.

EXAMPLES OF DIFFERENT PHOBIAS

- Acrophobia – Heights.
- Agoraphobia – Open spaces.
- Arachnophobia – Spiders.
- Aviophobia – Flying.
- Claustrophobia – Enclosed spaces.
- Hydrophobia – Water.
- Latrophobia – Doctors.
- Nosophobia – Becoming ill.

Post-traumatic stress disorder (PTSD)

SEE ALSO
➤ Anxiety, p342

This condition may occur after a person has been exposed to a particularly stressful and upsetting event. Common trigger events include an assault, and witnessing or being involved in a serious accident or disaster. This disorder is more likely to develop in anxiety-prone people.

SIGNS AND SYMPTOMS

These symptoms can develop at any time after the trigger event and tend to persist for months or years afterwards:

➤ Preoccupation with the event and/or flashbacks.

➤ Anxiety and panic attacks.

➤ Depression and poor concentration, often with signs of withdrawal and detachment.

This condition has been more widely recognized in recent years. Effective support and/or counselling following involvement in a traumatic event can help to prevent it from occurring or at least minimize its severity. People with this disorder often respond well to a few months of counselling in conjunction with antidepressant medication. The support of family and close friends is an invaluable aid to recovery.

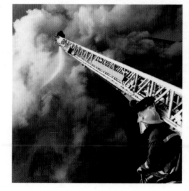

▷ Emergency workers such as firefighters are at risk from post-traumatic stress disorder because of the nature of their work.

Obsessive-compulsive disorder

SEE ALSO
► Learn to manage stress, p260
► Anxiety, p342
► Addictive behaviours, p350

This psychiatric disorder, or neurosis, is one in which a person experiences anxiety in connection with a persistently recurring thought, feeling or impulse. As a result of this there is often an irresistible urge (compulsion) to carry out rituals, such as the repeated washing of hands, excessive cleaning and constant checking of keys, gas controls or water taps. The affected person will very often understand that their behaviour is irrational but simply cannot control it. The rituals usually have an anxiety-reducing and containing function.

Obsessive-compulsive disorder is relatively common. Doctors believe it affects about 1 in 100 people in developed countries. However, the exact numbers affected are difficult to estimate because many people who suffer from this form of psychiatric disorder do not seek medical help.

WHAT TRIGGERS OBSESSIVE-COMPULSIVE BEHAVIOUR?

Many of us enact harmless rituals that often started in childhood – for example, always avoiding treading on the lines of paving stones or always taking precisely the same route home. This kind of ritualized behaviour is not a problem if it is not accompanied by extreme anxiety or fear of the consequences if the ritual is not carried out. It is only when the need to perform the ritual dominates a person's life and takes priority over other needs such as work that a person can be said to have this condition.

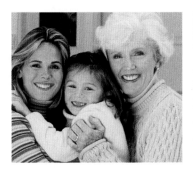

△ Some families are prone to obsessive-compulsive disorder, but it is unclear whether it is an inherited tendency or learned behaviour.

Obsessive-compulsive disorders often first appear in adolescence and many cases can be linked to stress or stressful events in a person's life. It sometimes runs in families. Some people are said to have an obsessive-compulsive personality, meaning that these people continually strive for perfection and disregard other people's feelings. People with such personality types are more likely to suffer from this problem.

WHEN TO SEE YOUR DOCTOR

In severe cases of obsessive-compulsive disorder, a person may perform rituals such as handwashing hundreds of times a day, which may interfere with everyday life such as going out to work or doing household chores. The anxiety that often accompanies the behaviour can be very distressing for the affected person. If you are worried about the fact that you are experiencing uncontrollable thoughts and are carrying out compulsive rituals, then it is a good idea to talk things through with your doctor.

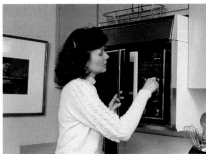

△ The excessive checking of switches or dials is a classic manifestation of an obsessive-compulsive disorder.

WHAT MIGHT YOUR DOCTOR DO?

Your doctor may suspect obsessive-compulsive disorder from a description of your feelings and behaviour. A range of psychotherapeutic approaches may be helpful – cognitive and behavioural therapies can be highly successful. Such therapy is designed to help you confront and control your compulsions to carry out rituals. You may find that things get worse for a short time before you start to experience an improvement in your condition. Your therapist or doctor may also prescribe a course of antidepressants.

WHAT IS THE OUTLOOK?

The majority of people with obsessive-compulsive disorder start to show substantial improvement once they are receiving appropriate therapy. Some people, such as those with an obsessive-compulsive personality, are prone to persistent or recurring episodes of such behaviour over many years.

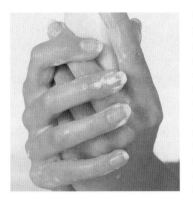

▽ The ritual of obsessive handwashing may be the result of an excessive fear of germs or a feeling of being unclean.

Depression

SEE ALSO

➤ Learn to manage stress, p260
➤ Eat healthily, p262
➤ Exercise for life, p266
➤ Sensible drinking, p270

Feelings of sadness are normal emotions that are experienced by all of us to some degree during our lives. Depression is a psychological state in which these feelings become intense and start to interfere with everyday activities. It is one of the most common mental health problems and affects twice as many women as men. Depression often clears spontaneously after a few days or weeks, but in other cases it requires professional help and support. Severely depressed people may need to be admitted to hospital to protect them from self-harm.

SIGNS AND SYMPTOMS

➤ General loss of interest and apathy.

➤ Low levels of energy.

➤ An inability to cope.

➤ Persistent low mood.

➤ Early morning waking.

➤ Loss of libido.

➤ Loss of appetite.

➤ Low self-esteem.

➤ Guilt.

➤ Anxiety.

➤ Morbid preoccupations.

➤ Thoughts of self-harm.

such as low levels of thyroid hormone (hypothyroidism) or the hormonal disruption that can occur after childbirth or around the menopause. In other cases lifestyle factors such as excessive alcohol consumption or drug abuse are the cause of the problem. However, depression may also develop suddenly in a person who has no clearly identifiable risk factors or who has not experienced any triggering life events. This is known as endogenous depression.

NON-DRUG TREATMENT

It is important to seek your doctor's advice if you are feeling persistently depressed. It is also vital that someone who has contemplated suicide obtains medical help as a matter of urgency.

You may find it helps to clarify things in your own mind by discussing your

△ Feelings of despair, futility and worthlessness are the hallmark of depression. Such feelings are more severe than just being "down".

situation with your doctor or, perhaps, a member of your church where this is appropriate. It is often therapeutic if a neutral person listens to your problems without being judgemental or critical.

Causes of depression are many and varied. There is evidence that some people inherit a genetic predisposition towards developing depression that may then be triggered by any or a combination of provoking events. Common triggers include:

• Loss and bereavement.
• Relationship problems and breakdown.
• Poor health.
• Acting as a carer for long periods.
• Financial worries.
• Work-related problems.
• Unresolved conflicts.

Sometimes depression develops when the accumulated load of problems becomes too much for a person to bear. In some cases depression is caused by physiological factors

JUST A BAD MOOD

Depression is part of the full spectrum of different moods that people experience – we all have our ups and downs in life and this is often reflected in how we feel. It is quite normal to feel sad every now and then, but if this becomes a persistent feeling, then that is depression, and there is something wrong with the balance of neurotransmitters in your brain that needs to be addressed. Likewise, everyone has periods of elation but if this became a permanent state of euphoria and excessive activity, known as mania, your mental function would suffer and you would need medical help to normalize brain function and behaviour. Below is a simplified medical interpretation of the full range of states of mind.

▬▬ Normal range of mood
▬▬ Abnormal range of mood

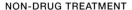

Mania
Depressive psychosis
Moderate depression

Mild euphoria
Cheery, hopeful, happy

Minor depression
Sad, gloomy, despondent

Your doctor may also suggest an assessment with a counsellor or a psychologist. A fair amount of overlap exists between these two disciplines. A counsellor tends to focus on your feelings and helps you to understand them, while a psychologist attempts to change negative patterns of thinking and channel them in a more positive direction.

Support from a range of sources is helpful. Immediate family and friends may be a ready source of day-to-day support, encouragement and help. However, not everyone is fortunate enough to have a supportive circle of people available to help them at such a time.

ANTIDEPRESSANT DRUG THERAPY

Your doctor may prescribe a course of antidepressants and you may take them in conjunction with psychological therapy. Antidepressants alter the balance of the chemicals in the brain and there are several different types. Your doctor will choose a drug suitable for your situation and needs. Although certain benefits, such as improved sleep, may be noticed immediately, it takes at least two weeks for most antidepressant drugs to start to lift mood. However, minor side effects may be noticed straight away. If

▽ Certain life-stages, such as leaving home to cope with the pressures of student life, often lead to stresses that in turn trigger depression.

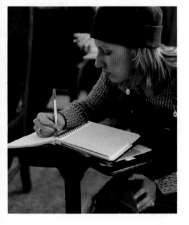

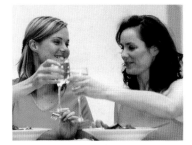

△ Talking to, and being around, friends can help to stave off depressive feelings, though medical help may also be necessary.

such side effects are troublesome you should contact your doctor, who may be able to find an alternative drug that is more suitable for you.

Once an antidepressant is working, initial improvements are often sustained and a person gradually becomes more able to cope with everyday life. Most doctors recommend that antidepressants are taken for at least four to six months. The decision to stop taking medication depends on how well you respond, along with a number of other factors. If the factors that caused the depression in the first place have not been resolved, or if a period of counselling is proving to be quite stressful, it is usually better to wait until things have settled down before discontinuing medication.

Antidepressants do not take away the ability to feel the natural spectrum of human emotions, and they are not addictive. People often confuse them with tranquillizers, which are addictive and are of no help in managing depression.

SELF-HELP

The effectiveness of any treatment for depression can be increased in many cases by attention to lifestyle and daily routine. It is important to establish that day to day you take plenty of exercise, preferably outdoors, and that your diet is healthy. Filling each day with interesting and enjoyable activities is important, although care should be taken not to take on too much too quickly.

SEASONAL AFFECTIVE DISORDER

Many people with recurrent depression tend to develop marked feelings of unhappiness and low mood during winter. This is known as seasonal affective disorder (SAD), and it is thought to be linked to low levels of light during the winter months.

Most people notice a lowering of mood in winter and this usually improves markedly with the brighter conditions of spring. Animals and plants are much less active during the cold months of winter and it may be that your body has a natural urge to slow down but modern lifestyles make no allowance for such reduced activity in winter.

Light therapy, which involves treatment with ultraviolet light, can improve the mood of people with SAD. If this fails, a course of antidepressant drugs may be prescribed.

▽ People who are affected by SAD often benefit from specialized treatment that involves being exposed to high-intensity light panels for several hours each day.

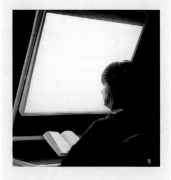

THE LONG-TERM OUTLOOK

In the majority of cases, depression either passes without any need for treatment or it is resolved with supportive therapy, counselling and/or medication. Some people, however, will continue to suffer from episodes of depression throughout their lives and often require long-term specialist treatment.

Bipolar affective disorder

Many people experience considerable swings of mood – episodes of low mood alternating with periods of elation and enthusiasm. Previously known as manic-depression, bipolar affective disorder is the condition in which this tendency to mood fluctuation becomes extreme. An affected person switches from periods of profound depression to episodes of extremely energetic activity (mania), often with very bizarre behaviour that may include excessive expenditure on unnecessary goods, personal neglect, and/or outbreaks of violence.

Bipolar affective disorder often becomes apparent during a person's early 20s. Researchers believe that some individuals may have a genetic predisposition toward developing this condition and that it may be triggered or unmasked by one or a number of adverse life events.

GETTING HELP

While in the depressed phase of this condition, the person may feel so despairing and demotivated that they can see no

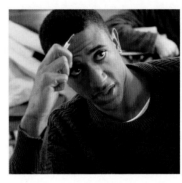

△ Inability to concentrate is a common symptom during the manic phase of bipolar affective disorder.

purpose in seeking help. They may feel so worthless that they do not believe that they deserve to be helped. At such times it is important for family and friends to make every effort to persuade the person to see their doctor.

During the manic phase, the person may feel completely well and have no insight into the abnormal nature of their behaviour or mood. They are likely to blame others for any difficulties that they are experiencing. In cases where the manic behaviour leads to aggression or violence, compulsory admission to hospital for treatment may be required.

TREATMENT OPTIONS

During the depressive phase, antidepressant drugs are usually prescribed. However, doctors must maintain a balance so that they control the depression without elevating the mood so much that a person becomes manic.

Treatment of the manic phase of this condition is more difficult because the person often does not accept the need for treatment. Severe mania is usually effectively controlled by treatment with antipsychotic drugs.

Individuals who are particularly prone to recurrent episodes of bipolar depression may respond well to lithium, a drug that tends to stabilize mood swings and prevent relapses. Certain anticonvulsant drugs also have mood-stabilizing properties and doctors sometimes prescribe these as an alternative treatment.

People with bipolar affective disorder need regular check-ups to monitor mood changes and fine-tune drug treatment.

▽ Periods of depression alternate with mania. As with other forms of depression, low mood is not helped by excessive alcohol consumption.

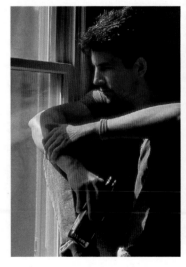

SIGNS AND SYMPTOMS

Bipolar affective disorder is characterized by alternating episodes of depression and mania. These episodes will last for varying lengths of time and are usually interspersed with periods of complete normality.

During the depressive episode, symptoms are the same as those experienced during depression and the severity of these symptoms will vary.

Episodes of mania are characterized by the following symptoms:

➤ High levels of energy and activity.

➤ Elation.

➤ Delusions of grandeur.

➤ Inability to concentrate.

➤ Lack of insight into the situation.

➤ Spending sprees.

➤ Lack of sexual restraint.

➤ Lack of self-care.

Schizophrenia

SEE ALSO
► Anxiety, p342
► Addictive behaviours, p350

This serious mental disorder affects about 1 in every 100 people and affects both men and women. Sufferers have a skewed view of reality and are unable to function socially. The causes of schizophrenia are uncertain but researchers believe that genetic factors may play a significant part in the condition's development. Adverse life events, such as a bereavement, may unmask a schizophrenic illness in someone with a genetic predisposition. Taking mood-altering drugs, such as Ecstasy, can also trigger schizophrenia in predisposed individuals.

SIGNS AND SYMPTOMS

The most common time for men to be diagnosed with schizophrenia is during the late teenage years and early 20s. Women tend to develop the condition later in life, during their 30s and 40s. The symptoms may become apparent gradually over many months but it is possible for them to appear suddenly in someone with no previous history.

Common symptoms include:

► Hearing imaginary voices.

► Paranoia.

► Having irrational beliefs.

► Becoming withdrawn.

► Agitation.

► Having rambling thoughts and ideas.

► Lack of insight.

Some of these symptoms, such as hearing voices, will often relate to a patient's personal belief system.

Schizophrenia is a serious form of psychological illness. Its name, meaning split personality, does not, in fact, describe this condition accurately. The characteristic features of this disorder are a loss of connection with reality, which leads to irrational beliefs, bizarre behaviour and emotional disturbance. Hallucinations, particularly hearing voices, are common in cases of schizophrenia. In many cases the person believes that their thoughts are being controlled by someone or something

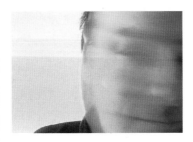

△ Disconnection from reality, isolation and inappropriate emotional responses are typical symptoms of schizophrenia.

outside themselves. He or she may ascribe unwarranted significance to minor events or things. The symptoms described above may occur in distinct episodes or be present continuously.

TREATMENT OPTIONS

A person with suspected schizophrenia needs medical help. Someone displaying signs of schizophrenia may be admitted to hospital for initial assessment and treatment. Investigations may include brain scans to eliminate other possible causes of the disturbed behaviour.

Once the condition is diagnosed, treatment with antipsychotic drugs is usually given, which in most cases helps to control symptoms and effectively prevent relapses. However, long-term treatment with such drugs can produce a variety of adverse effects such as tremors and other involuntary movements. These problems can sometimes be alleviated by an adjustment in dosage or the administration of other drugs to counter these effects. A range of newer drugs seem to have far fewer side effects than those associated with the older antipsychotic medications.

People living with schizophrenia usually require regular long-term follow-up care to ensure their wellbeing and to try to detect episodes of relapse before they become problematic. Family and friends prove invaluable in such situations. Supportive therapies such as counselling may help to reduce the levels of stress and anxiety triggered by this condition.

WHAT IS THE OUTLOOK?

About 20 per cent of affected people have one isolated episode of schizophrenic illness with no further episodes of the condition. For the remaining 80 per cent, however, the condition is a life long problem in which periods of apparent normality are interspersed with periods of schizophrenic illness of varying severity, which often require long periods of hospitalization.

▽ Schizophrenia requires doctors and other healthcare professionals to cooperate in working out the best long-term care strategy for the patient.

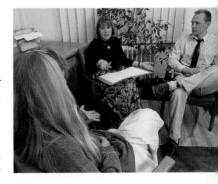

Addictive behaviours

Addiction is dependence on a particular substance or behaviour to the extent that fulfilling that dependence becomes a dominant preoccupation in a person's life. Substance misuse, most commonly involving alcohol and drugs, is an increasing problem worldwide. It causes a range of health problems as well as a variety of social problems, including the breakdown of families and increased levels of crime. Addictive behaviours, such as compulsive shopping or gambling, are likely to cause social rather than physiological problems.

For many people, obtaining and consuming an addictive substance or pursuing an addictive behaviour takes precedence over family relationships and breaks through social restraints, often leading to criminal behaviour. The addiction may be physical, in that withdrawal of the substance produces symptoms such as diarrhoea and vomiting, or the dependence may be psychological, producing craving and agitation if the consumption of the substance or behaviour is prevented. Most addictions to substances such as drugs and alcohol are a combination of both.

DRUG ADDICTION

Children and young people are influenced by parents, peers and role models. People who have difficulty dealing with anxiety and other emotions may find that drugs help control their symptoms and allow more effective social functioning. Children growing up in such an environment are vulnerable, and studies have shown that they are more at risk of succumbing to addictive patterns of behaviour.

DRUGS OF ABUSE

There is a wide range of illicit substances available. Commonly used stimulants are amphetamines, Ecstasy, crack and cocaine. These drugs stimulate the nervous system and induce a sense of power and energy. They allow the user to keep going for long periods without sleep but may also induce a sense of anxiety and paranoia. Exhaustion results from continuous use and there may be long-term psychological damage.

Many people believe that cocaine is a social drug with no potential for addiction, but crack and cocaine are extremely addictive. Cravings for crack are almost impossible to control and usually result in destructive behaviour designed to perpetuate the addiction.

Some drugs have a relaxant effect. The most commonly used is marijuana (cannabis) but heroin and the anaesthetic ketamine are widely used, too. Tranquillizers that are legally prescribed for the short-term treatment of anxiety may also be abused and have addictive potential. The long-term health risks of smoking cannabis are not fully known, but regular consumption may impair judgement and can induce long-term psychological

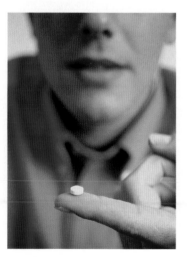

◁ The exact constituents of illicit drugs is usually unknown, which increases the risk of dangerous and unpredictable side effects.

SIGNS AND SYMPTOMS OF DRUG ABUSE

Tranquillizers such as benzodiazepine cause drowsiness, shallow breathing and a weak pulse. Stimulants such as cocaine and amphetamines cause extremely excitable behaviour and the shakes. Narcotics such as heroin cause confusion, tiny pupils and shallow breathing. Hallucinogens such as LSD cause sweating and hallucinations. Alchohol causes flushed skin, a weak pulse and, at worst, coma.

Withdrawal from any drug can cause a variety of symptoms including muscle aches and pains, diarrhoea and vomiting.

problems such as demotivation and depression, and it may also cause COPD (chronic obstructive pulmonary disease).

SOCIAL CONSEQUENCES

Users of drugs such as crack and heroin often develop physical dependence and become involved in crime to pay for their habit. Addiction has a destructive effect on relationships and employment. An addict may lose everything of value and face legal proceedings, often ending up in prison.

DRUG ABUSE HEALTH RISKS

People who inject drugs such as heroin risk contracting a range of infections. Where needles and syringes have been shared there is a high risk of catching:

• Hepatitis B.
• Hepatitis C.
• HIV.

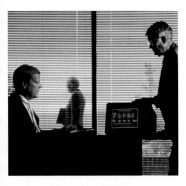

△ In much of the world today, work is a central part of many people's lives and long hours are the norm. In this climate, it is easy for work to dominate and turn into a kind of addiction.

Other common infections among injecting drug-users are:
• Septicaemia (blood poisoning).
• Endocarditis (infection of the valves inside the heart).
• Cellulitis (infection of the skin and subcutaneous tissues).
• Abscesses, especially at injection sites.

ALCOHOLISM

Alcohol is a central nervous system depressant that is an accepted part of everyday life in most societies around the world. Taken in moderation it can induce relaxation and ease inhibitions. In excess, it can severely impair judgement and coordination, and sometimes leads to violent behaviour. Regular heavy alcohol consumption may produce physical and psychological dependence, often preventing the person from working effectively and leading in some cases to loss of employment and severe disruption of family relationships The many health problems associated with heavy drinking include:
• Liver damage.
• Vitamin deficiencies.
• Peptic ulcers.

SIGNS OF ALCOHOLISM

It is not always easy to distinguish between regular social drinking and the excessive drinking that indicates alcoholism. The amount of alcohol consumed is only a rough indicator, although a person who drinks enough to be noticeably intoxicated several times a week is likely to have become dependent. Other indicators of a potential drinking problem include:
• Gradually increasing alcohol intake.
• A compulsion to drink and anxiety or physical symptoms if this is not possible.

TREATMENT OPTIONS FOR ADDICTION

It is very rare for any addictive behaviour, and particularly drug addictions and alcoholism, to improve spontaneously and addicts cannot begin their recovery programme until they admit that they have a problem and seek help. The addict may often need to be admitted to a special clinic where there is no access to the addictive substance or opportunity to pursue addictive behaviour. Supportive counselling and other specialized therapies such as cognitive and behaviour therapy also play an important part in the treatment process. The first step in the treatment of any addiction is to try to establish the root cause of the behaviour. Many specialists believe that there is such a thing as an "addictive personality", which might be partly genetic. However, there is also much evidence to support addiction as a learned behaviour.

If you know someone who has an addiction, you can go to your doctor to discuss how you should handle the problem

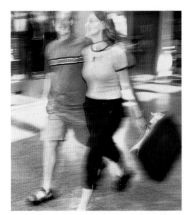

COMPULSIVE GAMBLING

Some people have an intense and compulsive desire to gamble and this urge dominates their lives. It more commonly affects men and often appears before the age of 25. Compulsive gamblers, also known as pathological gamblers, continuously increase the amounts of money they bet in order to experience the desired level of excitement. This kind of behaviour can destroy a person's life, affecting personal relationships, work, family and friends. In certain cases, gamblers lie, cheat or steal money for more gambling, regardless of the effects it may have on anyone close to them. Therapy via self-help groups, with encouragement from close friends and family members, can be successful.

▽ The motivation for compulsive gambling may be the "high" from the expectation rather than the win itself.

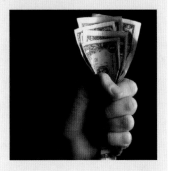

and how the addict can get help. Your doctor will be able to give you information and direct you to the many appropriate specialized services that have been developed to support and treat people with addictions.

However, the fact remains that any treatment can only be effective in the long term if the addict wants to stop and acknowledges their need for therapy.

◁ One form of addictive behaviour is obsessive "retail therapy", where shoppers feel highs and lows much like a drug addict. This can create all kinds of problems, including vast debt.

Eating disorders

SEE ALSO
➤ Eat healthily, p262
➤ Weight control, p264
➤ Depression, p346

Eating disorders are most common in Western cultures, which place great emphasis on being slim. Such problems are especially prevalent among the middle or upper social classes and are a particular occupational hazard for models, dancers, actors and certain athletes, who are required to maintain a slim body. There are two main types of eating disorder: anorexia nervosa and bulimia. About 1 per cent of teenage girls develop anorexia. Once considered a largely female problem, eating disorders are now seen increasingly in teenage boys and young men.

ANOREXIA NERVOSA

Anorexia usually affects teenage girls or young women. It is potentially life-threatening and 5 per cent of sufferers die from complications linked to severe weight loss. Women with anorexia even stop menstruating, as the condition affects their hormone balance. There may be muscle-wasting and loss of bone density. Depression is common. The affected person has a false body image, which makes them feel overweight and desperate to lose weight even when they are, in fact, very thin. Anorexics often hide their condition by wearing baggy clothes. They may show interest in food and cooking, while at the same time not eating.

BULIMIA

Bulimia is a less dangerous condition as it rarely leads to extreme weight loss. It tends to develop in young women who worry about their weight but, rather than diet

▽ Most sufferers of eating disorders are young women. This woman is being encouraged to look in a mirror in order to help her correct any distorted ideas she has about her body shape.

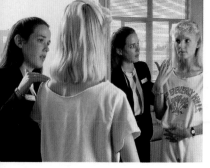

SIGNS AND SYMPTOMS OF EATING DISORDERS

Symptoms of anorexia nervosa include:

➤ Dieting and exercising excessively.

➤ Using laxatives and inducing vomiting.

➤ Using weight-reducing drugs, such as amphetamines.

Symptoms of bulimia include:

➤ Food cravings and binge eating.

➤ Eating induced by guilt and/or anxiety.

➤ Inducing vomiting.

➤ Excessive use of laxatives.

Other physical symptoms of eating disorders may include:

➤ Swollen ankles.

➤ Erosion of tooth enamel, on front teeth especially.

➤ Scars or bruises on the fingers from bouts of self-induced vomiting.

moderately, they follow an extreme regime of bingeing and starving themselves. There may be phases of anorexia and bulimia in the same person.

TREATMENT OPTIONS

Treating people with eating disorders can be difficult, especially when they refuse to acknowledge that they have a problem. Such treatment is highly specialized and is usually managed by a team of people with specific experience in dealing with eating disorders. Approaches that they use include:
• Counselling.
• Psychotherapy such as cognitive and behaviour therapies.
• Psychiatric support.
• Family therapy.

RECOVERY RATES

About 20 per cent of people with anorexia recover completely. But in two-thirds of patients, the condition persists or recurs.

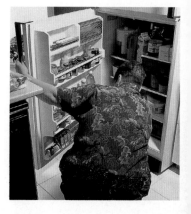

△ Secret binge eating is one of the key features of bulimia. A person with this condition is not usually underweight.

Symptoms often become especially apparent during times of stress and conflict. Bulimia can often be controlled – in four out of five cases the frequency of bingeing is reduced by therapy.

THE MUSCLES AND SKELETON

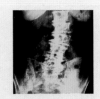

6

The bones of the skeleton provide the body with structural support, protection for the major internal organs and, combined with the muscles, enable our bodies to move. Each joint where bones meet allows flexibility and movement, and muscles are joined to bones at the joints by tough fibres called ligaments. Your muscles operate by contracting and relaxing to pull on the bones and so move the body around. Even a minor injury can cause major disruption to this complex structure, and regular exercise and a healthy diet will do much to keep the system functioning well.

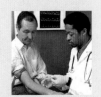

CONTENTS

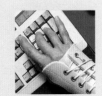

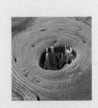

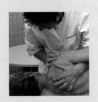

The musculoskeletal system

The musculoskeletal system is made up of the bones of the skeleton, joints that link the bones together and the muscles that enable the body to move. At birth, a baby has around 350 bones, some of which fuse together as it grows. Adults usually have 206 bones, though some have extra ribs and others have fewer. The body's largest bone is the femur in the thigh and its smallest is the tiny stapes in the ear. The muscles and ligaments act with the bones to produce a range of movements, from precision threading of a needle to the most vigorous exercise.

BONE STRUCTURE

There are two types of bone structure. Compact bone is smooth and hard. Spongy or cancellous bone has a honeycomb structure that makes it much lighter. A long bone has an outer layer of compact bone around a layer of spongy bone. Blood vessels run through cavities in the bone carrying oxygen and nutrients. Red bone marrow lies in the centre of flat and irregular shaped bones such as the ribs, vertebrae and skull.

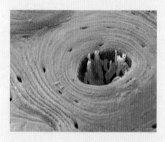

△ Blood vessels and nerves run through a cavity in a section of compact bone.

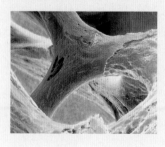

▽ Cancellous (spongy) bone from the femur. The cavities in the bone are filled with bone marrow.

Bone is a living part of the body that is constantly growing and changing. It has an immense and intricate blood supply, which is why major fractures can cause considerable blood loss. Bone consists of a mesh-like network of collagen, a protein that is the main building block of the body. Into this mesh, bone-making cells called osteoblasts deposit calcium and these give bone its hardness and strength. After death the collagen decays, and only the calcium element of the bones remains.

Most bone develops from cartilage (cartilage is the tough, gristly material found at the ends of ribs, in the outer ears and the tip of the nose). When a baby is still in the womb, cartilage starts to harden into bone in a process called ossification. As a child grows, the process continues. Bone growth occurs at the ends of the long bones as new cartilage is continually laid down before it goes through the hardening process. The skeleton is not fully formed until around 30 years of age.

THE FUNCTION OF BONES

The bones of the skeleton provide structural support for the body and work with the muscles to move it. Bones also have other functions:

• Some bones protect the vital organs. The skull acts as armour for the brain, and the pelvic bones keep abdominal organs from being damaged. The movement of the ribs aids the process of breathing and they also protect the organs of the chest, such as the heart and lungs.

• The bones of the ear help with hearing. They act as amplifiers when sound passes

PHYSIOTHERAPY

Treatment for many diseases affecting the musculoskeletal system involves physiotherapy. During physiotherapy the muscles, bones and joints are encouraged to recover through regular and systematic exercises, performed either by the patient or with manipulation by the physiotherapist. The trained physiotherapist also has access to ultrasound and heat treatments, as well as a range of supports and splints. The aim is to return the affected area of the body to health and get it working normally again as fast as possible.

from the outside world through the ear on its way to the brain.

• The bone marrow inside flat bones, such as the shoulder blades and breastbone, produces a range of blood cells.

THE JOINTS

A joint is the junction between two or more bones. Some joints are fixed, such as those of the skull, while others, such as the cartilaginous joints between the vertebrae of the spine, have hardly any movement. However, most joints in the body move freely and are known as synovial joints. The ends of the bones meeting at synovial joints are covered with a thin layer of cartilage to stop them grinding against each other. They are lubricated, to allow smooth movements, by a thin layer of fluid called synovial fluid. The ligaments are strong fibrous strips that hold bones together at the joint and stop them from moving too far apart.

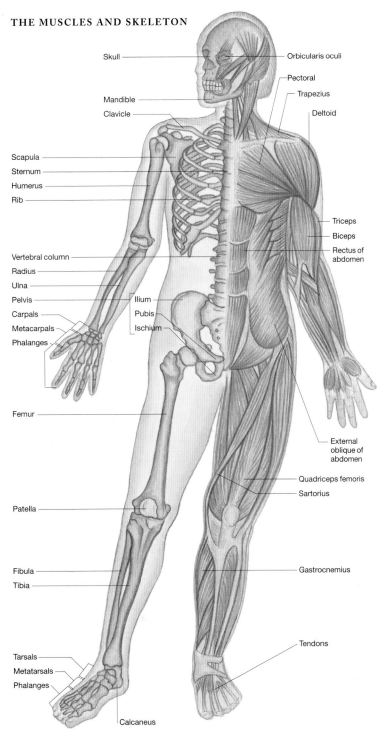

TYPES OF JOINTS

There are six types of joint and each joint has a different range of movement.

Type of joint	Where in the body
Ball and socket	Shoulders and hips.
Ellipsoidal	Links the radius to the wrist.
Hinge	Knees, elbows and fingers.
Plane or sliding	Links the carpal bones in the wrists and the tarsal bones in the feet.
Saddle	Base of the thumb.
Pivot	Links the first two vertebrae in the neck.

MUSCLE POWER

There are about 640 skeletal muscles in the body, forming up to half of the body's weight. Muscles cover the framework of the skeleton to give the body its shape. Skeletal muscles link two bones and pass across the joint between them. Each muscle is made up of muscle fibres that can be up to 30 cm (12 in) long but are thinner than a hair. There are three different types of muscle:

• Skeletal muscles – The bulk of the body's muscles are skeletal muscles, which move the body. Skeletal muscles are voluntary muscles – they do not contract on their own. In response to a nerve impulse from the brain, the muscle contracts, pulling on the bone and moving it. Muscles can only pull and never push so they work in pairs. When the biceps contracts it pulls the forearm towards the upper arm, bending the arm at the elbow. The triceps on the opposite side of the upper arm relaxes, allowing this to happen. When the triceps contracts, the biceps relaxes and the movement is reversed.

• Smooth muscles – Situated in the walls of the body's hollow organs, such as the digestive tract, they perform automatic tasks such as propelling food along.

• Cardiac muscle – This forms the non-stop pump that is the heart.

The labels on the figure read:

Skull — Orbicularis oculi — Pectoral — Trapezius — Mandible — Clavicle — Deltoid — Scapula — Sternum — Humerus — Rib — Triceps — Biceps — Rectus of abdomen — Vertebral column — Radius — Ulna — Pelvis — Ilium — Pubis — Ischium — Carpals — Metacarpals — Phalanges — Femur — External oblique of abdomen — Quadriceps femoris — Sartorius — Patella — Fibula — Tibia — Gastrocnemius — Tarsals — Metatarsals — Phalanges — Tendons — Calcaneus

Osteoporosis

Osteoporosis is a common condition in which the bone tissue loses calcium. This means the bones are brittle and more liable to fracture. Throughout life the body breaks down the bone and then builds it up again and this process promotes growth and repair. In young people the rate at which new bone is formed is faster than the breaking down process. This begins to change in early adulthood and from middle age onwards the breaking down process is accelerated and rebuilding slows down, so that bones become less strong and much lighter.

Osteoporosis affects one in twenty people, and it is four times more likely to affect women than men. This is probably because oestrogen levels fall in women after the menopause, often resulting in severe osteoporosis. Many people do not realize that they have osteoporosis until they have a minor fall that results in a fracture, most commonly of the wrist or hip. Other osteoporotic fractures are crush or compression fractures of the spine and fractures of the femur (thigh bone), which are a major cause of disability in elderly women and can be life-threatening.

WHO IS MOST AT RISK?

Age-related osteoporosis affects people with differing degrees of severity and the condition usually develops gradually over a period of 15 to 20 years. Postmenopausal osteoporosis takes only ten years to develop and is more common in women who have an early menopause.

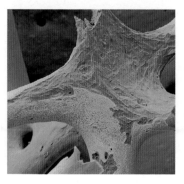

▽ A fractured femur from an osteoporosis patient. The dark areas show where the bone lacks minerals and fractures are likely.

BUILDING STRONG BONES

There are many strategies to keep your bones strong and healthy and prevent osteoporosis before a fracture happens.

➤ Avoid alcohol and stop smoking.

➤ A diet rich in milk, cheese and dark, leafy vegetables provides calcium which is vital for bone formation and can improve bone density.

➤ Depending on your BMD (bone mineral density), your doctor may advise low-impact activities, such as walking or yoga, rather than high-impact ones like jogging or aerobics. Weight training to tone and build muscle helps prevent osteoporosis by improving support to the joints.

➤ Hormone replacement therapy (HRT). If this is taken for five to ten years after the menopause, HRT can reduce the risk of fractures. It can slow down or halt osteoporosis and may help to prevent fractures.

Other risk factors include:
• Low body weight.
• Smoking.
• Excess alcohol consumption.
• Long-term corticosteroid drug therapy.
• Lack of exercise.
• Overactive thyroid.
• Family history of osteoporosis.
• Rheumatoid arthritis.
• Chronic kidney failure.

DIAGNOSING OSTEOPOROSIS

Your doctor may only detect signs of osteoporosis when examining an X-ray of a fracture. The patient will be sent for a scan to test bone mineral density (BMD) – the level of bone density is measured in the femur and wrist to confirm the diagnosis.

TREATMENT OPTIONS

You may be referred to a physiotherapist, who will advise on bone-building exercises. If you've had a fracture due to osteoporosis, you may receive the following treatments:

• HRT (hormone replacement therapy). This may halt the condition in women.
• Calcium tablets combined with a special drug, to encourage the bone to take up extra calcium.
• Vitamin D supplements can be effective, but their use must be monitored with blood tests.

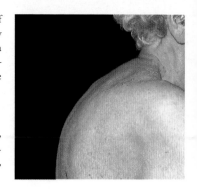

▽ Many osteoporosis sufferers develop a "hunchback" appearance. Their excessively curved spines are the result of crush fractures.

CALCIUM AND BONE HEALTH

An inadequate supply of calcium over a lifetime is believed to play a significant role in the development of osteoporosis. Studies show that low calcium intakes appear to be associated with low bone mass, rapid bone loss and high fracture rates. National nutrition surveys have shown that many people consume less than half the amount of calcium recommended to build and maintain healthy bones. Good sources of calcium include:

- Dairy products, such as low-fat yogurt, milk and cheese.
- Dark green, leafy vegetables, such as broccoli, watercress and spinach.
- Tinned fish with soft, edible bones.
- Tofu.
- Almonds and sesame seeds.
- Fresh parsley and thyme.
- Foods fortified with calcium, such as orange juice, cereals and breads.

Depending on how much calcium you get each day from food, you may need to take a calcium supplement, but most people do not need supplements so always check with your doctor or pharmacist first.

Your body's need for calcium changes as you get older. The need is at its greatest during childhood and adolescence, when the skeleton is growing rapidly, and during pregnancy and breastfeeding, when a mother passes calcium to her baby. With age, the body becomes less efficient at absorbing calcium. Older men and postmenopausal women need extra calcium because they lack adequate vitamin D, which is required for calcium absorption. Older adults with chronic medical problems may be taking drugs that impair calcium absorption.

THE EFFECT OF GRAVITY ON BONES

Having to support your own body weight against the effects of gravity stimulates bone growth. If you have a period of immobility due to illness your bones become temporarily weaker. Astronauts have great problems with loss of bone mass during space flights, although NASA has now developed a series of resistance exercises to counteract this effect. The exercises simulate gravity's bone-stimulating effects.

Osteomalacia and rickets

SEE ALSO
➤ Osteoporosis, p356

Osteomalacia is a weakening and softening of the bones that can lead to severe deformity. It is due to a vitamin D deficiency which causes a lack of calcium and phosphorus – minerals essential for bone growth. In children, the disease is known as rickets.

The commonest cause of osteomalacia is a shortage of vitamin D. Essential to enable the body to deal with calcium and phosphorus, vitamin D is found in green vegetables, fortified margarines, milk and fish. It is also made in the skin by exposure to sunlight.

A lack of vitamin D may occasionally occur in people on a vegetarian diet who do not eat dairy products or in people who are lactose intolerant (have trouble digesting milk products). Symptoms of osteomalacia are bone or muscle pain and tenderness.

Rickets is fairly rare. It is most likely to occur in young children around 6 to 24 months old, where the body demands high levels of calcium and phosphorus. Symptoms include forward projection of the breastbone (pigeon chest) and bow legs.

Both conditions can be confirmed by blood tests and X-rays. Treatment aims to increase intake of vitamin D and encourage increased exposure to sunlight.

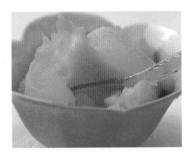

◁ Most margarines are fortified with vitamin D. This vitamin is essential in allowing the body to absorb calcium and phosphorus.

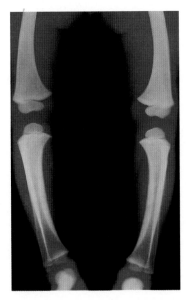

▷ Bow-leggedness caused by weakening of the bones in a child with rickets. Walking may be painful and the bones are prone to fracture.

Bone cancer

SEE ALSO

➤ The musculskeletal system, p354
➤ Lung cancer, p384

Cancers that originate in the bone, called primary bone cancers, are very rare. They most often occur in children and adolescents. Cancerous tumours in the bone "eat" their way through surrounding structures and spread quickly around the body, so early diagnosis is essential. If detected early, surgery can be carried out to remove the tumour, and most patients have only a slight chance of the disease recurring within five years, and after that recurrence is not likely. However, most cases are not diagnosed early and the prognosis is not good.

The causes of primary bone cancer are not yet known, but there may be a genetic link because it often seems to run in families. This form of cancer most often occurs in the leg, with a painful swelling just above or below the knee. The pain may be worse while standing or while in bed at night.

HOW IS IT DIAGNOSED?

Patients will be referred to a specialist to have X-rays taken and further tests such as a computerized tomography (CT) scan or magnetic resonance imaging (MRI) will be carried out so that the diagnosis can be confirmed. The most common primary bone cancer is called osteosarcoma.

Tumours are highly malignant and the disease will often spread to the lungs, so patients may also be sent for a chest X-ray.

TREATING BONE CANCER

In most cases the tumour is surgically removed and any bone that is taken away is replaced either by artificial bone or by a section of bone from elsewhere in the body or from a compatible donor. Radiotherapy or chemotherapy is normally given after surgery to get rid of any remaining cancer.

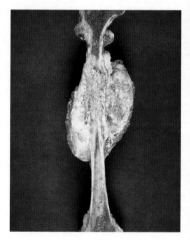

▷ This specimen of a femur – thigh bone – shows a cancerous growth. Bone tumours are highly malignant and the cancer often spreads quickly to the lungs.

Bone metastases

SEE ALSO

➤ Bone cancer, above

Bone metastases or secondary bone cancer are terms for tumours that have spread from other parts of the body. Cancers prone to metastasize to bones include breast, lung, thyroid, prostate and kidney cancers. Bone metastases are more common than primary bone cancers.

Bone metastases tend to occur in elderly people and most often affect the ribs, pelvis, skull and spine. There is a tender swelling of the area and severe bone pain, which is usually worse at night. The affected bones are weakened and may easily fracture.

Patients who have already been diagnosed with cancer elsewhere in the body may have an X-ray or radionuclide scanning to discover if the cancer has spread to the bones. If this is the first sign of cancer, further such tests may be necessary to locate the site of the primary cancer from which the metastases developed.

Treatment focuses on the primary site. A bone fracture may be fixed with metal plates or screws. Once cancer has spread to the bone any treatment is palliative not curative – chemotherapy, radiotherapy or hormone therapy may relieve pain only.

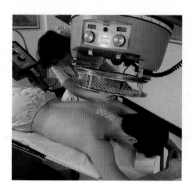

▷ A patient with secondary bone cancer has radiotherapy. The machine can be positioned very precisely so that the area to be treated is targeted accurately.

Arthritis

Arthritis refers to a group of conditions characterized by inflammation that causes pain and stiffness in one or more of the body's joints. The condition may be acute – typically sharp, severe and short-lived pain – or chronic – a constant dull ache. Arthritis may be linked to other complaints such as Crohn's disease or psoriasis. Treatment will largely depend on the severity and type of arthritis. Most treatments rely predominantly on painkillers to relieve the discomfort but as yet nothing can be done to cure the condition.

There are several different types of arthritis, and each type has its own characteristics:

- Osteoarthritis – The cartilage at the ends of bones is worn away and replaced by bony growths. It affects weight-bearing joints such as knees and hips and also the hands. It tends to occur in people over 60 and is twice as common in women.
- Rheumatoid arthritis – This causes the synovial membranes to become inflamed. The joints become swollen and stiff and ultimately deformed. It is most common between the ages of 40 and 60 and is four times as likely to affect women than men.
- Gout – This arthritis is due to deposition of uric acid crystals in the joints. The base of the big toe is most commonly affected. Gout is 20 times more common in men.
- Pseudogout – This is similar to gout in that crystals are deposited in the joints, but in pseudogout the crystals are formed from a chemical called pyrophosphate. This is more common in women.
- Psoriatic arthritis – The skin disease psoriasis can cause a form of arthritis similar to rheumatoid arthritis.

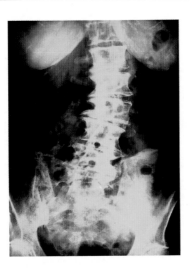

△ The spine of an 80-year-old woman with osteoarthritis shows a prominent curve and the growth of osteophytes – bony projections – between the vertebrae (upper left of picture).

- Ankylosing spondylitis – This arthritic condition can affect joints and may be associated with inflammatory bowel diseases such as Crohn's disease and ulcerative colitis. Ankylosing spondylitis is four times more likely to occur in men than in women.
- Septic arthritis – This type of arthritis results from infection in a joint, caused by a wide variety of bacteria. The joint involved is hot, swollen and painful to move. Young children and older people are most likely to develop this condition.

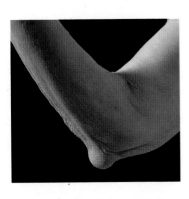

◁ A rheumatoid nodule on the arm of an elderly patient with rheumatoid arthritis. The soft nodule has been formed as a result of physical stress on the elbow joint.

- Irritable hip – In young children, a viral infection such as a cold can sometimes cause hip discomfort, difficulty walking and a limp which resolves spontaneously over a few days. However, a doctor should be consulted as there may be a problem with the hip joint called Perthes' disease where the blood supply to the joint can be affected, and a different treatment is required.

SELF-HELP FOR ARTHRITIS

A doctor will often prescribe strong drug treatments to relieve the pain but there are other treatments and self-help therapies that you may wish to consider:

- Consult a complementary practitioner in osteopathy, chiropractic or acupuncture, especially electro-acupuncture.
- Low-impact exercises such as yoga, t'ai chi and qi gong have all been shown to benefit arthritis sufferers.

▽ A finger-diameter gauge being used to measure arthritic knuckle joints. This helps to assess if a particular course of drug treatment is successfully reducing the painful swelling.

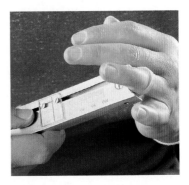

Osteoarthritis

SEE ALSO
➤ Weight control, p264
➤ Exercise for life, p266
➤ Complementary therapies and their uses, p492

Osteoarthritis is the commonest form of arthritis. It is due to the thinning and wearing away of the smooth cartilage at the ends of the bones at joints. It tends to affect the major weight-bearing joints such as the hips and knees, but very mobile joints, such as the shoulder and neck, can also be affected. Doctors once thought that osteoarthritis was simply wear and tear. However, the current theory is that it is a disease of the cartilage itself, and so new drug treatments to prevent a loss of cartilage are now in development.

If a joint has been damaged by infection or fracture, or an injury has caused damage to the cartilage pads, it is much more likely that osteoarthritis will develop in that joint later in life.

DIAGNOSING OSTEOARTHRITIS

It is possible that your doctor might suspect osteoarthritis straight away simply by taking note of your symptoms. However, in the over-55 age group, eight in ten people will probably have osteoarthritis but will not have any symptoms. No single test can confirm the diagnosis, so your doctor will want to know about pain, stiffness, and joint function, and how this has changed over time. It is also important for the doctor to know how the condition is affecting the patient's work and daily life. The patient may then be sent for an X-ray of the affected joint. X-rays can show such things as cartilage loss, bone damage and bone spurs. An X-ray will not necessarily give an accurate idea of the level of pain and disability being experienced by the patient. Your doctor may recommend a blood test to rule out other types of arthritis, such as rheumatoid arthritis.

SIMPLE SELF-HELP MEASURES

Your doctor may suggest a few simple measures to help ease osteoarthritis:
• Carrying extra body weight puts added pressure on the joints, so a healthy diet to lose weight is often recommended.
• Low-impact exercises, for example swimming, yoga and walking can be beneficial. Studies have shown that exercise improves mood and outlook. It also increases suppleness and flexibility, as well as easing pain, and improving heart function and blood flow. It helps maintain a healthy weight and boost general physical fitness. If done correctly, it should have no negative side effects. The amount and type of exercise will depend on which joints are involved, how stable those joints are, and whether a joint replacement has already been carried out. Some doctors recommend t'ai chi, a Chinese form of exercise that is gaining popularity in the West. It is easy to learn and easy to practise at home, and it involves slow, rhythmic movements that improve balance and concentration, which will help to reduce the risk of falls in the elderly. The weight-bearing aspects of this exercise have the potential to stimulate bone growth and strengthen connective tissue. Studies have shown that it also lowers blood pressure and reduces pain and inflammation.
• Wearing well-fitting, supportive shoes gives increased comfort when walking.
• Regular massage sessions bring relief.
• Warm baths, ice packs or heat pads can soothe joint pain.

HOW THE HIP JOINT IS AFFECTED

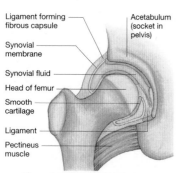

Ligament forming fibrous capsule
Synovial membrane
Synovial fluid
Head of femur
Smooth cartilage
Ligament
Pectineus muscle
Acetabulum (socket in pelvis)

△ In normal hip joints the ligaments, membrane and fluids work together to keep the joint moving smoothly.

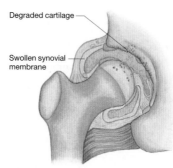

Degraded cartilage
Swollen synovial membrane

△ In an osteoarthritic hip joint, the swollen synovial membrane bulges outwards and smooth cartilage is degraded and worn away.

CERVICAL SPONDYLOSIS

This form of osteoarthritis affects the upper spine. As the cartilage between the backbones degenerates, bony growths develop on the neck vertebrae, which may press on spinal nerves in the neck. This causes pain in the neck and sometimes down the arms. Inflamed joints may restrict neck movement. It mainly affects people over the age of 45 and appears to be more common in men.

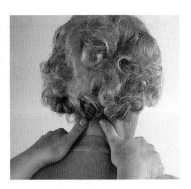

△ A neck massage provides relief. However, it is important to seek professional advice about this because massaging arthritic areas can cause damage if it is not properly done.

HOW IS IT TREATED?

Most successful programmes involve a combination of treatments tailored to the patient's individual needs, lifestyle and health. There is no cure for osteoarthritis and so treatment has four main goals:

- To control pain through drugs and other measures.
- To improve joint care through resting and gentle exercise.
- To maintain an acceptable body weight.
- To achieve a more healthy lifestyle.

There are a number of treatment options and these include:

- Taking simple painkillers.
- Taking anti-inflammatory painkillers. These drugs can cause stomach ulcers if used long term, so are combined with other drugs that protect the stomach.
- Glucosamine and chondroitin sulphate dietary supplements are among the latest treatments for osteoarthritis. These nutrients are found in small quantities in food and are components of normal cartilage. Studies have not yet shown that they affect the disease, though they may relieve symptoms in some patients.
- Physiotherapy.
- Walking aids, including walking frames.
- Steroid injections into the joint.
- Surgery to replace the joint.
- Many people find that osteopathy or

JOINT REPLACEMENT

Surgery may be required in cases where the damage to the joints is severe. A range of operations is available and they include fusing the joint, removing and replacing the affected joint and correcting any deformity. Joint replacement is the most advanced treatment. Hip and knee joints are routinely and successfully replaced. Elbow and shoulder joints can be replaced but are generally less successful.

In a hip replacement, a metal ball and stem is cemented into the top of the femur to recreate the "ball" of this ball-and-socket joint, while a plastic "socket" is cemented into the pelvis. This operation is very successful and replacement hips last approximately 15 years.

Knee replacements tend to be slightly less successful than hip replacements. A new metal end is attached to the lower end of the femur (thigh bone) and a plastic top to the tibia (shin bone). Knee replacements can last up to ten years.

Further operations to insert new replacements when the originals have worn out are much more difficult. For this reason surgeons operate as late as possible in a patient's life to minimize further operations.

▽ This is a prosthetic (artificial) hip joint. Hip-replacement operations can transform the lives of osteoarthritis sufferers, although the artificial joint may loosen with time.

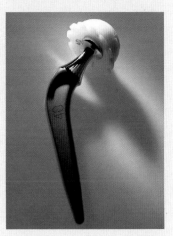

chiropractic manipulation helps ease pain and keep them mobile.

- Research shows that acupuncture is effective in some osteoarthritis patients, reducing pain and improving mobility. Licensed acupuncture therapists insert very fine needles into the skin at various points on the body. The needles are believed to stimulate the brain to produce natural painkilling chemicals.

THE IMPORTANCE OF REST

Regularly scheduled rest is important for good joint care. Patients must learn to listen to their body's signals, and know when to slow down or stop to prevent pain caused by over-use. Some patients benefit from using splints or braces to provide extra support for weakened joints during sleep or while active. Splints are used for limited periods only because joints and muscles must be exercised to prevent stiffness.

SIGNS AND SYMPTOMS

The symptoms are generally mild at first and slowly worsen over the years. The number of joints affected dictates the level of pain, discomfort and restricted mobility. Often only one or two joints are affected but it can be more widespread. The main symptoms are:

➤ Pain and tenderness, which worsens during periods of activity.

➤ Swelling around the joint.

➤ Joint stiffness.

➤ Restricted movement.

➤ Crackling noise on moving the joint, which is known as crepitus.

➤ The joints become increasingly immobile and deformed.

Rheumatoid arthritis

SEE ALSO

➤ Joint replacement, p361

➤ Anaemia, p450

➤ Autoimmune diseases, p459

Rheumatoid arthritis is a chronic inflammation of the synovial membrane that lines the joints. It is an autoimmune disease, a condition in which the body produces antibodies that attack its own tissues. This joint-destroying disease develops slowly and damages the ends of the bones and the cartilage that covers them within a joint. Continued inflammation results in damaged tendons and ligaments, which make the joint unstable and, ultimately, deform the joint. This condition can run in families and more commonly affects elderly women.

Rheumatoid arthritis is a serious disorder where symptoms may be set off by illness, stress or injury. Symptoms vary in severity and often worsen gradually.

Any joint in the body can be affected by rheumatoid arthritis, but the fingers, wrists, knees and ankles are most susceptible. There may be rheumatoid nodules (lumps of tissue under the skin), but the main indicators are pain and stiffness in the joints. Most people find that the pain and stiffness is worse in the morning but gradually improves during the day. Eventually, the damage may be so great that the joints develop characteristic swelling and deformities.

Other tissues of the body, including the eyes, skin, lungs, nerves and brain, kidneys,

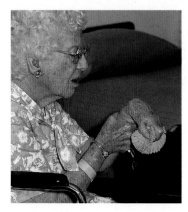

△ An elderly lady exercises her arthritic hand during a physiotherapy session. Gentle exercise can help ease pain and prolong mobility.

heart and spleen, can also be affected by rheumatoid arthritic inflammation.

SIGNS AND SYMPTOMS

The main symptoms are pain, swelling and stiffness of the joints. Other symptoms may include:

➤ Fever.

➤ Pallor.

➤ Anaemia.

➤ Loss of appetite and energy.

The joints of the hands and feet are often affected first. Rheumatoid arthritis commonly affects the wrist and many of the hand joints, but usually not the joints closest to the fingernails, except the thumb. It can also affect the elbows, shoulders, neck, knees, hips and ankles. Both sides of the body are usually affected to the same extent.

TREATMENT OPTIONS

There is as yet no cure for rheumatoid arthritis, but doctors can prescribe a range of highly effective drug therapies. Disease-modifying drugs, that act on the auto-immune disease, are usually the first line of treatment. Nonsteroidal anti-inflammatory drugs may be given to relieve pain and reduce swelling. These treatments decrease the inflammation and the deformity, and slow down the progress of the disease. Regular check-ups are advisable to monitor the drug's action and any possible side effects, which may include slight ulceration of the stomach.

In addition to drug therapy, your doctor may recommend wearing a brace or splint to support a troublesome joint and to slow

DIAGNOSIS

It is important to diagnose rheumatoid arthritis early in the disease in order to be able to treat it most effectively with disease-controlling drugs. The usual methods of diagnosis are to perform a physical examination and check X-ray images. A blood sample will be taken to test for the presence of certain antibodies known as rheumatoid factor. Rheumatoid factor is present in about 80 per cent of rheumatoid arthritis sufferers, but it can also be found in other conditions such as gout.

down the development of deformities. Patients may also be referred to a physiotherapist for guidance on regular gentle exercises to help keep symptoms at bay and joints mobile during periods of disease remission.

In the case of an acutely painful joint, the doctor may ease the pain using a corticosteroid drug, which is injected into the joint. Where joints are severely damaged, surgery may be necessary to release contracted tendons, allowing greater movement, or the inflamed synovial membrane is removed in a process called synovectomy. Sometimes joint replacement surgery is carried out on severely deformed, immobile and painful joints.

THE OUTLOOK

Many people with rheumatoid arthritis learn how to cope with the disease and lead normal lives but about 10 per cent of sufferers become severely disabled.

Gout

Also known as crystal-induced arthritis, gout is an extremely common condition, particularly in the developed world, affecting men more than women. Gout is an inflammation of the joints caused by high levels of a waste product called uric acid. Formerly a leading cause of painful and disabling chronic arthritis, gout has been all but conquered by advances in research. Unfortunately, many people with gout continue to suffer because knowledge of effective treatments has been slow to spread to patients and their doctors.

SIGNS AND SYMPTOMS

Gout can cause a very painful arthritis of any joint, but for reasons that are not yet fully understood, it tends to affect the base joint of the big toe. The joint becomes hot, red, swollen and extremely tender to touch. In some cases gout can affect the earlobes and the skin around a joint, especially the finger joints or the back of the heel.

Gout is the result of an excess of uric acid in the body. This excess can be caused by a failure of the kidneys to eliminate uric acid or by increased intake of foods containing substances called purines, which are metabolized to uric acid in the body. Purines are found in certain meats, seafood, dried peas and beans. Drinking alcohol may also significantly increase uric acid levels and trigger gout attacks.

In most people there is no immediately obvious cause for a sudden attack of gout, although it does tend to run in families. It is more prevalent in cases of obesity, where people eat a high-fat diet or drink large amounts of alcohol. It is also common in people with heart disease or high blood pressure. The incidence of gout tends to increase with age but is most common between the ages of 30 and 50.

Other conditions, including kidney disease and hypothyroidism, as well as diuretic drugs, may also lead to gout.

With time, as levels of uric acid in the blood rise, deposits collect around joints. Eventually, the uric acid forms needle-like crystals in the joints, leading to acute gout attacks. Uric acid may also collect under the skin in pockets called tophi, or in the urinary tract as kidney stones.

HOW IS IT DIAGNOSED?

The diagnosis of your condition may be obvious from your symptoms, but it is not always easy to distinguish gout from other types of arthritis. The definitive diagnosis depends on a blood test to confirm the presence of uric acid crystals in the joint

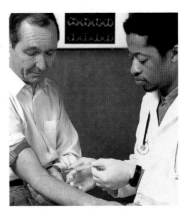

△ A blood sample is taken to confirm diagnosis of gout. The test will confirm if there are high levels of uric acid in the blood.

fluid during an acute attack. However, uric acid levels in gout sufferers are not always significantly high, and the diagnosis is made more complicated by the fact that a blood test for a non-gout sufferer may also show high uric acid readings.

TREATMENT FOR GOUT

Fortunately, an attack of gout will usually settle rapidly following a course of treatment with nonsteroidal anti-inflammatory drugs (NSAIDs), and this is the only treatment that most people require.

In patients who have suffered from multiple gout attacks, or who have developed tophi, the doctor may prescribe a drug to help the kidneys eliminate uric acid or to block its production in the body. This treatment must be started with care as it can cause an acute attack of gout when it is first used.

▽ This patient's left knee is affected by an attack of gout, causing pain and swelling. Gout is sometimes associated with other complaints, such as kidney stones and diabetes.

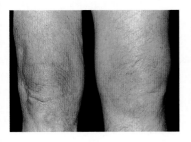

▽ This light micrograph shows uric acid crystals in a gouty joint, where they are causing an intensely painful attack of arthritis. Gout usually occurs in a single joint in the body.

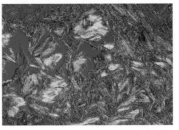

Ankylosing spondylitis

Ankylosing spondylitis primarily affects the pelvis and lower spine. It causes chronic, progressive inflammation of the joints and ligaments that normally permit the spine to move. The vertebrae may fuse and grow together, causing the spine to become rigid and inflexible. Other joints, such as the shoulders, knees or ankles, may also be involved. Men and women are affected equally, mainly in young adulthood, but the disease is usually more severe in men. There may be an inherited factor as ankylosing spondylitis can run in families.

SIGNS AND SYMPTOMS

Symptoms appear most commonly in men between the ages of 16 and 35. In women, the disease is often milder and is therefore more difficult to diagnose. The first symptoms are usually pain in the pelvis, knees, heels and big toes, followed by back pain and stiffness. Fatigue, mild fever and weight loss are also common.

Ankylosing spondylitis may take the form of intermittent back pain throughout life, or it may be a severe chronic disease that attacks the spine, peripheral joints and other body organs. It can eventually result in severe joint and back stiffness, loss of mobility and deformity.

▽ An X-ray of the pelvis and lower spine of a person with ankylosing spondylitis shows the joints in the pelvis are fused. Inflammation begins here and moves up the spine.

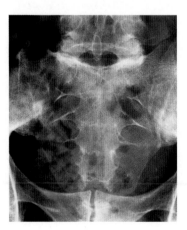

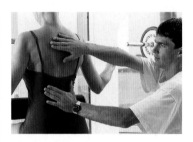

△ A physiotherapist adjusts the posture of a woman learning back exercises. Good posture while walking and standing minimizes pain.

The cause of ankylosing spondylitis is not yet known, but 90 per cent of people with the disease share a common genetic marker, called HLA-B27. In some cases, the disease is believed to be triggered in these predisposed people after exposure to infections of the bowel or urinary tract.

Symptoms usually first appear in late adolescence and early adulthood and then gradually develop over the course of months or years. In severe cases, bone starts to grow between the bones of the spine so that the vertebrae fuse together. In the long term, this leads to loss of mobility and a hunched-over appearance.

HOW IS IT DIAGNOSED?

Diagnosis of the disease is often delayed because symptoms may be attributed to more common back problems. A sudden and severe loss of flexibility in the lumbar region of the spine is an early symptom of ankylosing spondylitis.

Back problems may be followed by the development of inflammatory bowel disease, and sometimes by fever, exhaustion, weight loss, anaemia and inflammation of the eye. Malfunction of the heart valve is involved in some severe cases.

A diagnosis may be confirmed by an X-ray examination of the pelvis and spine. Blood tests can help determine the severity of the inflammation and detect the presence of genetic factor HLA-B27.

TREATMENT OPTIONS

The severity of the disease varies widely from one patient to another. Early, accurate diagnosis and treatment may spare years of suffering and disability.

Treatment is usually with nonsteroidal anti-inflammatory painkillers. These help control the symptoms, while physiotherapy sessions strengthen back muscles and help prevent stiffness and deformity of the spine.

Even with the best care and treatment, some patients will develop a permanently stiff or ankylosed spine. However, they can still retain mobility if the fusion keeps the spine upright. Ankylosing spondylitis is a lifelong problem and continuing care is essential if permanent posture and mobility losses are to be avoided.

SELF-HELP

Those with ankylosing spondylitis need to take proper rest and exercise. A physiotherapist will help with correcting a patient's posture and walking position as well as providing abdominal and back exercises to maximize joint flexibility. Deep-breathing exercises improve lung capacity and general health, and swimming offers gentle aerobic exercise.

Backache

SEE ALSO

► Weight control p264
► Exercise for life, p266
► Prolapsed disc and sciatica, p334
► Osteopathy and chiropractic, p494

Human beings are particularly prone to back pain, especially pain of the lower back because this is the part of the spine that supports most of the body's weight. This tendency may be explained by the fact that human beings walk upright when their spines are designed for moving around on all fours. After the common cold, backache is the cause of the most lost work days in adults under 45. Four out of five adults experience low back pain at some point, and it is one of the most frequent problems treated by orthopaedic surgeons.

The lower or lumbar spine is an important structure because it provides both mobility – allowing turning, twisting or bending movements – and the strength to stand, walk and lift. Smooth functioning of the lower back is vital for practically all the activities of daily life. Pain or stiffness in this area can severely restrict normal functioning, reduce work capacity and degrade quality of life.

DIAGNOSING BACK PAIN

Most types of back pain can be diagnosed by questioning and physical examination in the doctor's surgery. If the pain is severe and unresponsive to treatment, or if there is serious leg pain, imaging tests may be needed. For conditions that involve soft tissues such as the lumbar disks or nerves, a CT (computerized tomography) scan or MRI (magnetic resonance imaging) may be needed to make a diagnosis. A bone scan can assess bone activity and EMG

SIGNS AND SYMPTOMS

Pain in the lower back can be sharp and sudden or it can be persistent and dull. Backache is sometimes called lumbago, while a pain in the back that also sends stabbing pains down the leg is referred to as sciatica. Backache can be caused by damaging the back muscles when lifting something heavy incorrectly but it is more commonly due to long-term wear and tear of the ligaments, joints and discs and the softer bone tissue between the vertebrae.

PREVENTING BACK PAIN

Back pain is a major cause of disability and the options for treatment are limited, so prevention is crucial.

► Never bend or stoop forward to pick up something. Bend your knees and lift by using your thigh muscles while keeping your back straight.

► Sit for short periods only. Sitting puts great strain on the back and can be compounded by bad posture. Keep your back straight and if you have to sit for a long time, while driving for example, support the lower back with a pillow.

Special "Mackenzie D rolls", available from physiotherapists, provide excellent lumbar support.

► Lose excess weight. Your lower back supports most of the weight of your upper body, so less weight equals less stress on your back.

► Sleep on a firm, supportive mattress. Sleeping on a soft, sagging mattress will often lead to back problems.

► Practise regular stretching and bending exercises, such as yoga.

(electromyography) tests can detect nerve or muscle damage.

HOW IS IT TREATED?

In most people lower back pain settles in a few days. Contrary to popular belief, bed rest or lying on a hard surface are not recommended. Rest simply stiffens the back and prolongs the healing process. It is better to continue with gentle activity combined with painkillers to relieve the symptoms.

In cases of recurrent backache the best treatment is physiotherapy, though many people consult alternative practitioners such as chiropractors, osteopaths or cranial osteopaths. In some cases combined local anaesthetic and corticosteroid injections to affected joints may be necessary. Surgery on the lower back can remove the pressure from a prolapsed disc when it causes severe nerve and leg pain.

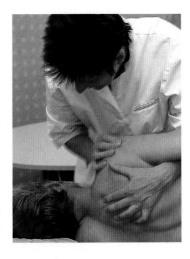

▽ An osteopath manipulates the back and shoulder of a patient. Osteopathy also involves stretching and applying pressure to affected parts of the body.

Frozen shoulder

SEE ALSO
➤ Diabetes, p314
➤ The musculoskeletal system, p354

A frozen shoulder is a chronic inflammation of the tendons and synovial capsule around the shoulder joint. In many cases the condition develops for no obvious reason, but it may be the result of an injury. The joint can also freeze up if the shoulder has been kept immobilized for a period of time, such as after a stroke. The pain is long-standing and gets worse on moving the shoulder. Movement is severely restricted. The condition occurs more often in people over 40 and affects more women than men. People with diabetes are particularly susceptible.

The ball-and-socket joint at the shoulder is prone to injury because of its huge range of movement. Any injury or damage to this joint can cause a frozen shoulder.

In a frozen shoulder, the capsule around the joint contracts and reduces movement at the joint. Movement becomes more and more restricted, and there is severe pain whether the joint is moved or not.

SIGNS AND SYMPTOMS

Pain is slight to start with and gradually worsens. Movement is difficult and it may be impossible to lie on the affected shoulder. In time, the pain may subside but the joint becomes increasingly stiff.

HOW IS IT TREATED?

Treatments that may help to ease stiffness and improve mobility of a frozen shoulder include a course of physiotherapy or manipulative treatment carried out by an osteopath or chiropractor. Nonsteroidal anti-inflammatory drugs may be prescribed to relieve pain and reduce inflammation. Your doctor may inject the shoulder with corticosteroids and this can act quickly, and may sort out the problem completely. However, in severe cases an injection may only give temporary relief and further manipulative treatments may be necessary.

Many cases of frozen shoulder eventually settle within three months, although it is possible for residual stiffness to last for much longer.

INJECTING A FROZEN SHOULDER

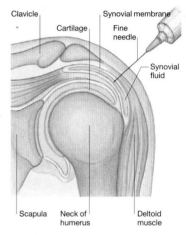

Clavicle
Cartilage
Synovial membrane
Fine needle
Synovial fluid
Scapula
Neck of humerus
Deltoid muscle

Bunions

SEE ALSO
➤ Osteoarthritis p360

A bunion is a thickened lump of soft tissue and bony overgrowth at the base of the big toe. This deformity is also known as hallux valgus. Bunions are painful and can affect either sex. They are more common in women and may be a result of wearing pointed, high-heeled shoes.

Bunions can often become inflamed and painful, making shoes uncomfortable and walking difficult. Underlying the bunion is a deformity of the bone that forces the big toe to point inwards towards the other toes. The cause of bunions is not yet known. They sometimes run in families and may be due to wearing tight shoes. Well-fitting shoes, and walking barefoot as often as possible, may ease the discomfort.

TREATMENT OPTIONS

For painful bunions the only solution is surgery in which the joint is straightened and fused. People normally make a full recovery within six weeks. Untreated bunions increase the risk of developing osteoarthritis in that joint in later years.

▷ A bunion can cause the big toe to point inwards and crush its neighbour. A cotton wool pad between the toes can help to correct this.

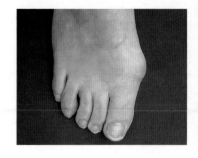

Repetitive strain injury

SEE ALSO
➤ Exercise for life,
  p266
➤ Rheumatoid arthritis,
  p362

Repetitive strain injury (RSI) is a common condition among people who do repetitive work, or play regular sport, that places strain on a particular part of the body. This painful condition is especially common in the muscles and tendons of the arms and hands and is caused by repeating the same movement over and over again, especially if that movement is rapid and forceful. RSI affects people in a range of occupations that place stress on joints and muscles – from keyboard operators and assembly line workers to musicians and athletes.

SIGNS AND SYMPTOMS

The symptoms of RSI develop gradually and include pain, aching and tingling in the affected limb during the key activity. In the early stages the pain often disappears during rest periods, though in the later stages, it is constant and severe.

Repetitive strain injury is much easier to treat in the early stages of the disease, so it is vital to act on symptoms as soon as they appear. If untreated, RSI may worsen, leaving the patient with permanent damage and unable to use the affected limb to work or play sport. This may mean an enforced change of lifestyle and, if symptoms are related to occupation, a change of jobs.

HOW IS IT DIAGNOSED?

Diagnosis is by questioning the patient and examination of the tender muscles or joints. There may be a blood test to rule out other diseases, such as rheumatoid arthritis.

TREATMENT FOR RSI

In many places of work, advice is given on posture and most will organize special equipment to reduce the likelihood of repeated symptoms. In all cases, there are steps to take to minimize the effects of RSI, or to prevent it in those at risk. Simple exercises such as swimming, walking, yoga and stretching routines can improve suppleness and mobility. Massage therapy is a relaxing way to reduce strain and prevent current discomfort from turning into chronic disabling pain.

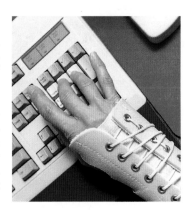

▽ Anyone working with computers is at risk from RSI because of the strain placed on the wrist by typing. If the disease has developed, wearing a wrist support may be recommended as well as exercises to avoid repetitive strain.

Fibromyalgia

SEE ALSO
➤ Learn to manage
  stress, p260

Fibromyalgia is a muscle disorder that causes sharp pains and aching all over the body. It has no obvious cause, but may be brought on by intense stress. Patients may also suffer from conditions such as chronic fatigue syndrome, irritable bowel syndrome and depression.

Fibromyalgia affects women more commonly than men, but is rarely diagnosed because it causes no visible abnormality in the muscle tissue. It is often misdiagnosed as chronic fatigue syndrome. No doctor would dispute that fibromyalgia can cause suffering, but medical opinion is divided as to the basis of physical and psychological factors.

WHAT MIGHT YOUR DOCTOR DO?

After a physical examination, a blood test may be taken to rule out other disorders, such as rheumatoid arthritis.

TREATING FIBROMYALGIA

Pain may be treated with therapies such as deep tissue massage and locally applied heat, or an injection with a local anaesthetic.

Painkillers must be used sparingly. Low-intensity exercise is recommended, such as walking, yoga or t'ai chi. Any related conditions, such as depression and irritable bowel syndrome, are treated accordingly. Psychological treatments, such as cognitive therapy, are often very helpful and many patients are able to make a complete recovery.

Fractures

SEE ALSO
➤ The musculoskeletal system, p354
➤ Osteoporosis, p356

Any bone can be fractured (break or crack) if enough force is applied to it, but fractures tend to occur at weaker spots in certain bones. Fractures are more likely to occur in children and the elderly. Children's bones are softer and tend to crumple on one side – a greenstick fracture – rather than snap. In the elderly, especially elderly women, bones can become brittle (osteoporotic) and even a minor injury can smash the bone into fragments. Spontaneous fractures in bones affected by cancer tumours are called pathological fractures.

There are two main types of fracture and these are closed (a simple fracture), in which the bone does not pierce the skin, and open (a compound fracture), in which the bone is exposed by piercing the skin. Open fractures are more serious because of the damage to nerves and blood vessels and the risk of infection.

Fractures are most often caused by an injury such as a twisting movement or impact after falling.

THE BONES OF THE ARM

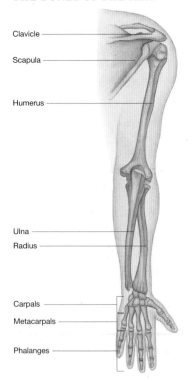

Clavicle

Scapula

Humerus

Ulna

Radius

Carpals

Metacarpals

Phalanges

ARM BONE FRACTURES

If a person trips and puts out a hand, the force that travels up the arm from impact can break any of its bones. There are a number of different fractures of the arm:

• Distal radius (or Colles' fracture) – This fracture, which often occurs in the elderly, takes about six weeks to heal. The end of the radius, near the wrist, breaks and is forced backwards. In children, greenstick fractures are common, but these usually settle within three weeks.

• Scaphoid – This fracture, of the small carpal bone in the wrist, most commonly occurs in young adults. Fractures may be slow to show up on an X-ray, so if a doctor suspects a fracture the wrist may plastered and X-rayed ten days later, by which time any fracture should be clear. This fracture heals in about six weeks.

• Radial head – In this fracture, which can happen at any age, the top of the radius, (at the elbow) fractures. It usually heals if the arm is kept still and supported in a sling for a few weeks.

• Base of the humerus (above the elbow) – This fracture occurs in children and as it may be close to a major artery, doctors will check the pulse.

• Shaft of humerus – The midpoint of the humerus can break. An important nerve is close to this bone so the fracture may need to be stabilized surgically. This fracture is most likely occur in the elderly.

• Neck of humerus – The top of the humerus can be smashed in the elderly. The fracture may appear horrific on X-ray images but it heals well with a collar and cuff support after a few weeks.

GREENSTICK FRACTURE TO THE RADIUS OF THE ARM

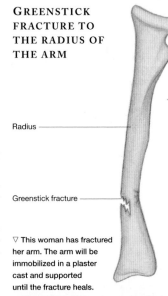

Radius

Greenstick fracture

▽ This woman has fractured her arm. The arm will be immobilized in a plaster cast and supported until the fracture heals.

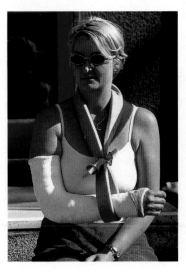

- Clavicle – The middle of the collarbone is easily broken but it heals well with a sling for support.

OTHER COMMON FRACTURES

The commonest fractures caused by a fall from any height are:
- Ankle fractures.
- Fractures of the heel bone.
- Fractures of the tibia and femur around the knee.
- Crush or compression fractures to the vertebrae in the spine.
- Pelvic fractures.
- Fractured neck of femur – This fracture of the top end of the femur (thigh bone) is common in the elderly. It often requires surgery and a half or full hip replacement may be needed. It is a major injury at any age but especially for the elderly, because they have to remain immobile for so long.

Turning over on the ankle produces two main types of fracture:
- Lateral malleolus fracture – The lower end of the fibula (one of the bones in the lower leg) is broken off and the ankle needs to be put in a cast for six weeks. Sometimes, the lower end of the other shinbone – the tibia – may also break. This usually needs to be fixed with metal screws and plates.
- Base of fifth metatarsal fracture – The end of the fifth toe bone can be snapped off, needing a cast for six weeks.

TREATMENT OPTIONS

Fractures will heal and most need only minimal treatment, which may include:
- Immobilization – Most fractures need to be immobilized to reduce pain. This may be done with a cast or traction. Traction is where the limb is held in place, during bed rest, with weights and pulleys.
- Reduction – Occasionally manipulation under anaesthetic is required to realign the bones.
- Fixation – Some fractures need surgery. Internal fixation involves inserting metal pins and/or plates under the skin to fix the bone. In external fixation, metal pins are inserted through the skin into the bone. Pins are held in place by a metal frame, the limb can be used in a few days and pins and frame are removed under anaesthetic once the bone has healed.

For all types of fracture, rehabilitation is vital for a return to normal function and physiotherapy sessions will strengthen the weakened joints and muscles.

DISLOCATION

If a large amount of force is applied to a joint, it can become dislocated with or without an associated fracture. A joint that has been dislocated once is more likely to be dislocated again in the future. It is common to sustain a dislocated shoulder when falling on to an outstretched hand. It is very painful but can usually be popped back in by a doctor with the help of pain relief and sedation. A support-strapping bandage is worn for about six weeks afterwards.

HOW BONE HEALS ITSELF

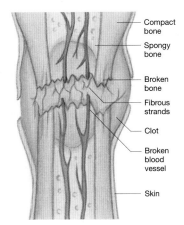

Compact bone
Spongy bone
Broken bone
Fibrous strands
Clot
Broken blood vessel
Skin

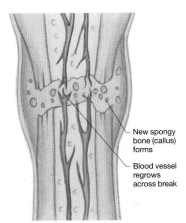

New spongy bone (callus) forms
Blood vessel regrows across break

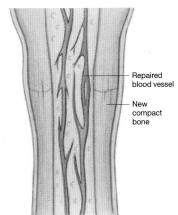

Repaired blood vessel
New compact bone

1 Broken bones have a huge capacity to repair themselves – they must simply be immobilized so that they knit together correctly. First, broken blood vessels heal and a mesh of new fibrous tissue forms.

2 In the second stage of healing, new spongy bone called callus is produced to make a tough temporary fix. Broken blood vessels regrow through the callus, allowing the flow of blood through the new bone.

3 Over the subsequent months and years this temporary repair is gradually replaced by compact bone. Any slight deformity is overlaid with new bone. Finally, it is difficult to tell that a fracture has ever occurred.

Knee injuries and disorders

SEE ALSO
➤ The musculoskeletal
  system, p354
➤ Osteoarthritis, p360
➤ Joint replacement,
  p361

The knee is the body's largest joint. The femur joins the tibia and the kneecap (patella) sits over this joint to help protect the knee. The knee is a hinge joint and because it has to bear heavy loads and constant pressure, it risks being twisted out of its plane and damaged. Injuries to the knee are common. They may be caused by activities such as jogging on hard pavements, which stresses the knee and damages cartilage, and skiing, where the constant bending of the knee can tear cartilage and strain the hamstring muscles that allow the knee to flex.

Damage to the knee can cause great pain. Treatments range from ice packs (a bag of frozen vegetables is a useful standby) to anti-inflammatory drugs. Rest followed by special exercises to strengthen the surrounding muscles is vital. Injury to one joint puts pressure on other joints of the body, and assessment of the damage and corrective treatment may be necessary.

TORN OR DAMAGED CARTILAGE

Inside the knee joint are two half-moon-shaped pieces of cartilage called menisci. If you twist awkwardly on a bent knee the menisci can be torn or damaged.

THE KNEE JOINT

▽ This picture shows the inside of the knee joint. Note that the kneecap (patella) has been removed for clarity.

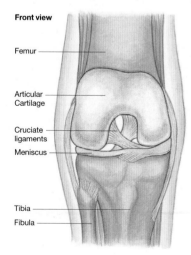

Front view

Femur

Articular Cartilage

Cruciate ligaments

Meniscus

Tibia

Fibula

Tearing the cartilage is extremely painful. The knee often swells up and cannot be straightened fully. The pain and swelling usually settle but can recur even when subjected to very slight trauma.

This condition is usually referred to an orthopaedic surgeon, who will examine and treat the knee via a telescopic viewing device called an arthroscope. This process is performed under a general anaesthetic. The arthroscope is inserted into the joint through a tiny incision in the skin and transmits pictures of the inside of the knee to a screen. Delicate surgery is carried out to shave the surface of the kneecap or remove damaged tissue.

Patients make a good recovery, but the joint may be prone to arthritis in later life.

RECURRENT DISLOCATION OF THE PATELLA

Any dislocation should be treated as an emergency, and medical assistance should be summoned immediately. The foot on the injured leg should be checked for blood flow by monitoring for coldness.

Some people, especially girls, are prone to repeated dislocation of the patella caused by minimal injury. The kneecap usually relocates itself, but it can be painful. Resting the joint in a cast, then exercising to strengthen the thigh muscles can stop the problem, but an operation may be required.

PAIN BEHIND THE KNEE

This condition is common and is usually due to overload of the joint between the kneecap and the femur. The knee is painful

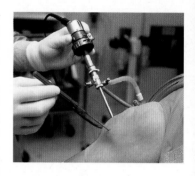

△ Torn cartilage in the knee is treated via an arthroscope. Pictures are transmitted to a monitor while the surgeon corrects the problem.

and may be swollen. Most people recover with rest, painkillers and physiotherapy. Occasionally, the kneecap will not move properly as it slides over the femur while bending the knee, and surgery is required to correct the problem.

CHONDROMALACIA

This condition causes pain in front of the knee and is due to an abnormality of the cartilage at the back of the kneecap. It occurs most commonly in adolescents of either sex and sometimes runs in families.

Chondromalacia can be triggered by a growth spurt, by sports or other injuries, or by putting too much strain on the knee joint while exercising.

The main symptom is pain in the knee when the leg is bent and straightened, for example going up or down stairs. There may be a crackling noise called crepitus when the knee joint is exercised and the joint may get stiff after sitting still.

The doctor may prescribe nonsteroidal anti-inflammatory drugs and advise ice packs for pain relief. Exercises to strengthen the muscles and reduce stress on the joint lessen the risk of developing osteoarthritis in later life. A knee support can provide temporary relief.

BURSITIS

Bursae are fatty sacs found around the joints. They act as cushions to reduce friction as the joint moves. Bursitis is inflammation of the bursae, which become swollen and painful, restricting movement.

The most common form of bursitis is found in the knee and is sometimes known as housemaid's knee, because it may be the result of frequent kneeling. Ice packs will provide some relief and your doctor may prescribe anti-inflammatory painkillers and, if there is a bacterial infection, a course of antibiotics. The condition will usually settle with rest after a few days but if pain and swelling persists, it may be necessary to drain the bursa.

KNEE JOINT REPLACEMENTS

Where damage to the knee joint is severe, through injury or by a condition such as arthritis, a joint may be replaced with an artificial one made of metal or plastic. This involves shaving off damaged bone ends before fitting the new parts.

OSGOOD-SCHLATTER DISEASE

This disease is common in adolescence. It is when the tendon from the muscle on the thigh (quadriceps) pulls on the growing part of the tibia. It causes pain and there may be a tender swelling on the front of the tibia. The pain settles with rest and by avoiding running and cycling. The condition disappears once the teenager stops growing.

LOOSE BODIES

The knee is a large and complex joint and is prone to pieces of bone and cartilage floating freely within it. These usually cause no problems, but if they cause problems they can be removed using an arthroscope.

Sprains

SEE ALSO
➤ Fractures, p368

A sprain occurs when a joint is wrenched, causing stretching or tearing of a ligament. Ligaments are flexible, fibrous connective tissue that attach bones to each other at the joints. Sprains most commonly occur in the ankles, wrists and knees, and can be extremely painful.

Sprains cause intense pain, swelling and discoloration in the affected area. A mild sprain settles with rest in a couple of days, but a more serious ligament tear may require surgery, especially if it has splintering to the bone to which the ligament is attached. An X-ray will confirm whether this is the case.

It is difficult to differentiate between a sprain and a muscular strain. Both involve severe pain, swelling and restricted movement of the limb. Both sprains and strains may recur if not allowed to heal fully. The joints most commonly sprained are:
• Ankles – This sprain occurs when the ankle is twisted, for example by walking on uneven ground.
• Knees – Sporting accidents may tear the ligaments on the inside of the knee.

▷ To avoid sprains while walking and climbing, it is important to wear strong, comfortable boots that provide support around the ankle.

Crutches may be needed to rest the joint.
• Wrists – Commonly sprained when the hand is put out to break a fall.

The ligament should heal in about eight weeks with rest and supportive bandaging – stretchy tubular bandages are easier to put on and are available from pharmacies. In some cases nonsteroidal, anti-inflammatory painkillers are prescribed.

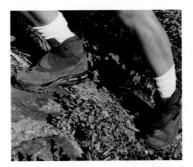

SIMPLE SELF-HELP MEASURES

While waiting to see a doctor, a sprain should be treated with the "RICE" procedure:

➤ Rest – Keep the injured limb still and support it on a cushion or footstool.

➤ Ice – Apply an ice pack (a packet of frozen peas will do) to the affected area for several minutes. This will reduce the swelling and bruising and also helps to relieve pain.

➤ Compression – Wrap the injured limb with a thick padding of cotton wool secured with a bandage wound in a figure of eight.

➤ Elevation – Make sure that the injured limb is supported and raised.

Tendon and muscle injuries

SEE ALSO
➤ The musculoskeletal system, p354
➤ Sprains, p371

Tendons are the tough, fibrous bands that link muscles to bones. They can tear and snap, especially during strenuous sporting activities, or they can be lacerated or cut, as a result of an accident, for example with a knife. Tendons are prone to becoming inflamed. This condition, called tendinitis, usually occurs in conjunction with tenosynovitis, the inflammation of the sheath of tissues that surrounds the tendon. Similar injuries of varying severity can result from overstraining or tearing a muscle, especially as a result of athletic sports or weight-training.

The most common symptoms of tendinitis and tenosynovitis are exacerbated by movement, and include pain, swelling and stiffness, and restricted mobility in the affected area. The skin may be hot and red and there may be a crackling sensation, called crepitus, when the joint is moved.

COMMON TENDON INJURIES

• Snapping of the Achilles tendon – The Achilles tendon links the calf muscle to the heel. It can snap under stress, especially when a middle-aged person does unaccustomed exercise. It causes severe pain around the lower calf and heel. Treatment involves surgical repair of the tendon or wearing a cast for six weeks. In either case, physiotherapy is required to restore mobility.

• Mallet finger – The tendon that is used to straighten the finger can snap off the bone if the end of the finger is bent suddenly. If the finger is splinted for six weeks, it may make a complete recovery.

THE ACHILLES TENDON

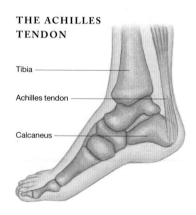

Tibia

Achilles tendon

Calcaneus

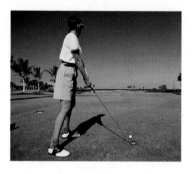

△ The sudden and powerful swing of the wrist involved in a golf stroke can cause golfer's elbow, a common form of tendinitis.

• Cut tendons – Hand lacerations on sharp objects can easily damage the tendons. Urgent surgical repair is needed to preserve their function.

TENDINITIS

All forms of tendinitis need rest and in some cases will heal faster if they are splinted. Physiotherapy is often helpful. Your doctor may prescribe nonsteroidal anti-inflammatory drugs or even an injection of a corticosteroid drug, and these will usually bring fast relief. Types of tendinitis include:

• Achilles tendinitis – Splinting is often recommended to resolve inflammation of this tendon at the back of the heel. Gentle exercises to stretch the tendon may also be helpful.

• Rotator cuff injury – The tendons that lift the arm out to the side can tear, making shoulder movement painful. The pain usually occurs at a certain point as the arm is lifted as the damaged tendon rubs underneath part of the shoulder blade. It is called painful arc syndrome.

• Plantar fasciitis – The flat tendon that covers the sole of the foot becomes inflamed and is painful when standing or walking (also called policeman's heel).

• Golfer's and tennis elbow – This painful condition occurs where the muscles that work the wrist are attached to the elbow – golfer's elbow affects the inner (medial) elbow and tennis elbow affects the outer (lateral) elbow. Rest with ice packs is recommended and for acute pain, a steroid injection can provide relief.

MUSCLE TEARS

Muscle injuries are common at any age, though older people performing unaccustomed movements or exercises and sportspeople are most at risk. Most sports depend on muscle strength and suppleness, and damage can easily be caused by sudden forceful movements or strain when lifting heavy weights. The muscles most often affected are those of the calf (gastrocnemius and soleus), the front of the thigh (quadriceps) and back of the thigh (hamstrings).

On pulling a muscle, you may feel a sharp pain and sometimes a tearing sensation. Bruising later appears and the area will be painful to the touch.

Such injuries usually settle with rest and treatments, such as heat pads or ice packs, over the course of a couple of weeks. Anti-inflammatory painkillers can be especially effective in severe cases. Physiotherapy is occasionally needed.

7

THE RESPIRATORY SYSTEM

The body fulfils its energy needs by burning up the fuel in food. Like a fire in the grate, this process of combustion (called metabolism) requires a ready supply of oxygen. Supplying this oxygen is the job of the respiratory system. The lungs are rather like a system of bellows, drawing oxygen from the air and delivering it through the blood to each cell in the body. The cells use up the energy in various ways: supplying power to muscles, rebuilding tissue, maintaining body temperature. When the oxygen in each cell is used up, the blood carries the waste – mostly carbon dioxide – back to the lungs, where it is expelled like smoke from a chimney when we breathe out.

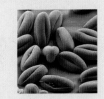

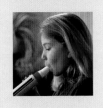

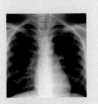

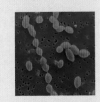

The breathing process

Every cell in your body needs a constant supply of oxygen and at the same time needs to get rid of its principal waste product – carbon dioxide. The respiratory system works with the blood circulation system to meet your body's energy demands. The respiratory system delivers oxygen from the air you breathe to the blood system and then transfers carbon dioxide from the blood into the air you breathe out. Your lungs have a network of branching tubes that become ever smaller, maximizing the surface area available for the transfer of oxygen and carbon dioxide.

With every breath, you inhale about 500 ml (roughly 1 pint) of air, and you breathe between 12 and 15 times a minute. The air travels through the upper respiratory tract – first through the mouth or nose, then into the throat and the trachea (windpipe).

From the trachea, air travels down one of the two main bronchi (airways) and into the ever-smaller branches – the bronchioles. At the end of the bronchioles are tiny air sacs called alveoli. The smallest functional units of the lungs, they carry out the sophisticated process of gaseous exchange – exchanging oxygen for carbon dioxide.

GASEOUS EXCHANGE

Each alveolus has a network of tiny blood vessels (capillaries). During gaseous exchange, oxygen from inhaled air diffuses into the walls of the alveolus through the capillaries and binds to haemoglobin

▽ X-rays are often used to diagnose problems in the respiratory system. The lungs are the dark areas at the right and left. They are enclosed and protected by the ribs, which show up here as pale bands.

BREATHING IN AND OUT

Breathing is an automatic action controlled by the respiratory centre in a part of the brain called the medulla. The medulla adjusts the rate at which you breathe in response to your body's constantly changing requirements to absorb oxygen and eliminate carbon dioxide.

Receptors in the arteries monitor levels of carbon dioxide in the blood. They relay this information to the brain, which adjusts the rate of inhalation and exhalation to maintain a balance of gases in the body. When you exercise and use up oxygen more quickly, the brain sends out a message to speed up breathing and get more oxygen to the lungs.

The mechanics of breathing are controlled by the intercostal muscles (found between the ribs) and the diaphragm. They work to create different pressures in the chest.

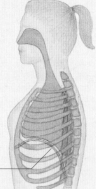

▷ Inhalation – When you breathe in the intercostal muscles contract to lift your ribcage as the diaphragm contracts and flattens. This expands the chest cavity and lowers pressure to draw air into the lungs.

Diaphragm

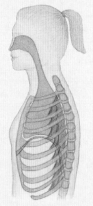

▷ Exhalation – As you breathe out the intercostal muscles and diaphragm relax. This reduces the chest cavity and increases the pressure so that air is forced out of the lungs.

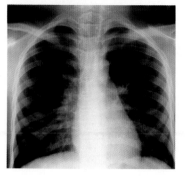

pigment in the red blood cells. This process transports oxygen around the circulation system to power the body's energy-making metabolic processes. At the same time, carbon dioxide, the waste product of the metabolic processes, diffuses from the blood into the alveoli and is expelled from the body during exhalation.

RESPIRATORY DEFENCES

The respiratory tract has different ways to protect itself from infection and irritation:

- Tissue – Protective tissue lines the upper and the lower respiratory tracts. In the upper tract, the protective tissue is concentrated in the tonsils and adenoids, which destroy agents before they can reach the lungs.
- Mucus coating – This sticky, protective coating lines the airways and traps any foreign particles.
- Cilia – These are tiny hair-like projections in the airways, which sweep any foreign particles up and away from the lungs.

HOW THE LUNGS WORK

▷ The unconscious act of breathing sends air down a system of ever-narrower airways and into the bloodstream. The respiratory system is a complex mechanism that also involves the ribcage and various different muscles.

Nasal passages
Air is warmed and moistened as it is inhaled through the nose and the mouth.

Trachea
This tube is held open by a series of cartilage rings and divides into the two bronchi.

Ribs
The ribcage aids the process of breathing, and protects the lungs and heart.

Bronchi
Two tubes, serving the left and the right lung, lead from the trachea and fill the chest cavity with ever-smaller branching airways called the bronchioles.

Intercostal muscles
These muscles, found between the ribs, move the ribcage during respiration.

Bronchiole
These branch off the bronchi. At the end of each bronchiole is an air sac called an alveolus.

Diaphragm
This major breathing muscle works with the intercostal muscles. It contracts and relaxes to increase and decrease the size of the chest cavity.

Pleura
This two-layered membrane separates the lungs from the chest wall. A thin layer of fluid – surfactant – helps the layers move smoothly as the lungs inflate and deflate.

Alveolus
Each alveolus is covered with tiny capillaries to create the maximum surface area for gaseous exchange.

Membranous wall
Alveolar walls allow oxygen from air to diffuse into the haemoglobin in red blood cells. At the same time, carbon dioxide from the red blood cells diffuses into the alveolus and is breathed out.

INVESTIGATING THE RESPIRATORY TRACT

Your doctor has various ways to diagnose respiratory problems, including:

➤ Listening to you cough and examining your chest.

➤ A chest X-ray can confirm the presence of infections or more serious diseases, such as lung cancer.

➤ A peak-flow meter measures exhalation to give an indication of any obstruction in the airways. It is also used to find out if asthma patients need to make any adjustments to their medication.

A range of investigations may be used by a hospital specialist including:

➤ Lung function tests measure how much air you can inhale or exhale, and how much air your lungs can hold.

➤ Two lung scans are taken to measure blood and air flow through the lungs.

➤ Bronchoscopy – A narrow tube with a camera at its tip is passed through the mouth or nose into the lungs so that the bronchi can be viewed. A local anaesthetic is given.

• Coughing – A cough reflex is triggered by irritation in the airways or the lungs to expel foreign particles from the body before they can do any damage.

Colds and flu

Colds and flu (influenza) are viral infections of the upper respiratory tract, and are among the most common reasons for people to visit their doctors. There are more than 200 different viruses that cause the common cold and three main flu types, A, B and C. Approximately half the population catches a cold once a year, most often in the colder months of autumn and winter. Flu affects fewer people and tends to occur in epidemics in winter. The most effective way to fight colds and flu is to ensure that your body is fit and healthy as possible.

Colds and flu are extremely contagious. They are spread by airborne droplets of mucus, expelled when an infected person coughs, sneezes or breathes into the air. The viruses can also be passed on by physical contact if the recipient picks up the virus on their hand and rubs their eyes or nose – which provide entry points for the virus. One infected person can pass on the virus to many others, and you are probably most infectious a day before symptoms develop.

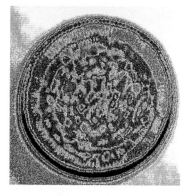

△ The common cold virus, shown here as a computer graphic, is easily spread by airborne droplets and by hand-to-hand contact.

SIGNS AND SYMPTOMS

Both cold and flu produce symptoms a day or two after you've been infected. They share some symptoms but flu symptoms tend to worsen dramatically in a few hours and are more severe.

The usual cold symptoms are:

➤ A runny nose in which the mucus becomes thick and greeny-yellow.

➤ Sneezing.

➤ Sore throat and cough.

➤ Wild fever and headache.

Very often people think they have flu when they have a bad cold. However, flu symptoms sometimes include a blocked nose, a cough and a sore throat but you are more likely to suffer from:

➤ High fever, sweating and chills.

➤ Aching muscles.

➤ Headaches.

➤ Severe exhaustion and weakness.

➤ Loss of appetite.

WARNING!

If you have a cold or flu and you experience difficulty in breathing at any time, or if a fever lasts more than a few days, see your doctor urgently. You can develop a chest infection, such as pneumonia, or other infection, such as sinusitis or ear infection. In such cases, your doctor may prescribe antibiotics to treat the infections; antibiotics do not, however, have any effects on the viruses that cause colds or flu.

Since many different viruses can cause the common cold, having one cold does not provide immunity from another. Adults are less susceptible to colds than children because they have developed some immunity to the most common forms, and children spend more time in large groups – at school or in nurseries – where viruses can spread rapidly from child to child.

Flu is principally caused by infection with virus types A or B, particularly the more severe type A virus. However, the flu viruses are continually mutating into new strains. Having one attack of flu will not provide you with immunity against an attack by a new strain. If you are concerned about developing flu, you can be immunized against the strains that are predicted to be most prevalent each year. Immunization is strongly recommended for certain groups of people who are at greater risk of developing complications (see box on flu jabs opposite).

SELF-HELP FOR TREATING COLDS AND FLU

All you can do for a cold or flu is make yourself more comfortable during the worst of the infection. The following may help to soothe the symptoms of a cold or flu:

• Drinking plenty of cool fluids will help to reduce a fever.

▽ A sneeze blasts a jet of tiny droplets into the air, which may be inhaled by anyone close by. This is usually how cold and flu viruses spread.

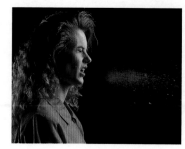

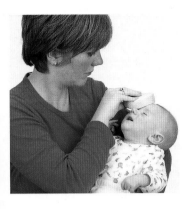

△ The symptoms of a cold can be particularly uncomfortable for a baby so anything you can do to soothe them will be helpful.

- Take painkillers (taking care to follow the directions on the packet) to help to reduce any fever and relieve the pain of a sore throat.
- Keep warm and have plenty of rest.
- Take decongestants to clear a stuffy nose.
- Avoid alcohol and smoking.
- Make sure that rooms are well ventilated and avoid spending time in stuffy, smoky or polluted atmospheres.

COLD AND FLU REMEDIES
A range of medicines are available over the counter and these usually combine a strong painkilling element with various decongestant drugs, caffeine and other ingredients. It is important to check each packet or bottle to find out what the remedy contains (check with your pharmacist if you are doubtful). This is particularly important if you are taking any other medication regularly. Levels of painkiller, especially paracetamol, must be monitored carefully.

Cough medicines simply provide some relief from the pain and irritation of a cough and sore throat. A hot honey and lemon drink contains vitamin C to help the body to fight a cold, and the honey and soothing effect of the hot drink will provide some relief.

A cold should only last a few days but the symptoms of flu can last up to a week. However, the worst symptoms of flu are likely to pass after two to three days, as long as no complications develop. After a bout of flu, you may feel depressed or tired for a while, and a cough may last for a couple of weeks or more.

WHEN TO SEE YOUR DOCTOR
Arrange an appointment with your doctor if you have an infection that seems to be lasting longer than usual or if the symptoms seem to be worse than you would usually expect. Flu can lead to some life-threatening complications and it is important to see your doctor if you suspect that you have a serious infection and if your symptoms are not showing any sign of improvement after two or three days.

WHO IS MOST AT RISK?
Certain individuals are at greater risk of developing complications if they contract flu. These complications include bronchitis, a bacterial infection that affects the airways, and pneumonia, an infection of the lungs. Deaths from pneumonia are common during flu epidemics.

Those most at risk from complications as a result of flu are:
- Newborn babies and infants that were premature or had a low birthweight.
- The elderly.
- Smokers.
- Asthmatics.
- People with weakened immune systems due to, for example, diabetes or AIDS.
- People with poor nutrition and poor general health.

If anyone in the at-risk groups develops the symptoms of flu, they should not be treated at home, but should consult their doctor as soon as any symptoms appear. Antiviral medication is available, but is effective only if taken within the first 36 hours. Your doctor may also prescribe antibiotics as a preventive measure against complications. If complications such as

FLU JABS
People who are at high risk of becoming seriously ill if they contract flu are now recommended to visit their doctor for a flu jab each autumn to protect themselves through the winter months. The immunization is different each year because it targets the strains predicted to be most widespread that winter. Flu jabs are recommended for:

➤ People aged over 65 years.
➤ People with diabetes.
➤ People with asthma.
➤ People suffering from cardio-respiratory disease.
➤ People taking immunosuppressants.

pneumonia are suspected, you may be sent for a chest X-ray to confirm the diagnosis. In very severe cases, you may be admitted to hospital for treatment.

▽ Making sure that you have plenty of rest, keep warm and drink plenty of liquids will enable your body to concentrate its energies on fighting the infection.

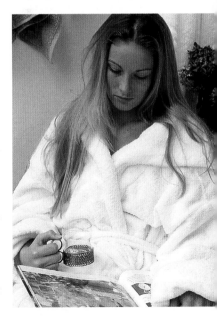

Asthma

Asthma is a condition where intermittent narrowing of the airways results in breathing difficulties. In mild cases, the person may suffer only sporadic bouts of wheezing and shortness of breath, but some people can have disabling and potentially life-threatening attacks almost every day. Asthma has become better recognized over the past two decades and cases are believed to have doubled in that time – although it is thought that this increase may be due to the fact that more people with mild symptoms are classified as asthmatics.

SIGNS AND SYMPTOMS

➤ Wheezing and coughing that is often worse at night, in the early hours of the morning and after exercise.

➤ Tightness in the chest.

➤ Shortness of breath.

➤ Panic and anxiety.

➤ Difficulty breathing out.

Asthma can develop at any age but generally it occurs first in childhood. The condition is often associated with allergies, and common triggers for allergic asthma are house-dust mites, pollen, mould and pet hair. Some of the more common food allergens (see box on asthma triggers) can also trigger an asthmatic attack. Children who are affected by allergic asthma often also develop eczema or hayfever.

Most adults who suffer from asthma first developed the condition as children. However, asthma can also start in adulthood, usually after a respiratory infection. Smoking, polluted or cold air, and stress may all trigger asthma attacks.

MAKING A DIAGNOSIS

Some people suffer only occasional attacks of asthma while others may have frequent and severe attacks in response to a range of triggers. It is not always easy for doctors to diagnose the condition, and the only clue that a child has asthma might be a cough that occurs at night or the fact that their breathing becomes wheezy during or after a bout of activity.

If your doctor suspects that you have asthma, you may be sent to hospital for further investigation. Tests that help with the diagnosis of asthma include spirometry and lung volume tests, which measure and monitor the rate and depth of your breathing. You may also be tested for allergic reactions to different substances, to pinpoint the likely trigger for your attacks. Sometimes, blood tests may be carried out to check the level of oxygen in your blood.

ASTHMA TRIGGERS

In any one individual, it is possible that there is more than one factor that initiates an asthmatic attack. Asthma may be triggered by:

➤ Upper respiratory tract infections, such as colds and flu.

➤ Lower respiratory tract infections, such as pneumonia and bronchitis.

➤ Allergy (allergens include house-dust mites, pollen, hair and saliva from furry animals, such as cats and dogs).

➤ Exposure to cold air.

➤ Dampness and mould.

➤ Anxiety and stress.

➤ Air pollution.

➤ Cigarette smoke.

In rare cases, certain foods – such as milk, eggs, nuts and wheat – prompt an attack. Many people with asthma are sensitive to aspirin and taking tablets can initiate an attack.

CAUSES OF ASTHMA

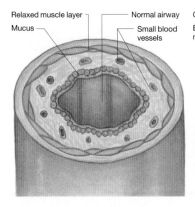

Relaxed muscle layer — Normal airway
Mucus — Small blood vessels

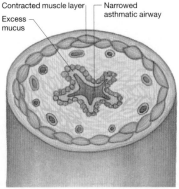

Contracted muscle layer — Narrowed asthmatic airway
Excess mucus

△ In asthma, the muscles in the bronchi constrict, causing them to narrow. At the same time, the mucus that protects the airways from infection is produced in excess and the lining of the airways become inflamed. This means that very little air can get into or out of the lungs.

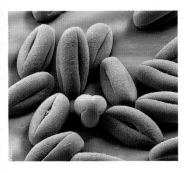

△ This picture shows a magnified image of flowering horse chestnut pollen. Pollen is a common trigger for attacks of allergic asthma.

MANAGEMENT OF ASTHMA

As yet, there is no cure for asthma. However, it can be managed extremely well with both drug therapy and by avoiding triggers – most people with asthma lead normal lives. In addition, many cases of

SEVERE ASTHMA ATTACKS

A severe asthma attack can result in respiratory failure and coma. More than 5000 people a year in the US and nearly 2000 a year in the UK die as a result of an asthma attack. Most of these deaths could be prevented if the severity of the attack had been recognized and treatment had been sought. If an asthma attack becomes severe, you will have some of the following symptoms:

➤ Silent wheezing because breathing is very shallow.

➤ Severe breathlessness.

➤ Blue lips, fingers and toes – due to a lack of oxygen.

➤ Pale, clammy skin.

➤ Exhaustion and confusion.

If your inhaler is not providing any relief, try to keep calm and call for an ambulance. Sit upright in the most comfortable position you can find but do not lie down. Try to slow your breathing, if possible, until medical help arrives.

childhood asthma become less of a problem with age and many cases disappear by the age of 20.

Doctors usually ask people with asthma to monitor their symptoms. Depending on the severity of your condition, you may be asked to perform self-assessment peak-flow measurements every day in the morning and evening. This involves breathing into a peak-flow meter which measures the quantity of air you exhale per minute. Plotting these measurements on a graph helps to show whether you are on the correct dose of drugs and how effectively your asthma is controlled.

Almost all asthma drugs are inhaled in vapour form so that they are taken directly into the lungs and get to work instantly. A "spacer device" can be used to make the lungs take up the vapour even more effectively.

There are two main kinds of inhalers - those that relieve an asthma attack and those that prevent future attacks:

• Reliever inhalers – These inhalers are normally blue in colour and contain drugs called bronchodilators. They relax and widen the airways and provide short-term relief.

• Preventer inhalers – These are usually low-dose corticosteroid devices and are normally brown in colour. They are used twice a day on a regular basis and have a protective effect upon the lungs by reducing any inflammation and the production of mucus.

Corticosteroids may also be prescribed as tablets, usually to relieve severe attacks or for people with long-term severe asthma.

LIVING WITH ASTHMA

If you have asthma, you should always carry your medication with you in case of an attack. You should avoid known triggers, such as smoky or polluted atmospheres or exposure to cold air, and should not keep furry pets if you are allergic to them. Smoking is known to make the condition worse and therefore is not advisable. It is also a good idea to exercise regularly since

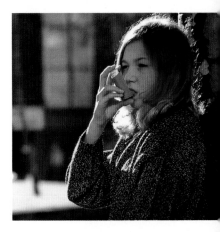

△ Asthma drugs act quickly to widen the airways and relieve symptoms. People with asthma should always carry their inhalers with them so that they can deal with a serious attack.

▽ People with asthma monitor their own condition from an early age. This young girl is breathing into a peak-flow meter, to measure her rate of exhalation.

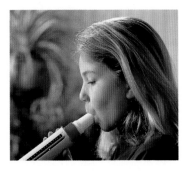

this improves lung capacity and makes breathing easier. You may have to take preventive medicine from an inhaler to make this possible; if in doubt, discuss this with your doctor. Swimming is a particularly good exercise for people with asthma, because of the humid environment, but in theory any sport is possible.

If you find that your asthma is worse when you are stressed, try relaxation techniques or a form of yoga to control levels of stress, which will in turn cut down the risk of an asthma attack.

Chronic obstructive pulmonary disease

Chronic obstructive pulmonary disease (COPD) is a progressive respiratory disease that causes severe shortness of breath and wheezing. The term is used to cover chronic bronchitis and emphysema – bronchitis is the inflammation of the bronchi, the large airways that lead to the lungs, while emphysema means permanent damage to the air sacs (alveoli), which lose their elasticity. People with COPD usually have both conditions, with one being dominant. COPD is almost always caused by smoking and is twice as likely to affect men as women.

COPD is a debilitating condition. As it progresses, people become so short of breath that they are increasingly unable to carry out everyday tasks – eventually they often become housebound.

COPD is almost entirely caused by smoking, although industrial pollutants may exacerbate the damage to the lungs. The condition is often not diagnosed until the damage has been done – many of those affected put early symptoms down to "smoker's cough" and do not seek help. Male smokers who live in industrial areas are most likely to be affected. Some sources estimate that up to one-quarter of all those affected are not diagnosed at all.

SIGNS AND SYMPTOMS

➤ A chronic cough, which is usually worse in the morning.

➤ Gradually increasing production of sputum (phlegm).

➤ Progressive shortness of breath.

➤ Ever-increasing susceptibility to acute lung infections.

➤ Symptoms that get worse in winter.

Some people who have COPD breathe rapidly to get more oxygen into their blood and will often have a rosy glow to their skin. Others can develop a barrel-shaped chest because the lungs have become distended.

If you are a smoker and have any of the above symptoms, it is advisable to make an appointment to see your doctor as soon as possible.

WHAT MIGHT YOUR DOCTOR DO?

If you are a smoker, your doctor is likely to suspect COPD following an initial consultation and examination. In order to determine the extent of lung damage, you may be referred to hospital for specialized tests so that your lung function can be assessed. These specialized tests may include spirometry, in which your rate of inhalation and exhalation is measured, and lung volume tests, which are carried out to measure the volume of air inhaled in one breath and volume of air left in the lungs when you have exhaled.

There is a range of other tests that can confirm the diagnosis, and these may include giving samples of blood in order that the levels of oxygen and carbon dioxide in your blood can be measured. An X-ray may also be taken so that any other underlying causes can be ruled out.

TREATMENT OPTIONS

The first and most important treatment for COPD is for the person to give up smoking immediately since this is the only way of preventing further damage to the lungs.

SELF-HELP MEASURES

➤ Giving up smoking is the only action that can delay the progression of your COPD. Cutting down will have little effect on your lung function. You should also avoid smoky and polluted atmospheres.

➤ Make your home environment free from smoke, dust, pollution, damp and cold – all can exacerbate COPD.

➤ Taking gentle exercise may help to improve your tolerance to exertion.

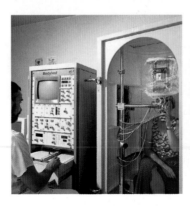

▽ In this spirometry test, a woman blows into a bag connected to a monitor unit, which draws a graph of her rate of exhalation. People affected by bronchitis will have a low rate of exhalation.

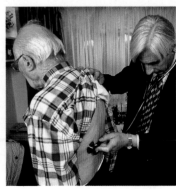

▽ A GP listens to the sound of the patient's heart and lungs through a stethoscope. This simple procedure can often be enough to make an initial diagnosis of serious lung disorders.

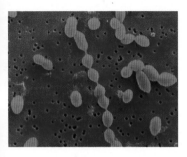

△ *Streptococcus* bacteria, above, are a major cause of pneumonia, which may be fatal in those suffering from COPD.

Unfortunately, it is not possible to reverse the damage that has been caused by COPD. However, there are various drug treatments available that can help to relieve the symptoms.

Your doctor may prescribe any of the following drugs:

• Antibiotics to treat acute infections.
• Bronchodilating inhalers, which help to open up the airways and thus make breathing easier.
• Inhaled steroids to reduce inflammation.
• Diuretics to reduce fluid build-up if you have swollen ankles.
• Continuous low-dose oxygen therapy to raise your blood oxygen levels and reduce the strain on the heart. This treatment is usually given in more advanced cases, and can be organized at home.

In terms of preventive measures, your doctor may recommend a flu jab each winter and another vaccination against *Streptococcus pneumoniae* bacterium. If someone suffering from COPD develops flu or pneumonia, the consequences can be life-threatening.

THE OUTLOOK

If the illness is diagnosed at an early stage and you give up smoking straight away, you may be able to avoid severe lung damage. However, most people with COPD are not diagnosed until their condition has reached an advanced stage and the damage has been done. If this is the case the outlook is not encouraging – increasing breathlessness and a limited exercise tolerance mean that those affected may find it more and more difficult to carry out everyday activities. Heart and respiratory failure may ultimately result. In most cases, those affected are unlikely to live longer than ten years.

Acute bronchitis

SEE ALSO
► Colds and flu, p376

Acute bronchitis is a short-term infection of the larger airways, the bronchi. It occurs either in young adults, when it is usually the result of a viral infection, or as a complication of chronic obstructive pulmonary disease, when the cause is usually bacterial.

Bronchitis often occurs as a complication of a respiratory infection, such as a common cold that has spread into the bronchi from the nose, throat or sinuses. People who smoke or those who are exposed to high levels of pollutants in the air are more susceptible to attacks of bronchitis. People with existing COPD may experience several bouts of acute bronchitis during the winter. The inflammation resulting from the infection produces excessive amounts of mucus, which triggers the cough reflex to remove it from the lungs.

HOW IS IT TREATED?

An otherwise healthy adult will expect to make a complete recovery within a week or so. In such cases, simple supportive treatment is all that is required – that is, plenty of fluids, rest and over-the-counter painkillers such as paracetamol. If you smoke, you should stop immediately.

Older people with COPD or those who have suffered a particularly severe attack of bronchitis will normally require a course of

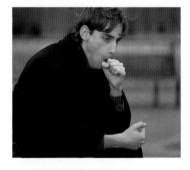

△ An irritating cough is one of the main symptoms of acute bronchitis, which is often associated with smoking.

antibiotics to aid recovery. More severe cases may require hospitalization. If the condition persists for longer than two weeks, you may need to have a chest X-ray to check for any underlying cause.

SIGNS AND SYMPTOMS

The symptoms of bronchitis tend to develop rapidly in one to two days, and may include:

➤ An irritating cough that may produce clear sputum (phlegm).

➤ Chest pain.

➤ Wheezing and tightness in the chest.

➤ Breathlessness.

➤ Mild fever.

Pneumonia

SEE ALSO
➤ Smoking and your health, p268
➤ Sensible drinking, p270
➤ Diabetes, p314
➤ Pleurisy, p383

Pneumonia is a serious chest infection that affects the air sacs (alveoli) in the lung, causing them to become inflamed. Because oxygen needs to pass through the walls of the alveoli in order to reach the bloodstream, this is a potentially life-threatening condition – especially if both lungs are affected. Pneumonia is the most common form of fatal infection acquired in hospital and is particularly dangerous for the elderly. In most cases, however, effective treatment with antibiotics leads to a full recovery with no lasting effects.

SIGNS AND SYMPTOMS

Pneumonia may develop gradually, particularly if the cause is viral. Bacterial pneumonia usually develops rapidly over the course of several hours. Symptoms of pneumonia are:

➤ A cough with mucus, which may be bloody.

➤ High fever.

➤ Breathlessness even when resting.

➤ Chest pain on breathing in (inspiration).

➤ Delirium and/or confusion.

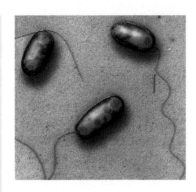

△ These bacteria, *Legionella pneumophila*, cause Legionnaire's disease, a form of pneumonia which can be fatal.

Pneumonia occurs most frequently among the very young and the very old, although it can occur at any age. The offending micro-organism can be a virus, a bacterium or a fungus – but in the majority of cases of pneumonia the cause is bacterial.

Certain factors make a person more likely to develop pneumonia – these include smoking, being malnourished or drinking excessive quantities of alcohol over a long period. People who are suffering from a long-term disorder such as diabetes are more at risk, as are those who have impaired immunity as a result of AIDS or because they are undergoing treatments such as chemotherapy or taking immunosuppression drugs.

Pneumonia used to be a common cause of death but effective antibiotics mean that most people now make a full recovery. But despite the best medical attention, the disease can still be fatal, particularly among the elderly and those already suffering from another serious disease.

TREATMENT FOR PNEUMONIA

Otherwise fit and healthy adults are often treated at home with a course of antibiotics. Painkillers help to lower fever and control pain, and plenty of fluids are required.

Children, elderly people and adults who rapidly become severely ill will normally be referred to hospital for immediate treatment. There they receive intravenous fluids and antibiotics. Sometimes, they need oxygen via an oxygen mask. Occasionally someone affected by pneumonia will need to be connected to a ventilator to maintain adequate levels of oxygen until they recover.

WHAT IS THE OUTLOOK?

People usually recover within a few weeks, although young children often make a full recovery much more quickly. However, pneumonia is associated with a number of complications. The pleura may become inflamed, leading to pleurisy. In some severe cases, the danger is that the infection may enter the bloodstream, causing septicaemia. And in the elderly and those with weakened immunity, the infection can spread deep into the lungs, causing respiratory failure.

HOW IS IT DIAGNOSED?

Your doctor may suspect pneumonia from your medical history and a chest examination. You may be referred to the hospital for a chest X-ray, and a blood test. A sputum (phlegm) sample may be sent for analysis to establish the cause.

▽ A chest X-ray will show the extent of infection. In this coloured X-ray, the infection shows up as a red patch at the base of the blue lung on the right.

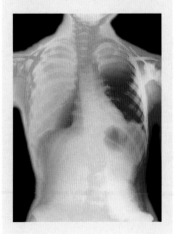

Pleurisy

EE ALSO
► Colds and flu, p376
Pneumonia, p382

Pleurisy is an inflammation of the pleura – the double-layered membrane that surrounds the lungs and separates them from the chest wall. When you are in good health, the two pleural layers slide smoothly over one another as you breathe in and out, which in turn allows the lungs to inflate and deflate. In pleurisy, the inflammation prevents this smooth movement and the layers rub over one another causing intense pain when you breathe in. Pleurisy usually occurs as a complication of other diseases, such as pneumonia.

SIGNS AND SYMPTOMS

Symptoms appear gradually and include:

➤ A sharp pain in the chest, usually located to one side or the other, made worse by breathing in deeply.

➤ A frightening feeling of being unable to breathe.

Pleurisy may be caused by a viral infection such as flu, but is usually due to pneumonia that has spread from the lung tissue. You should seek medical advice within 24 hours if you suspect you have pleurisy. Doctors can often diagnose pleurisy by using a stethoscope to listen for the sound of the pleura rubbing together. A chest X-ray will usually reveal the underlying cause.

TREATMENT OPTIONS

Any underlying cause is treated first and then doctors will want to control the symptoms of the pleurisy itself. This may involve taking an antibiotic to treat any infection in the lung as well as anti-inflammatory drugs to relieve pain and reduce the pleural inflammation. Most cases of pleurisy clear up within a week to ten days of the start of treatment.

HEALTHY AND INFLAMED MEMBRANES

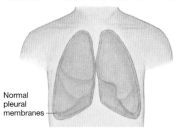

Normal pleural membranes

△ The pleura is a double-layered membrane surrounding the lungs. Fluid between the layers helps them move smoothly as you breathe.

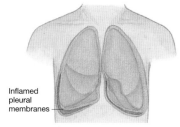

Inflamed pleural membranes

△ Inflamed pleural membranes rub together, causing pain. A pleural effusion is when the space between the layers fills with excess fluid.

Pneumothorax

EE ALSO
► COPD, p380

Pneumothorax occurs when air enters the space between the pleural layers which surround the lungs. The underlying lung may then collapse. A pneumothorax is generally a medical emergency and may be fatal if not treated quickly. Usually only one lung is affected.

SIGNS AND SYMPTOMS

➤ Shortness of breath, which may be very severe.

➤ Tightness across the chest.

A pneumothorax is when the lung is collapsed and it can occur as the result of a rupture of a small bubble of tissue (bulla) on the surface of the lung. This may occur during a bout of exercise but may have no apparent cause. A pneumothorax may be a complication of lung disease, such as chronic obstructive pulmonary disease. A fractured rib piercing the lung or any chest injury that allows air to pass from outside the body can also result in a pneumothorax.

TREATING A PNEUMOTHORAX

Most mild cases disappear without treatment. However, a larger pneumothorax needs to be treated urgently in hospital. Doctors insert a hollow tube into the affected side of the chest to release excess air and to allow the lung to reinflate. Most people recover fully, but the condition recurs in about 20 per cent of cases.

Lung cancer

SEE ALSO

➤ Smoking and your health, p268

➤ Bone cancer, p358

➤ Acute bronchitis, p381

➤ Pneumonia, p382

Lung cancer is the second most common form of the disease (after skin cancer) and the most common cause of cancer deaths. It is most likely to affect people who are aged between 50 and 70. Lung cancer is largely preventable – the main risk factor is smoking. It has always been more common in men but in recent years the gap has closed as more women have taken up smoking. People who spend a lot of time in a smoky atmosphere – bar staff, for example – are also at risk of developing lung cancer through passive smoking.

SIGNS AND SYMPTOMS

➤ A chronic (persistent) cough, sometimes containing sputum (phlegm) streaked with blood.

➤ Shortness of breath.

➤ Unexplained weight loss.

➤ Chest pain.

➤ Wheezing.

➤ Episodes of bronchitis or pneumonia.

Some forms of lung cancer produce no symptoms until they are well advanced.

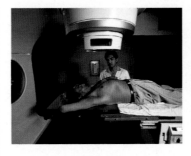

△ This man is about to receive radiotherapy treatment. The machine is being set up so that the X-rays target the affected area in his lung.

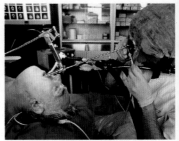

△ A bronchoscope is passed into the lungs under general anaesthetic to enable the doctor to view the airways and remove a tissue sample.

Lung cancer can develop very slowly, taking many years to produce symptoms. Also, some types of lung cancer do not cause any symptoms until they are in the final stages. As a result, lung cancer may be diagnosed only when it is well advanced, when treatment options are limited.

If your doctor suspects that you have lung cancer, you will be sent for a chest X-ray – an abnormal shadow on the lung may confirm the diagnosis. Your doctor may want to send a sputum (phlegm) sample for analysis, so that it can be checked for the presence of cancerous cells, or refer you for a bronchoscopy. In this procedure, a tube is passed through the mouth into the lungs to view the bronchi.

TREATMENT OPTIONS

There are three kinds of treatment and the nature and extent of the cancer will govern which one is used:

• Surgery – A tumour can be removed surgically only if the cancer has not spread to other organs. If there isn't any spread, surgeons will remove all of one lung or a major part of it.

• Chemotherapy – A course of chemotherapy drugs usually follows any surgery to remove a tumour, and it is also used to target highly malignant tumours.

• Radiation therapy – This treatment slows down the growth of a tumour but does not destroy it completely. It is often used to treat the tiny tumours – metastases – that have spread from the lungs to the brain, bones and liver. An initial course of radiotherapy is often followed by a course of chemotherapy.

THE LONG-TERM OUTLOOK

The prognosis is best for those whose cancer is detected early – people can and do survive lung cancer. But overall the outlook is poor: as few as one person in twenty survives longer than five years after treatment. In cases where the disease has spread, active treatment usually achieves only symptom control and improved quality of life, but may not extend life expectancy.

PREVENTING LUNG CANCER

Giving up smoking substantially reduces your risk of lung cancer. Research has shown that ex-smokers are only slightly more at risk of developing the disease than non-smokers.

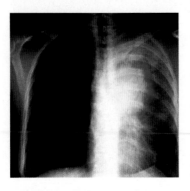

◁ This chest X-ray shows a large cancerous tumour in the lung of a 50-year-old woman. The tumour has been highlighted in red.

THE URINARY SYSTEM

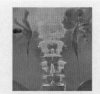

The urinary system, also known as the urinary tract, is a complex filter and drainage unit. This system separates useful by-products in the blood, which it keeps and reabsorbs, from unwanted waste substances, which it passes out of the body in the form of urine. Urine, which is mainly composed of water, is stored in the bladder until it can be passed out of the body. The fact that the urinary tract passes waste out of the body makes it vulnerable to attack by infection. Disease or infection in the kidneys and other parts of the urinary tract can result in a range of problems, from mild cystitis to chronic renal failure, so it is vital to keep this system in good working order.

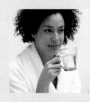

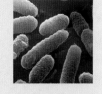

CONTENTS

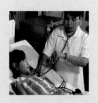

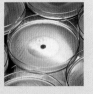

The urinary organs

SEE ALSO

➤ Urinary tract
  infections, p390

➤ Urinary incontinence,
  p392

➤ The roles of blood
  and lymph, p448

The urinary system is a sophisticated filtration unit which maintains fluid and chemical balance within the body. Many chemical reactions occurring in cells all over the body produce unwanted by-products and the kidneys filter these from the blood and excrete them in the form of urine. The urinary system is made up of a pair of kidneys, two ureters, a bladder and a urethra. As well as their important excretory function, the kidneys also produce hormones that control red blood cell production and help to regulate blood pressure.

The kidneys are the main organs of the urinary system, with many vital functions:

• Removing toxic waste products from the blood and excreting them as urine.

• Returning useful substances to the body's circulation.

• Regulating water balance. Your kidneys conserve water at times of relative dehydration and eliminate any surplus.

THE KIDNEY IN DETAIL

Your kidneys are about 12 cm (5 in) long and 6 cm (2.5 in) wide and are at the back of your abdomen, just in front of your spine. The kidney has several regions, each with a different function:

• The cortex – This outer layer houses filtering units called nephrons.

• The medulla – The next inner layer is full of cone-shaped urine-collecting ducts.

• The renal pelvis – This is at the heart of the kidney and is where urine collects before passing on to the bladder.

FILTERING THE BLOOD

Blood is transported to each kidney through the renal arteries. These blood vessels stem from the body's main artery, the aorta, and carry a rich blood supply that accounts for a quarter of the blood pumped by the heart.

Blood passes from these arteries through a sophisticated filtration system. The principal unit of the system is the nephron, which is made up of a glomerulus and a renal tubule.

URINARY CONTROL

The muscular wall of the bladder has an extensive nerve supply, which allows you to control when it is emptied. As your bladder fills your brain receives impulses from the nerves in the bladder wall. When your bladder is full your brain instructs it to contract and, at the same time, your bladder relaxes a ring of muscle at it's lower opening to control the release of urine through the urethra. This process requires a mature nervous system and such voluntary control of urination is not acquired until a few years after birth. Loss of this voluntary control can occur for various reasons in adults and is known as incontinence.

The glomerulus is a collection of tiny capillaries that allow small molecules to pass into the renal tubules. Only fluid in the blood is filtered, blood cells are not able to cross the membrane. The fluid (filtrate) passes through the tubules and useful substances, such as glucose and sodium, are reabsorbed into the bloodstream while harmful ones, such as urea, are retained.

The renal tubules have three sections:

• Proximal convoluted tubule – Most of the water and nutrients are reabsorbed here; unwanted substances are also secreted into the fluid at this point.

• Loop of Henle – More water and salts are reabsorbed in this section and waste products are secreted into the fluid here.

• Distal convoluted tubule – Fine-tuning of the water content of the urine is performed here.

THE STRUCTURE OF A KIDNEY

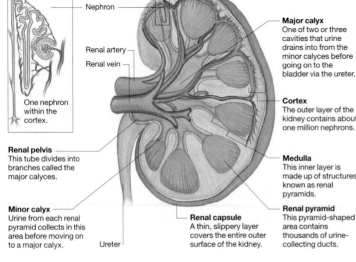

One nephron within the cortex.

Nephron

Renal artery

Renal vein

Renal pelvis
This tube divides into branches called the major calyces.

Minor calyx
Urine from each renal pyramid collects in this area before moving on to a major calyx.

Ureter

Renal capsule
A thin, slippery layer covers the entire outer surface of the kidney.

Major calyx
One of two or three cavities that urine drains into from the minor calyces before going on to the bladder via the ureter.

Cortex
The outer layer of the kidney contains about one million nephrons.

Medulla
This inner layer is made up of structures known as renal pyramids.

Renal pyramid
This pyramid-shaped area contains thousands of urine-collecting ducts.

THE FEMALE URINARY SYSTEM

▽ The bladder and the urethra in the male and female urinary systems have a different structure but apart from these differences the two urinary systems are the same.

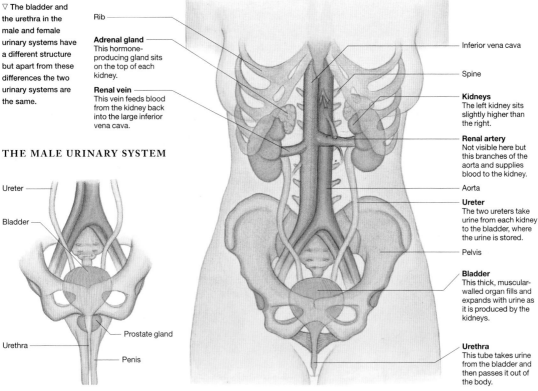

Rib

Adrenal gland
This hormone-producing gland sits on the top of each kidney.

Renal vein
This vein feeds blood from the kidney back into the large inferior vena cava.

Inferior vena cava

Spine

Kidneys
The left kidney sits slightly higher than the right.

Renal artery
Not visible here but this branches of the aorta and supplies blood to the kidney.

Aorta

Ureter
The two ureters take urine from each kidney to the bladder, where the urine is stored.

Pelvis

Bladder
This thick, muscular-walled organ fills and expands with urine as it is produced by the kidneys.

Urethra
This tube takes urine from the bladder and then passes it out of the body.

THE MALE URINARY SYSTEM

Ureter

Bladder

Prostate gland

Urethra

Penis

THE STRUCTURE OF A NEPHRON

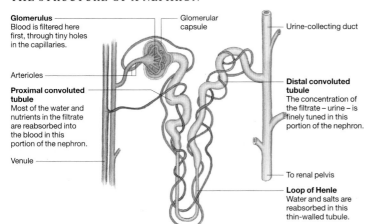

Glomerulus
Blood is filtered here first, through tiny holes in the capillaries.

Glomerular capsule

Urine-collecting duct

Arterioles

Proximal convoluted tubule
Most of the water and nutrients in the filtrate are reabsorbed into the blood in this portion of the nephron.

Venule

Distal convoluted tubule
The concentration of the filtrate – urine – is finely tuned in this portion of the nephron.

To renal pelvis

Loop of Henle
Water and salts are reabsorbed in this thin-walled tubule.

△ The nephron is part of the filtration unit through which the blood passes in the kidneys. Through this filtration system useful substances are reabsorbed into the bloodstream, and waste substances become urine, which is eventually passed from the kidneys by the ureter.

PASSAGE OF URINE

Once fluid reaches the end of the renal tubule it is urine. Urine from the nephrons travels via collecting ducts in the kidney's medulla to storage areas that feed into the renal pelvis. Each kidney is drained by a ureter, which is a thin muscular tube about 30 cm (12 in) long. Ureters carry urine to the bladder, which stores the urine until it is emptied. The bladder has a highly folded lining that smooths out as it expands and fills with urine. A healthy adult excretes 0.5–2 litres (1–3 pints) of urine every day.

WHAT IS URINE?

Urine is 95 per cent water and 5 per cent uric acid, urea, salts (such as sodium, potassium and chloride) and creatinine.

Kidney stones

SEE ALSO

➤ Eat healthily, p262
➤ The urinary organs, p386

Normally, waste products from the body pass out in the urine, which is produced in the kidneys. If the urine becomes saturated with waste chemicals, these can crystallize and form stone-like deposits in the kidneys. Kidney stones come in varying sizes: small ones may travel down the urinary tract and simply pass out in the urine; larger stones tend to stay within the kidney but can move into the ureter, where they can lodge and cause severe pain. Half of all people affected by kidney stones will develop further stones within seven years.

Kidney stones occur more frequently in young to middle-aged men. People living in a hot climate have a higher chance of developing kidney stones if they don't drink enough fluid to replace that lost through sweating. Some individuals may inherit a predisposition towards the condition.

HOW IS IT DIAGNOSED?

Your doctor may suspect kidney stones after taking your medical history. Then you may be referred for further investigations, including a plain X-ray and/or intravenous urography, to identify the presence and

SIGNS AND SYMPTOMS

Small stones may cause no symptoms whatsoever. However, larger stones are usually very painful because they cause the ureter to go into acute spasm. This is known as renal colic and the symptoms of renal colic are:

➤ Intense pain that radiates from the back (usually on one side) to the groin. Sometimes it can be felt in the genitals as well.

➤ Frequent, painful urination.

➤ Blood in the urine.

➤ Nausea and vomiting.

Renal colic subsides as soon as the offending stone is passed. An episode of renal colic may be an isolated incident, but some people are more prone to the condition and they may experience repeated attacks of kidney stones and renal colic.

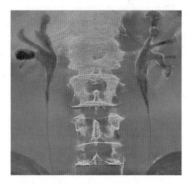

△ An intravenous pyelogram (IVP) image, which shows drainage of urine from the kidneys. Here, a stone can be seen in the right kidney (coloured orange, on the left of the picture).

location of stones. Some kidney stones are made from calcium salts and show up well on X-ray images. Other stones, made from oxalate, phosphate or uric acid, can be more difficult to see. More tests may be done on urine to check for secondary infection, any presence of blood in the urine and to measure kidney function.

TREATING KIDNEY STONES

Treatment for the condition depends on the size of the stone.

• Small stones may pass with rest, plenty of fluids and some appropriate pain relief. Occasionally smaller stones may become lodged in the ureter, and these can be removed during examination with an instrument called a cystoscope.

• Larger stones can cause more problems. They may not pass spontaneously and are more likely to become lodged in the kidney. These stones are usually treated

PREVENTING KIDNEY STONES

➤ Drink plenty of fluids, approximately 2–3 litres (3½–5 pints) a day.

➤ Increase your fluid intake during hot weather and after exercise.

➤ Avoid too much rhubarb, spinach and asparagus, as these promote the formation of oxalate stones.

➤ Check with your doctor in case you should limit your intake of calcium-rich substances, such as dairy products or calcium-based antacids.

▽ People who are prone to kidney stones may be advised to avoid, or reduce their consumption, of dairy products such as butter and cheese.

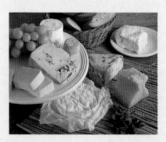

through a process known as lithotripsy. This method uses high-energy shock waves to break the stones down into a powder, which can then be expelled in the urine.

• In some cases, stones have to be removed surgically, although this is rare and generally only used as a last resort.

Kidney failure

EE ALSO
➤ High blood pressure, p278
➤ Diabetes, p314
➤ Enlarged prostate gland, p408

In kidney failure, the kidneys are no longer able to carry out their normal function of filtering the body's by-products from the blood. As a result, waste products and excessive fluid build up in the body. Kidney failure may happen very suddenly (acute renal failure) but more commonly the kidneys fail gradually over a period of many months, sometimes years – this is known as chronic renal failure. The degree of kidney failure depends on its cause in each individual. The main text here will focus on kidney failure of the chronic kind.

SIGNS AND SYMPTOMS OF CHRONIC RENAL FAILURE

Apart from a general tiredness and malaise, symptoms can include:

➤ Infrequent passage of urine.

➤ Shortness of breath.

➤ Nausea.

➤ Muscle cramps.

➤ Back pain.

Chronic renal failure develops gradually and symptoms may not appear for many months. It can be caused by:
• Acute renal failure (see box, right).
• Any chronic kidney disease that impairs function, e.g. polycystic kidney disease.
• High blood pressure.
• Diabetes mellitus.
• Prolonged urinary-tract obstruction, e.g. one caused by an enlarged prostate gland.

WHAT MIGHT YOUR DOCTOR DO?

Your doctor will probably ask for a sample of urine for testing. Other tests may need referral to a hospital specialist and include intravenous urography, ultrasound scanning, cytoscopy and kidney biopsy.

TREATMENT OPTIONS

Chronic renal failure may progress slowly. Renal failure can be limited by treating causative factors. Good management of patients with diabetes, high blood pressure and/or prostate disease is vital, and is carried out by a team of specialists.

When deterioration in kidney function is progressive and advanced, a person may consider dialysis or a kidney transplant.

There are two types of dialysis, peritoneal dialysis and haemodialysis, used to treat acute and chronic renal failure.
• In peritoneal dialysis, the peritoneum (a membrane that surrounds the abdominal organs) acts as a filter, instead of the kidneys. It can be carried out anywhere several times a day and the fluid is changed every four to six hours.
• In haemodialysis a machine does the work of the kidneys. Blood is taken from a vein in the arm to the dialysis machine, where waste is removed. The blood is returned via a cannula (a plastic or metal tube used to withdraw or introduce fluids). Patients are attached for up to four hours at a time, about three times a week.

PERITONEAL CATHETER

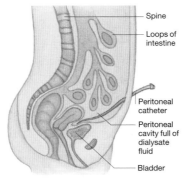

— Spine
— Loops of intestine
— Peritoneal catheter
— Peritoneal cavity full of dialysate fluid
— Bladder

△ Peritoneal dialysis uses the peritoneum (a two-layered membrane lining the abdominal cavity) as a filter. The blood passes through the membranes, which allows waste such as urea to pass out, but keeps proteins in the system.

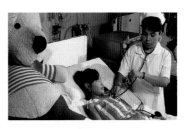

△ In some cases of kidney failure, renal dialysis is used. This is where a machine performs the function of the kidneys, filtering waste products and returning purified blood to the system.

ACUTE RENAL FAILURE

Acute renal failure is a medical emergency that can be fatal without immediate attention. It can be caused by:

➤ A dramatic fall in blood pressure due to severe infection, blood loss or heart attack.

➤ Acute disorders of the kidney.

➤ Drugs that are toxic to the kidney.

➤ Acute obstruction of the urinary tract.

Symptoms include:

➤ Dramatically reduced urine output.

➤ Vomiting.

➤ Drowsiness and headaches.

As long as the damage to the kidneys is reversible and causative conditions are managed, normal kidney function can return within several weeks. If the kidneys have sustained irreversible damage, they may not recover and the condition may progress to chronic renal failure.

Urinary tract infections (UTIs)

The urinary tract includes the kidneys, ureters, bladder and urethra, and the most common infection is cystitis, which affects the bladder. The bacteria most likely to cause a urinary tract infection are *Escherichia coli* (*E. coli*), normally found in the bowel. If a large number of *E. coli* get into the urethra, parts of the urinary tract can be infected. If the infection remains in the urethra it is called urethritis, and if it spreads to the kidneys it is pyelonephritis. Infection can take hold in a number of ways, including poor toilet hygiene, sexual intercourse and childbirth.

Urinary tract infections are less common in men and in childhood. Urinary tract infections more commonly affect women, and this is partly because a woman's urethra is shorter and nearer the anus and so is more vulnerable to infection.

CAUSES OF UTIs

Normally, urine is sterile – it contains no bacteria or fungi. However, sometimes bacteria from the digestive tract can find their way into the opening of the urethra, where they start to multiply. This causes infection and inflammation. These bacteria are usually *Escherichia coli* (*E. coli*) organisms, normally found in the bowel, where they are harmless. Occasionally, bacteria can make their way even further up the urinary tract and travel up the ureters into the kidneys, where they cause an infection known as pyelonephritis. Other organisms can be responsible for causing cystitis and other urinary tract infections, such as those acquired during sexual intercourse, for example chlamydia and mycoplasma.

Generally, the urinary unit works to prevent infection, stopping urine from backing up to the kidneys and washing bacteria out of the system through urination. Urinating immediately after sexual intercourse can prevent infection.

THOSE AT RISK

Groups that are at risk from urinary tract infections include the following:

- Postmenopausal women – Women who have been through the menopause are more prone to cystitis because the lack of oestrogen in their bodies causes the lining of the urethra to become thinner, making it vulnerable to bacterial attack.
- Someone with an abnormality of the urinary tract – An example would be a man with an enlarged prostate gland, which increases the risk of infection.
- People who are more prone to infections in general – Older people, those with diabetes and anyone taking drugs to suppress the immune system.

CYSTITIS

Your doctor will probably ask for a sample of your urine so that it can be tested for a variety of substances – white bloods cells, red blood cells and protein. Such tests are usually done quickly and simply using different dipsticks, and the results are usually available immediately.

Your doctor may want to send the sample to a laboratory to determine which

RECURRENT CYSTITIS
Recurrent episodes of infection in a woman or a single episode in a man or young child need further investigation. Your doctor will probably arrange for blood tests to check kidney function, an ultrasound scan, a cystoscopy (in which the bladder is viewed directly) and an intravenous urogram. You will probably be referred to a specialist known as a urologist. Such investigations aim to identify structural abnormalities that predispose to infection and assess the functional capacity of the bladder and how effectively it empties, because this affects its susceptibility to infection.

types of bacteria are growing and which antibiotics will be most effective. As this process takes a minimum of 48 hours, your doctor may decide to prescribe an appropriate antibiotic immediately rather

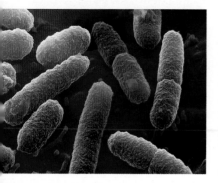

▽ E. coli bacteria are normally found in the human intestine and are generally harmless. Sometimes, however, they increase in number and find their way into the urinary tract, where they cause infections such as cystitis.

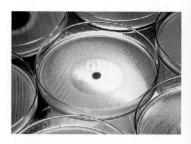

△ This picture shows how antibiotics are tested to find out how effective they are against different bacteria. The clear area around the antibiotic in this dish shows that it is killing the bacteria. Antibiotics are usually the most effective way of treating urinary tract infections.

PREVENTING CYSTITIS

➤ Drink plenty of fluids, particularly in hot weather.

➤ Empty the bladder frequently.

➤ Urinate promptly after sexual intercourse to prevent infection.

➤ Avoid using bubble baths and vaginal deodorants.

➤ Wipe yourself, after a bowel movement, from front to back.

➤ Avoid using a diaphragm and spermicide cream for contraception.

▽ Drinking plenty of fluids throughout the day is always a good idea, and it is also an effective way of avoiding cystitis and halting it at an early stage.

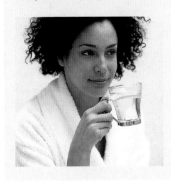

than wait for the results. The antibiotic can be changed once the bacteria's identity and sensitivity are known.

If an infection does not clear up within a few days, your doctor may recommend a test known as an intravenous pyelogram (IVP), a form of X-ray that shows the bladder, kidneys and ureters.

PYELONEPHRITIS

This is an infection that affects the kidney and it has similar symptoms to cystitis. These symptoms include difficulty in urinating accompanied by a burning sensation, and a pain in the back and below the ribs which may also spread to the abdomen. In extreme cases, it causes vomiting and high fever. The infection causes inflammation in the part of the kidney that collects urine, the renal pelvis, often accompanied by abscesses. It can be treated with antibiotics, but your doctor may advise further investigation to ensure there are no other underlying causes. If pyelonephritis is not treated, it may turn into a more serious condition called pyonephrosis or a larger kidney abscess. Both may require surgery to correct them.

In pyonephrosis, the kidney fills with pus and enlarges, causing great pain and a swelling that can be seen in your side. The infection can be a result of untreated pyelonephritis or hydronephrosis – distension of the kidney because of an obstruction in the ureter, which prevents urine flowing to the bladder; it can also be caused by kidney stones.

TREATMENT OPTIONS FOR UTIs

Infections of the urinary system can become worse very quickly, causing great discomfort and other potentially severe problems, so never hold back on seeking advice – especially if you are pregnant, suffer from

SIGNS AND SYMPTOMS OF URINARY TRACT INFECTIONS

The classic symptoms of a UTI are:

➤ A burning sensation whenever you pass urine.

➤ The need to pass urine urgently and frequently.

Accompanying symptoms are related to the bacterial infection, and may indicate a more serious kidney infection. They may include:

➤ Fever and chills.

➤ Lower abdominal pain.

➤ Lower back pain.

➤ Discharge.

➤ Cloudy or bloody urine.

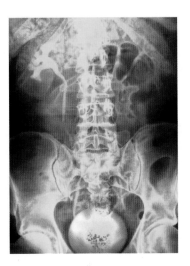

△ This X-ray shows a full bladder plus the ureters and the kidneys' branched collecting ducts. Images like this are produced by injecting a substance that shows up on X-rays into the blood. The kidneys automatically perform their filtering function and filter this substance from the blood – at which point the image is taken.

diabetes, or have high blood presssure or kidney disease. Treatment is often very straightforward. With cystitis, for example, it is vital to drink a great deal of extra fluid as soon as an episode starts. Many women find that cranberry juice eases discomfort, and simple painkillers and anti-inflammatory drugs are often effective in reducing any fever and dulling the pain. A mild cystitis episode may pass off quickly with a high fluid intake, but if the condition does not settle within 24 hours or if it worsens at all (and also if it recurs regularly), help should be sought. The infection will usually respond well to a short course of antibiotics.

Apart from cystitis, infections caused by other organisms, such as chlamydia and mycoplasma, will probably require a longer course of treatment. Your doctor may perform a urinalysis at the end of the course of drugs to ensure that the system is free from infection. The patient may feel better, but there is a chance that the infection may not be fully cleared up.

Urinary incontinence

There are four main types of urinary incontinence – stress, urge, overflow and total. The most common type is stress incontinence, in which small amounts of urine are expelled during exertion, coughing, sneezing or laughing. Urge incontinence is involuntary contractions of the bladder, which release large amounts of urine suddenly and without control. Overflow is a continual dribble of urine caused by the bladder's inability to empty properly, causing it to overflow. Total incontinence is the total loss of control over bladder function.

Complete or partial loss of control over bladder function can be an extremely distressing condition. Incontinence becomes more common in older age and occurs more frequently in women. It is also caused by:

- Any condition affecting the muscles at the neck of the bladder, such as those caused by a difficult labour and delivery.
- Weakness of the urethra and pelvic floor muscles, common during and after pregnancy and after the menopause; also caused by gynaecological conditions such as a prolapsed uterus.
- Bladder outlet obstruction, such as an enlarged prostate or bladder stones.
- Excessive bladder irritability, which may occur as a result of recurrent infection, nervous disease and/or anxiety.
- Abnormalities of nervous control, because of diabetes, spinal injury or spina bifida.
- Abnormalities of brain function, due to a stroke or dementia.

MANAGEMENT OF INCONTINENCE

There are several ways to manage incontinence. Bladder muscle problems may respond to pelvic floor exercises (see chart), physiotherapy or surgery aimed at restoring

INVESTIGATING INCONTINENCE

Urodynamic studies are used to investigate problems with bladder control, such as incontinence. These tests take place in a hospital outpatient clinic using X-ray monitoring and electronic probes to measure bladder filling and emptying.

HEALTHY AND POOR BLADDER CONTROL

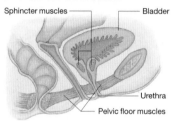

Sphincter muscles — Bladder

Urethra
Pelvic floor muscles

△ A healthy bladder has a firm pelvic floor and strong sphincter muscles.

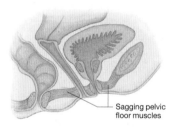

Sagging pelvic floor muscles

△ This picture shows how a sagging pelvic floor means that the neck of the bladder drops. This causes loss of bladder control.

bladder control. Hormone replacement therapy may help postmenopausal women to counteract any loss in pelvic floor muscle tone. Sometimes, however, the only options are to drain the bladder using a catheter (a long, thin tube) on an intermittent or permanent basis.

Where the incontinence is caused by a neurological problem, treatment can be much more problematic. Anticholinergic drugs are often used to help relax the muscles situated in the bladder wall and reduce the urge to urinate.

EXERCISES TO STRENGTHEN THE PELVIC FLOOR

Identify your pelvic floor muscles by imagining that you are urinating and that you have to suddenly stop the flow.

Feel the muscles tighten around your vagina, urethra and rectum. Then contract these muscles again and hold for ten seconds.

Relax the muscles slowly and then repeat. This exercise will be most effective if you repeat it five times, preferably two or three times a day.

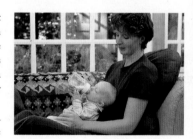

△ Incontinence can sometimes develop as a result of pregnancy and childbirth, because the pelvic floor is weakened. Exercises can be done to strengthen these muscles.

9

THE REPRODUCTIVE SYSTEM

The reproductive system is one of the most intricate areas of the male and female body, with all of the different parts – ovaries, Fallopian tubes, uterus and vagina in women; testes, prostate gland and penis in men – cleverly designed to function together towards the ultimate goal of reproduction. Understanding how the system works is crucial to coping with the various problems men and women can experience at particular times of their lives: from painful periods to prostate cancer, from puberty to menopause.

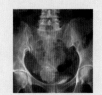

CONTENTS

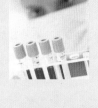

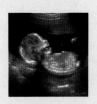

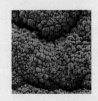

The reproductive organs

SEE ALSO

➤ Pregnancy and
   health, p396
➤ Menopausal
   complaints, p399
➤ Sexually transmitted
   infections, p411

The body's reproductive organs are developed in babies before they are even born. In fact, a baby girl is born with all the ova (eggs) that she will release during her adult life. Puberty is the major developmental stage for the reproductive systems of both genders. It is at this time that hormonal changes in the body bring great physical and mental changes, readying the reproductive systems for their adult role. Both the male and female systems are perfectly designed for their unique ultimate functions – sexual activity and reproduction.

THE FEMALE REPRODUCTIVE SYSTEM

The female reproductive organs are situated in the pelvic cavity and so are enclosed and protected by the pelvic bones. The ovaries are central to the female reproductive system because they hold all the female ova (eggs). The ovaries release one egg during the process of ovulation, and this happens first at puberty. Once released, the egg passes along the Fallopian tube to the uterus (womb) a hollow, muscular organ capable of considerable expansion to accommodate a growing fetus during pregnancy. The neck of the uterus, known as the cervix, projects in to the vagina. The vagina is a muscular organ that is able to expand greatly during sexual intercourse and childbirth.

HORMONES AND THE MENSTRUAL CYCLE

The ovaries produce two hormones – oestrogen and progesterone. These two hormones are controlled by the pituitary gland, which produces follicle-stimulating hormone (FSH) and luteinizing hormone (LH), which regulate the menstrual cycle.

During the first half of the menstrual cycle the pituitary produces FSH, which causes an egg to mature within the ovary in preparation for release. Towards the middle of the cycle, LH levels start to rise and trigger the release of the egg (this usually occurs about 14 days before the onset of menstruation). The hormone progesterone causes the uterine lining to thicken during the second half of the menstrual cycle, in preparation for possible implantation of a fertilized egg, should fertilization take place. Whenever fertilization does not occur, the uterine lining is expelled – menstrual bleeding.

When a woman's ovaries stop responding to the effects of FSH and LH (usually between the ages of 45 and 55), she starts to produce less oestrogen and progesterone; this is the start of the menopause, when menstruation gradually fades out and fertility ceases.

THE FEMALE REPRODUCTIVE ORGANS

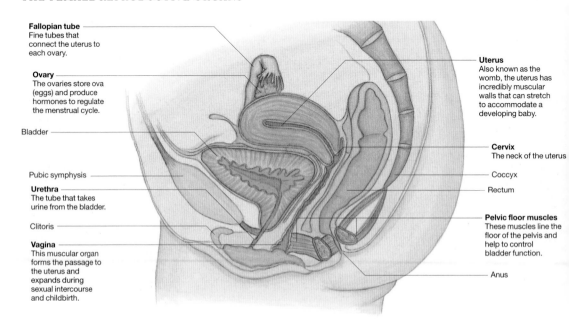

Fallopian tube
Fine tubes that connect the uterus to each ovary.

Ovary
The ovaries store ova (eggs) and produce hormones to regulate the menstrual cycle.

Bladder

Pubic symphysis

Urethra
The tube that takes urine from the bladder.

Clitoris

Vagina
This muscular organ forms the passage to the uterus and expands during sexual intercourse and childbirth.

Uterus
Also known as the womb, the uterus has incredibly muscular walls that can stretch to accommodate a developing baby.

Cervix
The neck of the uterus

Coccyx

Rectum

Pelvic floor muscles
These muscles line the floor of the pelvis and help to control bladder function.

Anus

INTRODUCTION

Forty-seven years ago I was ordained into the Ministry of the Gospel at Faith Baptist Church, Stoughton, Massachusetts—a recently started church, affiliated with the Baptist General Conference. The course of my ministry took me from this small church in New England to an established and vibrant church on the Pacific Coast Highway in Redondo Beach, California, followed by a twenty year tour of duty as a Chaplain Officer in the United States Army. As I reflected on my years of ministry, I realized that people inside the established churches and outside the church had a common need: they needed creditable tools by which to build a sure foundation for the living of life on a successful plane and which would prepare them for all the challenges and contingencies of life. Church creeds and catechisms are certainly helpful to get initiated into the Christian life, but unfortunately, for too many people these often become an end in themselves; they fail to add to that foundation with fresh knowledge and insight from which to draw strength and spiritual vitality for daily living.

For others, they have been wonderfully enriched by their church going experiences and their reading of Christian literature. They are interested in helping others to find the same Christian experience for themselves but they feel unprepared for the challenge of sharing about their Faith. Some have resorted to loaning or giving a book to a friend in hope that this will stimulate their interest in the things of the Lord. A trip to any good Christian bookstore will show anyone interested in finding material to share with others to be in abundant display. Many start reading a good book but fail to finish reading it for lack of interest in staying with it to the end.

With this in mind, I began to write some essays that were much shorter than a book but which developed a Biblical theme or principle that would answer to some of the basic needs of many people—Christian believer and the non-church going person, as well. These articles were made into multiple copies which I distributed to family members and friends in hopes they would find the material stimulating and helpful in grasping some of the most powerful and enriching themes of the Bible and the Christian Faith. To my delight, these articles were very much appreciated and people were telling me they shared their copy with their sons or daughters and with some of their friends. Some shared them with their pastors and they in turn shared portions of them with their congregations. In a matter of a few months these articles were circulating in California, Texas, Ohio, Georgia, Massachusetts and Connecticut. This type of response was far more than I could have anticipated.

It was one of my older brothers that cherished each of the articles so much that he persuaded me to look into getting them published so they could be available to people everywhere in the country who would love to have these articles also. My brother was so convincing, I began investigating the prospect of compiling these articles and adding to them in the form of a book that would be published and marketed across the nation.

My goal was to begin the book by getting to the essentials of fruitful Christian living and getting to the heart of the matter right away. This resulted in the first chapter and the title for the book: Brass Tacks Christianity, and Beyond! Since each chapter deals with a different theme, the book does not have to be read from cover to cover in order to get the sense of it. One can read one chapter without taking too much time and skip around in the book taking different chapters as they appeal to the interest of the reader.

There are abundant resources to help the Christian understand the foundations for their Faith in Jesus Christ, the Son of God, and our Lord and Savior. This information will also fortify the believer for sharing the Faith with others about whom they care and whom they would like to make the discovery of the love and power of God for themselves. My hope is similar as the

Apostle Paul's hope for young Timothy, his son in the Faith. Paul wrote to Timothy, "***Do your best to present yourself to God as one approved, a worker who does not need to be ashamed and who correctly handles the word of truth*** (2 Timothy 2:15)."

All the Scripture references used in this book are from the New International Version of the Bible, unless otherwise stated.

CHAPTER ONE

BRASS TACKS CHRISTIANITY

Of all the questions one might be asked in his or her lifetime, the most important question of all is this: "Are you a Christian?" I can remember the first time this question was asked of me. A total stranger approached me one day and simply asked, "Are you a Christian?" I was surprised at the directness of his question because it seemed to come out of nowhere and I was placed on the spot to give an answer for something I had considered to be quite a private matter. Nevertheless, I replied, "Yes, I am." The young man smiled broadly, said he was happy about that, and quickly moved on. I could not escape processing this brief encounter in my mind and I concluded two things about this young man. In the first place, I thought he was a courageous person to approach a stranger and ask a question that could easily have led into an argument of sorts. My reply might have been, "That is my business, and I am not going to give you an answer." I am assuming he was prepared for almost any answer I might have given or he would not have had the boldness to approach me with the question. The second thing I concluded about the young man is he must have cared about me to have asked me a question which has profound implications regarding my eternal destiny after my time in this life is finished! He got right to the point and simply asked a question which made me think of my relationship with God. I thought it quite amazing what that man accomplished in a few seconds of time.

Personally, I like it when people get to the nub of things instead of beating around the bush. This is one reason I don't like to listen to politicians being interviewed. It seems you hardly ever hear an answer to the question that is asked of them. The politician simply takes over and says what he or she wants to say that sounds acceptable and safe to the public ear. You could talk to some political figures for hours and never get a straight answer to a direct question! I would rather hear an honest answer with which I disagree than to be lied to by a politician who thinks his answer is satisfying John Q. Public, as if Mr. Public could not discern his true colors.

Before retirement from my former job as a Licensed Marriage and Family Therapist at the Naval Air Station, Lemoore, California, I can remember some staff meetings in which we were tasked to formulate our mission statement. All ideas were out on the table as each person tried to identify the major reason for our existence as an organization on the military base. The Fleet and Family Support Center was the name of our organization and we provided many functions for the military members and their families—both active duty and retired. Boiling all we did down to a succinct and brief mission statement was a lot more daunting a task than one might imagine. The exercise forces one to get down to the core of what we are all about. This is very important, because it translates into all we do every day on our jobs. It gives us a vision as to where we fit into the scheme of things in assisting the military base and its squadrons to accomplish their missions. The same holds true of any other organization or business that is geared for success. It needs to know in clear terms the purpose of its existence.

By the same token, why should not our life on earth pass through the same scrutiny? Have you ever asked yourself what the core purpose of your life is? Perhaps the best mission statement for a human life is found in the Westminster Shorter Catechism. The very first point made in the Shorter Catechism is this: "What is the chief end of man? The chief end of man is to glorify God and to enjoy Him forever." There is a world of meaning in those words. Just think about it! Think of how your life would be lived should you envision that mission statement every day of your life: "My chief aim today is to glorify God and to enjoy Him forever."

Return with me to the young man who approached me out of the blue and asked, "Are you a Christian?" That surely is an important question because the answer to that question determines our eternal destiny. Only people, who have received the Lord Jesus Christ into their lives by faith, repenting and renouncing their sins, are saved from the wrath to come by the grace of God. Salvation is never achieved by the doing of good works or by obeying the Ten Commandments. Neither does salvation come by membership in any church, nor by subscribing to any creed or any set of religious doctrines. The fact is that we could never become good enough to merit God's heaven by our achievements nor even by our acts of charity or deeds of kindness to other people. Were this at all possible, there would have been no need whatsoever for Jesus to come into this world and to suffer and die upon the cross of Calvary. His shed blood would have been wasted blood; His suffering would have been pointless masochism. Salvation was purchased by Jesus when he laid down His life on the cross. Listen to the words of the Apostle Paul: "***For the wages of sin is death, but the gift of God is eternal life in Christ Jesus our Lord*** (Romans 6:23)."

Jesus died for our sins. He became our substitute to take the penalty of our sins upon Him, nailing our sins to His cross. Once our salvation from sin was purchased by Jesus, He offers forgiveness and eternal life to any who would believe in Him and would receive Him by faith as their God-provided sin-bearer. Jesus Himself stated this clearly in His discourse to Nicodemus, a ruler of the Jews, who came to Jesus by night to enquire of Him. Among other truths, Jesus said to Nicodemus: "***Just as Moses lifted up the snake in the desert, so the Son of Man must be lifted up, that everyone who believes in him may have eternal life. For God so loved the world that he gave his one and only Son, that whoever believes in him shall not perish but have eternal life. For God did not send his Son into the world to condemn the world, but to save the world through him. Whoever believes in him is not condemned, but whoever does not believe stands condemned already because he has not believed in the name of God's one and only Son*** (John 3:14-18)." Salvation cannot be earned by any man. It comes only as a gift from God in response to faith in God's own son, Jesus Christ. A gift stems from the goodness of the giver, not in the worthiness of the recipient. Paul writes to the Ephesians, "***For it is by grace you have been*** *saved, through faith,—and this not of yourselves, it is the gift of God—not by works, so that no one can boast* (Ephesians 2:8-9)."

The sum of this is plain: the man or woman, boy or girl, who places faith in Jesus alone for their eventual entrance into heaven, will be saved and becomes a child of God. The child of God is called a "Christian," which I like to think of meaning, "Christ inside." Such a person could happily answer the question "Are you a Christian?" in the affirmative.

There is a vital second question, however, which will be much more difficult to answer. The question is: "Are you living the Christian life?" Being a Christian means you belong to Christ and He belongs to you. You are a part of God's family. This speaks to your status. No one can take you away from God once you are His. Jesus affirmed this truth in His discourse of the Shepherd saving His sheep. He said, "*My sheep listen to my voice; I know them, and they follow me. I give them eternal life, and they shall never perish; no one can snatch them out of my hand. My Father, who has given them to me, is greater than all; no one can snatch them out of my Father's hand. I and the Father are one* (John 10:27-30)."

Why then, is it so important to ask the second question? Why does it matter to determine if one is living the Christian life? It is the point of this chapter to answer that question. Simply put, accepting Christ by faith establishes your place in God's family and seals your eternal destiny. When you leave this world, you will enter the presence of God and will enjoy eternal bliss. Living the Christian life while here on earth will not affect your destiny but it will affect the quality of your life on earth and it will determine the reward you will receive when you get to heaven.

Let me suggest an example. I could board an airplane in Atlanta, Georgia that is scheduled to fly to Salt Lake City, Utah. En route to Utah the plane could encounter bad weather patterns and experience severe air turbulence. Passengers could be jostled and tossed around in their seats and could become extremely uncomfortable—possibly even get sick from such a rough and choppy flight. The plane may eventually arrive at Salt Lake City and may land safely on the runway. Few passengers, if any, however, would have considered it an enjoyable flight, even though they had reached their destination.

This analogy can be applied to our life on earth. Living a Christian life assures us of a good flight. Not living a Christian life can bode for a rough ride and a lot of misery and suffering on the way to the final destination. In fact, by one not living the Christian life, one invites into the course of life hardship, physical and emotional suffering, personal losses and miseries of almost any kind. Even though prayers may be offered up out of desperation, they may go unheard and may not bring favorable responses. One might hear someone quote the adage, "He made his own bed, now he must lay in it." In other words, one could be a Christian—a child of God—and be living a miserable and painful life. The reason is because that person is not aligning the decisions and choices of daily living with the will of God. Not considering God's will as it is expressed for us in the Bible—God's blueprint for Christian living—a person may get stuck in an ill-suited job or career, get paired off with the wrong person as a marital partner, or suffer the tortuous ordeal of dealing with wayward and rebellious children. They may even become trapped in a succession of their own vices and experience poverty, addictions, failures, shame and yes, may even suffer imprisonment, as part of the journey of life en route to heaven! The question is really "How do you choose to travel?"

The Apostle Paul sought to help young Timothy, his son in the faith, in his journey through life. He wrote to him and outlined a course for Christian living and Christian service that would assure success and guarantee the blessings of God. In the passage, 2 Timothy, Chapter 2, the Apostle cuts through the fluff that characterizes a lot of modern day preaching and gets down to the brass tacks. The expression, "get down to the brass tacks," usually means clearing out confusing details or extraneous verbosity and finding out the real basic facts about something. It was the brass tacks separated by exactly 36 inches on the wooden counter of fabric stores by which yards of material were quickly measured for the customers. It was brass tacks that furniture makers and upholsterers of the 17th and 18th centuries used to secure the initial layers of tightly-stretched cloth which formed the foundation of the padded seats in fine furniture. Therefore, "getting down to the brass tacks" implied stripping away the many layers of covering and padding atop the foundational layer to expose this first layer of construction. Another possibility for the use of the term can be found in the 1860s when the United States government issued boots for its soldiers that were constructed using brass tacks to hold the leather soles on to the bottoms of their boots. As the boots wore down, the tacks would protrude through the sole and in to the bottom of the soldier's feet. "Getting to the brass tacks" could then mean to get to the bottom of things.

Getting down to the brass tacks, then, what exactly does God expect of us after we have made a commitment to receive Him as our Savior and Lord and decided to live the Christian life? The very first step for walking the Christian walk is to acquire a strong awareness of who we are. We are no longer the same as before we came to Christ by faith. The Apostle Paul writes to Christians at Corinth: "***Therefore if anyone is in Christ, he is a new creation; the old has gone, the new has come!*** (2 Corinthians 5:17)." What the Apostle refers to as "the old" was the natural man. It is the unsaved man. It is a person who, by human nature, is a sinner and though living with the elements of body, mind and soul, is spiritually dead. Spiritual death is separation from God –just as physical death is separation of the soul from the body. What brought spiritual death to man is sin. It was like the title to a famous movie: "it started with Eve." God spoke to Adam and Eve in the Garden and gave instructions that they could eat of any tree except from the tree in the midst of the Garden. When God gave the prohibition to them, the first couple were innocent and had never known sin. God forewarned them: "***but you must not eat from the tree of the knowledge of good and evil, for when you eat of it you shall surely die***. (Genesis 2:17)." Eventually, through Satan's prompting, Eve ate from that forbidden tree and she invited Adam to do the same, which he did. They both became sinners by the act of disobeying God. The consequence of sin, among other things, was that they were banished from the Garden and were cut off from fellowship with God. This truncation from God was the beginning of spiritual death. At a later time, Adam and Eve would also die physically. The natural course for them and for everyone born after them would be to live in the natural environment on earth with no spiritual connection with God—man, the sinner, would live and die without ever knowing spiritual life. Their capacity for spiritual life would lie dormant unless and until such spiritual life would be awakened in them by an act of God. The Apostle Paul wrote in great detail in Romans, chapter 5, about this phenomenon that Adam's sin brought on spiritual death and Christ, the second Adam, died that sinners might be saved from their spiritual death and be given life in Him. Being given spiritual life is being saved from sin.

I like to think of it this way: before I accepted Christ as my Savior, I was the *natural* me. After accepting Christ, I am the *spiritually-activated* me. This speaks to the principle of the driving force inside every person; the force that governs the choices we make as to how we are going to behave in any given situation. From birth onward, we are a growing person with a developing mind that will give us the capacity to deal with the environment in which we live. From birth to age 5, one is learning the rudiments of life, a major portion of which is provided by interaction with our primary care-givers and play-time peers. By age five, one's personality is roughly 85% determined—the personality that will unfold and manifest for the balance of one's life! We learn how to judge people's vulnerabilities and how to manipulate them to get what we want. We learn both compliance with rules and instructions from the authority figures in our life and how to disobey to advance our selfish interests and pursuits. We learn how to assess what it will take to get what we need and to be what we choose to be. Constantly we are stuffing our brains with ever increasing knowledge of every imaginable sort and developing myriads of skills for the living of life. Part of our learning is the development of a moral compass and a conscience that acts as a governor over internal impulses to gratify and express purely selfish desires. That moral compass is to a great extent developed in accordance with the behaviors and the examples for living set by the key role models in our lives—usually our parents and siblings. All this is the development of the *natural* me.

The natural I will continue functioning along the same plane of learning and acting from hour to hour, day to day, year to year, through all the stages of life until from sudden causes or physical illness, we reach our final moment and die. Natural life and natural death is what is in store for every person born under the sun. There is no way of changing it; it is like the coursing of a mighty river that will not be stopped until it reaches its final destination. We live and die being bound by the laws of nature. That is why it is the *natural* me and the *natural* you. The only way a basic change in our nature can be made is by the interposing of Divine power, the intersection of the *natural* man with *supernatural* He—God almighty. God is the author of nature and the only source capable of changing nature. At such moments, when God chooses to change nature, a miracle takes place. That's what a miracle is—it is the abrogation of natural law to serve God's purposes.

Turning cisterns of water into fine wine is not natural; it is a miracle performed by Jesus at the wedding in Cana of Galilee. Feeding five thousand people with 5 loaves of bread and two small fishes is not natural, but Jesus performed this miracle to suit His purposes. When Jesus gave sight to the man who was blind from birth, it was not done on an operating table with fancy surgical devices; it was done with the gentle touch of His fingers and the command of His voice! It was a miracle. There is no need to go on to list the countless other miracles performed by Jesus, the Son of God. The point is clear: only God can change nature and the laws of nature to advance His purposes in this world. Without God's purposeful intervention, nothing on earth could be changed, because all of life follows a natural course. It follows then, that no one can live the Christian life as opposed to the natural life unless God institutes a change in the nature of a person. That change—that miracle—occurs instantaneously at the moment a person exercises his free will and chooses to receive Jesus into his or her life, electing in the process to evict "self" from the driver's seat, and asking Jesus to do the driving and directing, the leading and the empowering required for living life on a higher plane. It will be on a plane of God's choosing, in accordance with God's will. No longer being the *natural* me living my life, with Jesus inside it is the *spiritually-activated* me that is living my life and informing my values, revamping my moral compass to conform to His requirements and standards. Just as I require physical food to nurture and sustain my natural life, as a *spiritually-activated* person, I will need to ingest spiritual food to sustain spiritual life. The spiritual food is provided by God because He alone can sustain spiritual life because it is on a higher plane than natural life. Spiritual nourishment comes by reading and meditating on the Bible, which is food for the soul. The Bible is not a book, it is THE book! It is God's Word. It is the book that is authored by God, directing prophets and apostles to pen the words. Spiritual food also comes from prayer, which is communion with our source of spiritual life. It comes through worship, Christian instruction, Christian music, Christian art, and Christian poetry, to name a few more sources for spiritual nourishment.

Getting down to the brass tacks, the *spiritually-activated* life is initiated by Divine power released into a person's life in response to the person choosing to receive Jesus Christ as Lord and Savior of his or her life. It is not achieved by the *natural* me. There is nothing the *natural* me can do to advance anything in a supernatural or spiritual realm. That is God's realm only. Therefore, conversion from *natural* me to *spiritually-activated* me is nothing other than a mighty act of God in my life, resulting in a transformation from the inside out! Since there's nothing the *natural* me could do to earn or merit this transformation of character and personality, it is an act of God's grace. His grace is His unmerited favor. His grace is what God chooses to do simply because He wants to do. To be forgiven of all my life's sins is a gift of God's grace. Jesus paid for my sins through His dying on the cross. "**The wages of sin is death** (Romans 6:23a)." "**but the gift of God is eternal life** (Romans 6:23b)." What separates Romans 6:23a from 6:23b is God's grace! "**For it is by grace you have been saved, through faith** (Ephesians 2:8)."

This elemental truth is so important to grasp that the Apostle Paul begins his instructions to young Timothy by telling him to "**be strong in the grace that is in Christ Jesus** (2 Timothy 2:1)." One cannot live the Christian life other than by the grace of God. The first truth that needs to be embedded in the mind of the believer is that he or she is a Christian by the grace of God. My security as a believer hinges on what Jesus has done for me and what He has imparted to me the moment I believed in Him and received Him as my Lord and Savior. That instant, the Divine pierced the plane of the natural and made me a *spiritually-activated* person. I experienced the second birth! The first birth was the natural birth and what followed was my natural life. When Christ came into my life, I experienced the New Birth and began my spiritual journey which will carry me ultimately into God's eternal presence. Wow! Can you beat that?

John Newton captured the significance of this miracle of the new birth beautifully when he penned the words for the hymn, entitled Amazing Grace:

> "Amazing grace! How sweet the sound,
> That saved a wretch like me!
> I once was lost, but now am found,
> Was blind but now I see."

The Apostle Paul wanted Timothy to be strong in the grace that is in Christ Jesus because he knew it was God's grace that would sustain him in every contingency of his life! Becoming a Christian and living the Christian life is all by the grace of God. Our sins cannot separate us from the love of God; His grace holds on to us with an eternal grip! God accepts me on the terms of His grace. That is my strength. That is where I will draw the power to overcome the *natural* me and live the *Christ-inside-me* life! When Paul's son in the faith, young Timothy, becomes strong in the grace that is in Christ Jesus, he will not be a target for self-doubts or unbelief. God will never cast off anyone after He has performed the miracle of the New Birth in him or her because His grace has accepted them into the Divine family on the merits of Christ's atonement for their sins on the cross of Calvary. *"**Be strong in the grace that is in Christ Jesus**"* and you will see that Christianity is not a matter of do's and don'ts. What you do or what you don't do will in no way affect your relationship with God; you are His by grace, not of works. To believe that you could sin after becoming a child of God and consequently, fall from grace and become a lost soul again is a pitfall prepared by Satan to entrap and weaken the resolve and the commitment of many a Christian. But it is an untruth! Satan is God's arch-enemy, and he is the arch-enemy of every child of God. The devil wants to get the Christian to doubt his status with God because it will weaken his testimony for God and it will disconnect the Christian from the power connection with God. It will thereby render the Christian less likely to live the Christian life. Satan knows that when a believer is weak in grace and doubts his relationship with God, even though that relationship has not and cannot be broken, the deceived believer will think it has been broken, will become discouraged, and stop trying to live the Christian life. Chalk up another victory for Satan! He cannot defeat God. He cannot separate the Christian from God. The only thing he can do is to con the Christian into failing to believe in the mighty grace of God!

How vital it is, then, that Paul would urge Timothy at the outset of his instruction for living the Christian life to be "**strong in the grace that is in Christ Jesus**." He wants Timothy to know himself—to know who he is—he is a person for whom Jesus died to save from his sins—a person who has been born again by faith in Jesus Christ and due to that fact, will never perish, but will live forever in the family of God and in the Kingdom of God. Grace places you into the family of God and grace secures all your future in Him!

The second thing God wants every believer to do after being born again by the grace of God is to share the story of God's grace with others. Paul writes to Timothy: "**And the things you have heard me say in the presence of many witnesses entrust to reliable men who will also be qualified to teach others** (2 Timothy 2:2)." The message is to pass it on! What has enriched and transformed your life can do the same for others as you pass it on. What is great about this mandate is that whatever you pass on is becoming more deeply imbedded in your own thinking, causing you to grow even stronger in the grace that is in Christ Jesus. Can you recall an assignment you were given in school or in college where you had to learn something and then present it to the class? Perhaps it was a briefing you had to give to your boss or to colleagues on the job. It may have been a class you volunteered to teach. Whatever the case, you probably will agree that you always learn something better yourself when you are preparing to pass it on. Paul introduces Timothy to the time-tested truth of the value of Christian training. It is the means of spreading the Gospel and of deepening the faith of Christians, enabling them also to live the Christian life.

It is important to spend time with the individual Christian whenever possible. This is because Christian nurture is best administered as a one-on-one situation because it maximizes personal attention to the individual's growth capability. One Christian organization that is built around this principle is the Navigators. They specialize in a seasoned and experienced Christian meeting with the new believer on a regular basis, helping the believer to learn Bible verses and gain knowledge for the successful living of the Christian life. By the same token, parents are key persons to pass on the faith to their children, for there can be no better teacher than a devoted mother or father in a growing child's life. In any event, whether through instruction from Christian parents or from another Christian, the brass tacks teaching is not to hoard God's grace to you; pass it on! All who are saved become members of God's family and God's family is God's army. We are not saved to soak up but to serve. The usefulness of a sponge is not just in the soaking up; it is also in its emptying out. Pass it on.

After urging Timothy to become an instructor of the faith, Paul challenges him to "*Endure hardship with us like a good soldier of Christ Jesus* (2 Timothy 2:3)." The Apostle uses the illustration of the hard and disciplined life of a soldier to show how a Christian life consists of a struggle with adversaries. Living the Christian life will be an up-hill climb; it will be a spiritual warfare. A good soldier endures hardship. Things are not going to be easy for him. Jesus did not have it easy and He said: "*No servant is greater than his master. If they persecuted me, they will persecute you also. If they obeyed my teaching, they will obey yours also* (John 15:19-21." The Christian can count on having hard times to deal with because the ways of the world are contrary and opposed to the ways of Christ. The ways of the flesh will war against the ways of the Spirit. In the hymn, "Must Jesus bear the cross alone?" one question is raised: "Is this vile world a friend of grace to help me on to God?" It is, of course, a rhetorical question. As Christian, we will get no help from the world. The unsaved person does not help the Christian to live the Christian life. The Christian life is meant to exceed the natural life. Unfortunately, too few Christians are much help either. This is because only the growing Christians are drawing power from God to handle the challenges of life. One will have to draw his or her support and courage, for the most part, from a personal walk and fellowship with Jesus. Only His ever-present help can enable the Christian to be strong in grace and become able to endure hardship as a good soldier of Jesus Christ.

When I was serving as a chaplain in the United States Army, I can vividly remember meeting a soldier one day in front of the base bowling alley. He seemed from his appearance and the expression on his face to be the very picture of loneliness itself! He appeared to be starving for an understanding friend. Since I was not in uniform, there was no way the soldier could know who I was. He was the one who started up the conversation. The young man spilled out his anguish over the hardship he was dealing with in the barracks environment. He said almost all of the soldiers in his barracks were smoking grass and were urging him to do the same. He kept telling them he "wanted no part in that garbage." He said he was not going to start messing up his life just to please the crowd with which he was living. I did not find out of the young man was a Christian or not, but I know that he had his work cut out for him if he intended to buck the crowd! A good soldier of Jesus Christ is willing to pay the price of being faithful to the Lord and the price will often come in the opposition and ridicule of his peers. The Christian soldier will endure hardship rather than to give in to the folly and sinful ways of the world! There is no room for compromise on the moral issues of life. It is hard to be honest in a society that is characterized by cheating, lying and dishonesty of every imaginable sort. It is hard to be totally faithful to God's principles of what's right and what's wrong when one is dreadfully lonely and starving for companionship!

"**Endure**," says Paul to Timothy. "**Endure**," God says to you and to me. Endure hardship! Persevere in the face of opposition. Persist, even when you may feel like caving in or giving up. Plug away at being true to your Lord; He is counting on you! He is your commander, and you are His soldier. Life is a battle. Coping with sin requires a fight. It is hard going. Yet, a good soldier will do it! It may be hard to put church attendance above an early start for the mountains or to the beach on a Sunday morning. It may be hard to get out of bed when your body tells you it is not a work day and you can sleep in. God would have you get on with it! Endure hardship as a good soldier of Jesus Christ.

Unfortunately, the portrait of a Christian to many people is that of a placid, smiling face of contentment. I would rather think it should be of one who is gritting his teeth to muster inner strength to tap into self-control so that he may be able to resist and overcome temptation. It might be the picture of one choking back his or her tongue when tempted to curse or to spread a vicious rumor about someone else. Or, perhaps, it would be the picture of one saying "No" to wrong when he would like to say "Yes," and have a play with sin. Believe it! A Christian is not always a placid individual because he is a soldier who is in a struggle—waging spiritual warfare nearly every hour of his life! The soldier needs to put his roots into Christ so that he can draw strength for the hard times he faces nearly every day. Jesus said to His disciples, "***Remain in me, and I will remain in you. No branch can bear fruit by itself; it must remain in the vine: neither can you bear fruit unless you remain in me*** (John 15:4)." These same words can equally be applied to the situation of the Christian soldier. Christians cannot endure hardship by themselves, apart from God's active help. The soldier needs to remain in Christ—keeping in touch with God and being in tune with God's spirit—so that he can draw the strength and the resolve to stand and endure hardship. On another occasion, Paul said, "***I can do everything through Him who gives me strength*** (Philippians 4:13)." That is brass tacks Christianity! Develop closeness with Jesus if you want to be able to endure hardship as a good soldier of Jesus Christ.

Paul adds another qualification for the Christian as a good soldier: he says, "***No one serving as a soldier gets involved in civilian affairs—he wants to please his commanding officer*** (2 Timothy 2:4)." With this statement, the Apostle advances the principle that God expects our commitment and service to Him to be wholehearted. We cannot be effective for Him if we become entangled in a web of other allegiances and concerns. Again, he gives the example of a soldier. A paraphrase of these words might be like this: "**No soldier on active duty gets himself entangled in the business pursuits of civilian life, since his sole aim is to please the officer who enlisted him**."

War is serious business. Often, it is a matter of life and death, not only for the individual soldier, but of entire nations, kingdoms and governments. The enemy would have a decided advantage were he engaging a soldier who did not have his mind on the battle—whose attention was being diverted to other interests and pursuits. If a soldiering person should pursue a business on the side—one that would really absorb his interest—he would not be able to give himself to his appointed task as a soldier. Similarly, every true believer and faithful servant of Jesus Christ will actually devote himself wholeheartedly to his soldiering in order to please his master. These very thoughts must have been on the Apostle John's mind, also, as he writes in an entirely different context these words: "**Dear friends, if our hearts do not condemn us, we have confidence before God and receive from him anything we ask, because we obey his commands and do what pleases him. And this is his command: to believe in the name of his Son, Jesus Christ, and to love one another as He commanded us** (1 John 3:22-23)."

Each Christian must investigate his own commitment to Christ and weigh the other concerns of his life against that commitment. It is important to decide for ourselves how deeply we will become entangled in the pursuits of the world. The question we ask ourselves is: "Will my involvement in this become a hindrance to my complete devotion to serving Christ?" "How much of my time and attention will this venture demand?" "Is this activity of high enough priority to come before other activities I might be doing instead, that would increase my effectiveness in serving the Lord?" Sometimes it is not other commitments but other people who entangle the believer and derail the Christian from living the Christian life. How easily are some people prevailed upon to set aside important things simply to join others in activities of their choosing? How easily are students drawn away from their studies, workers drawn away from their jobs, athletes diverted from their practice sessions, by the siren call of friends who say they need their companionship? Much too easily, duty is cast aside in order to indulge in fun! Sometimes we become so entangled in lesser things that we forget for long periods of time that we have a job to do for God! We forget that there is a spiritual warfare being waged and God is counting on us to be prepared to exercise vigilance to soldier for Him!

As you can readily see from this context of 2 Timothy, chapter two, Paul has appealed to Timothy with the analogy of being a good soldier for the living of the Christian life. The brass tacks lesson for the soldier is to endure hardship for the Lord and avoid ulterior entanglements that would detract from fighting the battle. From the analogy of the soldier, Paul advances to the use of another analogy to further drive home his guidance for Christian living. Paul writes: "***Similarly, if any one competes as an athlete, he does not receive the victor's crown unless he competes according to the rules*** (2 Timothy 2:5)." Wholehearted commitment is not all that is required for Christian living; rules must be obeyed, also. In this respect, the best figure is always that of a person competing in an athletic event. Paul pictures the Christian in the very act of competing. When competing, rules for the contest must be obeyed or the contender is disqualified. Illustrations of this point are numerous. When bowling in league competition, for example, the foul line is activated on all lanes. Whenever a bowler's foot slips across that line, an "F" for "foul" is printed in the score box, and the bowler receives no credit for the pins he has knocked down on that ball. Some major horse races have been lost by a jockey committing a foul on an opponent while struggling for position in a turn or when heading down the home stretch. Breaking the rules on the football field may result in a five, ten or fifteen yard penalty just when the game may be on the line. The offending hockey player is sent to the penalty box. The foul on the basketball court sends an opposing player to the free throw line. The examples of this principle are exhaustive to cite.

The brass tacks lesson is that, unless the Christian who performs service for Christ, observes the rules established by God and revealed to us in His Word, the Bible, we cannot obtain the prize for our efforts. God not only requires us to do things for His glory, He requires that we do them in accordance with His standards of excellence. We won't know His standards until we read and know His Word! The Christian needs to study and to know the Word of God so that he can be sure he is observing the rules that God has established for the living of the Christian life.

Along this line, the Christian would do well to take self-inventory regarding his or her motives as they do their service for the Lord. An act may appear to be well and good on the surface, but if it is done for the wrong reasons it may violate the spirit of God's law—it may not be according to His rules for the Christian. One can give money, for example, but if it is done grudgingly or to be seen by others, it is not according to the rules, and one has lost his reward no matter how great the sum of money he has given! This is because the Bible teaches: "***Each man should give what he has decided in his heart to give, not reluctantly or under compulsion, for God loves a cheerful giver*** (2 Corinthians 9:7)." If one does his or her Christian service with an eye to receiving recognition from others, the ministry or service is done out of pride and selfishness, and it is not according to the rules that require the honor and the praise be given to God for what He enables us to do!

There is a marvelous progression that the Apostle Paul is using to give instruction to young Timothy for living the Christian life. He uses the example of the soldier who must endure hardship and must fight wholeheartedly for the good cause of serving Christ. He follows this up with the example of the athlete who must be diligent in competing for the faith but must do so by following the rules. Now, he summons the example of the Christian needing to toil energetically and faithfully, like the hard-working farmer. We have a triad of metaphors to show how a brass tacks Christianity is to be lived: the soldier, the athlete, and now the farmer.

Paul says to Timothy: "***The hard working farmer should be the first to receive a share of the crops*** (2 Timothy 2:6)." Hard work should be rewarded. The writer of the book of Proverbs makes a pertinent reference to this principle. He said: "**A sluggard does not plow in season; so at harvest time he looks and finds nothing** (Proverbs 20:4)." In another text, the lesson is driven home powerfully: "**I went past the field of the sluggard, past the vineyard of the man who lacks judgment; thorns had come up everywhere, the ground was covered with weeds, and the stone wall was in ruins. I applied my heart to what I observed and learned a lesson from what I saw: a little sleep, a little slumber, a little folding of the hands to rest—and poverty will come on you like a bandit and scarcity like an armed man** (Proverbs 24:30-34)."

The Christian is to be the exact opposite of the sluggard! He is to pattern himself after the diligent farmer who tends to the business of raising a good harvest. If the farmer works hard—prepares the soil, sows the seed, waters the field, digs out the weeds, applies fertilizer, sprays for pests and daily checks on his crop for early signs of disease or other problems—he will enjoy a good harvest. Paul says to Timothy that such a farmer should be the first to benefit from his labor. Similarly, any worker in God's vineyard who exerts himself to the full performance of his God-given spiritual task will be the first to be rewarded by God. Not only will his own faith be strengthened, his hope quickened, his love deepened, and the flame of his devotion enlivened, but "**He will be blessed in what he does** (James 1:25)." Additionally, he will see how his hard work for the Lord has blessed others—the beginnings of reaping the fruits of the spirit: "**But the fruit of the Spirit is love, joy, peace, patience, kindness, goodness, faithfulness, gentleness and self-control** (Galatians 5:22-23)." In the Lord's service, one's work is never for naught—labor for Christ is never in vain. God has promised that the results will come if we remain faithful in sowing the seed! One of my most favorite passages in the book of Psalms depicts the reward for farming for human souls: "**Those who sow in tears will reap with songs of joy. He, who goes out weeping, carrying seed to sow, will return with songs of joy, carrying sheaves with him** (Psalms 126:5-6)." There will be untold numbers of people rejoicing in heaven some day because of the patient, loving and hard work of other Christians who cared to farm for their souls—who shared God's Word with them, who checked up on them and was a good friend to them, who laughed with them and cried with them, who checked up on them and was a good friend to them, assisting them on the path of Christian living! Can you imagine how great a church you would have and how blessed would be the community in which you live if you had a troop of Christians who were serious about their commitment to God and were living daily with a loving zeal—farming for human souls? Would not you like to be such a person on whom God could rely to live your life like that?

Paul now says to Timothy in our text: "**Reflect on what I am saying, for the Lord will give you insight into all this** (2 Peter 2:7)." This approach is rare in Biblical writing, to state, "**Reflect on what I am saying**." It is not the type of phrase often used—it is used only when a very special emphasis is being made. In the Old Testament, the prophets used the expression, "**Hear the word of the Lord**." In the account of the birth of Jesus to the Virgin Mary, many signs and wonders were manifest. The Christmas story is replete with amazing events that were set off by the advent of Christ to earth from heaven come down: Angels appearing to shepherds tending their flocks in the fields by night, the glory of the Lord shining all around them, the Angelic announcement that on this day in the town of David a Savior has been born, the sudden appearing of a great company of the heavenly host, praising God. The shepherds left their flocks and travelled to Bethlehem and found the holy family in the manger and the shepherds worshipped the baby Jesus. The Bible says, "**But Mary treasured up all these things and pondered them in her heart** (Luke 2:19)." This is the feeling Paul is conveying now to Timothy: "These things I have just been telling you are of supreme importance—they are getting down to the brass tacks, so consider them well."

It's as if Paul was saying, "Think on these things often!" "Chew them over in your mind!" "Remember them by thinking of the three examples I have just given to you—the soldier, the athlete, the farmer: as a good soldier, endure hardship without bellyaching or griping—it is the cost of fighting a war!" He would also say, "And remember the athlete: be sure to go by the rules given by God, so that you won't become disqualified after all your effort. You cannot compromise with the rules and win God's approval." Furthermore, the Apostle would remind us, "And the farmer is a good example of toil and hard work; work at mastering sin in your life—eliminate sins like the farmer eliminates the weeds that might choke out the crop! Farming demands that a lot of attention be given, but the rewards are sure to come if you remain faithful. You must be the opposite of the sluggard who thinks things will take care of themselves, and that life owes him a living!"

At this juncture, Paul hits the proverbial nail on the head by citing one of the most foundational truths of the Christian faith: **"Remember Jesus Christ, raised from the dead, descended from David. This is my gospel, for which I am suffering even to the point of being chained like a criminal** (2 Timothy 2:8-9)." The Apostle realizes that what he has just said to Timothy amounts to a big order; getting down to brass tacks living is going to require a lot of personal dedication, followed by continued effort.

The single mindedness and hardness of a soldier, the faithful obedience of an athlete, and the diligent persistence of a good farmer—these requirements are going to take a person's best effort! One might ask, "Is it worth it?" "Can it really be done?" "Will it actually pay off in some tangible way?" Paul addresses these thoughts now, in the next six verses (verses 8-13). For brass tacks living, Paul cites some brass tacks theology! He goes back to the basic core of Christian Faith, which is our Lord and Savior, Jesus Christ, and Him crucified, risen and reigning!

"Remember Jesus Christ, raised from the dead, descended from David," he proclaimed. Why do you suppose Paul included the statement, **"descended from David?"** My sense of this is because Paul is intending to show that Jesus is the promised One! He is the descendent of King David, of Israel. He was promised by the prophets of old. The prophets stated that the seed of David would one day rule the world. They prophesied that David's Righteous Branch would come and bring salvation to His people. Christ is that Messiah Who was promised by the prophets of Israel! Jesus is the descendent of David, Whom God has sent in answer to His promises! God has kept His word! The promised One has come, has offered Himself as atonement for our sins, has been raised from the dead by God's almighty power, and He has inherited the rule of the world at the seat of God's right hand, in glory.

Imagine the conviction in his voice: "**Remember**!" "You serve this Christ!" He continues, "At times you may have to suffer for His name, but His Word which you believe and which you proclaim, will never be hindered; it will always prevail and do its perfect work! Just look at me! I am in prison and in bonds; but the Word of God is not bound! It still goes forth and has power to bring many to faith and salvation through the risen Christ!" The same God who promised the Savior would come, of the seed of David, has fulfilled that promise in sending Jesus into the world, and He is the same God who now is making promises to you! God will never let you down when He has promised to sustain you. God keeps His promises to men! God has promised to sustain us as we live the Christian life for Him, and He has promised to reward us for our faithfulness. Notice the self-sacrificing attitude of the Apostle Paul as he speaks to Timothy: "***Therefore I endure everything for the sake of the elect, that they too may obtain the salvation that is in Christ Jesus, with eternal glory*** (2 Timothy 2:10)."

Paul shifts gears at this point and decides to share with Timothy the brass tacks equation for Christian service; everything boils down to four courses of behavior, which can be practiced by any believer, and he describes what God's response would be to each behavior. First, he cites two positive behaviors, followed by two negative behaviors. The positive behaviors are (1) to die with Him, and (2) to endure. The negative behaviors are (1) to disown Him, and (2) to be faithless. Much can be learned from analyzing each of these possible behaviors in turn. First, he says, "***Here is a trustworthy saying: if we die with Him*** (2 Timothy 2:11a)." Have you thought of what dying with Christ might mean? It means that the life you are living when you commit to living the Christian life—your personal plans and desires, your self-interests and long-term goals are plowed under, *as if you had died*, so that Christ might fill the void, live in you and have total control! It is as John the Baptist said of Jesus: "***He must become greater; I must become less*** (John 3:30)." To die with Christ mans to die to our sins. This is exactly the way the Apostle Peter framed it: "***He himself bore our sins in his body on*** *the tree, so that we might <u>die to sins</u> and live for righteousness; by his wounds you have been healed* (1 Peter 2:24)." Every believer is called upon to put to death the sins of his former life so that the fruits of the new life in Christ might be obtained! Paul wrote to the Galatians: "*I have been crucified with Christ and I no longer live, but Christ lives in me, the life I live in the body, I live by faith in the son of God, who loved me and gave himself for me* (Galatians 2:20)." That, my friends, is brass tacks Christianity! Crucified with Christ! This is what Jesus expects of all who would follow Him. That does not sound to be an easy path to walk. It is a path of self-denial. It is a path of total surrender of my will to His will. It is no longer my will to live as I choose to live, but it is Him living in me as He chooses me to live! Our Lord said to His disciples, "*If anyone would come after me, he must deny himself and take up his cross and follow me. For whoever wants to save his life will lose it, but whoever loses his life for me will find it* (Matthew 17:24)."

Now notice the response God gives to this course of Christian commitment—being willing to die to ourselves in order to follow Jesus. The brass tacks equation is this: "*If we died with Him we shall also live with Him* (2 Peter 2:11a)." What a marvelous promise this is! We shall live with Him! When one considers the fear and uncertainty many feel when they face the reality of their own demise, hoping but not knowing what comes next, these words come as a tremendous comfort. In another passage of Scripture, Jesus describes what is in store for those who are willing to live the Christian life: "*Do not let your hearts be troubled. Trust in God; trust also in me. In my Father's house are many rooms; if it were not so, I would have told you. I am going there to prepare a place for you. And if I go and prepare a place for you, I will come back and take you to be with me that you also may be where I am* (John 14:1-3)." This is the brass tacks message to any who are questioning if it is really worth it to put all on the line and live only for Christ in this life: when we are willing to place ourselves last and Jesus first—when we are willing to be crucified to sin and to the world—then we are assured we shall live forever with Jesus! Is not that a really good deal?

The second possible positive behavior Paul speaks about to Timothy is this: "*If we endure*... (2 Timothy 2:12a)." In the King James Version of the Bible, the word used here is "suffer," that is, "*If we suffer with Him*." Put the two words together and it approximates the real meaning Paul is conveying to young Timothy: "When you are willing to die with Christ, you are willing also to endure suffering for Him." Again, like Jesus said, "*Take up your cross and follow me,*" implies this enduring suffering. It is a living death, you might say—we continue living our lives, but not as WE will, but as HE wills! It is not me that is in control of my life; it is He that is in control. When Jesus is in control, our lives will conform to God's principles or righteousness. And when this is the case, we may see that we are alienating some people who used to be important in our lives. We alienate them, because they are not comfortable sharing our values now that we are dedicated to a higher plane of living than they are willing to own for themselves. We will incur enemies from those who do not want to live for God! When a person lives for Christ and adopts the Bible's blueprint for Christian living, he or she will find they have stirred up resentment in some of their former acquaintances—perhaps even people in their own family—aroused their jealousy, envy and hostility, because they are opposed to our righteous ways. That is because by your walking in the light of God's Word, you are flashing a bright ray upon their sins and they may want to bring you down to ease their discomfort. They will want you to suffer for being different from them! Think about it. If the world crucified Jesus, Who lived in perfect love to everyone He encountered, what do you think they will do to the followers of Jesus? Jesus, Himself, warned His disciples of this: "*If they persecuted me, they will persecute you, also* (John 15:20b)." When citing Moses as a person of great faith, the writer of Hebrews says of him, "*By faith Moses, when he had grown up, refused to be known as the son of Pharaoh's daughter (which would have been a protected position). He chose to be mistreated along with the people of God rather than to enjoy the pleasures of sin for a short time. He regarded disgrace for the sake of Christ as of greater value than the treasures of Egypt, not fearing the king's anger; he persevered because he saw Him who is invisible* (Hebrews

11:24-26)." Moses had his priorities straight! He made sure he was on God's side in the contest of life and morality! Most people just see the human beings who may oppose them and retreat from righteousness out of fear of being rejected and ridiculed. Moses calculated the same choice. What enabled Moses to stand his ground and not compromise his principles was the fact that he saw Him Who is invisible. How did he do that? He did that through the eyes of faith! When you believe wholeheartedly in Jesus Christ, you will see Him Who is invisible in every situation where your dignity and your values are tested. You will make the right choices when you know He is with you!

What is God's response when we are willing to endure? Paul says to Timothy, "**We will also reign with Him** (2 Peter 2:12b)." Think of it this way: you have time and you have eternity; one is limited and relatively brief, the other is endless existence in a new realm—spiritual life. There is an eternity awaiting everyone. It will be eternal life, or it will be eternal death; eternal tranquility and joy, or eternal suffering and sorrow. Would you consider it a good bargain to enjoy freedom to live life as you please by disregarding the rules of God and making up your own rules as you go along—making money and having fun wherever you may find it, only to die in a few years, stand at the Judgment Seat of Christ, and find yourself banished from heaven and sent to an eternal hell? Or, would you rather abandon your life of sin where self is all that matters and submit to the authority and will of God in this brief life, and enjoy a warm welcome into God's heaven with the words, "**Well done, good and faithful servant! You have been faithful with a few things; I will put you in charge of many things. Come and share your master's happiness** (Matthew 25:21)." It is now and then; life now and life to come. Perhaps there may be some sacrifices in life, in order to live for Christ. Joy and blessing are waiting for you in the life to come! Remember, when you receive Christ into your life by faith, you become a child of God! There's no way you can understand in this life what fantastic events are waiting for you, simply because you are God's child. Listen to this astounding passage of Scripture: "**However, as it is written: no eye has seen, no ear has heard, no mind has conceived what God has** *prepared for those that love Him* ((1 Corinthians 2:9)." The brass tacks fact is "*We will reign with Him*."

To summarize where we are at this point, we have just considered the first two of four possible behaviors and the response God makes to each: If we die with Him, we shall also live with Him; if we endure, we shall reign with Him. At this point, the Apostle Paul introduces the first negative behavior and describes God's response. He said, "*If we disown Him* (2 Peter 2:12b)." Some, who claim to be Christians, may disown Christ, but when they do this, they only reveal the fact that they were never Christians at all! Paul is making the same point here that he also made to Titus. Listen to his unvarnished words: "*To the pure, all things are pure, but to those who are corrupted and do not believe, nothing is pure. In fact, both their consciences and their minds are corrupted. They claim to know god, but by their actions they deny Him. They are detestable, disobedient and unfit for doing anything good* (Titus 1:15-16)."

Atheists disown God, but I do not believe people who think they are Christians will set out to disown Christ. What usually happens, however, is that Christ is disowned at a point where it would cost a person something important to affirm allegiance to the Lord. Perhaps it is easier for someone to disown the Lord than to stand on some principle that might alienate them from their co-workers, employer or friends. At such times, the person in question may feel more comfortable agreeing with worldly-minded people than he or she would feel affirming faith in Christ. It may be to save one's own skin, so to speak, as did Peter when he denied the Lord three times in one night as the Lord was being subjected to a mock trial and rustled out to be crucified! The brass tacks fact is this: when you find it is prudent to conceal the fact you are a believer in Jesus—for whatever reason there may be—you are dangerously close to disowning Him!

What is God's response to this? Paul says, "*If we disown him, He will also disown us (*2 Timothy 2:12c)." Disowners of Christ are unbelievers. They never knew Him in the first place. Whatever religious behavior they may have displayed was only an outward shell with nothing but hollowness on the inside! There was no substance to their claims of being Christian. They were near but distant at the same time. They may have even said the right words, but they only fell from the lips and did not emanate from the heart! The lips must be able to affirm the Lord, it is true, but it only counts when it is backed up by the heart. Listen to Paul's words to the Romans: "*That if you confess with your mouth, Jesus as Lord, and believe in your heart that God has raised him from the dead, you will be saved. For it is with your heart that you believe and are justified, and it is with your mouth that you confess and are saved* (Romans 10:9-10)." Jesus died for your sins and for my sins in an open and public way. He was out there on Golgotha Hill, nailed to a wooden cross, in full public view. He was not bleeding and dying on that cross for sins He had committed. He was taking our place, paying for our sins that He might redeem us for Himself! If you believe in Him, He expects you to be public about it! You must be willing to confess your faith in Jesus! One may by nature be timid and shy, but that's not an excuse for not confessing faith in Him openly! That is the price of the ticket that will take you to heaven. There is no other entrance, except by faith in Jesus Christ. Jesus, Himself, stated this with utmost clarity: "*Whoever acknowledges me before men, I will also acknowledge before my father in heaven. But whoever disowns me before men, I will disown before my Father in heaven* (Matthew 10:32)."

The final possible behavior of which Paul speaks to Timothy is this: "*If we are faithless* (2 Timothy 2:13)." This is the second negative behavior. We may disown Him and we may not keep faith with the Lord. There is no remedy for disowning Him: it is clear He will disown anyone who should do this. It is not the same with the second behavior—to be faithless. Just as people make New Year's resolutions and fail to keep them, no matter how well-intentioned they were when they made them, people can make promises to God and later go back on those promises. Consider, for example, the man who is stricken with a heart attack and is rushed to the hospital emergency room in an ambulance. He still may be conscious while doctors are diagnosing the damage and considering life-saving options. It is not far-fetched to imagine a man in such a predicament to turn to God in a prayer of utter desperation and say such things as "Lord, let me live through this and I will serve you the rest of my life!" Subsequently, the man receives a coronary bypass surgery to restore the blood flow to his heart and he survives the ordeal. He thanks the Lord and begins his rehabilitative recovery. Months later, he is back on his job and is beginning to forget the promise he made to the Lord when he was in danger of dying. Now, watching Sunday morning football is more important than going to church and watching a movie on TV is more inviting than reading the Bible or praying to God. The man is demonstrating what is warned about here in Paul's words to Timothy: he is being faithless! He does not disown Christ; He is ignoring Him! Were he asked if he believed in Jesus, he would say loudly and clearly, "yes, I do." He holds faith in his heart, but it is being crowded out by a lot of other interests in his heart. You might see him in church at Christmas or Easter. He is proving to be unreliable. He is faithless.

One may be willing to bear any burden and pay any cost to fight the good fight against sin in his life, like the soldier waging battle with the enemy. One may study God's Word, pray and exercise his faith in any way possible, like the dedicated athlete who obeys the rules and strives for the mastery in sports competition. One may attend diligently with the strenuous toil of righteous living, like the farmer who tends to the business of his fields or crops. Those behaviors will bring wonderful responses and rich blessings from God. The word of caution is sounded, however, as Paul concludes his instructions to Timothy for living the Christian life: one may get in the habit of cutting corners out of self-interest and fail to obey the rules of the Christian life. Such behavior is faithlessness. There is a very interesting conclusion to this, however. What do you suppose God's response will be when a person loses his commitment to Christian living and becomes faithless? We might suspect He would respond in kind, but JOYFUL SURPRISE! The parallelism stops right here! The truth is that God cannot do what we can do! We may be faithless to Him, BUT HE CANNOT BECOME FAITHLESS TO US! Paul says to Timothy: "*If we are faithless, He will remain faithful, for He cannot disown Himself* (2 Timothy 2:13b)."

God will always keep His sayings, no matter whatever we do. God will fulfill His promises, no matter how weak we may become in our Christian living. God will always remain faithful! If you need a proverbial "shot in the arm" to enliven your esteem for your God, listen to Paul's words to the Christians at Corinth: "**And God is faithful; He will not let you be tempted beyond what you can bear. But when you are tempted, He will also provide a way out so that you can stand up under it** (1 Corinthians 10:13."

The Christians in Thessalonica heard similar words from the Apostle Paul. He wrote to them: "**And pray that we may be delivered from evil and wicked men, for not everyone has faith. But the Lord is faithful, and He will strengthen and protect you from the evil one** (2 Thessalonians 3:3)."   God is faithful—not because of what we do to please Him; He is faithful because He is God! Even when we sin, He is faithful. This is what we hear from the Apostle John: "**If we confess our sins, He is faithful and just and will forgive us our sins and purify us from all unrighteousness** (1 John 1:9)." The brass tacks message is that God will remain faithful; He cannot deny Himself!

Timothy has been skillfully and lovingly advised in this brief discourse of the Apostle Paul. Paul cuts directly to the core of what it means to live for God and to serve Him with our lives. He sketches out the parameters for productive Christian living and he does this by getting down to the brass tacks! May God help us to live up to the challenge!

CHAPTER TWO

THE LAW OF SPIRITUAL LIFE

Many people who read the Bible like to pay special attention to the words and teachings of Jesus. They hang on every word, expecting to get understanding and infallible guidance for the living of their lives. The publishers of the Bible realized the popularity and importance people place upon the words of Jesus and made accommodation to them by printing what has been called the "red letter" edition of the Bible. That is, the words of Jesus are all printed in red so that they stand out distinctly from the rest of the text. There is historical precedence for giving special attention to the words and teachings of Jesus: in his public ministry, crowds of people followed Jesus everywhere he went so that they could drink in the wisdom and insight he dispensed in his discourses. Many of His sayings were very simple expressions that carried profound truth. Such is the case, for example, with what has been called the golden rule: "*So in everything, do to others what you would have them do to you, for this sums up the Law and the Prophets* (Matthew 7:12)." There is a whole system of ethics bound up in that simple saying!

Not all of Jesus' sayings are so easy to understand. Some of his teachings are very difficult to comprehend and very hard to accept when taken at face value or at first glance. Not long before Jesus made his final entry into Jerusalem on Palm Sunday to begin the final week before His suffering and death on the cross, Jesus entered the city of Jericho. It was on that day that he encountered a man named Zacchaeus, a wealthy chief tax collector, who also was quite short of stature. Wanting badly to get a view of Jesus, Zacchaeus ran and climbed up into a sycamore-fig tree to see him.

The Biblical account explains how Jesus came to the place where the curious Zacchaeus was perched up in the tree, and Jesus looked up at Zacchaeus and ordered him to come down from the tree, using these surprising words: *"**Zacchaeus, come down immediately, I must stay at your house today** (Luke 19:5)."* The tax collector came down from the tree at once and welcomed Jesus gladly. The on-lookers were stunned by this encounter and began to criticize Jesus for his interest in a man the public had come to despise for his relentless shaking down of even the poor to gather the taxes from them. They began to mutter, "***He has gone to be the guest of a sinner** (Luke 19:6)."* They soon, however, had egg on their faces when they heard Zaccheaus behaved as a totally transformed man by this simple gesture of Jesus. The text states: *"**But Zacchaeus stood up and said to the Lord, 'look, Lord! Here and now I give half of my possessions to the poor, and if I have cheated anybody out of anything, I will pay back four times the amount** (Luke 19:8)."* In response to Zacchaeus' tremendous change of heart and purpose, Jesus uttered an astounding declaration: Jesus said to him, "***Today salvation has come to this house, because this man, too, is a son of Abraham. For the son of man came to seek and to save what was lost**. (Luke 19:9)."* Zacchaeus backed up his faith with changed behavior; he went from being greedy to being gracious and generous. The irony in this lies in the fact that while Zacchaeus was giving up his earthly wealth to help the poor, he was simultaneously really laying up treasure in heaven, that would prove infinitely more rewarding than any earthly gains he may have made! He was one of the lost souls Jesus came to save!

Following this incident with Zacchaeus, Jesus began to talk to the crowd following him, using a parable that is most difficult to understand, in order to convey a very important spiritual concept. The Bible says they were getting near Jerusalem, and because the people were assuming Jesus was going to establish the kingdom of God at once, Jesus spoke in the parable about a noble man who was about to go on a journey to a distant country where he would have himself appointed king and then to return. The man called ten of his servants and gave them ten minas—one to each, instructing them, "***Put this money to work until I come back** (Luke 19:13)."*

In terms of the currency of that day, one mina was equal to three months' wages. Each was entrusted, therefore, with considerable wealth to manage in the master's absence. As the parable unfolds, the noble man was made king and returned home. He called for his servants to come and report what they had done with the mina he had entrusted to them. The first servant had multiplied his mina to ten times its original worth. He was praised and told he would be appointed ruler over ten cities. The second servant gave account and said he had gained five times the original amount. He, too, was praised for his stewardship and was given charge of five cities. The third servant had nothing to report except to say that the mina he was given was secure and he was giving it back to the noble man. For an explanation, the servant said: "*I was afraid of you, because you are a hard man. You take out what you did not put in and reap what you did not sow* (Luke 19:21)."

Because the reply of Jesus is so critical to understanding a major spiritual principle, I would like to cite His exact words: "*His master replied, 'I will judge you by your own words, you wicked servant! You knew, did you, that I am a hard man, taking out what I did not put in, and reaping what I did not sow? Why then didn't you put my money on deposit, so that when I came back, I could have collected it with interest?' Then he said to those standing by, 'Take his mina away from him and give it to the one who has ten minas.' 'Sir,' they said, 'He already has ten!' he replied, 'I tell you that to everyone who has, more will be given, but as for the one who has nothing, even what he has will be taken away. But those enemies of mine who did not want me to be king over them—bring them here and kill them in front of me* (Luke 19:22-26)."

Many scholars believe Jesus was using an historical event that would have been familiar to the Jews of his day as a vehicle for his parable. Both Herod in 40 B.C. and Herod Archelaus in 4 B.C. went to Rome to receive ruling authority from the emperor. In both of their reigns over the Jews there was a lot of bloodshed at the outset. In the case of Archelaus, the Jews sent a fifty member delegation to Rome to try and persuade the emperor Augustus not to send Archelaus to rule over them. When Archelaus was selected anyway, he purged his detractors when he arrived to rule in Palestine. This historical footnote helps to explain the language Jesus used at the close of his parable.

More important than the details of every phrase in the parable is the basic truth the parable was fashioned to advance. The key is the phrase, *"**To everyone who has, more will be given, but as for the one who has nothing, even what he has will be taken away.**"* It is a simple statement of fact in regard to some who had little that even the little they had was taken away from them. The spiritual principle involved can be stated in just 3 words: <u>use or lose</u>! This brief statement represents an elemental truth which runs all through God's physical and spiritual universe. A person does well to become acquainted with the reality of this basic law because it can have a profound effect upon one's life. In fact, use or lose can be described as <u>The Law of Spiritual Life</u>.

Consider that the entire universe is built on this principle. Way out in the middle of the Pacific Ocean, for example, is a lonely little spot called Canton Island—one of the loneliest places anywhere until World War II. It was still the home of the Frigate bird back then. Centuries previous, the Frigates sought food like any other sea bird, flying out across the ocean and diving for fish. Then the Frigates discovered that the Gannets or Boobies were returning to the island with gullets loaded. If they were chased, the smaller birds would disgorge their fish, saving the Frigate birds a considerable amount of trouble searching for their own food. In time, however, the Frigates lost their capacity to search for food and relied completely on the Gannets. If the Gannets failed to return, the Frigates starved.

There are hundreds of examples of the "use or lose" principle in nature. In certain caves in Newfoundland, there are fish which have lived so long without light that, although they have eyes, the eyes no longer see. Naturalists tell us that long ago both the Kiwi of New Zealand and the Emu of Australia were capable of flying, but from long disuse their wings have now reached a point that they are useless.

In my high school days, I was very much interested in sports—especially soccer. When in training, I could run up and down the field for half of the afternoon, feeling no ill effects after such grueling exercise. On one occasion in college, however, I participated in a one-mile race on an Olympic day, without any preparatory training. The distance was only one mile, but I had to drop out before its completion from sheer exhaustion and was days in recovering! Everyone knows what happens to muscles that are not used.

One minister friend told of a lady he had in one of his congregations who was remarkably spry even when approaching her 90th year. She had since gone far beyond that point. The pastor asked her one day what was the secret of her good health? She explained that when she was young she became much impressed by a doctor who pointed out the need for every muscle, joint and organ of the body to be kept in continual use if the body's efficiency is to be maintained. Even in her eighties, this lady was still doing regular exercises daily and the results were certainly impressive!

"Use or lose" is a principle which we see operating daily in the financial, economic, or business world, also. In every major city we see great new buildings rising. In the past twenty years the skylines of many prominent cities have completely changed. Where are these great new structures being erected? For the most part, they are built on sites which were not being used sufficiently in relation to their present market value. Life seems to say to many people, justify your existence, or get out of the way.

In his parables Jesus was primarily concerned with moral and spiritual lessons. It's therefore important that we consider the "Use or Lose" principle at these vital levels. God has given each of us some capacity to resist temptation. A person may be tempted to do something dishonest. If the individual fails to use this capacity to resist such temptation, he or she will find it harder to resist the next time. Eventually, more and more opportunities to resist temptation will end in the same result—giving in to the temptation and failing to do the honest thing. Once the trend gets established, it will finally result in habitual dishonesty. Will-power not used will turn into will-power totally lost!

Another example can be found in the matters of prayer and worship. Every child is born with this capacity, but nothing is more certain than losing this capacity when it is neglected for a long time.

Prayer will become increasingly more difficult and unreal. Worship will become unappealing and boring instead of being the highest and most satisfying of spiritual experiences. The more one loves in a pure and unselfish manner, the greater becomes that person's ability to love. But let a person turn inward on himself or herself, live selfishly and refuse to exercise compassion for others, and that person's soul will shrivel and will lose this God-given ability. Many a married love is lost when separations occur, such as during deployments in military service, simply from the lack of exercising care to communicate by letter, by e-mail, or by making a phone call. Lacking in conscious expressions of love to each other, the love actually dies. Whatever the spiritual activity you name, the same principle applies: "*To him that has more will be given, and from him that has not, even what he has will be taken away from him*."

One spiritual phenomenon that is well known to many pastors, missionaries and evangelists is seeing people making public decisions to accept Jesus Christ as Lord and Savior. In any given Billy Graham crusade, for example, hundreds of people from all walks of life make their way to the altar during the invitation at the close of the sermon. There is scarcely a greater joy to anyone in the Lord's work than to see these converts to Christ grow in knowledge and grace and proceed to acquire a spiritual maturity that becomes a blessing to many others. On the other hand, one of the heartbreaks is to see some who make these commitments to Christ fail to follow up on their decision and do nothing to nurture and expand on their new-found faith. Many such individuals look back to their commitment with embarrassment and have no sense of conscious gain. They have learned the hard way the full force of the spiritual law: "Use or Lose." Any new convert to Christ needs to get into the reading and the study of the Word of God in order to feed his soul and nurture his faith.

Even as a young child learning to advance from riding a tricycle to riding a two-wheel bicycle, needs a supportive and steadying hand until the child develops the confidence and balance to ride unassisted, every new Christian needs the attention, support and caring contact from other Christians while they are learning how to read the Bible and to attend church services on a regular basis. Not to give the new-born Christian caring attention as they begin living a Christian lifestyle would be like planting a beautiful flower in your garden and expecting it to grow without giving it any water! The results will be no surprise to anyone who understands the law of spiritual life: "Use or Lose."

In spiritual matters, we can't stand still or "mark time." We go back or we go forward; we degenerate or we accelerate; we slip back a pace or we grow in grace. What you don't use by way of spiritual discernment you will lose. It is God's infallible law of spiritual life! God will not continually pour rich spiritual blessings into willfully idle hearts! If God gives spiritual light and insight to a person who will not use that insight in revamping his attitudes and his behavior accordingly, God will take from that individual even the little light and discernment he already has been given. It is "Use or Lose." It cannot be stressed enough the importance of possessing an inquisitive and thirsty spirit after the things of God! Jesus taught, **"Blessed are those who hunger and thirst for righteousness, for they will be filled** (Matthew 5:6)." The individuals who are receiving God's choicest spiritual blessings are those who most appreciate the ones God has already bestowed upon them. Look again to the text of Luke 19:26 and you will notice two important sides to this Law of Spiritual Life. The first side is, IF YOU DON'T USE, YOU LOSE MORE THAN THE ORIGINAL GIFT. This was true of the ten servants of the noble man who was about to embark on a long absence. They each would be entrusted with a mina to manage and each would be called to account upon his return. The one who didn't expand his mina failed to satisfy his master and ended up losing all he had. The same fate can be seen in nature neglected, in economics, and in many other directions. Many people have studied foreign languages only to find that they have totally forgotten all they had learned just a few years later. They lost the capacity for the language through disuse of it! I can't believe that I once figured out geometry and trigonometry problems in school. Since I never had to use these skills in any job or profession I followed, I lost any facility I ever had with higher math. Fortunately, I can still add, subtract, divide and multiply!

When I was in the Army and counseling soldiers there were many occasions where a soldier was seeking counseling because he was in a bind, not being able to perform his job to which he had recently been assigned. The soldier had been trained in a specific military occupational specialty (MOS), but for some reason was not allowed to work in that specialty right away because he was needed for a different job. A year or more later, the soldier had been assigned to fill a slot which called for his MOS. Not having done that job specialty for over a year caused the soldier to forget the skills he had learned when he acquired that MOS. He had lost the skill due to disuse. Moldy bread, rotten fruit, and spoiled meat all testify to the validity of the truth that things are lost when they are not used on a timely basis.

I remember talking with a young man once who, some years previously, made his decision for Christ but after a brief time, he fell by the wayside, turning his back on religion after getting in with the wrong crowd. Later, the young man became troubled because he feared he had committed the unpardonable sin. From his reading of certain passages of Scripture, mainly taken out of their context, it seemed clear to him that since he went back on his commitment to Christ, there was no second chance for him and this haunted him. I tried to explain to him that the church is full of people to whom God has given a second chance, just as Jesus did to Peter after his denial. The passages which troubled him were the Biblical expressions that cautioned against "**hardening your hearts**" to a point where one would not be able to respond to spiritual promptings any more.

It is commonly recognized that the hardest people to win to a decision for Christ are those who have been inoculated with a little religion until they have become immune to the real thing! To bring this back to our original theme, if we fail to nurture what little faith we have, not only will we lose that faith, but we may reach a state in which we are deprived of all the blessings and joys of the spiritual life.

Again, the point of the parable of the ten minas is clear: if you use what God has entrusted to you, you will be rewarded and given more responsibilities; if you fail to use what He has entrusted to you, you will lose it. The servant who failed spent much time meditating on the nature of his master, but that did not save him. Action was required. There is, no doubt, a place for theoretical theology, but unless we put our theology and our faith into practice the day will come when we will hear words from Jesus that will sting us to the bone. Listen to Jesus' words as he describes the future day when he will judge all men for what they did with the opportunities to practice genuine Christian faith. He said: "***When the Son of Man comes in his glory, and all the angels with him, He will sit on his throne in heavenly glory. All the nations will be gathered before him, and he will separate the people one from another as a shepherd separates the sheep from the goats. He will put the sheep on his right and goats on his left.***

"***Then the King will say to those on his right, 'come, you who are blessed by my Father; take your inheritance, the kingdom prepared for you since the creation of the world. For I was hungry and you gave me something to eat, I was thirsty and you gave me something to drink, I was a stranger and you invited me in. I needed clothes and you clothed me, I was sick and you looked after me, I was in prison and you came to visit me.'***

"***Then the righteous will answer him, Lord, when did we see you hungry and feed you, or thirsty and give you something to drink? When did we see you a stranger and invite you in or needing clothes and clothe you? When did we see you sick or in prison and go to visit you?'***

"***The King will reply, 'I tell you the truth, whatever you did for one of the least of these brothers of mine, you did for me.'***

"***Then he will say to those on his left, 'depart from me, you who are cursed, into the eternal fire prepared for the devil and his angels. For I was hungry and you gave me nothing to eat, I was thirsty and you gave me nothing to drink. I was a stranger and you did not invite me it, I needed clothes and you did not clothe me, I was sick and in prison and you did not look after me.'***

"***They all will answer, 'Lord, when did we see you hungry or thirsty or a stranger or needing clothes or sick or in prison, and did not help you?'***

"***He will reply, 'I tell you the truth, whatever you did not do for one of the least of these, you did not do for me.'***

"Then they will go away to eternal punishment, but the righteous to eternal life (Matthew 25:31-46)."

Let none of us forget that one day this life on earth will be over and there will be the Day of Judgment of which our Lord spoke in this passage. Each of us will have to look into the eyes of the living Christ and give account of our stewardship. The Law of Spiritual Life will be confirmed: "Use or Lose."

The second side of the Law of Spiritual Life is this: IF YOU DO USE, MUCH MORE WILL BE GIVEN TO YOU. It is the positive and encouraging note of this text which is just as true as the "Use or Lose" principle. This is what happened to the first servant in the parable of the minas; he multiplied his mina by tenfold and then received the mina taken from the unfaithful servant. In another parable, Jesus talked about a farmer who went forth to sow his seed: "*As he was scattering the seed, some fell along the path, and the birds came and ate it up. Some fell on rocky places, where it did not have much soil. It sprang up quickly, because the soil was shallow. But when the sun came up, the plants were scorched, and they withered because they had no root. Other seed fell among thorns, which grew up and choked the plants. Still other seed fell on good soil, where it produced a crop—a hundred, sixty or thirty times what was sown. He, who has ears, let him hear* (Matthew 13:4-9)."

The disciples were confused by the parable that Jesus used and did not understand how to apply the story to their lives. Jesus explained why he taught them using parables, then explained the meaning of the parable of the farmer sowing his seed: "*Listen then to what the parable of the sower means: when anyone hears the message about the kingdom and does not understand it, the evil one comes and snatches away what was sown in his heart. This is the seed sown along the path. The one who received the seed that fell on rocky places is the man who hears the word and at once receives it with joy. But since he has no root, he lasts only a short time. When trouble or persecution comes because of the Word, he quickly falls away. The one who received the seed that fell among the thorns is the man who hears the Word, but the worries of this life and the deceitfulness of wealth choke it,*

***making it unfruitful. But the one who received the seed that fell
on good soil is the man who hears the Word and understands it.
He produces a crop, yielding a hundred, sixty or thirty times what
was sown** (Matthew 13:18-23)."*

This entire parable reinforces the Law of Spiritual Life: he that
is faithful will receive much more than he was initially given—some
a hundred, some sixty or thirty times as much! The law is not only
"Use or Lose," it is also "Use and Gain."

A delightful story is told of the time that the artist Raphael
was painting one of his greatest pictures, the Sistine Madonna.
Raphael had almost finished his lovely portrayal of the Mother and
the Holy Child and was looking at a blank space at the bottom of
the picture. It needed something, but he could not think what to
do with it. As he pondered the problem, he heard a rustling in
the bushes outside his window. Two curly haired kids appeared.
Propping their arms on the window sill, they gazed with open-eyed
wonder at the painting and the artist. Who can resist the impulse
to watch an artist at work? Others might have been irritated at
their impudence, but Raphael seized this unexpected opportunity
and with superb skill, he painted their portraits into his picture,
capturing the look of wonder which was precisely what he wanted
for his sacred theme.

Raphael was unaware of the reason why the youngsters had
hidden in the bushes of his garden. In point of fact, they had been
up to mischief, ringing doorbells, stealing fruit, and throwing stones
at a horse until it bolted. Chased by some soldiers, they had taken
refuge in the bushes outside of the studio. Eventually, the soldiers
found the lads and began to haul them away for punishment, calling
them "young devils." Raphael intervened, saying, "You may call
them young devils, but I have made them angels forever." He then
showed the soldiers his canvas and the soldiers were so amazed
that the little rascals seized their opportunity and escaped again!

The artist who uses his talents is given more and more
opportunity to use them. The singer who develops his or her ability
to sing finds more and more open doors of opportunity to express
that gift. The truth is, when we are faithful with what God has given
us—even if the gift seems small in comparison to what someone

else may be given—the Lord will reward us beyond our imagination. God puts great emphasis on reliability and devotion to Him. Those who show God they are reliable will certainly discover that God is bountiful!

The servant who failed to use his mina and spent his time meditating on the nature of his master came to the conclusion that he was a hard man. The other servants, who used their mina and increased their value, came to know the real nature of their master, he was kind and generous! It is in taking action and in being consistent in our service for the Lord that we come to know the true nature of God. He is a God of graciousness and loving kindness, and He is a God of tremendous generosity. From the spiritual point of view, there is no doubt whatsoever that "**To everyone who has, more will be given, but as for the one who has nothing, even what he has will be taken away**." This is not a hunch, a guess, or a maybe—it is the Law of Spiritual Life!

Chapter Three

A COMMAND FOR TOMORROW

Should medical science ever discover a pill or a medicine that would be effective in dispelling anxiety and worry, it will have made a tremendous breakthrough for the health and wellbeing of mankind. Many of our most serious ailments are caused by uncontrollable apprehensions or debilitating fears concerning what we think might occur tomorrow or the next day. Many suicides, in fact, are brought on by advancing stages of depression. These periods of depression quite often center on events which may not have actually happened—they are events that are feared and are anticipated to happen in the near future. Only God knows of the pain and misery which countless individuals bring into their lives by the process of needless worry. It has become a major problem in our society in general, and more specifically, has taken on ominous dimensions with a recent turndown in our national economy. More and more people are becoming ill, suffer depression and are more suicidal in their thinking than has been the case for a long time. Hopefulness is giving way to despair, and people from all walks of life are searching for answers that might ease their burdens and lift their spirits.

The problem can be more vividly perceived by considering an illustration. What would you think, for example, of a man who decides to carry 6-7 large, brown, paper-wrapped packages with him wherever he goes, every day of the week? You would see him, perhaps, piling them into a small cart or wheel barrel before he leaves his house for work every morning. At work he piles them around his desk or his machine. When lunch time comes, back into the cart go the packages and they go with him to lunch. He puts them around his feet at the table, somewhat hindering his freedom to be at ease with those people who are eating around him. Even if he takes a bathroom break, the packages go there, too! Some times after work, he goes to a club and sits at the bar to have a few drinks so he might forget the packages he's been toting around all day. When the effects of the alcohol wear off, however, there are the ever-present packages! He dutifully picks up the packages and carries them off. To work, to town, to social events, the man is juggling and carrying all of these packages! You probably would think he was some kind of a "nut," wouldn't you?

Yet, if each of those 6-7 packages represented a burden, a worry or a problem, you might even imagine yourself as being not much different from that man! Many people carry their concerns and worries with them wherever they go, diminishing their effectiveness at their job, in their family life, even spilling over into their leisure time fun, hindering their involvement with other people and weighing them down continuously. One of the most favored weapons in Satan's arsenal to defeat the Christian is the weapon of anxiety, excessive care or worry. He uses it very effectively on even the most dedicated of God's children. Satan knows that once he can bring the Christian's frame of mind into despair, doubts may easily be implanted into his thoughts. Satan gains another victory because doubting is opposite of trusting!

You might ask yourself if you, perhaps, have been slipping into mental ruts recently, becoming obsessed or preoccupied with concerns about things on the horizon of your life. "Will the bank refinance my mortgage?" "Will my job remain secure as the company continues to downsize?" "Will we be able to afford the vacation we need so desperately?" "Will I be able to afford the tuition for finishing my schooling?" "I hope this pain is not something serious because my insurance has run out and I can't afford to go to the doctor." "Will there be enough money next month to fulfill my obligations?" The questions and concerns are endless! Simply examine your own thought processes and see if you haven't been troubled a great deal about the things of tomorrow. The unknown quantities of what might come our way or, perhaps, even of what won't come our way, tend to upset us and weigh heavily on our minds.

Jesus was fully aware of the way dreaded events and fears of the unknown become hindrances to faith and serve as stumbling blocks for the Christian. It was to address this dangerous weakness that becomes a hindrance to God's people and robs them of their confidence and joy in God that Jesus gave his disciples a brief discourse, which also contains a clear cut command for tomorrow. To set things up in your mind, I want to quote the brief discourse and it closes with the Command for Tomorrow:

"Therefore I tell you, do not worry about your life, what you will eat or drink; or about your body, what you will wear. Is not life more than food, and the body more important than clothes? Look at the birds of the air; they do not sow or reap or store away in barns, and yet your heavenly father feeds them. Are you not much more valuable than they? Who of you by worrying can add a single hour to his life?'

"And why do you worry about clothes? See how the lilies of the field grow. They do not labor or spin. Yet I tell you that not even Solomon in all his splendor was dressed like one of these. If that is how God clothes the grass of the field, which is here today and tomorrow is thrown into the fire, will he not much more clothe you, o you of little faith? So do not worry, saying 'what shall we eat?' or 'what shall we drink?' or 'what shall we wear? For the pagans run after all these things, and your heavenly Father knows that you need them. But seek first his kingdom and his righteousness, and all these things will be given to you as well. Therefore, do not worry about tomorrow, for tomorrow will worry about itself. Each day has trouble of its own (Matthew 6:25-34)."

"Take no thought for the morrow" —that is a command, and the implications for us are enormous. I would invite you to consider that when a Christian obeys this command, he eases himself away from a host of difficulties that otherwise would plague him, and he gains a healthy, happy confidence in the faithfulness and reliability of God. First, I suggest we examine the command itself, and then consider two reasons that Jesus gives for his issuing this important command.

In the first place, it is vital that a person understands a command in clearest terms if he is going to fulfill what the command requires of him. Using the military as an example, from the moment a soldier is inducted into the service, he is trained to listen to orders and follow them to the letter. If he slips up in the slightest, he will be called to task for it. This is part of military life because the soldier's very life and the lives of his buddies may someday depend on it! Leaders need to be taught how to give commands in a clear and understandable manner. This, of course, is because commands cannot be followed unless they are clearly given and easily understood by the soldier. When a soldier does not understand a command the way the giver of the command intends, the commander will not get the results he desires. We need to understand what Jesus is asking us to do in this verse of Scripture. Looking carefully, one will observe that this particular command of Christ requires both a definition and a distinction.

The definition embodies two distinct concepts: (1) "**Take no thought**," (2) "**For the morrow**." As to the first component, Jesus says "take no thought," which means "have no anxiety for tomorrow—it is not to be a worry or a burden to you today." Concerning the second component, Jesus says "the morrow." This expression can be understood in two ways: in the literal sense and the figurative sense. Literally, the morrow certainly involves the very next day—24 hours from now! Figuratively, however, in a very real sense, it encompasses the many tomorrows yet to come—even those things that lie in the more distant future. It could, in fact, pertain to all of one's life yet to come—all our futurity in this world. Indeed, the whole of our life time on earth is spoken of in the Scriptures as "**But a day** (Job 14:6)." Our childhood is the morning; our youth the afternoon; our adulthood is the evening!

You may recall the Epicureans reasoned: "*Eat, drink, and be merry, for tomorrow we die.*" They were right as to the fact that tomorrow—or, very shortly in a relative sense—they would die. But they were wrong in their implications. It should have been, "*Let us watch and pray today, we are to die tomorrow; let us labor for eternity because time is so short*!" The Epicureans could eat, drink and party their lives away because they did not believe anything follows death. Anyone who reads his Bible, however, knows for a certainty that we will all appear before the Lord in judgment following our death, and we will have to give an account of how we lived our lives on earth. Now that is a sobering thought!

Now that we've considered the definition of the command for tomorrow, it is important to see a distinction that is embodied in this command. When Jesus spoke of not having anxiety and forethought for tomorrow, he meant the THINGS of tomorrow. That is the distinction that is most important to make. Listen to his words: "***Tomorrow***," Jesus says, "***will worry about itself.***" The King James Version of the Bible phrases it: "***Take not thought for the morrow, for the morrow will take thought for the things of itself.***" In other words, we are not to suppose that the Lord wants us to ignore the duties of tomorrow—only its events.

Duty belongs to us, and there ought to be many thoughts as to how we might faithfully discharge our duty and obligations—whether to our jobs, our families, and to our God—in the days that lay before us. Our Lord is not asking for believers to have no forethought for tomorrow's duties! The events of tomorrow, however, are quite a different matter! They do not belong to us as duty does; they are entirely out of our control. To be worried over the events of tomorrow is to be concerned over those things over which we have no power to effect, either for good or for bad. We cannot determine what will or will not happen in the next day, next year or next decade! We must not, therefore, become anxious and fret ourselves concerning them. We must leave the <u>events</u> of tomorrow and thereby the events of the balance of our life on this earth, to the wisdom and discernment of God, our heavenly Father, Who rules over all. Our task, then, is to serve God today in the best way we can, and trust Him for each tomorrow He gives to us. He will provide!

Are we not to trust God with our lives? Is not this what faith is all about? If we could see the tomorrows like in a motion picture, what need would there be of faith? It is precisely because we cannot see what's in our future that we need to trust God! His command is to be not anxious about the events that shall come your way tomorrow, or at any other time in the future.

There are two reasons for this command. Using the example of the military again, when a soldier receives a command, an explanation is not required; he is simply to obey. A commander does not have to give the rhyme or reason to justify his every order. The soldier knows the commander has his reasons, and that is enough! In this case, however, our Lord senses how difficult it is to follow a command like this, so he chooses to give his reasons for issuing it. Jesus gives two reasons for why we are not to be troubled and burdened about the unknown events of tomorrow.

The first reason is explicitly stated: "(**For tomorrow will worry about itself (NIV)**," or "**For tomorrow will take care of the things of itself (KJV)**." That is to say, the events of tomorrow will come whether or not we anticipate or dread them. Furthermore, when the events of tomorrow come, we will handle them tomorrow because we cannot handle a problem until it comes upon us. We cannot change tomorrow's events, for good or for bad, so it is wrong for us to be troubled about them. Being troubled about what may come will only rob us of our strength and effectiveness for today's work and today's challenges and puts at risk the testimony we present to others concerning the Christian Life.

When Jesus says, *"Tomorrow will take care of itself,"* he means, "There is One that is quite capable of taking care of tomorrow, and He does not solicit your help or advice." When a Christian worries about things which have not yet happened, he is diverted from his present duty and is less effective in performing it. Just as having affection for anything which takes God's rightful place is called idolatry, so it is that anything detracting us from doing the will of God in the present, such as unwarranted fretting about the future, is very much wrong. It is herein condemned and forbidden by our Lord in His Command for Tomorrow.

Have you ever considered that, by erecting so many barriers such as fear or despair concerning future events, we are essentially limiting God? We are thereby making it difficult for God to impress us with His comfort and His assurance. How intolerably sinful a state it is when the soul is so filled and preoccupied with its own black thoughts, there is no room for better! Optimism cannot rule when pessimism is on the throne! What's more, these self-created clouds are so thick and dark that they resist the heavenly beams, and admit them not in the ordinary way to enter and shed their light upon our way.

A second reason for this command is implied, rather than explicitly stated. The implication is that we, as Christians, go about as living advertisements of what God is doing for us in our lives. Who would question the fact that a despairing countenance is a poor advertisement? That's why in commercials on television, the person smiles at the viewers—they don't scowl! It must be taken into account that a Christian's visible despondency is a poor witness to those who have not yet come to Christ! Any anxiety which tends to visible despondency and dejection of spirit is wrong, unless it is in the context of some tragedy or great loss for which the normal response is to grieve. Our thoughts are not always capable of being confined to the inside of our minds. It may be easily read in a person's countenance many times when that person is unduly thoughtful and depressed. Cares furrow the face and form the bearing of a person. One's looks, air, behavior and demeanor all show a thoughtful sadness. It should not be the case that a Christian's suspicions of future trouble should clothe his or her face with fear or disappointment. A fallen countenance reflects a heart that is sunk, so that we broadcast to the world that we despair of our cause and our God is no help! Is that the message we really want to give? Should our folly as believers serve to confirm the atheist in his stance? Should the Christian surrender the day to the skeptic and by countenance and demeanor proclaim to a very troubled world, THERE IS NO HELP FROM GOD?!

The fact of the matter is that our job is not to worry about what God will allow to happen, but to trust Him to do what is right! The writer of the Psalms had it right: "***Trust in the Lord and do good; dwell in the land and enjoy safe pasture. Delight yourself in the Lord and he will give you the desires of your heart*** (Psalm 37:3-4)." But far from complying with this statement of the Psalmist, many Christians are afraid that the condition of the land will be such as we shall not be able to live in it. God would rebuke such thinking! Do you think that by being anxious and apprehensive about the future, the Lord will respond and do something for you that He would not do in response to your simple faith and trust? Will worry avail more than faith? Will doubt win the heart of God while steadfast faith fails?

Actually, when all is considered, anxiety and fear is tantamount to unbelief! One's excessive care about tomorrow is an affront on God Himself, the Lord of all time, in whose hands all our times and affairs are held. Further, when we worry about the morrow, we not only do so without a call, we also do so against a prohibition. God distinctly says, **"Don't take anxious thought about the morrow."** That should be sufficient reason to quiet our minds right there! It is reckoned among men a rudeness to intrude into the affairs of another when not invited by them to do so; how much more rude is it if forbidden? It gives distaste and offense, and the reason is plain: it implies that God is not able to manage things without our help. Is God not likely to bring matters to any good state without us? Are we to look over God's shoulder, so to speak, and point out the moves He should make at every point?

It may seem ridiculous, but that's exactly what worrying about the events of tomorrow does! You see, the stress and strain of the affairs of this life do not lie upon us at all. The events that belong to tomorrow or the future time—whatever it be—will be brought about, whether we so care or care not. Our anxiety is needless in the case. Will not tomorrow come and carry all its events that belong to it, without us? This is exactly what Jesus meant when he said, **"The morrow will take care of itself."** Then Jesus adds the words, **"Each day has enough trouble of its own."** This is the second reason for taking no thought for the morrow. This is the other side of the coin. Side one says that anxiety can profit nothing; it is unable to bring about a change for the better. The reverse side of the coin says that anxiety is hurtful to us; it is more evil than we need to bear. It not only will do us no good; it is sure to do us considerable harm! This is what the Lord meant by these words.

Now, Jesus wants his followers to realize that there is enough in each day to bear as it comes along, and when excessive care and forethoughts are added, there may be enough extra cargo to overwhelm and sink us! There are four important facts about anxiety that we need to understand: anxiety multiplies suffering, it manufactures suffering, it magnifies suffering, and it misunderstands suffering. Let us consider each in turn.

In the first place, when we become anxious, it means we shall suffer the same thing over and over which we needed not to have suffered more than once, if at all. The Arabians have a proverb which states: *"An affliction is but one to him that suffers it, but to him that with fear expects it, double."* In other words, I shall be suffering the evil of tomorrow this day and tomorrow, too! What's more, this gets worse with habit, so that by this course I may bring the evil of all my future time into each passing day, and I may suffer the same afflictions a thousand times over, which God may have intended me to experience but once!

Secondly, I may by this means suffer in my own foreboding imagination many things that really I shall not suffer at all! The events may never happen which my forethoughts do suspect. What a foolish thing it is to be troubled beforehand at that, which for all I know, might never happen at all! This is nothing but self-made trouble, pure and simple, with nowhere to lay the blame except upon ourselves!

In the third place, this means that by forethought and anxiety I shall suffer hereby in a more grievous kind than if only the feared evil had actually happened to me. It is often the nature of outward evil to afflict us more severely in anticipation than in the actual experience. I've seen it happen many times, for example, that a well-intentioned nurse approaches a little child with a needle and says, "Now this may hurt." The poor child begins to scream and cry in anticipation of being inflicted with great pain. The actual puncture may prove more than a little annoying but not as terrifying as the introduction of the procedure may have engendered. How often do we find those evils in the bearing light, and to have little in them, which in our anticipation looked immense, formidable, and carried a dreadful appearance with them at a distance? What happens outwardly to a person is not nearly as devastating as the inward torture that springs from dread anticipation! It is almost inconceivable the evils we super-add to our days—beyond that which the Lord counts sufficient. Neither do we design our own good in the process as He does when he afflicts.

Fourthly, are we not also to consider that God establishes His laws in mercy to be for our own good? It is always the case that when we keep God's law, there is great reward. The Lord knows what trouble we would have by needless worry. It is, therefore, out of love and kindness that He forbids us to be anxious and fretful about tomorrow! Anxiety misunderstands suffering. When we become anxious about things that might happen we forget that God sometimes brings adversity in order to do a good work in us. Perhaps, it is to teach us patience. Perhaps, it is to melt our heart of stone so we can become more compassionate toward others. Perhaps, it is to destroy our pride and make us to be truly humble before the Lord. Perhaps, it is intended to strengthen our faith. If only we had a better understanding of the fact that troubles sometimes come as gifts of god to strengthen and perfect us, we would not worry and rebel at the unknown things of tomorrow! We could more easily walk with our hand in God's and trust in Him for keeping us safe each step of our way.

Consider the tenderness of God toward each of His children by noticing how many times He has given His injunctions against carrying the burden of needless care. The Apostle Peter writes in his epistle, "*Cast all your anxiety on him because he cares for you* (I Peter 5:7)." The Apostle Paul writes to the church at Philippi, "*Do not be anxious about anything, but in everything, by prayer and petition, with thanksgiving, present your requests to God. And the peace of God, which transcends all understanding, will guard your hearts and your minds in Christ Jesus* (Philippians 4:6-7)." Imagine that! By trusting in God for the outcome of all things, he will guard our hearts and our minds! Could worry or anxiety ever compare with those results? Finally, the Psalmist states, "*Commit your way to the Lord; trust in him and he will do this: He will make your righteousness shine like the dawn, the justice of your cause like the noonday sun* (Psalm 37:5-6)." My friends, if we neglect and disregard the Lord in these commands, we shall bring an evil into today that neither belongs to this day, nor to any other!

As we began this study, we saw that the Lord gives a command: "**Do not worry about tomorrow**." The response of every Christian should be that of ready obedience. To worry is sin! We would do well to strive at being in the temper of our spirits more indifferent about all future events that lie within the compass of time. Time will soon be over. Eternity should be the more vital concern.

The more important question does not concern tomorrow; it concerns our readiness to face God! Every person would do well to ask the most important question of one's life: "Am I prepared for facing God?" If a person is not certain of having received God's Son, the Lord Jesus Christ, as his or her personal Savior from sin— that person is definitely not ready to meet God! That person would be lost in sins and would never see the inside of God's heaven until turning to Jesus, and asking Him to become both Savior and Lord.

Additionally, it must also be acknowledged that every devout Christian, who loves and fears God, will be so taken up with devotion to Christ that he will have little cause to concern himself with passing events, which as to his part in the world to come, will not in any way alter the case. We are not more sure of heaven, or less sure, whatever the events of tomorrow! It must be remembered that anxiety does Satan's work. It always has a bad effect upon your life. Anxiety multiplies suffering. Anxiety manufactures suffering. Anxiety magnifies suffering. Anxiety misunderstands suffering. Someone has wisely coined a proverb, which we all would do well to memorize: "*be anxious for nothing, prayerful for everything, and thankful for anything.*"

The sum of the matter can be subsumed in this: Do not worry about tomorrow; instead, be much in prayer that this day shall find you zealous and true to your calling as a Christian—a child of God. Take each day in turn, as God sends it. Live one day at a time. There is a sweet serenity in trusting God in all things. Perhaps, we could learn to appropriate the attitude of the Psalmist who said, "**This is the day the Lord has made; let us rejoice and be glad in it** (Psalm 118:24)."

CHAPTER FOUR

PLACID TRUST IN GOD

For many, many, years people from every corner of the world have been drawing life-healing power and magnificent comfort from the 23rd Psalm, and it's not without good reason that this brief Psalm of David has been prized by millions of people and is recognized as one of the most precious passages of the entire Bible. A careful study of this Psalm will reveal just why this is so. Meditating on the words from this Psalm for a sufficient time will allow its dynamic truths to doctor your soul!

Ralph Waldo Emerson said, "*A man is what he thinks about all day long.*" Marcus Aurelius said, "*A man's life is what his thoughts make it.*" Norman Vincent Peale maintained, "*Change your thoughts and you change your world.*" The 23rd Psalm is a pattern of thinking, and when a person's mind becomes saturated with it, a new way of thinking and a new life are the result. It contains only 118 words. One could memorize it in a short period of time. The power of this Psalm lies in the fact that it represents a positive, hopeful, confident, and faith approach to life.

At the beginning of this Psalm, David introduces us to the person whom he calls his shepherd. He is the very best there is! David says, "**The Lord is my shepherd**." Who is the Lord? What do you think of when you consider the word, "Lord?" The word refers to the person holding the highest position of authority, the One who is ultimately in charge, the Sovereign. In European history, the Feudal System dominated for centuries. In that system, the king would be the sovereign and every subordinate would be his vassal or subject. The king was the owner of all the land in the kingdom and he would divide the land into fiefs and appoint a nobleman, possibly a family member, relative or friend to be the Lord over the fiefdom and would supply him with a manor. Each Lord swore allegiance to the King and provided one knight to the king. Also, the Lord of the manor sublet portions of his land to vassals, called Villeins. They managed but did not own the land. Under the villeins were the serfs, who were people of the working class, who could never own land but worked for the lord. As you can imagine, from this system there is enormous distance between the serf working for the lord of the manor and the King, who ruled over all the lords in the kingdom. It was a class system – the King at the top and the serf on the bottom. The livelihood of the serf depended on the villein. The fate of the villein rested in the hands of his lord. And the lord took his marching orders from the King. Yet, in this opening verse of the 23rd Psalm everything is in reverse! David, the serf, so to speak, identifies the King as his shepherd!

There is a very special relationship between David and his God, metaphorically similar to the special relationship between the sheep and the shepherd. In Biblical times, sheep were very valuable to the person who owned them. Well cared-for sheep would provide wool, meat, milk and cheese. One could derive a bountiful income from a well-managed flock of sheep. On the other hand, this result never comes easily because the sheep require constant attention and supervision in order for them to survive. They could not even survive if left on their own. The sheep would not be able to find the pastures on which to graze for their food because their eyesight is very limited.

They don't have a sense of direction that would keep them from wandering and getting lost. They require water to drink on a daily basis. They don't have the sense to lie down on their own so that they can digest the grass on which they have been grazing. Consequently, they could become very ill and die from undigested food. They have no physical defenses by which they can defend themselves from beasts of prey. They cannot outrun even the smallest of predators! You might say they are like "sitting ducks" out there on the field.

The optimal arrangement, as you can imagine, is for the owner of the sheep to be the shepherd of the sheep himself. This is seldom possible, however. The owner entrusts the sheep to a person he hires to do the job. Persons of character and integrity, who also happen to have a loving concern for the wellbeing of animals, might make good shepherds, indeed. Some, however, are in the job for the money it pays and do not really care for the sheep. They are known to bolt in the face of danger and will abandon the sheep to their fate. Not only are they unreliable in the face of danger, they will not put themselves out to make any extra effort to rescue a stray sheep or nurture a sick or wounded animal to health. Why should he care? He knows the loss will not be his, but the owner's loss.

I could not explain the issue any better than the picture that is given in the 34th chapter of the prophet Ezekiel. Here the matter is revealed with utmost clarity. In this chapter, the nation of Israel is depicted as sheep and the leaders of the nation are the shepherds. Here we have examples of bad or corrupt shepherds. Like a prosecuting attorney in a court of law, the Lord states the case against the shepherds of Israel: *"**The word of the Lord came to me: Son of Man, prophesy against the shepherds of Israel; prophesy and say to them: 'This is what the sovereign Lord says; woe to the shepherds of Israel who only take care of themselves! Should not shepherds take care of the flock? You eat the curds, clothe yourselves with the wool and slaughter the choice animals, but you do not take care of the flock. You have not strengthened the weak or healed the sick or bound up the injured. You have not brought back the strays or searched for the lost. You have ruled them harshly and brutally. So they were scattered because there was no shepherd, and when they were scattered they became food for all the wild animals. My sheep wandered over all the mountains and on every high hill. They were scattered over the whole earth and no one searched or looked for them** (Ezekiel 34:1-6)."*

Following this description of the bad shepherds that have ruled over Israel, the Lord reveals in the last part of Ezekiel 33 how the job of shepherding with loving devotion to the sheep would be done when the Lord, Himself, would take over the job in order to rescue the sheep from their fate. He says, for example, *"**I myself*** *will search for my sheep and look after them* (Ezekiel 33:11)." He goes on to describe other caring behaviors he will lavish upon the sheep: "*As a shepherd looks after his scattered flock when he is with them, so will I look after my sheep. I will rescue them from all the places where they were scattered on a day of clouds and darkness, I will bring them out from the nations and gather them from the countries and bring them into their own land. I will pasture them in a good pasture, and the mountain heights of Israel will be their grazing land. There they will lie down in good grazing land, and there they will feed in a rich pasture on the mountains of Israel. I myself will tend my sheep and have them lie down, declares the sovereign Lord. I will search for the lost and bring back the strays. I will bind up the injured and strengthen the weak, but the sleek and the strong I will destroy. I will shepherd the flock with justice* (Ezekiel 33:12-16)."

This is a picture of a perfect shepherd, who is the Lord, Himself! In this chapter we see the Lord shepherding the <u>nation</u>. We get the perspective of the entire flock in the care of the Shepherd. To get a perspective on the <u>individual</u> sheep in relation to his care-giver and protector, we need to turn to a study of the 23rd Psalm. This is called the Shepherd Psalm. For many, many years, people from every corner of the world have been drawing life-healing power and magnificent comfort from the 23rd Psalm, and it's not without good reason that this brief Psalm of David has been prized by millions of people and is recognized as one of the most precious and the most quoted passages of the entire Bible. There is life-healing power in this brief Psalm. The power, however, is not in just the words, but in thinking the thoughts. This Psalm should be read as though you were giving your own personal testimony, because that is exactly how David wrote it. It was his testimony of his relationship with his God.

At the beginning of this Psalm, David introduces us to the person who is his shepherd. He said his shepherd is the Lord. Who is the Lord? A good description of the Lord can be seen in the Apostle Paul's first letter to Timothy: "*I charge you to keep this command without spot or blame until the appearing of our Lord Jesus Christ, which God will bring about in his own time—God, the blessed and only ruler, the King of Kings and Lord of Lords, Who alone is immortal, and who lives in unapproachable light, whom no one has seen or can see. To Him be honor and might forever. Amen* (I Timothy 6:14--16)." As you can see, the Lord is called "the King of Kings and Lord of Lords!" He is the Omniscient, Omnipresent, Omnipotent and Immutable Supreme Being! Therefore, it follows all logic for David to announce, *"The Lord is my shepherd, I shall not be in want"* or *"I will have everything I need."* The Omniscience of God means He's all-knowing; I cannot have a problem, difficulty or need about which He does not know. The Omnipresence of God means He's everywhere; I cannot stray to where He cannot reach me or become lost to where He cannot find me. The Omnipotence of God means He is all-powerful; I cannot have any problem that would pose an insurmountable obstacle for Him. The Immutability of God means He can never change; I can rest assured that all that He has been to me in the past and is to me in the present, will also be the case in all my future days. He is the same yesterday, today and forever. He is indeed, an awesome Shepherd!

If anyone other than the Lord were my shepherd, I could suffer the loss or omission of some things I might need. My mother was loving, self-sacrificing and devoted to her children. She bore eight of us into this world—actually she bore nine, but one of my brothers had a twin who died at birth. My mother cooked, sewed, washed, dried and ironed our clothes, nursed and doctored us through illnesses. She comforted us in distress. She set a moral example and taught us skills that would enable us to become self-sufficient. When times were hard and there might not be coal in the cellar to keep the furnace going in the frigid New England winters and when food was scarce in the pantry and in the refrigerator, she got a job outside the home. She got up before sunrise, rode a bus across town and sewed in a factory to bring money home to provide those essentials. My mother was a good shepherd, but she had limitations. She could become ill herself. She could pray for a drought to end but she could not end it. If an intruder should break into our house while we slept at night, she could have been at risk as much as we. She would attempt to give her children everything they need, but there's a chance she could not deliver on her intentions. There were times we needed outside help. Perhaps it would be a doctor who had knowledge my mother did not possess, or a medicine that would control a life-threatening fever and drive it from my body when I was at death's door. Nor could she protect me from an automobile crash I had when I journeyed away from home to work. She could not save me from the perils of a war in a distant land to which I was taken as a soldier in the United States Army.

If loving me was enough, she being my shepherd would certainly suffice. But I could suffer loss. I could die of hunger or I could be lost in a wilderness and at mercy to the elements in their utmost ferocity and she could do nothing to rescue or protect me. Who on earth COULD provide for my every need in every contingency? The answer, of course, is NO ONE! But when I think of the one Being Who transcends all of nature, Who commands even the winds to cease and Who orders the waves of the sea to be still, I am comforted.

And there are historical examples of His sovereign power let loose to give His people everything they need. The Pharaoh of Egypt did everything his might and power could muster to keep Israel in bondage, but by God's miraculous and mighty hand the entire nation was safely delivered from his grasp. Even the Red Sea was parted so the nation could pass on dry land. In the wilderness, long before the invention of GPS systems, God led his people at night with a pillar of fire and by day with a pillar of clouds. When there was no water in the barren wilderness to drink, He commanded Moses to strike his rod against a rock and out poured all the water they needed. When there was no food to be found, God provided manna from heaven for everyone to eat.

Consider the wedding feast in Cana of Galilee, when the wine was insufficient for the needs of the guests. The Lord changed cisterns of water into cisterns of wine (John 2:1-11). When later, 5,000 souls had followed him into the wilderness, hanging on his every word of knowledge and wisdom they were all fed with 5 loaves and 2 small fish (Matthew 14:15-21). The lame were enabled to walk, the blind were given their sight and the sick were healed. Even the dead were raised to life again by His almighty power! See

Mark 5:22-24, 38-42; Luke 7:11-15; John 11:1-44. In fact, after He laid down His own life in death on Calvary's cross to deliver us from the consequences of our sins, even death could not hold him. On the third day, He arose and left the sealed tomb by the power of His Father in heaven! Could anyone having such a One as his personal shepherd have any concerns for which the Shepherd could not provide? That, my friends, is the grand rhetorical question of all time! No!! Because the LORD is my shepherd, I will have everything I need. *"The Lord is my shepherd....I will not be in want."* Could anything be more comforting and reassuring than this?

The opening sentence of this Psalm states a proposition which the rest of the Psalm will substantiate. The proposition is *"I shall not be in want "* or, *"I shall have everything I need."* The first need mentioned, is the need for rest. The human body is not like the Energizer Bunny that can keep on going without stopping. Many people live life at a relentless pace and scarcely slow down for anything. We are a revolving door society. It used to take hours to prepare a meal; but now some folks get impatient waiting for food to cook 3 minutes in a microwave oven! For many, they never stop until circumstances or illness puts them on their backs in bed at home or in the hospital ward. At such times, they are made to lie down! David says of the shepherd, *"He makes me lie down."* Can you recall a time when you were made to lie down? For me, it was coronary bypass surgery and kidney failure that followed. For my wife, it was when all treatment for cancer failed to cure her and she spent the last 4 months of her life in hospice care. Neither I nor my wife chose to lie down for so long a time; our illnesses required it.

It's important to notice where the Lord makes the sheep to lie down. David said *"He makes me lie down in green pastures."* Think about this: if I were to lie down in brown, dried up pastures where there would be nothing to eat when I got up, I might be worried and would not be able to rest. But, if the environment on which I depend for my food is green and verdant, my rest is certain. As a sheep, I am lying right on the green grass on which I can graze at leisure when I rise up to eat. Not only are the pastures sufficient to nourish my hunger, the shepherd doesn't leave it up to me to decide if I will rest or not. He knows when I need to rest, even if I might be thinking I could toil on longer. So he does not give me a choice: He makes me lie down.

Can you think of a commandment God gave to Israel that concerned their need for rest? You may recall that God gave Israel a command: *"Remember the Sabbath day, to keep it holy."* The Sabbath was the seventh day. God told Israel: every 7th day, stop your work; lie down! The commandment for the Sabbath was not for God's benefit; it was for man's benefit. Scientists long ago discovered that the biological and physiological needs of the human body require, for optimum performance and efficiency, one day's rest in a cycle of seven! Could it be just a coincidence that the scientific study determined the ideal cycle to be one day in seven instead of one in five or one in nine or ten? Not trusting man to have the wisdom or even the due regard for his own needs to take proper steps to secure periodic rest, God issued a command to guarantee it! He makes me to lie down.

We all need to draw apart for physical renewal and we need to do it for spiritual refreshment. It is in the quiet place that our souls are free to commune with God. The prophet Elijah found God, not in the earthquake or the fire, but in *"A still small voice."* Moses saw the burning bush when he was out on the hill side. Saul of Tarsus was on the lonely, quiet road to Damascus when he saw the heavenly vision that transformed his life. Jesus, Himself, took time apart to pray and commune with His Father in heaven. If you are not making time in your life for rest, reflection and prayer, your schedule needs revamping!

Again, the opening proposition of this psalm is *"The Lord is my shepherd, I will have no want,"* or, *"I will have everything I need."* I need periodic rest: *"He makes me lie down in green pastures."* Secondly, I have need of water to survive. If we all had to go without water to drink, we would all die in a VERY short time! This is so of man and it is so of sheep. In response to this need for life-sustaining water, *"He leads me beside the quiet waters."* I need water to drink, but don't lead me to Niagara Falls for my water. I could not muster the courage to attempt a drink from that powerful surge of water. Let me drink my water from a little fountain or from a glass tumbler! I am not fearful to drink from those sources.

The sheep will not attempt to drink from swiftly moving current. Instinctively, the sheep has a fear of rapidly moving water because the sheep knows it could lose its footing and fall into the water. This would be disastrous because the heavy coat of wool would become drenched and weigh the sheep down so heavily, it would not be able to get out of the water to safety. The sheep would die of thirst before it would drink from rushing waters. The shepherd knows this need of the sheep for still water, so he is constantly surveying the territory for quiet waters from which the sheep will be able to drink. If no quiet waters are obtainable, the shepherd will use rocks to fashion a little dam in the stream to create a quiet pool of water from which the sheep will drink. Sometimes, the shepherd would carry with him an empty pail so that he would be ready to scoop up water from a rushing stream and offer it to even the tiniest lamb to drink in peace and without fear.

This phrase from the 23rd Psalm speaks to us in an area of our deepest need—God accommodates to those concerns that make us most afraid! God will never make you to do what you fear to do. He will not laugh at your fears. He will not force you to confront your fears. He is your shepherd; He will take account of your fears and will deal with you accordingly. God knows our limitations and He does not condemn us for having weaknesses or fears. He does not force us where we feel we cannot safely go. God never demands of us work which is beyond our strength or abilities. Instead, God is constantly ministering to our needs. He understands the load you carry on your shoulders. He also knows where the places of nourishment and refreshment are located. It gives one confidence and assurance to know that, even while we may be sleeping, the shepherd is working to provide for tomorrow. Is there some paralyzing fear that you may have to deal with? Could you bring it to the Lord? Be assured He will go gently with you regarding your fear.

I can remember a time when I was serving as Family Life Chaplain at the Presidio of San Francisco—a job that involved a lot of individual and family counseling. On one occasion a female soldier revealed in a counseling session that she could never walk into a cemetery. She had lost her mother as a little girl and was made to go into the cemetery for the burial and the experience had traumatized her for life. Now that she was in the Army she was serving in a unit that on occasion had to pull duty providing honors at funerals and at the cemetery. She could not perform that duty and it jeopardized her career. As it happened, the chapel at the Presidio is situated adjacent to the Presidio National Cemetery. I explained to my client that I would help her to overcome her fear and resorted to a technique called "systematic desensitization." This involved walking her outside of the chapel and escorting her over to the side of the cemetery where there was a 2 foot high stone wall surrounding it. At first, just standing there and looking at the cemetery made this woman tremble and stiffen with fear and terror. By holding her by one elbow, I gently asked if she could at least put out her other hand and stretch it out over the wall and into the space of the cemetery. She did this, and began to cry, pulling back her hand. We went back inside and processed her experience. Each succeeding session involved a repeat of this behavior, each time adding a little more exposure to the cemetery itself. Finally, the day came when she was able to put one foot into the cemetery and then step back out. Feeling supported, or shepherded, if you please, this client was eventually able to overcome all her fear of the cemetery and could go in and out and walk in the cemetery! The transformation was beautiful to behold. It could not have been achieved without patience and gentleness. How like David's confidence: "*He leads me beside the quiet waters.*"

The first two areas of need are those that occur on a daily basis: the need for rest and the need for water. The third area of need is not on a daily basis but occurs on occasion when emotional and spiritual energy has become drained and depleted by the rigors, stress and disappointments of life. The mind of a person can be wounded just as the body can be wounded. In fact, mental wounds are harder to treat and take longer to heal than do the most usual physical injuries and wounds of the body. Some people, consequently, end up in psychotherapy treatment because they have become addicted to mutilating their own body with the mistaken belief that the physical pain will divert their minds from their internal mental anguish stemming from some traumatic experiences of their life. When the soul is injured, the cure is difficult to find. Many a drug or alcohol addicted person is a person whose soul has been injured by life experiences. Others, wounded in mind and spirit, have turned to a life of crime and have met untimely deaths or are residing in one of our penitentiaries or prisons. Some don't become casualties like others, but they are the walking wounded or the depressed. Like a squeezed lemon, they have lost their juice for living and are harboring a wounded, dying soul inside their body. Life can inflict pain. Life can hurt. There are enormous losses with which we must deal at some point in our life. What then is our need? It is a need for restoration. David exclaimed in this Psalm, *"**He restores my soul**."*

I remember vividly another client I had when I was Family Life Chaplain at the Presidio of San Francisco. A retired soldier came one day to get counseling because his wife had decided to leave him and she was taking the children with her. His wife was leaving him, I soon learned, because he had become a hopeless alcoholic. She kept telling him she could not handle his drunkenness and bad behavior and his many attempts to get a cure for his addiction always met with failure. He kept returning to his drinking. Now he was facing the loss of his marriage but even that could not cure him. Then, in one counseling session, I felt like I was searching in vain for the missing piece of the puzzle until a thought came into my mind-- as though put there by God Himself. I asked the man, "What did you do when you were in the Army?" He answered, "I flew helicopters." Estimating his age, I asked, "Were you in Vietnam by any chance?" "Yes," he answered, "I was a dust-off pilot." I knew immediately what that meant. A dust-off pilot would fly a Huey helicopter that came in to battle scenes to extract the wounded and carry them off to field hospitals where they could receive life-saving treatment. I was in Vietnam in 1968, which was the year of the Tet Offensive, and I witnessed the brave work of the dust-off pilots of the 1st Air Cavalry Division to which our Artillery Battalion was assigned. To me this man was a hero, but I sensed he did not see himself that way. I commented, "That must have been very difficult for you." At that simple word of understanding, the man bent over, buried his face in his hands and cried like a baby for about 5 minutes. I just let him cry because it was allowing him to release the poison within his soul.

When he was able to talk, I encouraged him to tell me what bothered him most. He began to tell of the times he was sent on a mission to extract the wounded. He could see from the air that they were still under enemy fire and he was ordered to turn back because the commander could not risk losing another helicopter and its crew. He felt guilty because he was "abandoning men to their death." He took no consolation in the hundreds of soldiers he successfully rescued and whose lives he saved. He only tortured himself over those he could not save! Now we had a focus for our counseling sessions. We worked on the realities of the situation. We considered what might have been his alternative options and what might have been the consequences. When all was said and done, this man was able to forgive himself for being human and for not being God. When that breakthrough occurred, he was no longer addicted to alcohol! His soul was restored. He was sick and guilty no longer. He was a different man! He would understand completely what David must have felt when he affirmed, "**He restores my soul**."

Is there a burden which you have been carrying that has been depressing you and depleting your vitality for life? Rather than trying to hide it away and live with the consequences, why not bring it to the shepherd of your life, and ask Him to restore your soul? The Bible says, "**If we confess our sins, He is faithful and just and will forgive us our sins and purify us from all unrighteousness** (I John 1:9)."

My shepherd will supply all that I need. I need periodic rest—"**He makes me lie down in green pastures**." I need water from sources I do not fear—"**He leads me beside the quiet waters**." At times, my soul needs restoration—"**He restores my soul**." A fourth need I have is to receive guidance when facing life's major decisions. David's answer to this is to state, "**He leads me in paths of righteousness for His name's sake**." On a plaque at Florida's Singing Tower you can read these words, "*I come here to find myself. It is so easy to get lost in this world*." How true this is! We come to junctures in life's journey and we often cannot decide which way to turn. The company you work for may be trying to downsize its work force and is offering early retirement buy-outs. You may be wondering if you should stay with the job you have or, because of ominous indicators on the horizon, perhaps resign your job now and get started in another job or in a different career field altogether. Should you sell your house or should you keep it and rent it out? Should you marry that person now, or wait until later? Should you continue suffering abuse from a partner or should you leave the relationship? The decisions of life are endless aren't they? A wrong turn at any point or an ill-considered decision could lead us down a strange path and we can become lost. We can become lost in selfish pursuits and wasteful living, also. Temptation feeds on loneliness, and if we are not careful, we can abandon our life-long values and indulge in practices that can ruin life completely and destroy what we have worked for all through the years!

Always there are decisions to be made and yet it is often difficult to decide what is best. We do get lost. We could use wise counsel and guidance at such times. David took counsel in the Lord. Confidently, he declares, "***He leads me in paths of righteousness,***" ***or, "in the right paths***." Doubtless, David remembered his own experiences in his profession as a shepherd. He knew that sheep have no sense of direction. A dog, cat, horse or other pet animal may become lost and still find its way home. They seem to have a compass within them. This is not the case with sheep, however. The sheep has very poor eyesight. It cannot see more than ten to fifteen yards ahead. Palestinian fields were covered with narrow paths over which the shepherds would lead their sheep to pasture. Some of these paths led to a precipice over which the sheep might plunge to its death. Other paths led to a blind alley, so to speak. But still other paths led to green and fertile pastures and refreshing still waters. The sheep get there by following the shepherd, knowing it is walking the right path. The paths were often steep and difficult, but by following the shepherd the sheep knew he would always end up somewhere good. The sheep is willing to trust the "somewhere" to the judgment of the shepherd. The hymn writer has captured this same thought in these words: "*Lord, I would place my hand in Thine, nor ever murmur nor repine; content whatever lot I see,* *since 'tis my God that leadeth me*." Perhaps David remembered his ancestors as they made their way across a trackless wilderness during their journey from Egypt to the Promised Land. God on that occasion sent a pillar of fire to lead them by night and a pillar of cloud to lead them by day. By following God's divine leading, the Israelites came to the land for which they yearned.

Your path way may not be easy at times. There may not be easy comfort or success to attend your way. There may even be outright hardship, deprivation, resistance or suffering. But, the shepherd of our souls promises us strength for every contingency, and what's more, He promises to accompany us in partnership along our way. He promises never to leave us or to forsake us. His words are like music to the ear: "***My grace is sufficient for you, for My power is made perfect in weakness*** (2 Corinthians 12:9)."

You will notice the Psalm says, "***He leads me***." God does not push or drive us. He does not force us. He leads us. He is climbing the same hill that we are climbing and makes sure we are not alone. If we could take life like we walk—taking one step at a time, we can walk with God and follow the right paths. Solomon in his wisdom said, "***In all your ways acknowledge Him and He will direct your paths*** (Proverbs 3:6)." That's a tremendous promise to claim! The person who sincerely seeks to do God's will in his life, whatever His will may be, will know the leading of eternal wisdom and unfailing goodness. God the shepherd will lead you to your promised land!

A fifth need I have is to have peace in the face of grieving over great loss. David said:

"***Even though I walk through the valley of the shadow of death, I will fear no evil, for You are with me***." There is a story about a mother during World War II who collapsed when news came to her that her son had been killed in battle. She went to her room, closed the door and refused to see any one. The minister of her church eventually came and she allowed him into the room but she continued to remain in bed and would not speak. For a little while all was quiet as the two just sat there. Slowly, the minister began saying the words, "***The Lord is my shepherd, I shall not want***..." Phrase after phrase, he gently spoke the words of the 23rd Psalm and the woman listened. When he came to that great phrase of comfort, she joined in and together they said, "***Even though I walk through the valley of the shadow of death, I will fear no evil, for You are with me***." A smile flickered on her lips, and she said, "I see it differently, now." Sometimes these words are directed to the person who himself is passing through illness, danger, peril or impending death and is afraid of the unknown. At other times, these words are directed to the loved one who is in danger of losing the loved one who is at death's door and is afraid to go on without him or her. In either case, these words of comfort are incomparable words in any language, for what could be more assuring than to hear from almighty God—the maker of heaven and earth, and the giver and sustainer of all of life, and the author of life eternal: "***Fear not, for I am with you***!"

Henry Ward Beecher said the 23rd Psalm is the Nightingale of the Psalms. The Nightingale sings its sweetest when the night is darkest. For most of us, death is the most terrifying fact of life! Of course, "***The valley of the shadow of death***" refers to more than the actual experiences of physical death. This phrase has been translated, "***The glen of gloom***." It might refer to every hard and terrifying experience of life. There is an actual valley of the shadow of death in Palestine. It leads from Jerusalem to the Dead Sea and is a very narrow and dangerous pathway through the mountain range. The path is rough and there is danger that a sheep may fall at any moment to its death. It is a forbidding journey that one dreads to take. The sheep is unafraid, however, because its only concern is to keep the shepherd in sight and follow him! There are dark and forbidding places in life through which circumstances compel us to pass, also. Death is certainly one of them. Disappointment can be another. Loneliness is another. There are many more.

I know what the valley of the shadow of death is like. I lived there for twelve months! My valley was a tour of duty in the Republic of Vietnam from February 1968 to February 1969. I was sent there as a U.S. Army chaplain, assigned to the 6th Battalion of the 33rd Field Artillery, 105 mm towed howitzers. This was my first experience with combat operations. We were deployed from Long Beach, California on a troop transport ship, the USS UPSHUR, and the advance party was setting up our base camp at Bear Cat, in II Corps, Vietnam. But while we were in the Indian Ocean, the North Vietnamese Army launched their TET offensive that devastated cities in the northern part of South Vietnam. Our ship was sent a message changing our destination from Bear Cat to Da Nang, because of the fierce fighting there. It was like an old John Wayne war movie when we disembarked the ship, climbing over the side, down rope netting, into LSTs that would deliver us to the beach. Fires were burning and shells exploding on the land right in the direction we were being delivered to the beach. Once we were ashore, we were rushed into cattle cars that took us through the city of Da Nang to Camp Books where the 3rd Marines were headquartered. The Marines put us in a tent city in the middle of their camp, but right under the radio tower that flashed a red light all night. The enemy honed in on the tower and sent in their rockets our first night in country and we dove into bunkers we had dug that afternoon, scared for dear life!

This was just the beginning of my walk through the valley of the shadow of death. I lived in a hole in the ground every night for the first 6 months in the country at our base camp on Landing Zone Sharon, in Quang Tri Province. We came under attack day and night nearly every day of the year. Our three firing batteries, Alpha, Beta and Charlie were deployed to strategic locations all over I Corps and my job was to travel by jeep with my driver to visit the troops and bring them moral and spiritual encouragement. I did not carry a weapon. My driver carried an M-16, but he was driving! At first, I was frightened and terrified every time we hit the road, fearing every pot hole might be concealing a land mine the enemy was fond of planting. Or, I trembled at the dense shrubs and growth that bordered the road, fearing the presence of an enemy sniper who might zap me as I sat there in my open jeep. I was tense, nervous and stressed. It was utterly exhausting. About the third day out, I began to have a chat with myself. I said, "Roger, you are a chaplain. The troops are looking to you for leadership and for setting an example of placing faith in God!" I bowed my head and prayed to God, asking Him to forgive me for my fears and I told Him that no matter what may happen, I was going to relax and trust in Him. If God wanted me to die in that war, I prayed, there's nothing

I can do about it. On the other hand, if God wants me to make it through unscathed, there's no power on earth that can harm me. For the rest of my tour of duty I had peace of mind. I lived, slept and worked in the valley of the shadow of death, but I did not fear evil because the shepherd of my soul was with me.

One important thing to do when going through your "valley of the shadow" is to get yourself apart to a quiet place. Give up the struggling. Forget the many details. Put your mind in idle, or shift into neutral. Stop trying to hurry on to the morrow, the next year or beyond. Just stop. In your quietness and in your "Glen of Gloom" you can discover a strange and powerful presence that you may never have felt before. By God's grace, you can feel the same power and comfort that many, many others have testified about, like hearing the Nightingale singing in the darkness. The keynote of the 23rd Psalm is the phrase *"For you are with me."* These words appear right in the very center of the Psalm: there are 58 words before them and 56 words after them! In the pastures of life, at the still waters, on the right paths, through the valley of the shadow of death, He is with me!! Wherever my pathway takes me, I will not be afraid, said David. He is not afraid of the unknown because he knows the shepherd and he knows He is with him. There is power and there is healing in His presence!

A sixth need I have is to be protected from dangers beyond my control. David affirmed, *"Your rod and your staff, they comfort me."* I heard of a man who was injured badly in a cyclone. From then on, much of the joy of life was gone from his life—not because of his injury—but because he was afraid that another cyclone might come. There was nothing he could do. He worried because there was still nothing he would be able to do if he saw another cyclone coming. This all changed for him one day, however, when his thoughtful children decided to build a cyclone cellar for the house. They completed the cellar and took their father to examine it. He looked at it with relaxed joy because he now realized he had protection should another cyclone come his way. It was a great comfort to him. In the 23rd Psalm we read, *"Your rod and your staff, they comfort me."* The sheep is a helpless animal. It has no weapon with which to fight for its survival. It is easy prey to any wild beast or predator of the field. It is afraid of being harmed. But the shepherd carried a rod, which was a heavy, hard, wooden club that usually was two to three feet in length. When David wrote this Psalm he probably remembered his own need for such a rod when tending his sheep. In I Samuel, chapter 17, David told Saul that he killed a lion and a bear in protecting his sheep. He did this with the shepherd's rod. The shepherd carried a staff, also, which was about eight feet long. The end of the staff was turned into a crook. Many paths in Palestine were along steep mountain sides. The sheep could lose footing and slide down the slopes or end up stranded on some ledge below. With his long staff, the shepherd could reach down, place the crook over the small chest of the sheep and lift it back up on to the pathway. The sheep instinctively is comforted by the sight of the shepherd's rod and his staff. They are visual symbols that the shepherd is prepared to meet any emergency to rescue and preserve them.

I have insurance on my automobile. I am not hoping for an accident to happen someday, but I am comforted by the fact of having it should it be needed. I regret my country has to spend so much money on military preparedness. Yet, when I see the condition of the world in which we live, my country's military might is, to a degree, somewhat comforting. There are needs in my life that I cannot meet by myself and, like St. Paul it comforts me to say, *"He is able to do immeasurably more than all we ask or imagine, according to the power that is at work within us* (Ephesians 3:20)." Seemingly, there is overwhelming evil in the world. We are a scared society. Many times we feel completely helpless to alter our circumstances. At such times we can find comfort in realizing anew the awesome power of God. Certainly, I don't think of God as being a cyclone cellar for emergency situations, or as an insurance policy for dealing with unforeseen disaster. Yet, I can say with James Montgomery who penned the words, *"God is my salvation: What foe have I to fear? In darkness and temptation, my Light, my Helper is near: Though hosts encamp around me, firm in the fight I stand, what terror can confound me, with God at my right hand?"* How much like David, who said, *"Your rod and your staff, they comfort me.*" These words take all of the dread and fear concerning the future out of my heart!

In the seventh place, I need peace of mind from the hidden dangers of life. David adds: *"**You prepare a table before me in the presence of my enemies**.*" Many years ago I was astounded to read in the paper one day that the State of Oklahoma had just passed a law forbidding the sale of alcohol to anyone under the age of forty! Of course, such a decision by a state legislature set quite a precedent and caused shock and uproar from many quarters. My own initial reaction was of dumbfounded surprise. I asked myself, "How do they ever expect to be able to enforce such a law?" I thought the Oklahoma law makers were being a little ridiculous! The more I reflected on this really courageous decision, however, I began to appreciate the motivation for their decision, at least. They were concerned for the wellbeing of their communities, families and their young people. While one method is to try to keep the youth from the bars and taverns, it seemed to the legislature to be easier and safer to significantly elevate the age for being legally able to purchase alcohol in hopes that it would succeed in keeping the alcohol from the youth. It sort of illustrates what David meant in the 23rd Psalm when he said, "***You prepare a table before me in the presence of my enemies**.*"

In the pastures of the Holy Land grew poisonous plants which were fatal fodder to sheep if eaten by them. Also, there were plants in abundance whose sharp thorns would penetrate the soft noses of the sheep and cause ugly and painful sores. Each spring time, therefore, the shepherd would take his mattock and dig out these enemies of the sheep as he walked the pastures, piling them up and later burning them. The shepherd was assuring that the pastures into which he would be leading the sheep would be a safe place for them to graze. The pasture became, as it were, a table prepared for the sheep. The present enemies of the sheep were extracted and destroyed.

We constantly must do this for our children. When children walk to school, a policeman or street corner guard stands at intersections or at crosswalks. They are positioned to protect the children. Oklahoma's concern for the abuse of alcohol is another example of preparing the table. Other localities are taking strong community action against the abuse of drugs and narcotics. Still others are waging a war on pornography, obscene literature and entertainment as well as against many other things that could harm and destroy lives. We must constantly crusade against the enemies of life!

To use another metaphor, it is never enough for the farmer to simply plant the seed. He must go through his crop again and again to destroy the weeds or exterminate the pests that infest the crop. It is the same principle when it comes to morality and spiritual life. The Spirit of God militantly crusades against evil in our world. It is not enough just to preach the Gospel and attend worship services; we must destroy the enemies! One time I heard of former Attorney General of the United States, Ramsay Clark, tell a gathering of students at New York University in 1975 that Child Abuse was rampant in America. Mr. Clark told the audience "*there are 20,000 to 30,000 children in danger of their lives in New York City just while I am talking with you.*" He pointed out that newspapers and the media have a responsibility to focus on child abuse as a menacing problem for society. Parents, scientists, government, society as a whole must all join forces to prepare a table, destroying the enemies so that all good life may be safely nourished.

In the book of Jude, verses 3 and 4, Jude opens with these solemn words, "***Dear friends, although I was very eager to write to you about the salvation we share, I felt I had to write and urge you to contend for the faith that was once for all entrusted to the saints. For certain men whose condemnation was written about long ago have secretly slipped among you. They are godless men, who change the grace of God into a license for immorality and deny Jesus Christ our only sovereign and Lord***." Jude continued to outline in the chapter of his one chapter length book the damage caused by evil men. Jude was calling for Christians to prepare the table in the presence of our enemies! We should thank God for His preparing the table for the believer. We do not know the hidden snares that surround us at any given moment. We do not know the dangers that lie ahead. We often do not know what can possibly do us irreparable harm as we carelessly experiment with new behaviors in life. But the shepherd of men is out ahead of his sheep, and we can be assured of his protection and of his strength. It is as John said, "**For everyone born of God overcomes the world. This is the victory that has overcome the world, even our faith** (1 John 5:4)." Blessed Savior! "**You prepare a table before me.**"

Next, David says: "**You anoint my head with oil; my cup overflows**." This speaks to my need for healing and renewal. A football coach tells his players on the very first day of practice that football is a rough game and if they are willing to play it, they must also expect sometimes to get hurt. So it is with life. If you live it, you must also expect some bruises and hurts. That is just the reality of things. David, thinking of this fact, said in the 23rd Psalm, "**You anoint my head with oil; my cup overflows**." Sometimes, as the sheep grazed, its head would be cut by the sharp edge of a stone buried in the grass. There were briars to scratch and thorns to puncture the flesh. Some days the sheep would have to walk steep paths under a relentlessly hot and merciless sun. By the end of such a day the sheep would be tired and spent. The shepherd would stand at the door of the fold and examine each sheep as it came in. If there were hurt places on the sheep, the shepherd would apply soothing and healing oil. Instead of becoming infected, the hurt would soon heal.

Also, the shepherd had a large earthen jug of water—the kind of jar which kept the water refreshingly cool through evaporation. As the sheep filed in, the shepherd would dip down into the water with his big cup and bring it up brim full. The tired and thirsty sheep would drink deeply of the life-quickening draft. Do you remember when you were a little child you would bruise a small finger or toe? You would come running to your mother, who would probably have kissed the hurt away. There was mystic healing in her loving concern. As older children, we still get hurt. A heart can be broken, a conscience can ache like an infected tooth, feelings can be crushed; the world can deal cruelly and harshly. One can become discouraged and tired. Sometimes the burdens of life can be nearly unbearable. The problems are certainly there, but so is the shepherd! Jesus is the tender shepherd Who understands the hurt of his children and He is ever ready and able to minister to that hurt. We only have to trot over to Him with our need!

You will notice that David said, "**You anoint _my_ head with oil; _my_ cup overflows**." He did not say "our" heads or "our" cup. It is the singular, personal pronoun that he uses. All day long the shepherd has been concerned with the entire flock. But as they go into the fold, He takes them one by one. The fact that my God knows me as an individual is one of the most comforting thoughts I know! I am not just another head in a crowd. Jesus said, "**I am the Good Shepherd; I know my sheep, and my sheep know me** (John 10:14)." I like that! I love also the words in another Psalm, "**For this God is our God for ever and ever; He will be our guide even unto the end** (Psalm 48:14)." Knowing Christ and living with Christ in one's heart and mind is to have a great shepherd taking care of us. He anoints my head with oil. He fills my cup to overflowing! No one or nothing else on earth can do those things for me, but Jesus. Can you remember a time when your "head was bruised" by some adverse life experience and you needed the "oil of healing?"

The ninth need I have is to have hope for my future. David did not know what was in his future, but he knew who held the future, and he said confidently**, "Surely goodness and love will follow me all the days of my life**." In the play, "South Pacific," Mary Martin sang a song that I think is wonderful. In that song she sang: "I'm stuck like a dope, with a thing called hope, I can't get it out of my heart." David said the same thing using different words: "**Surely goodness and love shall follow me all the days of my life**." David is not wistfully thinking. On the contrary, he says surely...surely... surely. By the time of this writing of the 23rd Psalm, David was an old man. He had seen tragedies and disappointments, but he also had come to know God. He came to know a God who understood the needs of His children and Who abundantly provided for all those needs. He was a God Who could restore life in him and take away all his fears. In spite of dark clouds on the horizon, David knew he had a God Who would cause the sun to shine tomorrow like He caused it to shine today. David, said "goodness and love shall follow me all the days of my life."

How do you experience God's goodness and love in your life? We hear a lot about the wickedness of men and the destruction of the world. We know there are bombs that can destroy cities with one awful blast. We sometimes tremble at dire predictions of a terrible vengeance unleashed by God in judgment of a wayward world. But somehow, when we let our minds become filled with the vision of the loving shepherd leading His sheep we feel confident that He who led us in the past will lead us through the dark valleys ahead. If affairs were entirely in our hands, we would have every reason to fear and every justification for predicting disaster and despair. But, thankfully, things are in God's hands, and when we know Jesus as Lord and Savior, we are in God's hands, too. Trusting in such a shepherd is no difficult task! Jesus said, "**Come to me, all you who are weary and burdened, and I will give you rest** (Matthew 11:28)." When we trust the Lord with all our future days, we can awaken each morning to say with the Psalmist, "**This is the day the Lord has made; let us rejoice and be glad in it** (Psalm 118:24)." Begin each morning with hope. Plant this firmly in your mind, "**Surely goodness and love will follow me all the days of my life,**" and they will!

My final and ultimate need is to gain entrance into God's presence when my time on earth is finished. David felt that same need but he closes this Psalm with a word of assurance: *"And I will dwell in the house of the Lord forever."* When I was serving in the United States Army in Thailand in 1971, it was always a thrilling experience to be at the Udorn Air Force Base terminal at about 6:00 p.m. when the C-141 airplane was on the ground. It was thrilling because people were going home to the United States of America. At a prior time, when in Vietnam in 1968, it was the "freedom bird," as we called it. What a joy it was to see scores of soldiers boarding that plane that would transport them from that dangerous place to the comforts of home.

John Howard Payne had been away from home for nine years. One afternoon he stood at the window watching the throngs of people, happy, hurrying, and going to their homes at the day's end. Suddenly he felt lonely there in a Paris boarding house room. Impatiently, he turned from the window. He had work to do. It was an important play he was writing. He had no time for sentimental dreaming. But the mood and the memories of a little town on Long Island would not leave him. He picked up a pencil and began writing: *"Mid pleasures and palaces though we may roam, be it ever so humble, there's no place like home."* There is one saddening note, however, to the scene of watching the crowds going home at day's end. I am afraid many folks have no home to which they can go. Some wander around our streets seeking a cheap bed for the night. Others can afford the nicest hotel suite in the city, but it still is not home! Much more heart-wrenching than seeing a homeless person at the end of the day is to find a person who is not sure of God and has no hope of the eternal home, who, at the close of life's day, can look forward only to some dark grave and oblivion!

David closes this Psalm with a mighty crescendo of faith when he declares, *"I will dwell in the house of the Lord forever."* David did not have the insights we possess today. He did not know the words Jesus spoke hundreds of years later when he said to Martha at the tomb of his deceased friend, Lazarus, *"I am the resurrection and the life. He who believes in me will live, even though he dies; and whoever lives and believes in me will never die* (John11:25,26)." David said, just because he knew the character of the shepherd he loved, *"I will dwell in the house of the Lord forever."* Just knowing intimately a God like he described in the 23rd Psalm gave David assurance that at the close of life's day he would go home. Do you have this assurance? This magnificent Psalm opens with the assurance that in all of life I will have everything I need, and the Psalm closes with the assurance that, at death I will not perish!

By now you should have judged that this is a tremendous passage of scripture. We would fail to catch its deepest significance if we did not notice that this Psalm depicts a relationship between a man and his God. It is "He" and "me" all the way through! One cannot mistake the fact that David knew his shepherd, and that the shepherd knew David. The bond between them was the bond of love. It is the story of a man who had come to the place of having placid trust in God!

Every Christmas season we are reminded of shepherds abiding with their flocks in the field when Angels announced the fact that the Shepherd Himself was just born in the little town of Bethlehem. Again, the Christmas event is the account of the God of our salvation making Himself personal, just as He did to David of old, who wrote the 23rd Psalm. I tried to capture what this gift of God meant to me in a poem I wrote some years ago while serving as an Army Chaplain. I titled the poem, <u>Christmas Mystery</u>. I would like to share it with you:

"To earth's cold crust now bending,
God stoops to condescend;
His heart aflame, His Son now sending,
Our God, the sinner's friend!

The babe now helpless and dependent,
God's gift to man—but just a child;
Yet, in Him a future gift resplendent;
Rebel hearts reclaimed—yes, reconciled!

In mercy Thy glory part concealing
Within that form so sweet and mild,
And yet Thy truth and grace revealing,
Oh glad mystery—this heaven-sent Son—a child!

Celestial songs borne by angel wings
To man, the creature poor;
Glorious tidings of redemption brings,
Christ our joy forever more!

Christian voices join in singing,
Where're the evangel's feet have trod,
The angel's word still heard, still ringing,
This infant son is infinite God!"

Many are the descriptions of this personal God! To Matthew, Jesus is the King, the Son of David, the long-promised Deliverer of His people. To Luke, Jesus is the Worker of wonders and the tireless Servant of both God and man, demonstrating His divinity and compassion by His mighty works of mercy and help. John sees Jesus in many roles, some of which are the Bread of Life from Whom we eat and never again feel hunger, the Water of Life of Whom we drink and never again thirst, the Light of the world, the Vine, the Resurrection and the Life. Paul, the Apostle, sees Jesus as the Lord of Glory, our Only Foundation, and Head of the Church. To the writer of the book of Hebrews, Jesus is the Captain of our Salvation, the Great High Priest, the Author and Finisher of our faith.

But I think it is Peter who comes closest to seeing Christ as David saw his Shepherd. Peter said, "**For you were like sheep going astray, but now you have returned to the shepherd and overseer of your souls** (I Peter 2:25)." This is David's sentiment when he says, "**The Lord is my shepherd, I shall not be in want.**" He then goes on in his Psalm to describe the shepherd as One providing, leading, guiding, restoring, protecting, healing, comforting and supporting right up until the day he enters God's presence in the heavenly pasture, forever. Through personal faith and trust in Christ, you can know the Shepherd and overseer of your soul, too! My Shepherd can be your Shepherd, too.

In the 10th chapter of the Gospel of John, Jesus delivers a discourse that states He is the gate by which people must pass to enter God's sheepfold. Trying to enter by any other means is the same as being a thief or robber for whom the watchman will not open the gate. Listen to the words of Jesus: "**I tell you the truth, I am the gate for the sheep. All who ever came before me were thieves and robbers, but the sheep did not listen to them. I am the gate: whoever enters through me will be saved. He will come in and go out and find pasture** (John 10:7-9)." Jesus is the gate into Eternal Life. To become that Gate, He had to lay down his life. Our salvation did not come cheap. It cost the Son of God His life's blood as he died on the cross of Calvary! Again, Jesus said in the same discourse, "**I am the Good Shepherd. The Good Shepherd lays down his life for the sheep** (John 10:11)."

Earlier in John's Gospel, Jesus had a conversation with Nicodemus, a Pharisee and a ruler of the Jews. Nicodemus was inquiring of Jesus because he believed no one could do the miracles Jesus performed unless God were with him. Jesus came right to the point and replied to Nicodemus, "*I tell you the truth, no one can see the Kingdom of God unless he is born again* (John 3:3)." Nicodemus was puzzled because he could not imagine a person re-entering his mother and being born a second time. Jesus explained the physical birth is how all of us come into this world, but to enter the Kingdom of God which is a spiritual realm, one needs to be born of the Spirit. Being born of the Spirit is the second birth. Therefore, Jesus said, "*You must be born again* (John 3:7)." The entire discourse with Nicodemus is fascinating and enlightening, indeed. The high light of the conversation, however is the 16th verse, often referred to as "the gospel in a nutshell": "*For God so loved the world that he gave his one and only Son, that whoever believes in Him shall not perish but have everlasting life.*"

Jesus is God's great Gift to man. We are all sheep who have gone astray and are lost in our sins. None of us would be able to enter God's sheepfold because our sins would keep us from entering. The only Gate is Jesus. And it is Jesus dying on the cross to take away the curse for our sins. Forgiveness for our sins comes when we believe Jesus died in our place, taking our sins on himself and paying the price for us. To appropriate what Jesus did for us on the cross, we must receive him into our hearts by faith. Faith is believing. Whoever believes in Him shall not perish but have everlasting life. What else can you do with a gift? You cannot pay for a gift or it is a gift no longer. All you can do with a gift is to receive it or reject it. What do you do with Jesus? You receive Him or you reject Him. There is no middle ground. To procrastinate and delay your decision is the same as rejecting Him. Until you decide to receive Jesus into your heart, you are still without the Shepherd and are lost in sin.

The apostle Paul set the matter plainly. He said, "*For it is by grace you have been saved, through faith—and this not from yourselves, it is the gift of God—not by works, so that no one can boast* (Ephesians 2:8-9**).**" The sum of the matter is simply this: God loves you like the Good Shepherd loves his sheep. He wants to take care of you and provide for all your needs in this life and He wants to keep you in His fold for all eternity if you will turn your life over to Him and submit to His authority. Make Jesus the Lord of your life! Confess your sins and unworthiness and ask Him to come into your life and save your soul on the basis of His promise: **"Whoever believes in Him shall not perish but have everlasting life."** Pray to God and receive Jesus into your life. When invited by faith, Jesus will surely come in. And when He comes in, He brings with him all the goodness of heaven into your soul. Only when that happens, will the life-healing power of the 23rd Psalm be yours. You will be able to say with David of old:

"The Lord is my shepherd, I shall not be in want.
He makes me lie down in green pastures,
He leads me beside the quiet waters,
He restores my soul.
He guides me in paths of righteousness
for his name's sake.
Even though I walk
through the valley of the shadow of death,
I will fear no evil,
for you are with me;
your rod and your staff,
they comfort me.
You prepare a table before me
in the presence of my enemies.
You anoint my head with oil,
my cup overflows.
Surely goodness and love will follow me
all the days of my life,
and I will dwell in the house of the Lord forever."

Chapter Five

LONELINESS

There was a captivating article in the Los Angeles Times on September 2, 1980 that really got my attention. It reported that a man and a woman were walking down Sunset Boulevard one night and they were suddenly approached by a neatly dressed teen-aged girl who had long blond hair. She had been sitting on the edge of a pillar that was supporting a billboard near the corner of La Cienaga Boulevard.

"Can I walk with you for a few minutes?" she asked, "I'm lonely."

The man studied her for a moment. He was thinking, is she a panhandler? Or worse, he wondered if she was a hooker. He looked over at his companion who simply smiled and shrugged her shoulders almost imperceptibly. "Sure," the man said, "Why not?"

The girl refused to give her name or even talk about herself as they walked. Instead, she asked the man and woman about their lives. After about fifteen minutes, the young girl stopped. She said, "I'm okay now. Thank you. It was very nice." Promptly she turned around and walked off in the opposite direction.

Loneliness is the gnawing agony of many, many people in our society. The lonely people are all around us and they are of every age group: young people, young adults, middle-aged and, of course, the elderly. For some, loneliness is but a temporary episode in life brought on by a strange or hard set of unwelcome circumstances. For others, loneliness is the name of their very existence. This is terribly sad because loneliness is not something to which one gets adjusted with the passing of time. Rather than to improve with time, the pain of loneliness grows increasingly worse as one gets more deeply mired in the hapless rut of feeling neglected, forgotten, overlooked, left out and unloved.

Loneliness must be differentiated from solitude if it is to be properly understood. Solitude can be an oasis of refuge for many people who lead full and busy lives, shouldering heavy burdens and many responsibilities. Hosts of people will pay dearly in dollars and cents for but a weekend of quiet solitude as a relief from mounting pressures of their busy lives. Solitude is often sought after; loneliness, on the other hand, is something from which some want to escape. A person can feel lonely in a crowd of people as easily as in a remote place of isolation. One can feel lonely in illness, lonely in their work when it cannot be easily shared with others, lonely because one's life style and personal values are diametrically opposed to the milieu in which they live and work, lonely because one has a burning conviction or a set of ideals which cannot be caught and shared by others.

One can feel very alone even when there happens to be a lot of people around and they are interacting with their companions and you are being ignored. I have had that feeling while serving in the Army. I remember a time when I was serving as the United States Army chaplain at the 7th Radio Research Field Station in Udorn, Thailand. One of my duties was to travel to the different cities or outposts in the country where we had a contingency of troops stationed. One such place was near the capital city, Bangkok. When I visited that group of soldiers I took a room at the Chao Phraya Hotel in down town Bangkok. The hotel dining room was spacious and elegantly furnished. One evening, I went down to the dining room for dinner and the Maitre De escorted me to a table. It was a beautiful setting--chandelier lights, candles glowing on every table and a room packed with people. Every table was occupied. After ordering my selection from the menu, I began to muse and survey the surroundings while waiting for my food. As I observed all the other guests visiting and interacting with each other, it suddenly hit me how utterly lonely I felt in that setting! I truly had been missing my wife, my daughter and my son for a long time but had been suppressing my longing for them by keeping active and occupied in my ministry to the troops. On this occasion and at this precise moment, however, my defenses were down and the tears flooded my eyes and coursed down my cheeks. I could not help myself. I felt terribly alone and forgotten. Fortunately, a voice in my head told me to stop feeling sorry for myself—yes, I miss my family and that is understandable. The voice continued: "I want you to know that I am with you and I will never leave you." It was like taking a sedative to hear that voice–perhaps it was me talking to myself; my super-ego communicating to my ego, or the nurturing parent in me comforting my inner child. In any event, the rest of my time in the dining room went much better as I communed and visited with the Lord through His indwelling Spirit. Jesus was at work, shepherding my soul! I wondered then, and I still wonder, what is it like for people who do not have the Lord in their life when they encounter similar situations?

Loneliness is part of the human condition for everyone at various times in life. A child can feel lonely when the parents are occupied elsewhere and there are no play mates available to interact with. For some children who have parents who work, the after-school time until the parent(s) get home from work can be very lonely time. A divorced person may feel the bitter pangs of loneliness as life takes on an entirely new and different dimension. With no one else to take care of you and you have to take care of yourself to survive, one can feel quite alone. The same is true for someone who has lost a partner or family member through illness, death, through some tragic accident or some other tragic cause. Losing the object of your deepest love and affection can lead to a devastating loneliness. It is a loneliness that is reflected in a phrase from the 23rd Psalm: "**Even though I walk through the valley of the shadow of death** (Psalm 23:4a)." The message in the Psalm, however, is a supremely comforting one, for the very next phrase says: "**I will fear no evil for you are with me; your rod and staff, they comfort me** (Psalm 23:4b)."

My daughter is a grown woman now and her job places her in Dayton, Ohio—about 2,000 miles from my home in Lemoore, California. Whenever I can fly to Ohio to spend a few days with her, I am overjoyed. The same is true on those occasions she flies out to visit with me. The time always seems to speed by like a super-sonic jet plane! There is always a lump in my throat and tears in my eyes whenever we must part and we give each other a final hug and a kiss before one of us gets on an airplane to return to our home. When I am buckled into my seat on the airplane, that familiar feeling of abject loneliness reappears and I have to fight myself internally to keep my emotions in check and not create a scene on the airplane. Again, what helps me regain equilibrium is the abiding presence of the Lord. He is always there, but we have to turn to Him with our thoughts to experience the comfort He supplies.

Loneliness often intensifies at certain junctures where the happiness of others soars, such as at Christmas, New Years or other times of special significance. We must remind ourselves that loneliness is a plight which many cannot tolerate for long. If their isolation lasts for too long a time, they may resort to alcohol abuse or drug addiction to dull reality. For still others, the way out becomes a total abandonment of their prized values while embracing the lesser values of those who would share their company in unchecked indulgences or careless living. Unfortunately, for some the path of escape from their loneliness and despair is nothing less than succumbing to the urge for suicide. They want to place a final period to the dreadful sentence of loneliness!

The pain of loneliness is all the more sharp and piercing to a person when one realizes it doesn't always need to be so. Just one person drawing close with genuine caring and concern can dissolve loneliness like a snow bank melting beneath a hot, early Spring-time sun. It is precisely at this very point that many who have relationships need to share with those who have not. The sharing need not be anything more than a few well-spent minutes of one's time, a few words of concern and encouragement, or, better still, some patient and intense listening to the emanations and heart-cry of the lonely person.

People need not be consigned to their loneliness by the sheer thoughtlessness of others whose path is well marked out with purpose and meaning. It is not very difficult for even the most active people to bring some lonely person along with them for at least part of their journey and thereby achieve a sort of double fulfillment in what they do and accomplish.

There is scarcely a more natural result of the Spirit-filled life of the Christian than to be reaching out with open and generous hand to the lonely folks of this world. Such folks are not hard to find when the believer channels God's compassion, remaining alert and empathic toward those who are trapped in the web of changeless loneliness.

The Bible says, "*Religion that God our Father accepts as pure and faultless is this: to look after orphans and widows in their distress and to keep oneself from being polluted by the world*" (James 1:27). To His disciples our Lord Himself spoke of the sick, the naked, the hungry and the poor of this world who need to be tended to, clothed, fed and assisted. Jesus said, "*For as much as you have done it unto the least of these my brethren, you have done it also unto me*" (Matthew 25:40).

Outreach is the by-word of practicing Christians who take their religious faith seriously enough to translate the guidance and heart beat of God into feet that go where the lonely are trapped, hands that reach out to touch them and help them, hearts that will find room for them and which will open channels through which the tender love of Christ can flow to the lonely, filling hearts with meaning and hope.

Ask yourself often the searching question: "Whom am I forgetting that I might be opening up my life to more fully?" Perhaps it could be a parent with whom you have lost contact and whom you have neglected to write a letter or call on the phone. Perhaps it is a son or daughter who has gone off to school or into the service whom you have allowed to drift out of touch because you have not persisted in keeping open the lines of communication. Could the forgotten person be a relative or a former friend who now may be in a home for the aged, in prison or some other institution? Would an evening visit or a Sunday afternoon drive be a welcome and refreshing stimulus to that poor soul?

Could the person you are forgetting be your own growing child right there in your home? The child may be regarded, you feel, as being too little to share the adult activities and the socializing which you have established as your life-pattern. If so, might your life pattern and practice bear scrutiny and realignment to provide time and activities that would wonderfully include and brighten the life of your child?

Could you be forgetting, perhaps, the most significant and important other person in your life: your husband or your wife? Are you failing to bring him or her into the dimensions of your life to share your moments of frustration as well as those gratifying moments of joy and triumph? Need your life's partner be excluded so much from your life only because you have been inept at communicating and sharing your thoughts and feelings? Have you felt this person could not understand or share your intimate disclosures? Let your conscience guide you into the arena of awareness where, with increasing sensitivity, you can more readily sense the presence of lonely people who surround you but have failed to elicit from you a helping or an attentive response.

The guidance of our Lord consists of a stern word of caution: "**He that saves his life (hoards it to himself) shall lose it, but he who loses his life (reaches out, gives and shares with others) for my sake shall find it** (Matthew 10:39). May we learn from the Lord the lesson that in loving we will be loved, in giving we will receive—even much more than that which we are capable of giving? When reaching out to the lonely in this world we are not only lifting their despair, we also are "**Laying up treasures in heaven where thieves do not break through and steal and where moth and rust do not corrupt** (Matthew 6:19)."

Someone you know may be lonely, and you could make a difference! Do for that person what you would want someone to do for you if you were in that person's place. The truth of it all is this: when you help to ease the burden of a lonely person, both of you are winners!

CHAPTER SIX

MAN'S RESPONSE TO GOD'S OVERTURES

One of the most astonishing miracles of Jesus' public ministry in the city of Jerusalem occurred on an occasion when He encountered on a Sabbath day a man who had been blind from his birth. The man was doing what he had done every day: he was seated by the road side begging for alms. He survived on the charity of those who would pass by and have compassion or sympathy for his predicament. He was obviously a very poor soul and most likely was scarcely educated, given his life of blindness. His was a boring but necessary routine, come rain or shine. No doubt, also, he was not very socially connected to other folks in the city. He was insulated from society, isolated from a meaningful relationship with others, immersed in begging and scrounging just to exist. No one would want to change places with that man, to be sure!

What the begging blind man could not know as he sat by the roadside on that Sabbath day was that this would be the day that would change his life forever. His boring routine would be shattered and his life would never be the same again. He would encounter Jesus! The account of this historic event was recorded in John's Gospel, chapter 9. The essence of the situation consists of Jesus journeying along, accompanied by His disciples. As they got to the place where they saw the man who was blind from birth, Jesus' disciples turned to Jesus and asked this question: "**Rabbi, who sinned, this man or his parents, that he was born blind?**" This was not a mischievous question. It was based on their knowledge of the teaching of the rabbis, based on Exodus 34:7, that if a person suffered from a physical ailment from birth, this must have been because the person's parents or grandparents had committed some grievous sin and the punishment for that sin would extend to their children unto the third or fourth generation. Remember, this is before the age of modern science that gives us an explanation regarding some inherited disabilities passed on through the DNA from generation to generation.

Rather than support this theory of the rabbis, Jesus shattered the myth that all who suffer from birth is attributed to some sin in the family! Instead, Jesus asserted that this man's plight was established by God so that God's Son could demonstrate before many witnesses that the work of God would be displayed in this man's life. The unforgettable lesson to the disciples and to anyone else who would encounter this man in the future is that God has the power to heal any malady of man, even if he owned that malady from birth! They would learn that with God, nothing is impossible! Sin is not the reason for the man's blindness from birth; the reason is that the power of almighty God might be displayed in the healing of the man of his blindness and giving him the gift of sight! God's overture to this man was to heal him of his blindness by His power working through His Son, Jesus.

The healing was not instantaneous. Jesus spit on the ground, made some mud with the saliva and put it on the man's eyes. Then, Jesus instructed the man to go and wash in the pool of Siloam, which was on the southern ridge on which Jerusalem was built and was part of the major water system that was developed by a former King, Hezekiah. The pool is still in existence today.

By sending the blind man to wash in the pool of Siloam the Lord was putting a condition on the man's healing: God would heal him as long as he obeyed the Lord's instruction and displayed his faith in Jesus. The Bible text says, "***So the man went and washed, and came home seeing*** (John 9:7)." The man had left his home in the morning as a shuffling blind man, but he came home as a man who was confident of his surroundings, enjoying the gift of sight! Could anything be more wonderful than that? And, it was Jesus Who made the difference!

As you would imagine, the man's neighbors were totally amazed and could not even believe that this was the same man they had known all along to have been a blind beggar. They resorted to telling one another, "that can't be him; it must be a man who looks just like him." But the man insisted that he was one and the same man but Jesus had healed him. The neighbors could not leave well enough alone; they took the man who had been blind from birth and went to show him to the Pharisees, who were the rulers of the Jews. The Pharisees questioned the man concerning the alleged miracle of healing. When they heard the man's story, some of the Pharisees immediately denounced Jesus as an imposter—he could not be from God since he performed "the healing" on the Sabbath. Others, however, would not denounce Jesus because they reasoned *"How can a sinner do such miraculous signs?"* So the Pharisees were divided.

Finally, the Pharisees turned to the man and asked him what he had to say about Jesus, since he claimed Jesus had given him his sight? The man replied, "He is a Prophet." The Pharisees were still not convinced so they sent for the man's parents and asked them, "Is this your son?" The parents replied, "We know he is our son and we know he was born blind." The parents added, "But how he can see or who opened his eyes, we don't know. Why don't you ask him, he is of age; he can speak for himself."

Now comes the really good part. The Pharisees a second time summoned the man who had been blind, and said to him, **"Give glory to God, we know this man (Jesus) is a sinner." He replied, "Whether he is a sinner or not, I don't know. One thing I know. I was blind but now I see!"** It was like a man being brutally interrogated at a police station after having been arrested and suspected of committing a crime. The Pharisees pressed the matter further, asking, **"What did he do to you? How did he open your eyes?"** The man answered, sticking to his story, **"I have told you already and you did not listen. Why do you want to hear it again? Do you want to become his disciples, too?"**

The Pharisees were far from believers, they were prototypical unbelievers! The very suggestion from the man who had been born blind that they might want to be disciples of Jesus, too, was infuriating to them. At this point, the text says, **"Then they hurled insults at him and said, you are this fellow's disciple! We are disciples of Moses!"** The man answered, **"Now that is remarkable!**

You don't know where he comes from, yet he opened my eyes. We know that God does not listen to sinners. He listens to the godly man who does his will. Nobody has ever heard of opening the eyes of a man born blind. If this man were not from God, he could do nothing."

To this they replied, "**You were steeped in sin at birth, how dare you lecture us!**" Then, they threw the man out of the temple. But this is not the end of the matter. The Bible text reveals that Jesus heard about the man being thrown out so he found the man and asked him, "**Do you believe in the Son of Man?**" Listen to what follows:

"Who is he, sir?' the man asked,'tell me so that I might believe in him."Jesus said, 'You have now seen him; in fact, He is the one speaking with you."Then the man said, 'Lord, I believe,' and he worshipped him.   Jesus said, 'For judgment I have come into this world, so that the blind will see and those who see will become blind." (John 9:36-39).

With this dialogue with the man he had healed of his blindness, the Lord gave a lesson about spiritual vision (the blind man believed—an act of faith in God) and spiritual blindness (the Pharisees who enjoyed physical sight displayed their spiritual blindness to God because they would not believe in spite of the evidence God had put before their eyes)!

When questioned by the Pharisees, the blind man could not vouch for the character of Jesus, nor could he explain the dynamics of the situation in which he was healed and was given his sight. One thing he could vouch for without equivocation, however, was that before the incident with Jesus he was a blind man, but now he can see. That fact was indisputable. His was an experience that was real and he could not be talked or argued out of it. He was blind, but now, no matter how it came about, he could see!

This response of the blind man who was given his sight is somewhat representative of what all Christians might say concerning their relationship with God. All Christians do not come to know God in the same way. A person may be unaware of the dynamics of his own conversion experience in which he or she came into a saving relationship with God. But one should be able to say, "One thing I know, I am a child of God and Jesus is my Savior—he died on the cross to take away my sins."

It is a mistake, however, to think that all who come to know Christ as Savior and Lord will have a similar experience. In the Scriptures of the Bible we find at least three different types of conversion experiences—three different types of response to God's overtures. I would invite you to consider these three possibilities.

The first possible response to God's overture can be seen in the example of the conversion of Saul of Tarsus, who became known after his conversion as Paul, the Apostle to the Gentiles. The record of Saul's encounter with Jesus is found in Acts 9:1-6. If called upon to tell of his experience, Saul would say something like this: "I was a Pharisee and a persecutor of the Christians. I believed that it was my mission on earth to seek out and destroy the Galilean heresy that sprang up in connection with Jesus of Nazareth. Beginning at Jerusalem, I made havoc of the church, entering into every house and arresting men and women and committing them to prison. When they were brought to trial, I gave my vote against them, and many were put to death. I punished them often times in every synagogue and compelled them even unto strange and distant cities."

Saul would go on to say, "Having completed my task at Jerusalem, I obtained from the High Priest letters to the synagogues at Damascus, authorizing me, if I should find any of this way, whether men or women, to bring them in chains to Jerusalem. Thus equipped, I was on my way to Damascus and almost there, when a marvelous thing happened: suddenly, there shone around about me a light from heaven above the brightness of the sun. I was overwhelmed as were my companions, and together we fell to the earth and I heard a voice saying, 'Saul, Saul, why do you persecute me?' And I said, 'who are you, Lord?' And then, though blind to the physical world around me, I saw what I had never seen before, that Jesus the Nazarene was both Lord and Christ; and trembling and astonished I threw myself at his feet in whole-hearted submission and cried out, 'Lord, what do you want me to do?"

Such is the story. Here is a clear case of a sudden conversion experience. Not only is it sudden, but also convulsive and overwhelming. So vivid were his impressions that Saul remembered the experience as long as he lived. Relating it to King Agrippa many years after, he tells just when and where it took place, and all the attending circumstances: it was at mid-day, it was on the way to Damascus, he was aiming to persecute the church, he saw a glorious light, and he heard an audible voice from heaven and had a vision of the Christ Himself! Could we read this account in the book of Acts and wonder that the Apostle had such an experience which filled him with wonder, surprise and unforgettable memories? The flood tides of emotion surged through him. The effect was dramatic: blinded and overwhelmed, laying prostrate on the ground and for three days afterward he had no desire for food or drink.

The sudden conversion of Saul of Tarsus was indeed a unique event. But it is by no means isolated in so far as many of its particulars are concerned. The history of the Christian church reveals many instances of wonderful, dramatic and amazing conversion experiences. Almost every Christian community has some member who can testify of a sudden, dramatic and unforgettable conversion experience. I have talked with individuals who were former drug addicts who had encounters with Christ that were completely overwhelming and just short of being completely miraculous. Theirs were sudden, dynamic and amazing conversion experiences even as was the Apostle Paul's.

One astonishing modern day example of this type of conversion experience, quite similar to that of Saul of Tarsus, was reported on Reverend Robert Schuler's service, The Hour of Power, broadcasted on Television on Sunday morning, 26 July, 2009. Doctor Sheila Schuler Coleman was interviewing Reverend Hananiah Zoe, a man born in Liberia and now serving as President of "The Ministry of Hope" there in Liberia. From 1989 to 1996 Liberia has experienced an awful civil war that has left 240,000 orphans!

Rev. Zoe reported that a particular Islamic element of the civil war really took advantage to execute pastors and key leaders, Christian leaders. Many pastors were executed in a very gruesome manner. We lost many pastors, he said. He said his own brother was one of the ones executed. He said even during the civil war when he was becoming very bitter a verse from the Apostle Paul in

II Corinthians 5:13-17 turned him around, particularly the phrase *"**The love of God compels us**."* He said thereafter the Christians were compelled by the love of God to pray for even those who were persecuting them.

He said a notable thing that God did was a leading Islamic militant general, General Muhammad Fufana went into the minaret, the highest part of the mosque during Ramadan to pray and as he went (speaking Islamic) which is "God is great," calling for prayers with thousands of worshippers pouring in. The General became mute and could not speak. It appeared as though his jaws were completely locked. He could not talk and the leaders led him down in the sanctuary of the mosque and asked him what's happening to you general? After a while of being in that state of shock, he opened his mouth and the first words he said were "Jesus is God, Jesus is the Son of God."

Rev Zoe went on to explain what had happened to him was what he said in his own words, that the Lord Jesus appeared right there before him in the mosque and said "I am the one that you are persecuting." And General Muhammad was very notorious for executing pastors and even as they were praying before the final bullets he would tell them "Go and tell Jesus, I General Muhammad kill you. He is not God." Rev Zoe said, "How awesome our God is, and I was privileged after some time to work with him and disciple him."

Here is a powerful Islamic general of Liberia's terrible civil war being transformed from being a persecutor and murderer of thousands of Christians in a most dramatic and memorable encounter with Jesus becoming a believer himself!

Yes, the first type of conversion experience is the sudden and dramatic and memorable type of experience. There is a second type of conversion experience: typified by the conversion of the disciple, Matthew. The account of Matthew's conversion is recorded in the Gospel of Matthew, chapter 9 and verse 9. If asked what happened, Matthew would say something like this: "I was a tax collector. My home was in Capernaum, that great Galilean city where Jesus spent so much of his time; where many of His mighty works were done. The whole city, as well as the country around them, was talking about Jesus. I had seen Him, and heard him many times. I had witnessed some of His miracles and had been thinking about His claims. Then, one day—I shall never forget it—as I sat at my desk writing tax receipts, I saw Him approaching, and as He reached my side, He paused, and looking at me in love He said in a quiet, yet powerful and persuasive voice, "Matthew, follow me." And realizing my need of Him, and convinced that He alone could satisfy my soul's desires and undying thirst, I rose up, left all, and followed Him. I've been following as best I could from then until now."

In some respects, Matthew's experience is just like that of Saul. He, too, remembered the time and the place and all the attending circumstances, and relating the story afterwards, tells where he was and what he was doing when he passed from death unto life—when he became a Christian! Yet, while Saul's conversion was convulsive and overwhelming, Matthew's was calm and quiet. No vision of glory was there. There was no voice from the heavens. There was no shock that blinded and convulsed him and threw him to the ground. Matthew simply rose up and followed Jesus just as quietly and dispassionately as he went about his daily task. If Saul's conversion can be likened to an earthquake shock or a stormy sea, that of Matthew was like a mountain bathed in the beauty of an autumn sunset, with scarcely a ripple on the surface of the waters and hardly a leaf rustling among the trees.

In exactly the same way, thousands of God's children through all the centuries have come to the saving knowledge of the truth in Christ. As a rule, they are people who are naturally quiet and undemonstrative—people who never lose their heads, who never become greatly excited or stirred up about anything—people who are in the habit of doing their own thinking and reaching their own conclusions. They have been reading the Bible and hearing sermons for years. Yet, on one memorable day they come face to face with Jesus and see Him as they never saw Him before, through the eyes of faith. By the help of God the Holy Spirit they yield themselves, surrender their wills and receive Jesus as their personal Savior and Lord. They follow this up with consecrating themselves to God's service. That holy hour they will never forget, but they do this as they do everything else: quietly and deliberately, with no whirlwind or tempest, no earthquake or ocean storm.

There is yet a third type of conversion experience: the experience of John the Baptist. The account of his conversion is recorded in the Gospel of Luke, chapter one and verses 13-15. If called upon to relate his experience, John would have to say something like this:

"I have listened to these experiences of yours with deepest interest, and yet, with wonder and amazement. They are marvelous stories, but they sound to me like one speaking in an unknown tongue. Conversion is an experience about which I know nothing. I have never had an experience of conversion so far as I know. As far back as I can remember I have been a child of God. I have heard my father Zacharias tell how the angel Gabriel appeared to him as he ministered in the Temple, and assured him that his prayer had been heard and that his wife Elizabeth should bear him a son who should be called John, who should be the forerunner of the Lord and be full of the Holy Ghost from his mother's womb. Through the agency of that Spirit, I must have become God's child before I was even born. At any rate, however it may be explained, I have no recollection of an experience that you call conversion. I have never known the time when I did not believe in the Lord my Savior and when I did not love and serve Him."

John had godly parents: he was the subject of many prayers, and we should never wonder that a prayer-hearing God answered those prayers so early in his life that he had no conscious experience of conversion. I am perfectly satisfied that this is the experience of countless thousands of God's children—those who, as a rule, have been brought up in Christian homes and were taught from infancy the doctrines and duties of the Christian faith.

Some who read this may be wondering right now if I believe in the new birth in such instances. Indeed, I do. Jesus said to Nicodemus, "***I tell you the truth, no one can see the Kingdom of God unless he is born again.*** (John 3:3)." The Bible clearly teaches the necessity of the new birth—being born of the spirit (unlike our first birth, which is being born of the flesh)—a necessity to which there are no exceptions. The Bible nowhere teaches, however, the necessity of our knowing when or where the new birth took place.

Regeneration is the act of God's Spirit, and the Spirit can work the new birth in the young child just as easily as in the grown adult!

Perhaps you have wondered, "How shall I know that I have been converted at all if I have no conscious experience to which I can point and say, that's when it happened?" Some reason, "Since I cannot put my finger on the time and place of my conversion, may it not be possible that I am cherishing a false hope in believing myself to be a Christian?" Let me respond to this with a question: How do you know that you were born the first time? Do you remember it? Have you a conscious recollection of the time and the place and all the attending circumstances? You, of course, would answer, "No." I would reply, "why then have you not been going about all these years with a long face and a heavy heart wondering if you have been born or not? " It is absurd, is it not? We reason that since we have a consciousness of our existence, we do not question the experience of our birth. It is as the philosopher, Rene Descartes, once said: "I think, therefore I am." That which is alive today must have been born somewhere and sometime. There is no way to life except through childbirth. Therefore, we are satisfied and we never question having experienced the first birth—being born of the flesh.

In exactly the same way, you may be certain and satisfied about the second birth—being born of the Spirit, as Jesus declared to Nicodemus, a ruler of the Jews. Are you spiritually alive and sensitive toward God right now? Do you have a feeling and a conviction of having Christ as your Lord and Savior from sin and are you now resting on Him alone for your salvation? Have you prayed to God and repented of your sin? Do you love God? Are you genuinely interested in supporting His cause? Are you seeking to walk in love toward Christian brethren and toward all men? Are you for the most part bringing forth the *"Fruit of the Spirit: love, joy, peace, longsuffering, gentleness, goodness, meekness, faithfulness, self-control"*? Do you believe you have been growing in grace and in the knowledge of Jesus Christ, your Lord and Savior?

These are some of the evidences of life through the Spirit of God. If you find these in your life, you do not ever need to worry about your conversion or the new birth. That is because the person who displays these attributes has surely been born of God even though the person may not know when, or where, or how this new life came about. Yours will be an experience like that of John the Baptist. Or your experience can be compared to the man whom Jesus healed of his blindness at the roadside in Jerusalem. You can say with that man who had been blind from birth: "I don't know much about it; I cannot explain it. But there is one thing I know for sure: before I met Jesus I was blind, now I can see!"

We have considered three basic types of response to God's overtures. God comes to us and confronts us in many different ways, seeking our believing response. Some people are hit with the reality of the love of Christ in a sudden and jarring manner, resulting in a sudden conversion experience of a most dramatic nature. It is vivid and unforgettable. Others, like the disciple Matthew, respond to the overtures of God by decisive obedience. They believe in Christ and set out to follow Him regardless of the cost or personal sacrifice. Still there are others, raised by godly parents in an environment of faith and never know a time in their life when they did not believe in Christ, love Him with their whole heart , pray to Him and serve Him as best they know how. Whichever the way or whatever the experience, the important point is that all of these are born again believers in Jesus Christ.

If, upon reflecting on these facts, you find yourself questioning your own relationship to God, you need to make time to settle this all important question immediately. Your eternal destiny hinges on whether or not you have been born again (born of the Spirit) and have Jesus firmly embraced in your heart of hearts. You can experience the new birth which Jesus demands of all who would see heaven and have eternal life. You can settle the question of your sins—whether or not you have obtained God's forgiveness. You can become a child of God for now and forever by simply confessing your sins to God in quiet but sincere prayer, and by inviting Jesus, God's own Son, into your heart and life, asking Him to be your Lord and Savior. The Bible promises: "***For God so loved the world (that includes you) that He gave his one and only Son, that whoever believes in Him should not perish but have eternal life.***" (John 3:16).

Perhaps God has made an overture to you. What will be your response to Him?

CHAPTER SEVEN

THE RESURRECTION OF JESUS CHRIST—FACT, WITH SIX IMMENSE IMPLICATIONS

Hours earlier, His lifeless, blood and water-drained body had been removed from the Roman Cross that had been erected outside the gates of Jerusalem on Mount Golgotha, also known as the hill called Calvary. Hundreds of eye-witnesses to His ignominious death had already retired to their homes. The 33 year-old body had released its final gasp of breath after suffering a most painfully agonizing ordeal of human suffering. He had been affixed to those wooden timbers by huge nails that had been driven through his outstretched hands and through his overlapped feet. His head bore the imprint of a crown of thorns that had been pressed upon his brow and encircled his skull, piercing skin to bone, forcing blood to ooze and trickle in rivulets of crimson down his temple and cheeks, painting red, jagged, vertical stripes upon His naked body. Loving hands had cleaned his body, prepared it with burial spices, enveloped it in layers of linen cloth, and had laid it on the shelf in the stone-hewn tomb of Joseph of Arimathea, which was located in his garden, also outside the gates of Jerusalem. Now that He was laid out in His final resting place, his faithful attendants departed from the tomb and a huge, circular stone was rolled into place to seal the opening to the sepulcher. A troop of Roman soldiers was posted as guards to ensure that no mischief could occur while the reality of the death of Jesus of Nazareth gained final acceptance by both the Jews and the citizens of Rome.

It had been a truly momentous day, perhaps the greatest day in all of history. A man Who had a brilliant public ministry of profound goodness, superlative teaching, tender and loving healing of the sick and suffering multitudes in the length and breadth of Palestine and who had attracted a large and loyal following, was finally opposed, captured by force, hurriedly tried and declared guilty of a single crime: He had uttered blasphemy by making claim that He was the Son of God! Not only this, He had come to Jerusalem a week before, riding on a young donkey and acknowledging the cheers of the throngs who lined his path and spread palm fronds along the way as a symbol of his majesty and of their adoration. It was a story of triumph to tragedy. That the crowds would shortly be calling out for his crucifixion was no surprise to Him for He had already prepared his disciples with the news that He would suffer and die in Jerusalem and after three days He would rise again. All of this drama was thoroughly documented by both sacred and secular historians. The essential elements of this unique, incomparable event are that Jesus was rejected, tortured and killed. His body was bound, sealed in a stone-hewn tomb and was guarded by Roman soldiers. The soldiers kept vigilance, knowing that if the tomb became invaded, they would have paid with their very lives. We are faced with incontrovertible fact: Jesus Christ was dead and buried.

The next day was the Jewish Sabbath, a Saturday. It was historically an uneventful, normal day, except for the fact that loved ones and friends, as well as a band of 11 disciples were ensconced in secrecy and were sadly grieving the loss of the one person they had admired and revered and believed to have been the almighty Son of God from heaven to earth come down. Their hopes had been dashed; their hearts had been broken. Jesus was gone.

On the third day, early on Sunday morning, while it was still dark, two women who loved Jesus—Mary Magdalene and Mary the mother of James-- came to see the sepulcher. They brought with them some sweet spices, hoping they might come and anoint the body of Jesus. An amazing thing then took place: an earth quake struck the area, shaking and dislodging the giant stone that had sealed the entrance to the tomb and rolled it away. Here is the description of the Biblical account: *"There was a violent earthquake, for an angel of the Lord came down from heaven and, going to the tomb, rolled back the stone and sat upon it. His appearance was like lightning, and his clothes were white as snow. The guards were so afraid of him that they shook and became like dead men. The angel said to the women; do not be afraid, for I know that you are looking for Jesus, who was crucified. He is not here; He has risen just as He said. Come and see the place where He lay. Then go quickly and tell his disciples: 'He has risen from the dead and is going ahead of you into Galilee. There you will see Him.' Now I have told you* (Matthew 28:2-7)."

What follows over the course of the next forty days are numerous public appearances of the risen Jesus and many infallible proofs of his resurrection from the dead. The Biblical record has Jesus appearing (1) to Mary Magdalene, (Mark 16:9-10) in the early morning, (2) to the other women, (Matthew 28:9-10), (3) to the two disciples, on the way to Emmaus (Mark 16:12-13, Luke 24:13-32), (4) to Peter (Luke 24:34) sometime that day, (5) to the eleven disciples in an upper room that night (Mark 16:14, Luke 24:36, John 20:19) with Thomas absent, (6) to the eleven a week later, with Thomas present (John 20:26-31), (7) to the seven, beside the Sea of Galilee (John 21), (8) to the eleven and a crowd of over 500 brethren on a mountain in Galilee (Matthew 28:16-20), (9) to James at a time and place unknown (1 Corinthians 15:7), (10) a final appearance and His Ascension into heaven (Mark 16:9, Luke 24:44, Acts 1:3). Later, Jesus made a special trip from heaven to make an appearance to the Apostle Paul (Acts 9:1-16).

The Easter event must be considered to be the most dynamic and powerful happening of all time, since the creation of the Universe. Almighty God, the Source of all life, had come from eternity to pierce time and space when he took on human form, miraculously implanted in the womb of the Virgin Mary and born in a humble stable in the little town of Bethlehem over 2,000 years ago. That infant child of Mary was the infinite Son of God, *"The Word became flesh and made His dwelling among us* (John 1:14)." He was Jesus—Savior; the long-anticipated Messiah of Israel, foretold by the prophets of the Old Testament, the Redeemer

Who had come on a mission to give His life to ransom sinners, save them from their fate, and build a Church that would endure for eternity and against which even the gates of Hell could not prevail. Jesus fulfilled His Divine mission. He died on the cross, was buried and rose in resurrection power on the third day. After 40 days of displaying Himself in His resurrection body, Jesus miraculously ascended back to heaven with the dazed and awed disciples staring in wide-eyed wonder. Within weeks, the small band of cowering and fearful disciples were marvelously transformed into bold and vigorous apostles, dispatched by the risen Christ, after being infused with power by the Holy Spirit on the day of Pentecost, went forth to proclaim salvation throughout the known world, making disciples from all nations. Shortly, the Apostles Peter and John would be summoned to appear before an audience of rulers, elders and teachers of the law who met in Jerusalem, and who had called them to account by what power or what name had they healed a cripple. "**Then Peter, filled with the Holy Spirit, said to them, 'Rulers and elders of the people! If we are being called to account today for an act of kindness shown to a cripple, and are asked how he was healed, then know this, you and the people of Israel: It is by the name of Jesus Christ of Nazareth, whom you crucified but whom God raised from the dead, that this man stands before you healed. He is 'the stone you builders rejected, which has become the capstone.' Salvation is found in no one else, for there is no other name under heaven given to men by which we must be saved** (Acts 4:8-12)." Occasions such as this marked but just the beginning of the stunning results stemming from the triumph of Jesus over sin and death and His mighty resurrection on Easter morning. The resurrection of Christ is fact. What are the implications of this momentous event?

I am certain that the fruits of the resurrection of Jesus are without number, but I would like to direct your focus to six immense implications of this glorious miracle. I would suggest that the resurrection of Jesus is a polemic for miracles, a proof of the atonement, a premise for validating all the promises and teachings of Jesus, a primer for the preaching of the Gospel, a picture of our resurrection to come, and a power over the clutches of sin in our lives. Could any solitary event ever yield such profound and extraordinary results? I think not.

In the first place, the resurrection of Jesus from being dead as a proverbial door nail to becoming the vibrant and ubiquitous risen Lord and Savior is nothing short of miracle of miracles! It has been said by many scholars that the uniqueness of the Bible as being the Word of God, thereby setting it apart from all other literature, is the fact that it rests primarily on two giant pillars of truth: the prophecies and the miracles. Neither of these two phenomena can be explained from Science or from a strict Naturalism. Naturalism allows for no happenings that do not accord with Natural Law. One would never be able to accept the Bible as being true if he were committed to a strict naturalism for he would stumble and fall over the prophecies and the miracles of the Bible. The core of the problem for the naturalist is the fact that the Bible is full of supernatural elements from cover to cover because it gives account of the mighty acts of God in human history and among men in order to deliver salvation from sin to the people of God.

It is impossible to disprove prophecy because the prophecies can be dated through scientific and historical methods and they can be dated and fixed in time. The subsequent occurrence of events that answer to the prophecies in minute details gives sterling verification to them. It is most difficult, also, to disprove miracles without impugning the reliability, honesty and character of the eye-witnesses that report them. The major strength of Biblical miracles lies in the fact that the incidents of miracle were never done in a corner or in obscurity, but they were performed in the open and in the presence of many, many witnesses—many witnesses, in fact, who were often hostile to the ones performing those miracles. They would have to have been convinced beyond a shadow of a doubt before they would agree that a miracle had taken place!

Additionally, from a logical perspective, one needs to prove that only one miracle ever was performed in order to open the possibility for accepting all the miracles of the Bible. Perhaps the most defensible of all miracles and the one which is logically impossible of successful refutation is the resurrection of Jesus Christ from the dead. The collaborating evidence is not a few falling stones that a stalwart naturalist might cleverly dodge; it is a cascading avalanche of circumstances and evidence that would crush any intellectual opposition. The reality is that the resurrection of Jesus, reported by the writers of the New Testament and historians of the times, is a tremendous polemic for all of the other miracles of the Bible because its accomplishment required a greater demonstration of Divine power and abrogation of the Laws of Nature than in any of the other miracles recorded in sacred history. This is what is known in philosophical parlance as an "a-fortiori argument"; an argument of the greater to the lesser. If a man can show that he can consume 40 wieners in a contest, then a-fortiori, he could eat 10 wieners at another occasion. If a woman can leap 12 feet in the long jump, a-fortiori, she could jump over a 3 foot puddle of water! Accept the resurrection of Jesus and you can believe His birth of a Virgin mother, His turning the water into wine, feeding the five thousand with five loaves of bread and two small fish, healing the blind, the lame and the crippled, walking on the water, and even the raising of the dead! Only God could do such things. And Jesus was God in the flesh! Listen to His own words: "**the words I say to you are not just my own. Rather, it is the Father, living in me, who is doing his work. Believe me when I say that I am in the Father and the Father is in me; or at least believe on the evidence of the miracles themselves** (John 14:9-11)."

Watching a superstar professional athlete make an amazing play that exhibits the utmost in dexterity, balance and skill, is a wonder to behold but it is no surprise. It is what we come to expect from such athletes. Admiring the latest painting of a Rembrandt or a Picasso is breath-taking to an Art aficionado, but it is no surprise. We have come to expect such masterpieces from those immortal artists. By the same token, as we consider that God is at work in human history to fashion events to fit His divine purpose for the redemption of a people for Himself, it should be no surprise when we are confronted with a miracle. Indeed, the surprise would be in not finding Him performing miracles! Miracles recorded in the Bible are the credentials that validate the prophets and the apostles as messengers and chosen representatives of the

Almighty God. The history of the early church in which we have the Apostles going about proclaiming the resurrection of Jesus and the urgent necessity of people to repent of their sins and embrace Jesus as Lord and Savior finds their ministrations attended by many miracles, signs and wonders. The miracles served to authenticate their message! Their message was from God. In other words, they spoke the truth. And when the truth of the salvation message is believed and a person opens his mind and heart to accept Jesus as Lord and Savior, nothing short of a miracle occurs in that person's life. There is a transformation from being bound by a sinful nature to being imbued with a portion of the Divine Nature. The Apostle Paul defined the miracle as changing from having only a worldly point of view to becoming the righteousness of God! How does this dynamic change take place? It cannot be that man can reinvent himself and decide to change. Through determined resolution, some behavioral changes can indeed be made. But the nature of the man remains the same—he is still a sinner. He's just a sinner that has made some good changes, but a sinner none the less. Paul is talking about a change that dumps the sinful nature in a man and takes on a part of the Divine Nature. The believer becomes a new person from the inside out! Listen to his words to the Corinthians: *"So from now on we regard no one from a worldly point of view. Though we once regarded Christ in this way, we do so no longer. Therefore, if anyone is in Christ, he is a new creation; the old has gone, the new has come! All this is from God, who reconciled us to himself through Christ and gave us the ministry of reconciliation: that God was reconciling the world to himself in Christ, not counting men's sins against them. And he has committed to us the message of reconciliation. We are therefore Christ's ambassadors, as though God were making his appeal through us. We implore you on Christ's behalf: Be reconciled to God. God made him who had no sin to be sin for us, so that in him we might become the righteousness of God* (2 Corinthians 5:16-21)." Yes, the resurrection of Jesus from the dead on that first Easter morning is a powerful polemic for miracles. The ultimate miracle is that a sinner may be saved and transformed by the grace of God, forgiven of his or her sins, and be given the hope of eternal life by simply repenting or turning from their sins, admitting they are sinners, and asking Jesus (the risen One) to come into the heart and transform the life, so that it can be a life to be lived for God, no longer for self!

Not only is the resurrection of Jesus a polemic for miracles, it is also a proof of the atonement. Resurrection presupposes death. Jesus really died upon the cross; he did not merely faint into unconsciousness and later revive. He bled from head, hands and feet for three hours as he was nailed to the cross. What little blood that may have been left was driven out when a Roman soldier jabbed his spear into His side as he hung lifeless on the cross. The Bible states that when his side was opened up by the piercing spear, out flowed blood and water. The mixing of the blood and water is medical proof of death. He was not in a swoon, as some unbelievers have guessed. He was not in a coma from which he might later become resuscitated. He was dead. The Apostle Paul proclaimed to people at Rome: "*The wages of sin is death* (Romans 6:23)." Christ was on that cross in the first place for only one reason: it was to offer his life for our sins. Since the wages of sin is death, he had to die in order to save us from that fate. The cross, therefore, is a place of substitution—Jesus took our place and paid the price we deserve to pay for our sins. He died to set us free from having to pay the wages for our sins! Life is in the blood. Since the wages of sin is death, blood would need be shed; life for sin. That is the meaning of atonement. The Old Testament sacrificial system was based on the slaying of the sacrificial lamb, bull or goat and the sprinkling of its blood on the mercy seat, offering atonement for the sins of the people; life for sin. Flash back, if you will, to the commencement of Jesus' public ministry. As Jesus approached the crowd to which John the Baptist had been speaking, John pointed to Jesus and said, "*Look, the Lamb of God, Who takes away the sin of the world* (John 1:29)!" The means by which he would save the world was becoming the sinless "lamb," bleeding and dying on the cross.

The fact is that Jesus had to pay the price for our sins to satisfy the justice of a Holy God. God's justice is what demands the wages of sin, which is death. The only way a Holy God could allow sinners into His presence is if a covering or atonement could be offered on their behalf—if a sinless substitute should bear the sinner's sins in himself and die on his behalf. The only possible sinless person who could take our place was Jesus. He was without sin, free of spot or blemish. He fulfilled the law of righteousness. He alone could satisfy the justice of God. His trek to the cross was His way of opening up the path to heaven for all who would embrace His sacrifice on their behalf! Had Jesus not been sinless, and had he not satisfied the justice of God by his death on the cross, there would have been no resurrection. God would have no grounds for raising him from the dead. When Jesus came forth in his resurrection, it was proof that his death had atoned for our sins. Paul said to the Romans, "**If Christ has not been raised, your faith is futile; you are still in your sins** (Romans 15:17)." The Apostle did not say, "If Christ is not raised, how should you know if your sins are forgiven?" With him, there is no question: "***you are still in your sins.***"

I cannot conceive of a greater waste than should Jesus have suffered such a tragic death, but to no avail. Without the resurrection, His effort to offer atonement for our sins would be for nothing and we would still be without hope. Happily, however, the resurrection of Jesus signifies the Divine acknowledgment of the efficacy of Christ's death on our behalf—that is, God accepted His atoning work. Perhaps, you can recall from reading the Old Testament the accounts of the high priest of Israel entering into the Holy of Holies of the Tabernacle on Yom Kippur, the Day of Atonement. None but the High Priest was ever allowed to enter the innermost chamber—the Holy of Holies, which contained the Ark of the Covenant and the Mercy Seat. The High Priest entered with the blood of the sacrificial animal to offer it as atonement for the sins of the people. If the offered atonement had not been found pleasing to God, the High Priest would have been struck dead and would not have come out of the Holy of Holies. The High Priest had bells sewn into the hem of his robe, causing a jingling that was audible to the worshippers waiting outside. As long as they heard the bells jingling, the people had confidence the High Priest was being successful in obtaining God's forgiveness of their sins with the sacrifice he was offering. The return of the High Priest from the Holy of Holies to the outer court of the tabernacle was a visible proof to the awaiting worshippers that God had been satisfied with the atonement that was offered.

In the same manner, Jesus' resurrection and visible appearances served to verify that what He did on the cross had satisfied the justice of God. It was proof of the atonement. The hymn writer has captured this wonder with these words: "**Jesus paid it all, all to Him I owe; sin had left a crimson stain, He washed it white as snow.**"

In the third place, the resurrection of Jesus is a primer for the preaching of the Gospel. Until the disciples had been confronted with the resurrected Christ, they had been cowering in fear and retirement from public view. They had absolutely no disposition for preaching. Their hopes and expectations for God's kingdom on earth were crushed. Jesus was taken from them and he was crucified. Even as a pump is primed with water in order to set it into action, so the disciples had to be primed on the news of the Lord's resurrection before they could begin the preaching of the Gospel that faith in Jesus would bring the forgiveness of sins and the gift of eternal life. Preaching was the essential format for spreading the news of Christ's victory over sin and death and the salvation that could be obtained through faith in Him. Paul wrote these encouraging words to young Timothy: "**So do not be ashamed to testify about our Lord, or ashamed of me his prisoner. But join with me in suffering for the gospel, by the power of God, who has saved us and called us to a holy life—not because of anything we have done but because of his own purpose and grace. This grace was given us in Christ Jesus before the beginning of time, but it has now been revealed through the appearing of our Savior, Christ Jesus, who has destroyed death and has brought life and immortality to light through the gospel. And of this gospel I was appointed a herald and an apostle and a teacher. That is why I am suffering as I am. Yet I am not ashamed, because I know whom I have believed, and am convinced that he is able to guard what I have entrusted to him for that day** (2 Timothy 1:8-12)."

Paul could preach, as could all of the other apostles, because Christ had risen from the dead! The resurrection event became the keynote of all the preaching of the apostles and was the main reason that thousands of people, both Jews and Gentiles, were converted to Christ and became the pillars of the churches that were established throughout world. One needs only to read the Acts of the Apostles to become convinced that the fact of the resurrection of Jesus was the one great truth which became the primer for the preaching of the gospel of redemption. Christians all over the world are meeting in churches and are celebrating their faith in Jesus Christ. For them, there is no other justification for preaching or worship. We serve a living Christ! One of the most beloved of Christian hymns has the words, "*I serve a risen Savior, He's in the world today; I know that He is living, whatever men may say. I see His hand of mercy, I hear His voice of cheer, and just the time I need Him He's always near. He lives, He lives, Christ Jesus lives today! He walks with me and talks with me along life's narrow way. He lives, He lives, salvation to impart! You ask me how I know He lives? He lives within my heart.*"

The implications of the resurrection of Jesus from the dead are truly enormous. As we have already considered, the resurrection is a powerful polemic for the miracles of the Bible. It is a proof of the atonement and it is a primer for the preaching of the gospel. Additionally, the resurrection is a premise for validating all of the promises and the teachings of Jesus. After Peter had made his great confession, "**You are the Christ, the Son of the Living God** (Matthew 16:16)," Jesus began to prepare his disciples for his impending death and his resurrection to follow. The Bible says, "**From that time on Jesus began to explain to his disciples that he must go to Jerusalem and suffer many things at the hands of the elders, chief priests and teachers of the law, and that he must be killed and on the third day be raised to life** (Matthew 16:21)." On the morning of His resurrection some women had come to the tomb very early in the morning and found the stone had been rolled away from the tomb, and when they entered the tomb they did not find the body of Jesus. The Scripture says, "**While they were wondering about this, suddenly two men in clothes that gleamed like lightening stood beside them. In their fright the women bowed down with their faces to the ground, but the men said to them, 'Why do you** *look for the living among the dead? He is not here, he has risen! Remember how he told you, while he was still with you in Galilee, 'The Son of Man must be delivered into the hands of sinful men, be crucified and on the third day be raised again.' Then they remembered his words* (Luke 24:4-8)."

That Jesus would predict that he would die in Jerusalem, where there was a lot of opposition to him because he was a threat to established religion, is quite creditable. But when he adds that he will be raised from the dead on the third day-- that is another matter. Everyone might expect the possibility of his own death. To say, however, that after being dead you would rise again in three days is a bold assertion and virtually impossible to believe. People in their right minds do not say things like that—that is, unless the person happens also to be God and knows He can do it! Jesus made many other promises, many of which are yet to be fulfilled. He taught many things that would be most difficult for us to accept unless we are sure they are truly the words and the wisdom of almighty God. How could we know this? Good logic would tell us that we can measure the truthfulness of a person by the way they have the habit of delivering on their promises. If a person is right on a hundred things, it is easy to believe he would also be right on the one-hundred and first thing. Again, we have the a-fortiori argument. When one can deliver on the most difficult things, it is easier to believe the less difficult. If you can show me you can play Chopin or Beethoven on the piano, then a-fortiori, you should be able to play "Mary Had a Little Lamb," or "Jingle Bells."

We need to apply the same reasoning and logic to the miraculous resurrection of Jesus from the dead. When Jesus foretold with precise detail that he would suffer many things in Jerusalem, would be put to death and would rise again on the third day, time would tell if he was right or not. Since everything happened just as He said, it would seem that everything else Jesus said must also be accepted as truth: that His blood was to be shed for the remission of sins, that He came down from the Father above, that the words He spoke had been given Him by the Father, that He and the Father are one, that He was the Son of God, that whosoever would believe on Him would be forgiven their sins and would receive everlasting life, and whoever refused to believe on Him would be eternally condemned. The empty tomb and the fact of the risen Lord should assure us forever that when Jesus said He was going to prepare a place for us and that He would one day return to receive us unto Himself, He was not whistling in the wind. When Jesus said that one day the dead in their graves would hear the voice of the Son of God and would come forth from their graves to face Him in Divine judgment, He was speaking the truth. It is impossible to accept the resurrection of Jesus and entertain any doubt about any utterance that ever came from His lips. It is no wonder, then, that the condition of saving faith is predicated on the fact that Jesus died for our sins and He was raised from the dead. The Apostle Paul was right on target when he declared, "*The word is near you; it is in your mouth and in your heart, that is, the word of faith we are proclaiming. That if you confess with your mouth, Jesus is Lord, and believe in your heart that God has raised Him from the dead, you will be saved. For it is with your heart that you believe and are justified, and it is with your mouth that you confess and are saved* (Romans 10:8-9)."

Men tell lies because they have a sinful nature. God cannot tell lies because He has a Divine Nature. God is perfect. With Him there can be no deceit or duplicity. The writer of the book of Hebrews in the New Testament declares this same fact: "*it is impossible for God to lie* (Hebrews 6:18)." Since Jesus is God's Son, He shares God's Divine nature. It is impossible, therefore, for Jesus to lie. The only question that could be asked is this: is Jesus really God? The answer is the resurrection. It is as Paul said when stating his credentials to the church at Rome, "*Paul, a servant of Christ Jesus, called to be an apostle and set apart for the gospel of God—the gospel he promised beforehand through his prophets in the Holy Scriptures regarding his Son, who as to his human nature was a descendent of David, and who through the Spirit of holiness was declared with power to be the Son of God <u>by his resurrection from the dead</u>: Jesus Christ our Lord* (Romans 1:1-4)." Yes, when a person believes in his heart that God has raised Jesus from the dead, he will be compelled to believe every other promise and teaching that Jesus ever uttered.

Another truly marvelous and stirring implication of the resurrection of Jesus is that it is a picture of the resurrection of every believer to come. His victory over death and the grave is our victory, also. This is because our victory is subsumed under His miraculous resurrection! For the Christian believer, death and the grave are not final. There is a destiny in store for the believer that will one day bring him or her out of the grave in resurrection glory and transports the believer into God's presence to abide with Him forever. We are benefactors of His amazing love and grace. This is a concept around which many people cannot wrap their minds. Many think this would be impossible—there will be no resurrection after death. It is to such persons the Apostle Paul addressed his words: "***But if it is preached that Christ has been raised from the dead, how can some of you say that there is no resurrection of the dead? If there is no resurrection of the dead, then not even Christ has been raised. And if Christ has not been raised, our preaching is useless and so is your faith. More than that, we are then found to be false witnesses about God, for we have testified about God that He raised Christ from the dead. But he did not raise him if in fact the dead are not raised. For if the dead are not raised, then Christ has not been raised either. And if Christ has not been raised, your faith is futile; you are still in your sins. Then those also who have fallen asleep in Christ are lost. If only in this life we have hope in Christ, we are to be pitied more than all men. <u>But Christ has indeed been raised from the dead, the first fruits of those who have fallen asleep</u>. For since death came through a man, the resurrection of the dead comes also through a man. For as in Adam all die, so in Christ all will be made alive. But each in his own turn: Christ the first fruits, then, when he comes, those who belong to him*** (I Corinthians 15:12-23)."

The first fruits are the beginning of the harvest and are a harbinger of the greater harvest to come. In His resurrection of Easter morning, Jesus was the first fruits and the guarantor of the resurrection of every believer in the great day of His second coming to earth. He will come to gather his people in a tremendous upsurge of resurrected souls, reunited with their new bodies that will prepare them for their new dwelling in God's heaven. They will be spiritual bodies, not bodies of flesh and blood. But they will bear their own original identity and people will be able to recognize those whom they knew in life on earth. Consider the resurrected Jesus. His disciples all recognized Him when he appeared to them in the upper room where they were in hiding. The apostle Thomas was absent the first time Jesus appeared to the disciples. When the other disciples joyfully told Thomas that Jesus was alive and back from the dead, Thomas doubted their disclosure. He said, *"Unless I see the nail marks in his hands and put my fingers where the nails were, and put my hand into his side, I will not believe it* (John 20:25)." It was a week later that Jesus returned the second time to the disciples, with Thomas among them. Listen to John's account: *"A week later his disciples were in the house again, and Thomas with them. Though the doors were locked, Jesus came and stood among them and said, 'Peace be with you!' Then he said to Thomas, 'Put your finger here; see my hands. Reach out your hand and put it into my side. Stop doubting and believe* (John 20:26-27)."

This encounter of the risen Lord to His disciples is highly instructional to us concerning our future resurrection bodies in which our departed souls will inhabit at Jesus' second coming. As already mentioned, we will bear the image of our earthly body but will be in a body that is not confined to the limitations of our physical bodies. Jesus appeared through locked doors to confront his disciples. Yet, he convinced Thomas he was the same Jesus he knew before he was buried in Joseph's tomb: he displayed the holes in his hands, his feet and his side. Remember, if you will, we are examining no ordinary person here; we are viewing God almighty in the person of His Son, Creator of the Universe and the only One who has the power to abrogate the laws of nature to accomplish His will! What we have, therefore, in the resurrection of Jesus, is a preview of what a spiritual body will be like as opposed to the natural bodies we now possess. We know a solid body cannot pass through a solid door without disturbing the composition of the door. Yet, Jesus was able to pass through the locked door or the walls of the room where the disciples were meeting and appear among them. He did this with a spiritual body. We cannot explain this from the laws of nature as we now know them. There is, however, a law of physics which states that matter cannot be either created or destroyed. What things happen when things are "destroyed" are a break-down of the existing molecular structure and a rearrangement of the molecules into different substances. Suppose it were possible to name or label every single atom in a structure or substance and a 3-D snapshot could be taken showing the structural and spatial relation of each individual atom to every other atom that comprises the object described. If one could hold absolute control over each atom and engineer its position in relation to all the other atoms, he could take the object apart and put it back together again, much like a person might put together a 1,000 piece puzzle, then break it down to its individual pieces again. Only, in the case of life-sized objects, such as a human being, we are talking about a puzzle with billions of atoms. For a human being to be able to deconstruct and then reconstruct an object into its identical form is currently impossible as far as current technology allows. But Almighty God, creator and sustainer of all that exists, who is bound by no intellectual or scientific limitations, would have no problem in doing whatever could be imagined. It is not beyond belief, therefore, that Jesus in His spiritual resurrection body operated by rules that man has not yet discovered, and was able to pass his "body" through a solid barrier such as a door or wall, simply by meshing the atomic structures of both during the "pass through" and putting everything back together as it was before the pass through. We see beams of light passing through panes of glass every day and do not wonder at all how this could be. You might say, "Yes, but light will not pass through a panel of wood like it passes through a panel of glass." That's correct. But this does not alter the premise. All you have shown is light will do certain things through translucent substances that it will not do through non-translucent substances. My premise in this discussion is that with God, nothing is impossible. We may not understand how it is done, but it is done none the less.

The foregoing reference to the atomic structure of all physical matter and the law of physics that asserts matter cannot be either created or destroyed presents a basis for believing God could witness our atomic destruction through any means possible, such as from decay or from fire, for example, and at His will could call each rearranged atom back into the position it held before the destruction took place. Blown to bits on the field of battle? Cremated in a raging fire or in a cremation oven? Drowned at sea and devoured by fish? It really does not matter what may have happened if the Power that put everything together as it is in the first place decides to reconstruct it after it has been "destroyed." He could with the voice of command or with an instantaneous thought in His mind order anything to happen. This is what happened in the beginning of creation! God spoke, and it was done! Is it reasonable to doubt that He could deliver on His promises— that even as He raised Jesus from the state of being dead for three days, He could also at a future moment of His choosing, give the command to order all who have died to come back to life in a form that would be consistent to occupy the realm for which He purposes—whether it be eternal life or eternal damnation?

While He was still living, before His crucifixion and death, Jesus was teaching his followers about His own powers as the Son of God and what will happen on a future day. Jesus said, "*I tell you the truth, the Son can do nothing by himself; he can do only what he sees his Father doing, because whatever the Father does the Son also does. For the Father loves the Son and shows him all he does. Yes, to your amazement he will show him even greater things than these. For just as the Father raises the dead and gives them life, even so the Son gives life to whom he is pleased to give it. Moreover, the Father judges no one, but has entrusted all judgment to the Son, that all may honor the Son just as they honor the Father. He who does not honor the Son does not honor the Father, who sent him. I tell you the truth; whoever hears my word and believes him who sent me has eternal life and will not be condemned; he has crossed over from death to life. I tell you the truth, a time is coming and has now come when the dead will hear the voice of the Son of God and those who hear will live. For as the Father has life in himself, so he has granted the Son to have life in himself. And he has given him authority to judge because he is the Son of Man. Do not be amazed at this, for a time is coming when all who are in their graves will hear his voice and come out—those who have done good will rise to live, and those who have done evil will rise to be condemned* (John 5:19-29)."

This is serious business, dear reader. It is clearly a matter of life and death. One day, all who are dead will be raised by the power of God and will experience one of two possible destinies: eternal life or eternal condemnation. If you are not absolutely certain you are a child of God, it would be wise for you to interrupt your reading of this paper right now, bow your head in prayer, and reach out to God. Confess to Him that you know you are a sinner for whom Jesus died. Ask Jesus to come into your heart, forgive you of your sins, and transform your life, that you might live for Him! Do this with deepest sincerity, and ask this in Jesus' name, Amen.

Jesus said, "*For God so loved the world that He gave his one and only Son, that whoever believes in him shall not perish but have everlasting life. For God did not send His Son into the world to condemn the world, but to save the world through Him* (John 3:16-17)." At the close of this chapter, John writes these words: "*The Father loves the Son and has placed everything in his hands. Whoever believes in the Son has eternal life, but whoever rejects the Son will not see life, for God's wrath remains on him* (John 3:35)."

In his great chapter on the subject of the resurrection of Jesus and our own resurrection to come, the apostle Paul gives a picture of what is in store for those who believe in Jesus. Here are his astounding words: "*But someone may ask, 'How are the dead raised? With what kind of body will they come?' How foolish! What you sow does not come to life unless it dies. When you sow, you do not plant the body that will be, but just the seed, perhaps of wheat or of something else. But God gives it a body as he has determined, and to each kind of seed he gives its own body. All flesh is not the same: Human beings have one kind of flesh, animals have another, birds another and fish another. There are also heavenly bodies and there are earthly bodies; but the splendor of the heavenly bodies is one kind, and splendor of the earthly bodies is another. The sun has one kind of splendor, the moon another and the stars another; and star differs from star in splendor. So it will be with the resurrection of the dead. The body that is sown is perishable, it is raised imperishable; it is sown in dishonor, it is raised in glory; it is sown in weakness, it is raised in power; it is sown a natural body, it is raised a spiritual body. . .I declare to you, brothers, that flesh and blood cannot inherit the kingdom of God, nor does the perishable inherit the imperishable. Listen, I tell you a mystery: we will not all sleep, but we will all be changed—in a flash, in the twinkling of an eye, at the last trumpet. For the trumpet will sound, the dead will be raised imperishable, and we will be changed. For the perishable must clothe itself with the imperishable, and the mortal with immortality. When the perishable has been clothed with the imperishable, and the mortal with immortality, then the saying that is written will come true: Death has been swallowed up in victory. Where o death is your victory? Where o death is your sting? The sting of death is sin, and the power of sin is the law. But thanks be to God! He gives us the victory through our Lord Jesus Christ. Therefore, my dear brothers, stand firm. Let nothing move you. Always give yourselves fully to the work of the Lord, because you know that your labor in the Lord is not in vain* (I Corinthians 15:35-44, 50-58)."

Finally, the sixth implication of the resurrection of Jesus from the dead is that it gives the believers power over the clutches of sin in their lives. Christ arises to become our bulwark against the forces of sin. He arises to abide with us! Jesus abides in the believer to enable the believer to win the battle over sin which binds him. It is the power of the resurrected Christ, indwelling the believer that gives the believer the ability to live on the plain of righteousness and obedience to His will. Before receiving Christ into one's life by faith, the person is bound by the law of sin and death. He is a slave to his own weaknesses. In Christ, however, all this is changed! The apostle Paul explains, *"Therefore, there is now no condemnation for those who are in Christ Jesus, because through Christ Jesus the law of the Spirit of life set me free from the law of sin and death. For what the law was powerless to do in that it was weakened by the sinful nature, God did by sending his own Son in the likeness of sinful man to be a sin offering. And so he condemned sin in sinful man, in order that the righteous requirements of the law might be fully met in us, who do not live according to the sinful nature but according to the Spirit* (Romans 8:1-4)."

The key to successful living is to let Christ live through us by His Spirit. Only as the believer maintains a fellowship with the risen Christ, and abides in Him by thought and intention, does he have the moral strength to resist temptation and have the power to live a life of victory over the sin that would otherwise defeat him. This is why the Lord instructed his disciples to pray and to include this plea: "*forgive us our debts as we forgive our debtors, and lead us not into temptation, but deliver us from the evil one* (Matthew 6:12-13)." When we live in a state of walking with God we can face any challenge and come up winning! It is not our strength that gives us the victory; it is His strength abiding in us. As we succeed, we cannot take pride, because what was accomplished was owing to His enablement. One of my favorite passages in the Bible contains the words of Paul: "*If God is for us, who can be against us? He who did not spare his own Son, but gave him up for us all—how will he not also, along with him, graciously give us all things? Who will bring any charge against those whom God has chosen? It is God who justifies. Who is he that condemns? Christ Jesus, who died—more than that, who was raised to life—is at the right hand of God and is also interceding for us. Who shall separate us from the love of Christ? Shall trouble or hardship or persecution or famine or nakedness or danger or sword? As it is written: 'For your sake we face death all day long; we are considered as sheep to be slaughtered.' No, in all these things we are more than conquerors through him who loved us. For I am convinced that neither death nor life, neither angels nor demons, neither the present nor the future, nor any powers, neither height nor depth, nor anything else in all creation, will be able to separate us from the love of God that is in Christ Jesus the Lord* (Romans 8:31-39)."

Our Lord and Savior, Jesus Christ, died upon the cross, offering his life as a sacrifice for our sins, so that we, lost in our sins, might be redeemed and given eternal life in Him. It is as the apostle declared, "*For the wages of sin is death, but the gift of God is eternal life in Christ Jesus our Lord* (Romans 6:23)." Listen to the words the angels spoke to the women who came to visit the tomb of Jesus on that first Easter morning, "**He is not here, He is risen just as he said** (Matthew 28:6)." The words spoken to those grieving women are words we need to hear whenever we have any concerns that weigh us down and burden our spirits. Jesus is not dead. He is risen.

The resurrection of Jesus from the dead is amazing fact, and because of that fact there are at least six immense implications: He is risen—it is a polemic for all the miracles of the Bible; He is risen—it is a proof of the atonement for our sins; He is risen—it is a premise for validating all of the promises and teachings of Jesus; He is risen—it is a primer for the preaching of the gospel; He is risen—it is a picture of our resurrection to come; He is risen—it is a power over the clutches of sin in our lives! Thanks be to God for the incomparable and wonderful gift of Jesus' resurrection!

Chapter Eight

THE MIRROR THAT CHANGES YOU

Most people are probably familiar with the warning to be careful and selective about the company you keep, because when you associate with the wrong kind of people for much of the time, you will soon be acting just like them. Of course, this saying is true if reversed, as well. This seems to be a basic truth about personal behavior. Being in close contact with another person for a lengthy period of time, one is soon practicing many of the same habits as the other—even similar mannerisms and patterns of speech. Often, one is not even aware that this is happening. Young people, for example, often readily adopt the habits of their parents, students their teachers and athletes their favorite stars, and so on.

This truth can be applied with good advantage to the area of Christian living. The problem comes, however, when trying to find a good model. This is because even Christians have problems with sin. The phenomenon of the transformed life after placing faith in Jesus Christ and asking him into one's life, and to make of oneself a new person, is dependent on a lot of variables for the process to move along. Reading the Bible, attending worship services, participating in Bible Study groups, developing a pattern of prayer and personal meditation are all activities that spur Christian growth and changes in behavior. Eliminate some or all of these features from one's life and growth will be slow indeed, if at all! Many, in fact, who consider themselves Christian, behave sometimes in a manner that would make others blush in confusion. They ask themselves, "How can one who claims to be Christian do things like that?" Unfortunately, anyone can be Christian and do unchristian things and sport unchristian attitudes. As long as there is a remnant of the old sinful nature in us, we are going to slip into sin and have a battle on our hands trying to say and do what is right—what God expects us to do.

We do not become perfected the moment we believe. We experience the new birth when we receive Jesus Christ into our hearts. Spiritual life springs up within us at the moment of conversion. We are started in a new direction—but we have started only; we have not arrived at perfection or anywhere near perfection! The balance of one's life after receiving Christ as Savior and Lord is a process of becoming what God wants us to become. Sometimes our progress or growth as Christians is rapid and exhilarating; at other times, it seems we are getting nowhere in the process of overcoming sinfulness that is within us. We already had the old nature before coming to Christ. After coming to Christ we have a new nature—a spiritual nature. The apostle Paul compares the two in his book to the Romans, chapter seven. He talks about the old nature and refers it to the carnal man. He talks about the new nature and refers it to the spiritual man. The non-Christian has one nature (the carnal nature) and the Christian has two natures (the carnal and the spiritual). Transformation of the person who becomes a Christian requires putting to death the old nature and indulging the new nature. It becomes warfare within as the Christian faces decisions all day long: the old nature in me wants to say or do one thing but the new nature wants me to react differently, so as to please the Lord. The more that the new nature wins out over the old nature, a change in moral tone occurs and equates to progress in achieving a transformed life. There are no shortcuts or crash courses. It will take time, and patience is a virtue that will assist the process.

The Apostle Paul had some great things to say on this matter of growth and change in the Christian life. To the Corinthians he wrote about this subject of personal transformation and explained how the believer in the Lord is totally changed into a new person by the power of God working within. Listen to his words: "***Therefore, if anyone is in Christ, he is a new creation; the old has gone, the new has come! (***2 Corinthians 5:17)." It is a fact of spiritual life, therefore, that the person who is in Christ will experience dramatic change. How this change actually takes place he describes in another passage of this letter to the Corinthians. He writes, "**Now the Lord is the Spirit, and where the Spirit of Lord is, there is freedom. And we, who with unveiled faces all reflect the Lord's glory, are being transformed into His likeness with ever-increasing glory, which comes from the Lord, who is the Spirit.** (2 Corinthians 3:17-18)."

The first thing Paul points out is that the change will come to believers simply because they have the Holy Spirit within them. Wherever the Spirit dwells, there is liberty—there is freedom. To use a paradigm, it is as though a person lives his or her whole life in a prison called "the sinful nature." That person knows nothing different because the sinful nature confines and limits both knowledge and experience. One momentous day, however, the Lord Jesus confronts that person in his or her prison and asks for that person to trust in Him and make a decision to follow Him no matter the cost. The person confined in the prison of the sinful nature exercises faith and receives Christ as Lord. At that moment, the Lord places the Holy Spirit inside that person and the Holy Spirit is the key that unlocks the door of the prison, setting the person free from that prison and gives the person a new nature—a spiritual nature—so that the person can begin living a transformed life.

We are no longer condemned for our sins when Christ enters our lives. Repentance from sin and acceptance of God's grace results in a miraculous change! Paul writes of this to the church at Rome: "**Therefore, there is now no condemnation for those who are in Christ Jesus, because through Christ Jesus the law of the Spirit of life set me free from the law of sin and death. For what the law was powerless to do in that it was weakened by the sinful nature, God did by sending his own Son in the likeness of sinful man to be a sin offering, And he condemned sin in sinful man, in order that the righteous requirements of the law might be fully met in us, who do not live according to the sinful nature but according to the Spirit.** (Romans 8:1-4)." There is no other way by which a person can rid himself of his sinful nature than by the liberating work of God's Spirit. The theological name given to this process of change in the believer's life is sanctification. It is the name for the process of reproducing the likeness of Christ in the believer. We who believe in Jesus and who receive Him as Lord and

Savior are made partakers of the glory of God by a gradual process of change—we are increasingly and incrementally transformed into the likeness of Christ, from one stage of glory to another.

Sanctification in the Westminster Catechism is said to be "the work of God's free grace, whereby we are renewed in the whole man after the image of God, and are enabled more and more to die unto sin and live unto righteousness." There is, however, a nuance that is missing from this definition. It is accurate in what it says when it defines sanctification as the work of God's free grace: it is not earned or deserved. It is not merited by good works we may do. But what seems to be missing is the fact that it is a cooperative effort between the believer and the Holy Spirit that brings about the transformation in the life of the believer. This principle is different from the principle that is at work in salvation. The soul's salvation from sin is NOT a cooperative effort—it is ALL the work of God in His Son, Jesus Christ. Jesus took our sins in His own body on the Cross and paid the price for our redemption. The hymn writer captured it in these words: "Jesus paid it all, all to Him I owe. Sin had left a crimson stain; He washed it white as snow." As far as our salvation from sin is concerned, we contribute nothing to that effort. It is all the work of God in Christ. Salvation comes to us as a gift of God's grace, totally apart from any good works on our part. Paul underscored this point when he wrote to Titus. He said: "*But when the kindness and love of God our Savior appeared, He saved us, not because of righteous things we had done, but because of His mercy. He saved us through the washing of rebirth and renewal by the Holy Spirit, whom he poured out on us generously through Jesus Christ our Savior, so that, having been justified by His grace, we might become heirs having the hope of eternal life* (Titus 3:4-7)."

Salvation is all the work of Christ, but the principle at work in our transformation once we have become children of God is a cooperative effort between the individual Christian and the Holy Spirit who dwells within him. How do we know this is the way it works? We discover this in the context of Paul's remarks in 2 Corinthians, chapter 3, beginning with verse 16: "*But whenever anyone turns to the Lord, the veil is taken away.*" This may not seem like much that a person does, at first, but actually it is a tremendous happening. The person cooperates in the process by turning to the Lord. It is a very simple statement about what seems to be a very simple act. The problem, however, is it is seldom simply done! If you leave one step out of a mathematic equation you will come up with a wrong answer. Look carefully at the process described in this text. (1) The individual believer turns to the Lord. (2) God takes the veil away (the veil which had obscured the vision and prevented the individual from capturing a full image of God's truth and grace). (3) With the veil now lifted the believer beholds the Lord's glory. (4) The believer is transformed into His likeness with ever-increasing glory, "**which comes from the Lord, Who is Spirit.**" The King James Version of the Bible renders this text: "**But we all with open face, beholding as in a glass the glory of the Lord...**" This rendering suggests the process as though we view God's glory as we gaze on him in a mirror, and in the process of looking into that mirror we ourselves are changed into His likeness, from one stage to increasing stages of glory.

Now, return with me for a moment to stage one of these processes. The text has a conditional clause that introduces the process of transformation. It says, "**But whenever anyone turns to the Lord** (2 Corinthians 4:16a)...**" Would you believe how difficult this simple act of turning to the Lord is for many people? It is difficult for many because they like to think of themselves as competent enough to take care of their own needs and they desire to be independent. They will almost die before they would ask anyone else for any assistance. If there's anything they cannot do for themselves, they will just go without, but they will not turn to someone else for help. People of this mindset are very difficult people to convince of God's grace—His unmerited favor! Others will not turn to the Lord because they have the mistaken idea they can earn God's forgiveness by amassing a life of righteous living and charitable giving. If we could earn our way to heaven by any means of our own contriving, the cross on which Jesus died would then be superfluous! But most people do not realize this or do not take the time to even think of such issues. Most people's lives are fairly programmed to routines of responsibility and habits of leisure that preclude church attendance, listening to religious programming or reading the Bible. Rarely do they even have the occasion when they are in a place where they will feel a tug on their heart and hear a still small voice of God's Spirit speaking to them in their minds of the need to repent from a life of sin and turn to Jesus for His salvation! The invitation to receive Christ as Lord and Savior is freely offered, but few are in the right spirit to turn to Jesus. Yet, that is the starting point for experiencing the transformed life of which Paul speaks to the Corinthians. Again, "**But whenever anyone turns to the Lord**,"—that's a major happening!

The first step is turning to the Lord. The first step is the most difficult to take because it means a person is making a major choice for his or her life. It is difficult because of one basic principle: ANY TURNING TO IS ALSO A TURNING FROM. When I am driving on an interstate highway and choose to turn on to an exit, I am immediately removed from the interstate. When a person chooses to enter college, that person is turning from a life of leisure or postponing the beginning of a career. A person falls in love with another person and this experience begins to realign all of the priorities in each person's life. Should they choose to marry, both would be turning from a single lifestyle to a married lifestyle. Such a change is usually far beyond what either might have anticipated unless either of them had been previously married. One could scarcely have a successful married life if he or she is truly not ready to abandon the lifestyle of a single person. All of this is because a turning to is also a turning from. It is a matter of choice. In fact, your entire life to this point is a story of your choices! Every path you chose to take was a turning from something else. If you chose to smoke, you chose to leave the lifestyle of a non-smoker. If you chose to have premarital sex, you chose to give up your virginity. If you chose to take something that belonged to another person you became a thief and turned from having a respect for the rights of others. If you turned to telling a lie to save your skin, you turned from honesty. Turning to secretiveness is turning from transparency. Turning to spontaneity could mean a turning from reliability and dependability. The examples are exhaustive; you could come up with hundreds of examples of this principle.

But there is a huge difference when one is confronted with Jesus. He does not want to be selected as extra baggage to tag along where you want to go with your life. He is God; and if selected, He expects to be Lord and in charge of your life. His values will replace your values. His will shall prevail over your will. It is as Paul wrote to the Colossians, "**So that in everything He might have the supremacy** (Colossians 1:18)." This means anyone turning to Jesus is choosing to make Him the focal point of all their main choices for the rest of life! It is every bit an act of commitment as a marriage ceremony where two become one! The potential for change is simply enormous as one joins forces with the King of Kings and Lord of Lords! It is the most profound and most intelligent choice any person could ever make—turning to Jesus! Immediately upon turning to Him, a veil has been lifted from covering our faces and we begin to view the glory of Jesus as if looking into a glass. Beholding His glory changes us from one stage of glory into another, and we gradually become transformed into the image of the living Christ! It matters not what you were like before you turned to Jesus. You may have had a really messed-up life. You may have brought to him a wreck of a life, but not to worry. It is not what you did with your life that counts. What counts is what He can do with what is left of your life! What matters is that you can post a new sign over your life for all to see; a sign which simply says, "UNDER NEW MANAGEMENT."

We see, then, that the Bible is like a mirror—but a mirror different from all others. Other mirrors show us what we look like on the outside; the Bible shows us what we look like on the inside. More than that, in fact, because the Bible also shows us what Jesus is like! As we compare what the Bible shows us about ourselves with what it shows us about Jesus, we develop a longing to emulate characteristics of Christ's divine life. The more we see Him for who he is the more we want to become like Him. This dynamic drives the process of transformation —the sanctification of the believer. To become like Jesus means we will think about things the way He thinks about them, we feel about things the way He feels about them, and we behave in ways we have observed Him to have behaved. Where can we possibly know how Jesus thinks, feels and behaves? We know these things only through His self-disclosure—in His Word, the Bible. As you read the Gospels of Matthew, Mark, Luke and John you construct a mosaic of the character and mindset of Jesus—how he viewed people as sheep needing a shepherd. You observe what he thought about the poor, the sick, the lost and the lonely. He had compassion on them. How did He respond? He constantly reached out to them with tenderness, caring and love and he met their needs. When the believer replicates these feelings of compassion for people and reaches out to them in their need, the believer is displaying a Christ-likeness in thought, feeling and behavior. By reading in the Gospels about the life and acts of Jesus, the believer is beholding Christ as in a mirror, and the image in the mirror begins to change the believer into the same image on a much smaller scale—but it is change none the less! It is sanctification in progress.

How a person reads the Bible can make a huge difference in what they get from reading it. Some people read the Bible like they are running through a curio shop; they could scarcely tell you what they have read after reading it because they were hurrying along to get through one chapter to get to the next! Hurrying may make perfect sense to a trained speed reader but it won't work for most people. A more helpful approach would be to slow down in the reading of the text, then take time to ponder the insights just revealed. Pondering is similar to the cow chewing the cud so that the grass can be digested when it is swallowed. The grass could not be digested if it was swallowed whole, without first grinding and chewing it between the teeth. The Christian will get the most benefit from Bible reading when he or she ponders the thoughts received in the reading of the Scriptures.

When Mary, the mother of our Lord, gave birth to Jesus by means of the miracle of the Holy Ghost and not from a seed planted by a male partner, she was clearly overwhelmed. It just never happens this way, she must have mused! Mary was greeted by a heavenly Angel who told her to not be afraid because she had found favor with God; she would conceive and give birth to a son, and she should call his name Jesus. The angel said her son would be great and be called the Son of the Most High and God will give

Him the throne of his father David, and He would reign over the house of Jacob forever; His kingdom will never end. When Mary asked how this could happen since she was a virgin, the angel answered, "**The Holy Spirit will come on you, and the power of the Most High will overshadow you. So the holy one to be born will be called the Son of God** (Luke 2:35)." Later, after the baby Jesus was born in the manger in Bethlehem, the Bible says there were shepherds living out in the fields nearby, keeping watch over their flocks by night when an angel of the Lord appeared to them, and the glory of the Lord shone round about them, and the shepherds were terrified. The angel calmed their fears and directed them to where they could find the baby wrapped in cloths and lying in a manger. The Bible text briefly describes a scene where shepherds come to the manger and find Mary and Joseph and the baby, who was lying in the manger. "**When they had seen him, they spread the word concerning what had been told them about this child, and all who heard it were amazed at what the shepherd said to them. But Mary treasured up all these things and pondered them in her heart** (Luke 2:17-19)." Mary pondered over these wondrous and miraculous happenings, like a cow lying on the grass chewing his cud so as to digest the grass. The significance of what was happening was too great to quickly pass on to some other thoughts or concerns—pondering allowed her to grasp its wondrous meaning. Mary would never be the same again!

In your Bible reading you will encounter passages that may hit you as having tremendous significance and hold great meaning for your particular life situation; you will see Jesus and the salvation He gives you by His grace and you may need to pause and ponder those truths until the significance bores into your memory bank in your brain. When this happens, you will undergo some spiritual change—you will be seeing Jesus as in a mirror and you will be changed a little more into His likeness—from one stage of glory unto another stage of glory. I like to think of pondering as a kaleidoscopic effect. You keep the different thoughts of a verse constantly turning in your mind until the pattern falls into place before your eyes.

An example may help to illuminate this principle. I recently had a "wow" moment when reading from 2 Timothy, chapter two.

When I read the fifteenth verse, it struck me as being pretty special. These are the words: "***Do your best to present yourself to God as one approved, a worker who does not need to be ashamed and who correctly handles the word of truth.***" I thought I would take some more time to simply analyze this verse, using the kaleidoscopic approach. First I jotted down on some paper the verbs of action: "Do your best," "present yourself," "approved," "correctly handles." Next, I wrote down the nouns: "God," "worker," and "Word of truth." Now, the words are turned around and danced around with the nouns just to see what might emerge. I started seeing things like "handling the Word of truth correctly...is hard work...but do your best ...you won't be ashamed of your effort...you will earn the approval of God when you present yourself to Him."

Coming up with that picture was rewarding in itself, but to give it my best shot, I decided to check out the meaning of one of the key words—"correctly handling." Checking a different translation of the verse, I noticed the KJV Bible had worded it "rightly dividing." The message is for the worker who works for God wins His approval when he correctly handles or rightly divides His Word of Truth. Carelessness won't win His approval. Jumping to immediate conclusions because they support our previously formed views on points of theology will not win His approval either. Now this is where the "worker" idea is further established: I took more time and looked up the meaning of the word used for "handling" or "dividing" and discovered that the word in the original Greek language—in which the New Testament is written—is "quarrying." A good Bible commentary might be pulled off the shelf at this point to see what can be learned about quarrying in New Testament times. I did just this and learned that the method of quarrying stone in Biblical times was to cut the stone at precise specifications right at the quarry so that when brought to the construction site it was a perfect fit with the stones already in place! Therefore, the worker in the quarry carefully measuring and accurately cutting the stone, adhering to all the angles specified by the blueprint would be presenting himself as unashamed and would win the approval of the architect of the building. The spiritual significance is profound: if we as God's quarrymen render a passage of Scripture accurately within its context, it can be taken to other passages of Scripture dealing with the same issue or theme and it will fit right in perfectly. Correctly rendered Scripture will mesh with correctly rendered passages elsewhere because God's Word will never contradict itself. This is why a good "worker" will compare Scripture with Scripture before forming a conclusion on major tenants of our Faith!

In addition to pondering, or mulling a text over and over in one's mind, one must be prepared to make a painstaking analysis of a Scripture text if he is to *"**behold the glory of the Lord**."* Whenever you do not understand the meaning of even a single word, you should not just pass it by. You may do this with a novel or with a biography and be none the worse for it. But the Bible is God's word and a misunderstood word can turn a meaning into quite a different matter. I would encourage one to study important Biblical passages using all the tools available: a dictionary, to determine the meaning of a word; a concordance, to see how the same word is used elsewhere in the Scriptures; good commentaries, to compare the hard work other scholars have already put into the matter of rendering a particular passage and which often sets forth all the competing theories on the interpretation of the given passage. Particularly helpful are commentaries that delve into the words and structure, including the grammatical rules of the original languages—Hebrew for the Old Testament and Greek for the New Testament.

Painstaking analysis requires more than delving into the passage itself. It involves considering the entire picture the author is painting, noticing what has been said before the verse you are analyzing and what is said after the verse you are analyzing. This way you obtain a feeling for the movement of the passage. Sometimes you may feel like you are wrestling with the passage until the light breaks through and you do understand. If you were declared to be a beneficiary in a person's will, you probably would find yourself reading a legally worded document with great patience and with steady concentration of thought. If you were the commander of a Brigade of soldiers on the field of battle, I cannot imagine you reading the Oplan (Operations Plan) in a hurry. You would be carefully examining its every nuance because it could mean life and death for hundreds of soldiers you are sending into battle with the enemy! Why should reading God's Word bring forth only a casual effort?

I remember a period in my military career when I served as the Station Chaplain at the 7th Radio Research Station in Udorn, Thailand, during the Vietnam War. The troops assigned there were both United States Air Force and United States Army. I was the only chaplain at the station and conducted all of the worship services and midweek Bible studies and prayer meetings. I also had a radio program that was broadcasted only to the radios on the station. Almost any night of the week I could be found in the chapel, hanging out with the soldiers and discussing their concerns and studying the Bible together. It occurred to me one day that all these Christian young men were depending on the digging I was doing to find the gems in the Bible. What I was able to come up with could be shared with them, but anything I might be missing, they would miss out on also. It is something like Mom making supper for the family every night–if she prepared a healthy diet, the family ate well, but if she had other things to do and cut corners on meal preparation, the family would go improperly nourished. So, one night I shocked everybody by acting like a college professor handing out assignments. I told the congregation of soldiers that I wanted them to each write an equivalent to a 15-20 page term paper on what the Lord had come to mean to them. I gave a deadline of three weeks in which to turn in their papers. I will never forget what joy came to my heart as I would walk into the station library or into company Day Rooms and see soldiers of all ranks with open Bible and books spread around them, pencil or pen in hand as they worked on their term papers. The greatest joy, however, was to see what it meant to each of them as they presented their finished products–recounting their personal experiences on their journey of faith, telling of the Scriptures that spoke to them, the people who played a part in their conversion to Christ, lessons they had learned from both negative and positive experiences in their lives. Instead of one "worker" correctly handling God's Word of truth, there were thirty-five or forty of them! Each had grown spiritually from the discipline. It bore out the adage, give a person a fish and you have given him a meal. Teach the person to fish and you have fed him for a lifetime.

Pondering and painstaking analysis will both serve one well in the reading of the Bible. A third and practical strategy is projection. This technique has the reader of the Scriptures projecting him or her right into the passage being read or studied. When reading in Luke 23, for example, the account of the two thieves who were being crucified on their crosses alongside Jesus, you can project yourself into the thief who is rebuking the other thief for taunting Jesus. Then you can imagine it being your words as the thief turns to Jesus and says, "**Jesus, remember me when you come into your kingdom** (Luke 23:42)." You will get a tremendous spiritual lift when you read Jesus' reply as though spoken directly to you: "**Truly I tell you, today you will be with me in paradise** (Luke 23:43)."

Try projecting yourself into this scene recorded in Mark's Gospel: "**Then they came to Jericho. As Jesus and his disciples, together with a large crowd, were leaving the city, a blind man, Bartimaeus (substitute your name here) (which means "son of Timaeus"), was sitting by the roadside begging. When he heard that it was Jesus of Nazareth, he began to shout, 'Jesus, Son of David, have mercy on me!' Many rebuked him and told him to be quiet, but he shouted all the more, 'Son of David, have mercy on me!' Jesus stopped and said, 'Call him.' So they called to the blind man, 'Cheer up! On your feet! He's calling for you. Throwing his cloak aside, he jumped up to his feet and came to Jesus. What do you want me to do for you? Jesus asked him. The blind man said, Rabbi, I want to see. Go, said Jesus, your faith has healed you. Immediately he received his sight and followed Jesus along the road** (Mark 10:46-52)."

As you can see, when you project yourself into these Biblical incidents, your heart warms up to Christ like it never has before. It is during these moments of deep love for Him, as your heart melts in compassion, that the Son of God shapes and molds the tender heart more to His liking. Pondering, painstaking analysis and projecting are just a few of the techniques a person can use to get more out of the mirror that changes you. There are many more techniques, as well. The key is to spend time with God—quality time, carefully reading His Word. This is the road to transformation!

The Apostle Paul has been telling us in this great passage of Scripture that we can expect to undergo steady change, from one degree of character improvement to another—from glory to glory, "**which comes from the Lord, Who is the Spirit** (2 Corinthians 3:18)." Let us remember that God expects this change of us. It is His will for each Christian. Paul reminds the Thessalonian believers of this fact, saying to them: "**It is God's will that you should be sanctified** (1 Thessalonians 4:3a)."

Most believers have a marvelous mirror. They have a copy of the Bible, which Paul reminds us is as a glass that reflects the beauty and the glory of Christ to us. Unfortunately, that mirror often collects dust on coffee tables, in book shelves, in footlockers or in desk drawers. We would do well to get out that wonderful mirror at every opportunity so that we might peer steadily into it. It will bring us into a closer fellowship with our Lord, and His Spirit will perfect the likeness of Christ in us—step by step, from glory to increasing glory. Think of your Bible as a mirror—the mirror that will change your life!

CHAPTER NINE

TEAM SPIRIT

The one thought that weighed most heavily upon the mind of our Lord and Savior, Jesus Christ, just prior to His going to the Cross to die for our sins, was the unity of the believers whom He would be leaving behind to carry on His work in the world when His work was finished and He would be returning to the Father on High. Jesus went apart from His disciples on the night of His betrayal for the purpose of pouring out His soul in prayer and communication with His Father in Heaven. The central theme of Jesus' prayer was that God the Father would build a working team out of all the believers He had given to Jesus. Jesus knew that the work of building His kingdom would require the talents of all His people. He prayed, therefore, that these followers of His would be welded together so as to forge a unity of spirit that would maximize their strength, magnify their testimony and make effective their witness to the unbelieving world. Jesus prayed for team spirit to prevail among believers. The prayer is so beautiful and the petitions so earnest and instructive of the mind and heart of our Savior, I want to present a key part of that prayer before commenting further:

"I have revealed you to those whom you gave me out of the world. They were yours; you gave them to me and they have obeyed your word. Now they know that everything you have given me comes from you. For I gave them the words you gave me and they accepted them. I am not praying for the world, but for those you have given me, for they are yours. All I have is yours, and all you have is mine. And glory has come to me through them. I will remain in the world no longer, but they are still in the world, and I am coming to you. Holy Father, protect them by the power of

your name—the name you gave me—so that they may be one as we are one. While I was with them, I protected them and kept them safe by that name you gave me. None has been lost, except the one doomed to destruction, so that Scripture would be fulfilled.

"I am coming to you now, but I say these things while I am still in the world, so that they may have the full measure of my joy within them. I have given them your word and the world has hated them, for they are not of the world. My prayer is not that you take them out of the world but that you protect them from the evil one. They are not of the world, even as I am not of it. Sanctify them by the truth; your word is truth. As you sent me into the world, I have sent them into the world. For them I sanctify myself, that they too may be truly sanctified.

"My prayer is not for them alone. I pray also for those who will believe in me through their message, that all of them may be one, Father, just as you are in me and I am in you. May they also be in us so that the world may believe that you have sent me. I have given them the glory that you gave me, that they may be one as we are one. I in them and you in me. <u>May they be brought to complete unity</u> to let the world know that you sent me and have loved them even as you have loved me (John 17:6-23). "

I was serving one time as a United States Army chaplain, assigned as Brigade Chaplain of the 1st Infantry Brigade (Lancers) of the 25th Infantry Division, home stationed on the Island of Oahu in Hawaii. The year was 1979, and the Brigade was chosen to be reinforced by other units within 25th Infantry Division to form Task Force Lancer which was to participate in Operation Team Spirit '79. Historical precedence was being established for this was the largest infantry deployment during peace time in the history of the Pacific Theater. It was a giant undertaking in many respects. The Task Force Lancer mission was to work under the operational control of the Commander of the 27th Division, Republic of Korea Army. Soldiers of the American and Korean armies were to be working side by side in <u>Operation Team Spirit</u> to accomplish a common military objective posed by a simulated enemy threat in South Korea. The effort was so successful, and the kindred spirit of the two armies working together was so well developed that a decision was made for the establishment of a permanent bond between 27th Republic of Korea Army and the American 25th Infantry Division of the United States Army. This was Team Spirit!

During this military exercise I was serving as the Task Force Chaplain, supervising the work of one Roman Catholic chaplain and two other Protestant chaplains, giving religious and spiritual coverage to thousands of soldiers in simulated combat parameters. This position gave me a seat in all the command staff meetings of the Task Force commander, where I learned of all the obstacles and challenges facing our contingent forces as they worked the battle plan. I also became intimately aware of how things were going down in the battalions and companies working the problems where "the rubber meets the road," because my job was to minister to the troops just as my other chaplains were doing. I mention this because it means I had a first-hand knowledge of how this tremendous team work was developed as our forces had to cope with a highly motivated enemy and frequent challenges posed by driving rain and mud-filled ruts that engulfed and imprisoned many of our vehicles, causing delays and problems of timing and coordination of battle elements. Further adding to difficulties was the fact that our troops were just air-transported from a tropical climate in Hawaii and interposed into a frozen winter terrain of South Korea. Believe me when I tell you it was no picnic!

What the American and Korean peoples achieved by way of a team spirit in a military context for defense against a common enemy is something like the team spirit our Lord must have had in mind in his Garden of Gethsemane prayer. Jesus prayed for the team play of His followers against a common enemy—the forces of evil that are at work in the world. Jesus was sending His people into the world where Satan's power is immense and He expected they would become victorious and be a testimony to God's righteousness and power. Jesus wanted the believers to model a spirit of love and have a unity that would cause the world to notice the greater quality of life available in Christ than anything possible within the world.

Every Christian has a personal responsibility for contributing to the unity of the believers for which Christ prayed to the Father.

There is a sense in which the oneness of all believers is already achieved—it is a fact not to be disputed that all in Christ are members one of another. In the Scriptures, there are many metaphors to accent this fact. In John 15, for example, Christ is described as the Vine and we are the branches bearing fruit to the glory of God. I never thought of it this way before, but the branches of a vine are all working together to produce the harvest of grapes. If every other branch decided to quit, the harvest would be substantially reduced!

In 1 Corinthians, chapter 3, the believers are chided for their quarreling and jealousy because it makes them "**worldly**" and Paul asks, "**Are you not acting like mere men**? (Verse 3)." He goes on to show them that they are "**God's fellow workers; you are God's field, God's building** (verse 9)." He then goes on in verse 16 to say, "**Don't you know you are God's temple and that God's spirit lives in you**?" In each of these metaphors the Apostle is appealing to the early Christians to act with team spirit!

In Ephesians 2, the Apostle addresses the division that existed between Jew and Gentile and reminded them that Christ's atoning work on the cross was powerful enough to dissolve any division between them and that all who are in Christ—no matter what they were before—are now united as brothers and sisters in Him. Listen to the powerful words of the Apostle to the Ephesians: "*For he himself is our peace, who has made the two one and has destroyed the barrier, the dividing wall of hostility, by abolishing in his flesh the law with its commandments and regulations. His purpose was to create in himself one new man out of the two, thus making peace, and in this one body to reconcile both of them to God through the cross, by which he put to death their hostility. He came and preached peace to you who were far away and peace to you who were near. For through him we both have access to the Father by one Spirit. Consequently, you are no longer foreigners and aliens, but fellow citizens with God's people and members of God's household, built on the foundations of the apostles and prophets, with Christ Jesus himself as the chief cornerstone. In him the whole building is joined together and rises to become a holy temple in the Lord. And in him you too are being built together to become a dwelling in which God lives by his spirit* (Ephesians 2:14-22)." If this is not an argument for team spirit, nothing is!

Again, in 1 Peter, chapter 2, believers are described as fitting together like stones forming a building. The description is almost breathtaking: "*As you come to him, the living Stone—rejected by men but chosen by God and precious to him—you also, like living stones, are being built into a spiritual house to be a holy priesthood, offering spiritual sacrifices acceptable to God through Jesus Christ* (1 Peter 2:4-5)."

Finally, in Ephesians, chapter 5 and verses 25-32, the Apostle Paul uses the lofty ideal of husband and wife to show the closeness that exists between Christ, bridegroom, and the Church–which is the bride of Christ. In other words, we are a team of believers UNITED TO CHRIST like a bride to her husband, to complement him in his work in the world, harvesting souls for his eternal kingdom! Since we are in Christ by faith, we are all partakers together of the Divine nature and are brothers and sisters in Christ. This picture does not define us according to our theological or doctrinal differences. We are not seen in God's eyes as being Roman Catholic, Anglican, Presbyterian, Lutheran, Baptist, Methodist, Congregationalist, Assembly of God, Church of the Nazarene, and so on. We are not viewed as to our differences; we are seen as to our unity as sinners who have been saved by God's grace and are fellow members of His universal Church—all of whom comprise the Bride of Christ! This is not a picture of how it is to be in the future when we get to heaven; it is reality right now!

There is nothing wrong with having our differences in style of worship because it allows for everyone to find a comfort zone in their worship of God. Some prefer a more formal approach with high liturgy while others prefer more informality and spontaneity in worship. None of these differences really matter as long as we still see ourselves as brothers and sisters in Christ. Even doctrinal differences should not really separate us. Whether or not communion is a sacrament or an ordinance, baptism is for infants or for adults, and many others. The bottom line is this: we are in the same family of faith and share a common responsibility for the oneness of spirit that needs to prevail within the Body of Christ if we, as His Church, are to accomplish the mission Jesus has given us to perform. The quality of our oneness in Christ is determined by the level of commitment each of us has toward one another. In Christ we all have the Holy Spirit. Since this is the case, it is incumbent on all of us to build a team spirit so that we can work together for the glory of God!

How best can Team Spirit be achieved? I believe there are four factors within the power of every person to exercise which would be their minimal contribution toward building Team Spirit among believers. I call them the DDTT of Team Spirit: Diversity of strengths, Dependency on others, Tolerance for weaknesses and Tenacity of effort. We will look at each of these factors in turn.

When you really think about it, all of God's creation points to the beauty and value of diversity. Uniformity would be a curse on humanity. From the stars in the heavens to the infinite variety of fish in the seas, from the fantastic array of birds in every habitat of the planet to the tiniest of insects that fly on the wing or that crawl on the earth, from mammals of every stripe to Homosapiens that walk on two feet, there is infinite, wonderful and staggering variety. It would take us a lifetime just to comprehend and appreciate what lies in the environment in which we live! We would not enjoy it any other way. The wisdom of God decreed it to be so. Certainly, the first factor in building a team spirit among believers is to recognize how vital the individual and peculiar strengths of each Christian are to the accomplishment of our total mission in the world–the way God envisions it.

Revisiting my experience as Task Force Chaplain in Operation Team Spirit in 1979, I learned that the military itself is a prime example of this principle. During the exercises in the frigid and rugged terrain of South Korea, the strengths and skills of literally hundreds of people were of paramount importance at one time or another. One Battalion executive officer was immobilized on a lonely road for many hours because of a vehicle failure. Being highly skilled in management, programming and planning did not equip this fine officer to get his jeep moving! He needed the skills of a mechanic! Indeed, it was simply that—the skills of a mechanical passer-by—that finally got the officer on his way and enabled him to deliver rations he was taking to a battalion of hungry soldiers.

Yet, who would put a vehicle mechanic at the Radio and Telegraph Rig where vital communications are handled? Time and again, during the scenario of a developing field problem the expertise of the Engineer Officer, the knowledge and skills of the Transportation Officer, the guidance of the Fire Support Coordinators, the tactical savvy of Commanders and Operations Officers, the timely input on weather and enemy movements from Intelligence people, the leadership and organizational skills of Staff Officers and Platoon Sergeants alike became crucial for the moving of our troops to the places required within the context of the simulated battle. Further, where would any of the team up front be were there not the skills of Food Service personnel to keep them nourished and fed, Medical people to treat their sicknesses and monitor for sanitation in a germ-laden environment, Supply people for the equipment and ammunition upon which everyone depended. Adequate space could not be given in the scope of this book to mention the many divergent strengths and skills necessary within a single Company of soldiers that enables them to function effectively on the battlefield!

What's even more amazing is the fact that all of this effort required for moving the United States Army Task Force effectively is that all their efforts had to mesh with the functions of an army of a different culture—the Republic of South Korea Army! I was eye-witness to complications posed by language barriers until the skills of brilliant interpreters were employed to assist American and Korean soldiers in communicating so as to synchronize movements of troops and taking of strategic objectives. I also learned the Army cannot maximize its force capability without the timely and adequate cover and support of the Air Force. The comparisons are endless.

The fact of the matter is clear: everyone does not do the same job; neither does everyone do a similar job in the same way. One person's method of performing a task may be comfortable and effective for him or her, but ineffective and awkward for the personality and skills of another individual. All commanders do not command with the same style of leadership; all chaplains do not perform with the same style of ministry. Team Spirit is built when we recognize and call into use the divergent skills and strengths of all individuals on the team.

This leads me to my second point: dependency on others. It follows quite naturally that, when the individual skills and strengths of others are recognized, there will be a need to be dependent upon one another. Some people will recognize their own strengths and put them to work in fine fashion, but soon they are caught up with their own importance and they fail to realize how much they really depend on the work of others. They may fancy themselves at times to be independent and self-sufficient, but actually are blinded in their own minds to the reality that they could not possibly stand alone. The Lone Ranger syndrome is terribly destructive of team spirit. If you will pardon another reference to the Operation Team Spirit exercise, I overheard a First Lieutenant boasting to a friend that his battalion proved itself far superior because it had managed to keep constant contact with the enemy. This assertion was stated as if that company had won the war all by itself! How preposterous! Contact with the enemy is important but it is only one variable in the assessment of victory. The fortuitous positioning of that particular unit gave them terrain and opportunity where the enemy was most likely to be present. Had another unit not been in sector and in strength, the enemy would not have been denied that terrain for movement and would not have been able to avoid being channeled into the area where the boastful Lieutenant was operating. What about the battalions in reserve? Were they to be considered less effective because their prescribed mission was different? How do you evaluate adequately the contribution of the elements that are employed in a reuse or fake maneuver to confuse the enemy? In matters of tactics, it is wiser to acknowledge inter-dependency on other units rather than to sound off about the singular greatness of a given unit.

The Bible has a lot to say on the subject of our dependency on one another. We are admonished not to forsake the assembling of ourselves together for worship in the book of Hebrews. We are told often of the need to uphold one another in strong and intercessory prayer. We are asked to bear with each other's infirmities, to assist each other in trouble, to encourage each other in distress and to contribute to supplying of each other's needs. The classic passage in the Bible that speaks to diversity into unity is Paul's words to the Christians at Corinth: *"The body is a unit, though it is made up of many parts; and though all its parts are many, they form one body. So it is with Christ. For we were all baptized by one Spirit into one body—whether Jews or Greeks, slave or free—and we were all given the one Spirit to drink. Now the body is not made up of one part but of many. If the foot should say, 'Because I am not a hand, I do not belong to the body,' it would not for that reason cease to be a part of the body. And if the ear should say, 'Because I am not an eye, I do not belong to the body,' it would not for that reason cease to be a part of the body. If the whole body were an eye, where would the sense of hearing be? If the whole body were an ear, where would the sense of smell be? But in fact God has arranged the parts in the body, every one of them, just as he wanted them to be. If they were all one part, where would the body be? As it is, there are many parts, but one body* (1 Corinthians 12:14-20)."

This dependency on others is very much a part of the Christian community as the Lord intended. We need one another. What if all Christians were singers but none could preach or teach? What if all could preach but none could sing, play an instrument or comfort the sick? What if all preachers were evangelists and none were pastors or expositors of the meaty passages of God's Word? What if all preachers were expositors of the meaty passages of God's Word but could not be effective at evangelizing, pastoring or bringing lost souls to a saving knowledge of Jesus Christ? Team Spirit is built when we realize and practice a dependency upon one another to do the work of Christ.

The first two elements in the formula for building Team Spirit have been explored: we need diversity of strengths and dependency on others. The third element is tolerance for weaknesses. Perhaps some readers are wondering about the value of having a tolerance for weaknesses in building team spirit. The reason this factor is so vital is because no person is all strengths; each of us has weaknesses. If we need and depend upon one another's strengths, then we had better be prepared to tolerate the weaknesses they bring to the job with them. God only knows how much the church has suffered the loss of the skills and talents of so many Christians because they have been literally ostracized from the fellowship of the church because of some personal weaknesses or shortcomings. The narrow mind-set of many of God's people over the years has been simply incredible!

The history of the church in America has many bright sides and many notable triumphs that are joyful to behold. There have been powerful ministries that have helped millions of people when taken together. There has been a tremendous commitment to world missions and the missionary successes owe a lot to a strong backing of folks in the churches throughout the United States of America. One could fill pages listing organizations and ministries that reach beyond our borders to the uttermost corners of the world that depend for their existence upon the charitable giving of believers of all denominations in our country. There have been outpourings of God's Spirit and the breaking out of revivals that have been accompanied by signs, wonders and miracles that leave no doubt as to the presence and mighty working of God in places one would scarcely suspect.

But to be fair in assessment of the history of the church in America, one would have to acknowledge the dark side. There have been communities where racial discrimination has reached inside the church and drawn many devoted believers into doing the work of the devil because of their rigid racial prejudices. Who would want to advertise and extol the deeds of the Ku Klux Klan? Many will have to answer to God for the people of other races and ethnicities who have been denied membership—even attendance—in their churches. Many will have to answer to the Lord for the unclaimed harvest of souls in communities where the Presbyterians could not work together with the Baptists and where the Lutherans and Methodists could find no common ground for ministry. Surely God will hold all of us to account for the terrible waste of manpower and spiritual power to build His kingdom on earth because of the isolationism and compartmentalization of His church into factions to the right and the left of center.

Are we all of Paul? Are we all of Apollos? No, of course, we are not. But surely, if Christianity means anything at all, we are all of Christ! If we are in Christ, we must think about His earnest prayer in Gethsemane where the Lord pleaded with His Father in heaven that the church would be one just as He and the Father are one. We have a responsibility to accept each other in the bonds of Christian love, to lose our consciousness of each other's faults or submerging them in a deep sea of Godly love which flows throughout the entire world, embracing Christians of every nation as brothers and sisters in Jesus! That, my friends, is the Team Spirit for which Jesus prayed when he uttered the words: *"I in them and you in me. May they be brought to complete unity to let the world know that you have sent me and have loved them as you have loved me* (John 17:23)."

The fourth and vital factor for the effective building of Team Spirit among believers is tenacity of effort. This principle speaks to the energy level that activates the other three principles. Diversity of strengths, dependency on others and tolerance for weaknesses will all be undergirded by tenacity of effort. A half-hearted or luke-warm application of any of the principles mentioned will never please the Lord or accomplish the job that God has set out for us to do. The greatest blight to the human race and its greatest shame is mediocrity of effort! It is absolutely amazing how little we will settle for from ourselves and from others when our capacity is so much greater than what we actually give.

"Go to the ant, you sluggard; consider its ways and be wise! It has no commander, no overseer or ruler, yet it stores its provisions in summer and gathers its food at harvest (Proverbs 6:6-8)." Here is a stern warning against laziness, indifference and mediocre attention to the needs of life. Tenacity of effort helps the bees in the hive, the ants in their colonies and thousands of other species in God's creation to survive and prosper. How utterly refreshing and encouraging it is to see someone putting forth a solid effort for the well-being of others. There were many notable examples of this high level of commitment on the part of soldiers

during our exercise of Operation Team Spirit. Personally, I attribute a lot of the success to the man at the top—the commander of 1st Infantry Brigade (Lancers) of the 25th Infantry Division, Colonel Pat Patrick. From the first day he set foot in the brigade headquarters he showed the stripes of what sort of a man and a leader he was. One of Colonel Patrick's first gestures was to summon me to his office so he could meet the man who was the chaplain of his troops. I will never forget his gesture of framing the eagle insignia on his shirt collar with his fingers and telling me, "Chaplain, I did not earn this rank that I hold today; my troops earned it for me. I am holding you accountable to take care of my troops because I love soldiers." It was a clear understanding that I was to take care of his soldiers and should I need anything to support that effort I was not to hesitate to come directly to him. I soon learned that these were not just words—this was his Modes Operendi!

Not long after taking command of Lancer Brigade, Colonel Patrick instituted what was known as "the Patrick shuffle." He came to believe there was too much "make work" to fill time during the week and troops were being brought back to work on Saturdays to meet objectives. He offered a different perspective to the brigade. He said he believed we could do better and to prove his point he promised that the troops could be released for the weekends on Friday noon if all their objectives for training had been completed. This brought out a superb effort from each battalion, every company and squad in the brigade. Everything was ship-shape by Friday mornings and hundreds of soldiers were spending quality time having fun with each other or relaxing with their wives and families. They could not wait to tackle duties on Mondays so that things would be wrapped up by Fridays. Every other brigade in the 25th Division was amazed that Colonel Patrick could send his troops home for long weekends and yet get better results on unit tests than the other brigades, even though they were working their soldiers on Saturdays and even on Sundays to try and catch up to him! Because he loved and believed in his soldiers, they returned to him their love and undying commitment. When he commanded Task Force Lancer in Operation Team Spirit it is no wonder that it was a success. Neither is it any wonder that Pat Patrick was promoted up to the rank of Lieutenant General by the time of his retirement.

Colonel Patrick set the tone and the example. His troops followed his lead. One sergeant labored the entire 12 days of the exercise in South Korea with a fractured hand, not complaining and not willing to turn back from his task. One sergeant E-9 would not admit to respiratory illness even when it was nearly full-blown pneumonia because he did not want to disrupt the morale of his troops who were depending upon him. Another soldier pressed on with his squad through days of marching and climbing hills and rugged terrain with a full pack on his back in spite of having two injured knees that would require full casts at the termination of the exercise in order for those knees to heal. These are just a few of the scores of cases where soldiers put forth a tremendous effort to do a top-rate job for the units in the field!

Christians can learn much from such sacrificial expenditure of energy on the part of dedicated soldiers. Paul exhorts the believers in Rome, "*Love must be sincere. Hate what is evil; cling to what is good. Be devoted to one another in brotherly love. Honor one another above yourselves. Never be lacking in zeal, but keep your spiritual fervor, serving the Lord* (Romans 12:9-11)." To Titus, Paul writes that Christians are to be "*a people who are his very own, eager to do what is good* (Titus 2:14)." In Jude, verse 3, he writes: "*I felt I had to write and urge you to contend for the faith that was once for all entrusted to the saints*." Jude wrote this because there were already many enemies in the world, many of which were infiltrating into the church to cripple the effectiveness and snuff out the witness of God's people in a very evil age. The times in which we live right now are too severely opposed to God for the Church to be able to survive on mediocrity of effort! The enemy is too strong. The work God has given us to do is too vital. The team spirit of Christ's people is calling for a tenacity of effort to meet the challenges of our times!

We need to heed the admonishment of the Apostle Paul who wrote to the Colossians, "*Whatever you do, work at it with all your heart, as working for the Lord, not for men* (Colossians 3:23)."

Were we to see everything we undertake to do as being for the Lord Jesus Christ, what team members each of us would be!

Dr. Martin Luther King, Jr. is going to be long remembered for one magnificent sermon he preached which eventually became a byword for all of his own efforts to end discrimination against his people and which inspired many, many others to join forces to attack the ills of society that Dr. King sought to eliminate. In that very moving sermon, Dr. King kept repeating the words "I have a dream..." and then he poured forth the content of his hopes with great eloquence that moved the hearts of millions. Martin Luther King, Jr. had a dream. Jesus Christ had one, too. It is that prayer which we have already alluded to and cited—his prayer in the garden of Gethsemane before he was to go to the cross, suffer and die for our sins. Jesus had a prayer for the unity of His followers. Jesus had a prayer that we who name the name of Christ would band together in love. Jesus had a prayer that His Church would have a powerful and compelling witness to His own divinity within the world in which we live. Jesus had a prayer that we believers would develop a Team Spirit so that we could help build His kingdom and hasten the day of His return.

How much do you become concerned about the prayer of Jesus? Can you feel something of His heart throbbing for our togetherness? I believe we need to listen to our Commander In Chief and march smartly to His orders. Let us recognize the diversity of strengths present in the Body of Christ. Let us practice a dependency on one another. Let us show tolerance for weaknesses; let us give a tenacity of effort for the cause of Christ. Eternity is the time for rest. Now is the time for work. Now is the time for Team Spirit!

CHAPTER TEN

THE WORDS WE LIVE WITH

To know the character of a person you only have to factor in two things: the person's words and the person's behavior. When you really come down to it, there is no other means by which to measure the character of an individual. Someone might offer that you can learn a lot about a person by looking at them. This would be true for forming first impressions, I grant you, but visual assessment can lead only to hints about a person's character. Visual plays easily to our prejudices but can lead us to conclusions far distant from reality. This is why people of different ethnic backgrounds become incensed with anger at being racially profiled by larger elements of society or by law enforcement personnel. The color of one's skin or the clothes on one's body have very little to do with character because we do not choose our skin pigmentation and our wardrobe choices are usually a matter of preference or personal taste. A person's behavior and the words they live with are the only reliable sources for assessing a person's character. We broadcast who we are by what we say and what we do. It is as simple as that——and just as profound!

There is a third way a person displays character: it is by what a person thinks. Unless you are psychic or administer a truth serum, you will not know what another person thinks until they speak or act to reveal what they were thinking. This, for practical purposes, leaves only our words and our behavior as the vehicles for showing the world what we are really like. Only God knows our thoughts. That's a good thing. If the world knew all one's thoughts, one could have a lot of problems on their hands because one has no control over thoughts that pop into his or her mind. It's what is done with the thoughts after they arrive in the conscious mind that reveals one's character. Scarcely would a wise person act on the first thought that flashes across the conscious mind; a lot of sifting, sorting, evaluating, estimating, calculating goes on in a split second of time. This is because the mind is faster than our best man-made computer. God is privy to this entire internal dynamic, but no one else has a clue. In fact, the person in question cannot even recall with any degree of accuracy the sequential mental machinations they used before they spoke or acted. A person can recall a lot of what they were thinking before they spoke or before they behaved as they did, but they cannot walk you through every thought and nuance of thought in the sequence in which it paraded through their mind. People are not held responsible for every thought they think. People are responsible for the words they use when they speak and for their behavior. If the conditions are right, either one could land a person in a court of law and, if found guilty of a felony, in a jail cell! By the same token, if the conditions are right, the person could be elected Governor of his or her State or President of the United States. To put it another way, exactly where you are in your life right this very moment is a direct result of your words and your behavior! This is to emphasize how crucially important these two features are in the revealing of one's character to the society and the world in which they live.

More solemn still, our words and our behavior are judged by God and He has given words of instruction and words of caution on this subject in His Word, the Holy Bible. I call to your attention one of the most puzzling yet revealing incidents in the entire life of Jesus as recorded for us in the Gospel of Matthew. It is puzzling and it is astounding because it is in this particular encounter with some Pharisees of Judaism that Jesus speaks of the only unpardonable sin. The unpardonable sin is not murder; it is not suicide, it is speaking words of blasphemy against God's Holy Spirit. Being this is so important a matter to understand correctly, I want to quote the passage at length:

"Then they brought him a demon-possessed man who was blind and mute, and Jesus healed him, so that he could both talk and see. All the people were astonished and said, 'Could this be the

Son of David?" "But when the Pharisees heard this, they said, 'It is only by Beelzebub, the prince of demons, that this fellow drives out demons." "Jesus knew their thoughts and said to them, 'Every kingdom divided against itself will be ruined, and every city or household divided against itself will not stand. If Satan drives out Satan, he is divided against himself. How then can his kingdom stand? And if I drive out demons by Beelzebub, by whom do your people drive them out? So then, they will be your judges. But if I drive out demons by the Spirit of God, then the kingdom of God has come upon you. Or, again, how can anyone enter a strong man's house and carry off his possessions unless he first ties up the strong man? Then he can rob his house. He who is not with me is against me, and he who does not gather with me scatters. And so I tell you, every sin and blasphemy will be forgiven men, but the blasphemy against the Spirit will not be forgiven. Anyone who speaks a word against the Son of Man will be forgiven, but anyone who speaks against the Holy Spirit will not be forgiven, either in this age or in the age to come."

"Make a tree good and its fruit will be good, or make a tree bad and its fruit will be bad, for a tree is recognized by its fruit. You brood of vipers, how can you who are evil say anything good? For out of the overflow of the heart the mouth speaks. The good man brings good things out of the good stored up in him, and the evil man brings evil things out of the evil stored up in him. But I tell you that men will have to give an account on the Day of Judgment for every careless word they have spoken. For by your words you will be acquitted, and by your words you will be condemned (Matthew 12:22-37)."

In this passage we are told that words can so negatively be used they can bring eternal damnation upon the person speaking those words. This is, of course, when one's heart is so cemented in unbelief that they can utter blasphemy against the Holy Spirit. Going so far as to blaspheme the Holy Spirit is an exercise very few would be evil enough to say and mean it. The Pharisees of Jesus' time were violently opposed to the wonder-working miracles of Jesus because they could not believe He was the Son of God. Jesus affirmed that He drove out demons from the man possessed of demons by the power of the Spirit of God. The Pharisees refused to believe this and said Jesus was using the power of Satan to drive out the demons. How could this be? Satan put the demons into the man to possess the man and ruin his life; Satan is not now driving himself out of whom he already possesses! That would be a house divided against itself! So, indeed, Jesus sets the Pharisees straight on this fact: a house divided against itself cannot stand. What the Pharisees are left with, therefore, is a situation they cannot defend unless they deny the Spirit of God had anything to do with the demons being cast out of the man. They cannot deny the man has been liberated from the tormenting demons that once owned his soul. If not God, they credit Satan with the act of delivering the man. In other words, blasphemy against the Holy Spirit is attributing to the devil what you know has been done by the Holy Spirit. This, warned Jesus, is the unpardonable sin! Many were the vile words and false charges that were hurled against Jesus, yet Jesus said anything said against Him could be forgiven. Even those who nailed Him to His cross and railed against him derisively were spoken of with marvelous grace. The Lord with dying breath cried out to heaven, **"Father, forgive them for they do not know what they are doing."** One can be terribly disappointed that God failed to answer their prayers as they hoped he would and have spoken angry words to God. These words can be forgiven. God understands the emanations from a wounded and suffering soul! Blasphemy against the Holy Spirit is another matter, completely.

Another lesson to draw from this event and the instruction the Lord gives to the Pharisees is that the words of blasphemy proceed from the heart of a person. The heart is set against Jesus to so great an extent, the Pharisees were using words to announce their opposition to Him; words not directed at Jesus the person but against the power by which Jesus claimed to perform this miracle. Jesus said the exorcism of the demons was by the power of the Spirit of God; the Pharisees could see from this that they faced a trap. If they agreed that the Spirit of God cast out the demons, they would be validating Jesus' claim to be the Son of God. They could no longer oppose Him! Their hearts were so set against Jesus, they attacked the power by which Jesus performed the miracle and attributed that act to the power of Satan. Those things which only the Spirit of God could do, the Pharisees made the blasphemous charge that they were done by Satan's power. This accusation only solidified their contempt for Jesus. That, my friends, is the unpardonable sin!

We also learn from this discourse of Jesus with the Pharisees that words come from what is inside a person. This is borne out by our Lord's reference to trees and their fruit. The good tree will bear good fruit. The bad tree will bear bad fruit. The nature of the tree is displayed by the fruit it bears! It is not what goes into a person that defines his character; it is what comes out of the person. It is what comes out by both words and deeds. Mentioning this presents a great opportunity to put in a plug for the value of effective parenting. The period from birth to age six in a child's life is critical to the forming of character. That is why this period of time is called the formative years. Physical development is firmly established by school age. Most any physical disability will have been displayed by then. The critical aspect is the formulation of sense of self and expression of self—building personality and character that will stay with that person for the rest of life. Once character is formed, out of that will issue all the decisions and behaviors of life, unless at some point the parentally-guided character is countermanded by peer pressures. Unless a child's companions are of a similar belief and value system taught by the child's parents, the child is at risk for exchanging acquired values and beliefs for the belief systems prevalent in the peer group with which the child has daily association. The values and mores of the peer group can be quite different from what was obtained in the family of origin. The child's home, therefore, is the child's school room for learning what kind of a person to become. The teachers are the parents, care-givers and siblings. What's done in the home, what's said in the home, how people are allowed to act in the home—these are all critical factors to determine formation of character.

How a parent speaks to a child, or how a parent speaks to another adult about their child within the range of the child's hearing can have a profound effect on the child's sense of self. Keep this in mind, because a child in the formative years will act according to what they are taught to believe about themselves. If a parent makes negative statements about his or her child, the child will be affected by this. One who says negative things should not be surprised if they have a misbehaving and very difficult- to-control child on their hands! As a Marriage and Family Therapist, I can remember a particular session I conducted with a mother who brought her two young children with her into the session. She was at her wit's end trying to control the behavior of her three year old son. She sat in a chair with a month-old infant on her lap and the three year old had some toys with him so he would be occupied as the mother talked with me. One of the boy's toys was a little airplane. He could see his mother's attention was now directed toward me and not toward him. The boy took the airplane and began roaming around the room pretending to be flying his plane. He was basically ignored. Soon, the boy flew his airplane right in the direction of the baby's face and then whisking it away. As you might suppose, the mother addressed the boy and said, "Don't do that, fly the plane someplace else." It was only a matter of seconds before the boy was back flying precariously close to the baby's and mother's faces. "Stop that! Don't do that again. I'm trying to talk with this man." What do you think happened next? In a very short time the boy was doing just what he was told not to do. This time the mother said, "Jimmy, you're a bad boy!" I suspect Jimmy expected this would be said and that he had heard those words before. They did not deter him nor improve his behavior. I finally spoke up and addressed the mother, not the child. I said, "Correction, he is not a bad boy. He is a sweet and loving little boy. He's just doing something right now that is unacceptable." Jimmy, hearing this, turned toward me with eyes as big as saucers, stunned with amazement and appreciation. He did not say another word. Neither did he misbehave another second for the rest of the mother's session. He behaved like an angel, as they say. The mother needed to get a different perspective on her son's worth and use words that supported his worth rather than words that detracted from his worth. His behavior was proof enough that he would behave in accordance with what people believed about him.

Most parents would probably defend themselves with rationalizations such as, "Of course I love my Jimmy; I told him he was a bad boy to try and get him to behave. He knows his Mommy loves him." Perhaps Jimmy does know his mother loves him, but he also heard her label him as being a bad boy. How can this not have an effect upon the little child? Are we to use words carelessly in order to manipulate people to do what we want them to do? Is there no way we are to be held to account for the words we use? Even as a bullet cannot be retrieved and placed back into the gun's chamber once it has been fired, our words once spoken cannot be withdrawn. Whatever meaning our words convey will have made an impression upon the hearer, and there is a chance that an apology or an effort to repair the damage will be successful. This is why the wisdom of the Proverbs is so timely: "*He who restrains his lips is wise* (Proverbs 10:19)." A further warning from the same book states, "*Whoever guards his mouth and tongue keeps his soul from troubles* (Proverbs 21:23)."

The Bible speaks often of the importance of the words we use—of the tongue, and how it should be carefully controlled. God regards the use of our words to be of such importance that He devoted two of the Ten Commandments to deal specifically with our words: the 3rd Commandment, "*You shall not misuse the name of the Lord your God, for the Lord will not hold anyone guiltless who misuses his name* (Exodus 20:7), and the 9th Commandment, "*You shall not give false testimony against your neighbor* (Exodus 20:16)." The Apostle James devotes an entire chapter (chapter 3) of his brief epistle to the all-important matter of controlling the tongue. Being this subject is regarded by God to be of high importance, why is it a subject carelessly neglected by so many people? We would be prudent indeed were we to evaluate and consider the words we live with. In doing such an analysis, I would suggest three things to be considered regarding the words we live with: words we need, words we do not need, and all the words we use will be held in judgment by almighty God.

A prime consideration ought certainly to be for the words which we all need, and heading this list is the Word of God. No words from any other source are more desperately needed to help each of us to build our lives and to guide us in the making of our every important decision than the words of God. His Word conveys His truth and His timely wisdom to us. In a day and age when there are so many different voices vying for the minds and consciences of people, we need more than ever to have a sure word from God. The Psalmist thought much of the Word of God and its importance for the living of life. He wrote: *"Your word is a lamp to my feet and a light for my path* (Psalm 119:105)." I never fully appreciated what this sentence meant until I was in Korea for Task Force Lancer on Operation Team Spirit. Camped out in the countryside on a pitch dark night, I could not see even the hand in front of my face. There was no moonlight or starlight to give even slight illumination. Suddenly, in the distant darkness I saw some little yellow lights moving slowly through the night. The lights seemed to zigzag as they moved along. When the lights got much closer to where I was located I could see little feet following the glow of the lamps that were dangling from a wooden bar that was held on one shoulder of each person in the small group that was safely navigating their way across a rice patty. They were Koreans walking the berms between flooded fields of rice plants. The light of their little lamps was sufficient to cast a glow for about two steps ahead of them at a time. The lamps marked where it was safe to plant the foot on the path, only one or two feet at a time! Without the illumination from those tiny lamps, any of them would have been tumbling off the berms and into the rice patties. This was a powerful example for me as I applied this picture to the verse just quoted. God's Word gives sufficient illumination to us as we make our way through life—with all its accompanying dangers and attending risks. We can safely walk under the guidance of His Word even though He may reveal only where to place our feet next, and not reveal to us what's coming a little farther down the path. When we get to that place farther down the path, His Word will be the lamp unto our feet!

Elsewhere, the same Psalm writer extolled other virtues conveyed by God's Word: *"The law of the Lord is perfect, reviving the soul. The statutes of the Lord are trustworthy, making wise the simple. The precepts of the Lord are right, giving joy to the heart. The commands of the Lord are radiant, giving light*

to the eyes. The fear of the Lord is pure, enduring forever. The ordinances of the Lord are sure and altogether righteous. They are more precious than gold, than much pure gold; they are sweeter than honey, than honey from the comb. By them is your servant warned; in keeping them there is great reward (Psalm 19:7-11)."
Oh, that more of us should have an estimate of the value and need for the Word of God as that displayed by the Psalmist! We must remember that no matter how brilliant and accomplished a person may become, the words of even the wisest of men are still mere opinions. Because that person's comments are usually right on target and very valuable to hear, we cannot trust that they are never wrong or misguided in their judgments. There are times when we need much more than opinions—we need to know it like it is! I will never forget what music it was to my thirsty ears when as a 13 year-old young man I was sitting in a little Baptist church in Springfield, Massachusetts on a Sunday evening in 1946. It was there that I heard God's Word preached in clarity, shedding light on my inquisitive mind concerning subjects about which I had often wondered—about sin, God's judgment of sin in our lives, hell, and heaven. I heard Scripture quoted that explained how salvation from sin's penalty can be had through personal faith in Jesus Christ, believing that His death upon the cross was for my sins and the sins of anyone else who would receive Him into their lives as Lord and Savior! The message I heard answered my life-long questions. I believed the message of the Word of God and received Christ into my heart by faith and it was a life-transforming decision. I felt immediate relief and I knew in a moment that I was now born again! I was a recipient of God's love and salvation from sin—a new member in the family of God!

In addition to God's Word, there are other words we need, also. We need words of hope. Many people spread words of doom and gloom and are broadcasters of pessimism. Our troubled world and struggling economy offer abundant support for negativistic banter. There is no dearth of comment on the evils of our time; what are needed more at such a time are words that will build hope rather than despair. Martin Luther King, Junior, used to stir the hearts of millions as he shared the words, "I have a dream. . ." What he was really saying is that he had hope for change. Jesse Jackson could not have picked a better slogan than his often repeated salutation, "Keep hope alive!" Hope is the great motivator when all else is failing. After a tornado has struck a community or a Tsunami has struck and wreaked unbelievable and devastating destruction, people have nothing left to hold on to. What makes them start to clean up the debris? What motivates them to press on to rebuild and repair the damage done when all that can be seen is chaos? The answer is hope. People who are survivors and rebuilders are people who have hope that their efforts will bring about change and improvement of their current state of affairs. Most people will invest both energy and vigor into their activities when they have hope! Words of hope are timely and uplifting. We need words of hope.

Some other words we surely can use are words of commendation or praise. Many people work hard and are faithfully devoted to their jobs, get paid for what they do and nothing more. It seldom occurs to some employers or supervisors that the worker could use some words of commendation on occasion. They may receive criticism when they've made mistakes, and perhaps it is needed, depending on the circumstances. Words of praise and commendation, however, are given over and above one's wages in order to convey to the employee the sense of value they bring to the organization. Who wouldn't work more cheerfully and productively when they know that they are appreciated for the quality of work they do? What's true for the employee is doubly true for children. The child is not getting paid money for the effort he or she is expected to give as a student in the class room or as a member of the family in the home. It is both good teaching and good parenting to give the child words of commendation when they have been earned through faithful and exceptional effort. Such words provide more incentive for the child to continue growing and producing what they are capable of doing.

Similar to words of commendation are words of appreciation. These can be given much more frequently to the people who surround us and serve to enhance the quality of our lives in so many ways. They labor for us because it is their nature to be loyal and supporting. It is the wife who does countless chores and duties to keep her husband from being inconvenienced and distracted from his primary focus. It is the husband who answers to anything the wife may need to make her work easier or more enjoyable–providing her with the tools of her trade, so to speak. Yet, it is more than this; it is finding ways to say "thank you." One can enjoy getting thanked for the meal well prepared and enjoyed by the family. One can enjoy words of appreciation for having set aside the ball game to fix the leaky faucet in the kitchen or to repair daughter's bicycle. What is being suggested by this is that anyone can spread more cheer than gloom when they give words of appreciation to those in their life who give so much, expecting nothing more than to be appreciated. Do you like donuts? Some people love those little snacks but they cannot eat them due to health considerations. Think of words of appreciation as "do nots," not donuts. Do not accept the kindness of others without giving thanks. Do not stop telling your children how much they mean to you. Do not pass up an opportunity to express your gratitude to those who try to enhance your life! Do not act like a sponge soaking up all that others give without giving in return. Do not accept the mindset that you are here on earth to be taken care of by others, to be encouraged by others, to be waited on by others, to be tolerated by others. Realize there is value and there is joy in giving more than in receiving. Do not be blinded from seeing what you could say to the important people at your job, in your school, in your circle of friends or in your family that would convey your appreciation. People need words like that.

No matter how hard we try to succeed at what we do, there will be times we run into obstacles that demand of us more than we can give. Life has its hurdles to get past, some walls that need climbing if we are to get to where we want to go. These are the low points in life. Sometimes they are ushered in by some great loss, such as through a break up in a relationship, a failure in a marriage or an untimely death of a loved one. Going forward seems impossible to do because we sense our life has been altered forever. When these hardships or reversals of fortune occur in our lives we could use words of encouragement. It takes courage to press on when there are attending risks of failure or losses to assimilate. The natural emotional response is discouragement—being robbed of our courage. What helps is an infusion of support from someone who cares and understands what we are experiencing but who believes we can succeed nonetheless. That support may come with tangible assistance or even with words of encouragement—conveying belief in our ability to achieve success in spite of the difficulties.

Close to words of encouragement are words of reassurance. These are words that build on what we already believe by reminding us of their validity. Words that dispel our doubts, calm our spirit and boost our confidence are words of reassurance. Parents must not get weary of responding to a child's questioning, thinking the child should have figured that out for himself. Much of a child's questioning is to gain reassurance. The Bible says, "***The tongue that brings healing is a tree of life, but a deceitful tongue crushes the spirit*** (Proverbs 15:4)." Here we are reminded that the words we use carry tremendous power to the person who is discouraged. Discouragement unabated is just a few steps from depression; discouragement relieved by words of encouragement may be steps to survival and eventual victory. The same passage in Proverbs has the words: "***A man finds joy in giving an apt reply—how good is a timely word!*** (Proverbs 15:23)." Perhaps the most beautiful analogy of timely words of encouragement is recorded in Proverbs 25:11: "***A word aptly spoken is like apples of gold in settings of silver.***" These are words we need.

While there are quite a few types of words that we all need, it is also true that there are many types of words that we can do without. Just as the Word of God heads the list of the words we need, there is something also that heads the list of the words we can do without. We have previously alluded to it already: it is blasphemy against the Holy Ghost. This is the worse sin that can be committed and it is called the unpardonable sin. It is knowingly attributing to the Devil what is the work of the Holy Spirit of God.

Another type of word we can do without is careless and evil language. Examples of evil language include poor choice of words, indecent speech, swearing and cussing, making light of sacred things, filthy communication and terminology. People who use such language are an offense to people who do not want to be exposed to such vulgarity. People who spit out garbage from their mouths do not beautify life; they only pollute it! Other words we could do without includes idle words, useless talk, senseless expressions, vulgar expressions which punctuate conversation even though they pour no meaningful content into what is being said. Jesus warned, *"**But I tell you that men will have to give account on the Day of Judgment for every careless word they have spoken. For by your words you will be acquitted, and by your words you will be condemned** (Matthew 12:36-37)."* Other words we could do without are words of gossip by which rumors are started or perpetuated that are meant to belittle or damage the reputation of others. Some gossip takes the form of slander or assassination of character. Someone has said "Make your words sweet because you may have to eat them!" Words that stir up strife and report things that may not be really true are devastating attacks on innocent people. These words are called false rumors. This is a violation of the ninth commandment, *"**You shall not bear false testimony against your neighbor (**Exodus 20:16**).**"*

Beside the damage that gossip may inflict on an innocent person, there is the destructive consequence of negative criticism. Fault-finding and criticism are as much a part of life as eating your lunch or taking a coffee break. This is because there is a lot wrong in society, in business, in government and in the workplace that earns the criticism people make. Sometimes it is useful to gripe and complain to a friend or close associate because it allows one to blow off some steam and release some pressurized discontentment that has been building up inside. Every day of the week, except on Sunday, in a million barbershops and hair salons across the United States, a litany of complaining takes place and opinions are freely given and eagerly shared and sometimes the value received from letting off steam is worth more than the price of the haircut or permanent. Often the one complaining not only releases pent-up emotions, he also gains a different perspective on the situation when the person they are complaining to offers a reply that, essentially, rolls the shades up some windows of the mind and lets more light inside. It helps to see a situation from other perspectives than the one that makes you so angry! This being said, it is the excessive use of griping or complaining that emanates from a person who is definitely on a railroad track heading to a collision with the goals and purposes of an organization that can wreak havoc. Like a virus that cannot be stopped, their negativism spreads to others and can corrupt the morale of the team, the unit, the work section or whatever else may be in question. I can remember sitting in many staff meetings with a new military commander when I served in the Army as a chaplain. I can still hear in my mind the commanders saying something like this: "Do not bring to me any problems without also offering some solutions or courses of action." We all need to be educated by this type of reasoning—complaining changes nothing. Ideas for change—that is a different matter! The complainer and griper is renouncing responsibility for the problems by deferring the blame to others. Words we need are words that identify weaknesses, injustices, inefficiencies and problems within the context of being willing to also work for change if others can be persuaded into agreement and taking dynamic team action to correct what is wrong.

Finally, when it comes to the words we live with, nothing we say—even if said in private—is off-the-record with God. We are all accountable to Him for the words we use. As previously quoted, "**But I tell you that men will have to give account on the Day of Judgment for every careless word they have spoken. For by your words you will be acquitted and by your words you will be condemned** (Matthew 12:36-37)." The memory of God is infallible; His memory does not fade with the passing of time as does the memory of mere mortals. His warning should be taken very seriously. Bad words are like weapons; they are fashioned to inflict pain and to destroy. Many who operate with a shallow conscience believe they can blast a partner or family member or work subordinate with nasty words that hurt, and they expect the person who is the object of their verbal assault will stop hurting as soon as the sound of their voice has ceased. This may or may not be the case, time will tell. Quite possibly, all they have given their victim is the raw material with which to build an emotional wall which some day may become impregnable! In any event, why live on the edge of propriety and take the risk of angering God for the mistreatment of others because we will have to give an account to him for every careless word spoken. Wisdom suggests persons would do well to refrain from evil speaking. Listen to the warning of the Apostle Peter, quoting from the Psalms on this subject: *"Whoever would love life and see good days must keep his tongue from evil and his lips from deceitful speech. He must turn from evil and do good; he must seek peace and pursue it. For the eyes of the Lord are on the righteous and his ears are attentive to their prayer, but the face of the Lord is against those who do evil* (1 Peter 3:10-12)."

The simple truth is that very few things reveal what the inside of a person is like as do the words they use. Medical science has discovered some truly ingenious ways to take a look inside the body of a person. We have all kinds of X-Ray machines, ultrasound equipment, electrocardiogram machines, gastro scopes, body scans and hosts of other techniques which give doctors a view on virtually every organ of the body, including the human brain. Yes, we have to go to stupendous scientific means to look into the body of a person, yet to see what a person is thinking and peering into mind and soul—looking into the very heart of a person, one scarcely has to do more than to listen to the words that person uses. That's what Jesus meant when he said, *"The good man brings good things out of the good stored up in him, and the evil man brings evil things out of the evil stored up in him* (Matthew 12:35)." Jesus uses in this context the illustration of a tree. We evaluate the nature of a tree by the fruit it bears. Good fruit means a good tree. Bad fruit means a bad tree. This is because the fruit, either good or bad, owes its origin to the nature of the tree which produced it. One can go just a little below the surface of the ground to note that the tree which is producing good fruit is drawing nourishment and refreshment from a healthy root system and a good source of supply—be it fertile soil or sub-surface springs of water. If not water in the soil, there is at least an irrigation system that provides the water the tree requires to be a healthy tree.

What is your life rooted in? From what does your mind draw its supply? A few moments of inventory taking might reveal to us our habits for focusing our attention in our moments of leisure.

The possibilities are staggering: how and what we read, what we take time to view on television or pay to see at the theater, how we use our personal computers, cell phones and other inventions that bring data and information into our minds. What we give our attention to contributes significantly to what we think, and what we think governs to a major extent what we speak. Our words are the fruit from what we have been taking in for a long, long time. It is just as true as are the laws of nature!

The only infallible source of supply for bringing forth the good fruits of a righteous life is in God almighty. Anyone who is in Christ is in God, and God is in that person! This will change that person's basic nature from bad to good. The nature of a person being transformed, the fruits of that person's life will be changed as well. The Bible says this will happen: "***Therefore, if anyone is in Christ, the new creation has come: The old has gone, the new has come!*** (2 Corinthians 5:17)."

Some might possibly wonder "How is it that a person can be a Christian and still have some evil fruits in evidence—his or her words are not very good?" The answer to that question must relate to the source of that person's supply. One can take a perfectly good tree, dig it up from its present location and transplant it. At the new location, the consistency of the soil may be different. There may be rocky soil or parched earth into which the tree had been transplanted. If the source of supply to the newly planted tree does not get changed, the tree may not be able to sustain good fruit. It would be a good tree with a bad source of supply.

Similarly, a Christian has the potential for bearing good fruit but he cannot ignore the requirement of getting a good supply by abiding in Christ! Continual fellowship with the Lord through meditation, prayers, reading the Word of God and finding companionship with other children of God will make the Christian well-supplied for a good life that will honor God. Further, there are warnings in the Bible concerning branches in the vine that do not bear fruit as expected. They will be cut back and otherwise corrected by the pruning hand of God.

Of course, the words of a person are just one aspect of the fruits of that person's life. All of their behavior is in the category of the fruit of their life. The words that a person uses are focused on here only because they are such prominent features that display the character of the person. The words of a person are fairly good indicators of the nature of the person and of the source of that person's supply. As we have already considered, there are words we need and there are words we can do without. A person can give careful thought to this issue and would do well to not let the words he lives with slip into a low level of meaninglessness. One should speak with sincerity and avoid vain flattering and deceitfulness. One should strive to bear the fruits of wholesome conversation that enriches the lives of others and should weed out of his speech those four-letter vulgarities that serve no useful purpose but are the products of sheer habit and carelessness.

Indeed, it would be far better for a person to choose silence than to speak poorly. We are reminded of this by the Apostle James: "***Those who consider themselves religious and yet do not keep a tight rein on their tongues deceive themselves, and their religion is worthless*** (James 1:27)."

What are the words you live with? Let your prayer ever be with that of the Psalmist, who said in all earnestness: "***Set a guard over my mouth, Lord; keep watch over the door of my lips*** (Psalm 141:3)." May each of us also pray with the Psalmist, "***May these words of my mouth and this meditation of my heart be pleasing in your sight, Lord my Rock and my Redeemer*** (Psalm 19:14)."

CHAPTER ELEVEN

THE POWER OF LOVE

Love is the most vital force at our command. It is the most powerful of all emotions. There are other strong motivators for human behavior. Fear is one. Desire for success is another. Avoidance of failure is also a strong motivator. Acquisition of wealth ranks right up there, also. Doing one's duty out of a sense of moral obligation is a powerful source of motivation as well. No matter what motivator you might name, nothing rivals the power of love. If you can convince a person that you love him or her, you have won that person's heart. People will literally work their fingers to the bone for the people they love. People will not only labor and give for the people they love; they will also make any sacrifice that will assure the survival and wellbeing of the beloved. Such is the power of love that noble souls have been willing to sacrifice limb or life to secure the freedom of the ones they love. There is absolutely no power on earth or in heaven above that is greater than love!

Dwight Lyman Moody was an American evangelist who was internationally famous during the late 19th century. Among other accomplishments, he founded the Northfield Schools in Massachusetts, Moody church and Moody Bible Institute in Chicago and the Colportage Association. You might say that Rev. Moody was to the 19th century what Rev. Billy Graham was to the 20th century. He was a tireless firebrand for God. Dr. Moody told of the time when he had led his people in Chicago in building a new church. Moody and his parishioners wanted to teach people the love of God. They felt if they could not preach into their hearts they would try to burn it in. So, they put right over the pulpit in gas jets these words: "GOD IS LOVE." One result of this showed up one night when a man was walking down the street and glanced through the open doors of the church and saw the flaming text. He was a poor prodigal—homeless, unkempt, bumming along on the streets to survive. As he passed on he thought to himself, "God is Love," "No!" He continued to think, "He does not love me because I'm nothing but a failure and a miserable sinner."

The man kept trying to rid his mind of that text, but it persisted to stay in his thoughts in letters of fire. He went a little farther, then turned around and went back to the church and into the meeting. He did not hear the sermon, but the words of that short text sank deeply into his heart, and that was enough. The man stayed after the first meeting was over and Dr. Moody found him there weeping like a child. Moody explained the Scriptures and told the man how God had loved him all the time even thought he had wandered so far from God. He said God is waiting to receive you and forgive you. The light of the Gospel broke into this man's mind and into his heart and he went away that night rejoicing.

There is nothing in this world that people prize so much as they do love. Show me a person who has no one to care for or to love him or her and I will show you one of the most wretched beings on the face of this earth. Why do you suppose many people commit suicide? Very often it is because this thought steals in upon them: "No one loves me; I would rather die than to live."

I cannot think of another truth in the entire Word of God that ought to come home to us with such power and tenderness as that of the love of God. There is no truth which Satan strives harder to blot out. For more than six thousand years the father of lies has been trying to persuade men that God does not love them. He succeeded in making Adam and Eve believe the lie, and he too often succeeds with everyone born thereafter. Satan wants people to believe that because they are sinners, God is angry at them and God will punish them for their failures. All one has to do is look at what the Bible says on this issue and they would find that nothing could be farther from the truth! God is in the business of loving sinners. He loves them because He knows their potential to love and serve him when they can come to believe that He loves them—He loves them with an indescribable love! The Apostle Paul wrote to Romans: "***You see, at just the right time, when we were still powerless, Christ died for the ungodly. Very rarely will anyone die for a righteous person, though for a good person someone might possibly dare to die. But God demonstrates his own love for us in this: While we were still sinners, Christ died for us (Romans 5:6-8).***"

What is this verse saying to you? It is saying that no matter what you have done in your life for which you are ashamed to even mention, all of your sins and trespasses against the commandments of God—however many or for however long a time they have been practiced—the forgiveness for all has been bought and paid for by the blood of Jesus Christ when He died on the cross of Calvary! His blood was shed to blot out our sins from the sight of almighty God. Instead of seeing your sins, God sees the blood of His precious Son and He sees no further! In Christ, a sinner is justified from all sin he or she has committed. Someone once defined justification in these terms: "Just as if I'd never sinned." One's moral slate has been wiped clean when Jesus has been received as Lord and Savior. This is the power of love! The Apostle John explains this in a beautiful fashion: "***This is how God showed his love among us: He sent his one and only Son into the world that we might live through him. This is love: not that we loved God, but that he loved us and sent his Son as an atoning sacrifice for our sins (1 John 4:9-10).***" Another verse that depicts this amazing phenomenon of God's love for the sinner can be found in a verse that has been called "the Gospel in a nutshell": "***For God so loved the world that he gave his one and only Son, that whoever believes in him shall not perish but have eternal life (John 3:16).***" This concept is unique to Christianity. No other religion in the world makes such a claim. All other religions are built on the concept of earning one's salvation. Christianity is based on the grace of God, which is his unmerited favor toward sinners. Salvation is never deserved—never possible to be earned by doing good works. It is too great to be earned. It can only be yours by God's grace. Salvation is a gift of God. A gift is never earned or it is no longer a gift. A gift is only yours as you receive it by an act of your will. A gift is offered to you, but it is yours only when you receive it! The forgiveness of your sins and eternal life is a gift that was purchased for you by the blood of Jesus when he died on the cross and it is offered to you by God; it is yours by receiving Jesus into your heart by faith. You might say faith is the hand that reaches out and receives the gift of God. This is precisely what the Apostle Paul wrote to the Ephesians: "*For it is by grace you have been saved through faith—and this is not from yourselves, it is the gift of God—not of works, so that no one can boast (Ephesians 2:8-9)*." We do not deserve God's love. If we got what we deserve we would receive His condemnation because we all are sinners. The word for sin means "missing the mark." We all fall short of what God wants us to be. Because of our selfishness and rebellious hearts, we fall short and we miss the mark. Jesus, on the other hand, never missed the mark in his entire life on earth. He was sinless. He achieved perfect righteousness. When a sinner receives Jesus into his heart by faith, Jesus comes into that life and His perfect righteousness covers that person's sins in the sight of God.

The heart of the issue is the difference between law and grace. When a person is measured by the law of God—the Ten Commandments, he or she is guilty of breaking the law. No one has ever been able to keep the law perfectly. God says, "*There is no one righteous, not even one (Romans 3:10*)." One can only be said to be righteous when they have kept the whole law. To offend in any one aspect of the law is to be a law-breaker. Breaking God's law earns for us the description of "sinner." The Apostle Paul clarifies this fact in his letter to the Romans: "*Now we know that whatever the law says, it says to those who are under the law, so that every mouth may be silenced and the whole world held accountable to God. Therefore no one will be declared righteous in God's sight by observing the law, rather, through the law we become conscious of our sin (Romans 3:19-20)*."

Were it not for the love of God, we would all perish because we have all broken God's law and none of us has achieved righteousness. But God wants to save us from our condition. The only way we can be accounted righteous in His sight is if the righteousness achieved by Jesus could be reckoned to be in our behalf. If the righteousness of Jesus could be transferred to us we would have standing before God; we would stand in the righteousness of Christ! God's solution to the problems is to exercise His divine grace and make the righteousness of His Son a free gift to anyone who would believe in Him! Faith in Jesus as God's provided sin-bearer through His death on the cross acquires for us the righteousness of Jesus in the sight of God. It is not righteousness from keeping the law; it is a righteousness received as God's gift to us in response to our willingness to repent of our sins and accept Jesus as Lord and Savior. No better explanation of this can be found than the words of the Apostle Paul: *"**But now apart from the law the righteousness of God has been made known to which the Law and the Prophets testify. This righteousness is given through faith in Jesus Christ to all who believe. There is no difference between Jew and Gentile, for all have sinned and fall short of the glory of God, and all are justified freely by his grace through the redemption that came by Christ Jesus (Romans 3:21-24)**."* The grace of God issues from the love of God. To save a sinner from his sins and give to him the gift of eternal life is a demonstration of the power of love!

Many have witnessed the power of love on the human level. Every time you see a newborn baby cradled in the arms of the infant's mother or father, you are quite likely to see a vivid image of love and tenderness in action. It is not hard to love members of your family—the product of your own flesh and blood. Loving someone outside your family is more difficult. Yet, as difficult as it may seem, it is happening all the time. Some teachers have a profound love for all their pupils. Some folks have an extraordinary love for animals and their own pets. Doctors and nurses have demonstrated more than their duty for their patients; they have often demonstrated profound love for them. When my late wife was suffering from her bout with stage four cancer, she elected to live her final days at home and I became her care-giver twenty-four-seven, as they say. Loving her gave me the stamina to carry on and strive to meet her needs. I witnessed tremendous love in action from the hospice nurse who came for regular visits to check up on my wife and to administer whatever assistance she needed. The hospice nurse's aide also came several times a week to help with personal care and bathing. Not only the ministrations of the nurse and the nurse's aide were the picture of love in action; it was also their sincere faith in God and infectious optimism that so often lifted my wife's spirit so much that she lived for their coming in to see her.

I have served in the United States Army and I had a tour of duty in the Republic of Vietnam during a very intense period of that war—in 1968. I served with the Field Artillery and with the Combat Engineers and gave chaplain support to the Marines who were stationed at the same locations as our Army troops were stationed. When the chaplain arrived at a base or at an outpost or landing zone, it was to minister to soldiers of all the services who happened to be deployed there. During my year in combat zones I witnessed first-hand the love a commander has for his troops and the love the troops have for a commander who puts their safety as his top priority. I saw the love one soldier would have for his buddies; the love that would lead some to bear the brunt of an exploding device in order to shield his buddies from the damage that otherwise would come to them. Many paid the ultimate price out of love for their comrades in arms and love for their country.

I believe there is no medicine stronger than love to help a severely ill person back to health. I can vouch for this from my own experience. A few years ago I entered the hospital to undergo a second coronary artery bypass surgery. It was going to be a more difficult procedure than the first bypass surgery I had experienced about ten years before. The difficulty was increased due to the scar tissue from the first surgery, and because I was now ten years older.

I survived the procedure on the operating table but my survival was much in question in the recovery room and in the Intensive Care Unit. My kidneys had shut down and I needed blood transfusions to try and keep me alive. I felt so weak and weary regardless of the tireless ministrations of a fabulous Intensive Care nurse. I can vividly remember feeling that my life was slipping away and I was losing the strength and even the desire to fight to hold on for another minute. I was telling myself that the struggle wasn't worth it; I should just let go and die and go to be with the Lord. I felt like I was hanging on a cliff by my finger tips and I could not hold on any longer. Right at that critical point of wanting to give up, I opened my eyes and looked up to see my daughter standing at my side, holding my hand with deep love and awesome concern for me written all over her face. She looked as though she was pleading to God to spare my life. That glimpse of her face placed a resolve in me to fight for all it's worth to hold on one more minute and keep fighting to hold on minute after minute; I did not want her to feel the pain of losing her Dad. Soon, it was morning and I was surprised to see that I was still alive! Yes, the blood transfusions helped to revive me. Yes, the dedication of the nurse was so marvelous that she refused to leave me even when her shift had ended. What really sealed the deal, however, was the love that emanated from my daughter at my side! It was both her love for me and my love for her that brought me through that terrible ordeal. I believe she wrestled with God and God answered her prayers.

Many reading this are finding my experience resonating with their own experiences of love in action. Love is the most powerful emotion a human being is capable of showing. It is revealed in countless acts of tender devotion and undying loyalty on behalf of the beloved partner or family member in their hours of greatest need. Some will spare no cost, give no less than their utmost strength, or make any personal sacrifice to rescue, attend, or nurture a loved one through sickness, setback or adversity. Love is not peculiar to any race, any nationality, and persons of any religion or to persons of any sex or any age. The youngest child or the oldest member of any family is capable of showing profound love in many tangible ways. I, myself, am just a member of a single family among the millions of families on this earth, and yet I have witnessed profound and awesome love being given by my siblings to their spouses and children and given by nieces, nephews and children to their parents.

Recently we had a prolonged heat wave in my area of central California. With temperature of 110 degrees on the outside, I chose to stay on the inside where there is an air-conditioning system. In the midst of this heat wave I heard the doorbell ring. I went to open the door to see who was there and to my surprise, I saw two young girls standing there with a can in their hands. On the can was glued a picture of a young man who had recently been killed in a tragic accident. These girls were hiking through the city neighborhoods in the intense heat, trying to raise funds to pay for the young man's funeral. Their devotion to the memory of a friend was a tribute to their capacity to care and to love. The same devotion has been replayed time and again in dozens of citizens laboring to wash people's cars for the cost of a donation to help their church or to help a family in need. It impresses me as being love in action—love with sun-burned faces, banged-up hands, aching backs and tired feet!

I have a friend who is the mother of two children—a boy and a girl, ages 11 and 6. She has a business cleaning houses for people and cleaning offices five to six days a week. She also has a husband who needs some of her time and she has a father who lives nearby, who calls on her regularly to help him in the office of his business. Like many mothers, she does shopping for food, cooking meals, making lunches, doing laundry and housekeeping duties, figuring the budget, making appointments and paying the bills. On every day of the week, it is one thing or another, on top of cleaning homes for her customers: transporting her son to flag football practice two times per week and to his games or taking her daughter to dance lessons and to soccer practice and her games. At soccer practice, she runs the show because she happens also to be the coach of the soccer team! During hockey season, she drives 70-80 miles round-trip two nights a week so her son can attend hockey practice at the nearest arena and drives him to games on week-ends. She is so involved with her children's lives to give them every advantage possible during their growing years that she is harder to reach than flagging down a race car driver into the pits at the Indianapolis 500! For her it is self-sacrifice out of love for her children and her family! Her devotion does not stop with her two children, either. She also is mother and confidant to her husband's two teen-age daughters and is going to the aid of any number of her friends, wedged between all her other commitments. She makes time—whether it is before going to her first job in the morning, at mid-day, or early evening—to visit her grandmother who is confined to a convalescent home and suffering early stages of Alzheimer's disease. She rarely misses a single day to visit her grandmother or take her out for an outing or a meal. How do you assess the value of a single person's awesome faithfulness and loyalty to all who depend on her? What could explain such total expenditure of energy for the needs of others if it is not a powerful love? I know it is love that drives her because love is at the very core of her character. Her character embodies the description of love that the Apostle Paul gives in his letter to the Corinthians: "**Love is patient, love is kind. It does not envy, it does not boast, it is not proud. It does not dishonor others, it is not self-seeking, it is not easily angered, it keeps no record of wrongs. Love does not delight in evil but rejoices with the truth. It always protects, always trusts, always hopes, always perseveres. Love never fails** (1 Corinthians 13:4-8)."

I have shared several examples of human love that exudes a power that almost defies description. These examples are from my own experience, and I suspect there are thousands of stories my readers could supply of similar portrayals of love in action from their own experiences as well. Newspapers and TV news broadcasts are dominated by the evils in our society—the crimes, murders, robberies and tragedies of life in America and around the world. Some times at the end of these national broadcasts, 90 seconds are devoted to highlight something that is positive! I believe there would be more hope and goodwill in the world were we to hear more stories of the loving behaviors of people every day in every city and every small town or out in the country at some farmhouses, where kindness and helpfulness are prominent features. Good and evil are both in full display! Each one of us must make a decision—perhaps a hundred times each day—whether we will choose to display the good or the evil in our behaviors. To love is not automatic; we choose to love. Love is not static; it is dynamic! Love is not weakness. Love is a force. Love is power like no other!

As strong as human love may be, however, it cannot match the love God shows even to sinners. Many have failed to grasp this truth and cling to the mistaken notion that God hates sinners—they break his laws, are mean and cruel to other human beings and some oppose him and blaspheme his name. The idea that God hates sinners comes from false teaching. Mothers make a mistake when they tell their children that God loves them only when they behave and do right. If you are a parent, you do not teach your children that when they do wrong, you hate them. Their misbehaviors do not change your love for them to hate. If it did, you would change your love a good many times in a single day! When your child is fretful or has committed some act of disobedience, you do not cast him or her out as though that child no longer belongs to you! No! That child is still your child and is loved by you! The same is true with God; if men have gone astray from him, it does not follow that God hates them. It is only the sin he hates; not the sinner.

I believe the reason why a great many people think God does not love them is because they are measuring God by their own small understanding. We love people as long as we consider them worthy of our love. When they are not worthy, we turn away from them. It is not so with God. There is an eternity of difference between human love and Divine love!

In the Apostle Paul's letter to the Ephesians, he describes the measure of God's love—the width, length, depth and height of his love. He writes: "***And I pray that you, being rooted and established in love, may have power, together with all the Lord's people, to grasp how wide and long and high and deep is the love of Christ, and to know this love that surpasses knowledge----that you may be filled to the measure of all the fullness of God*** (Ephesians 3:17b—19)." Many of us think we know something of God's love, but decades from now we shall admit we have never found out much of the truly matchless love of God. Christopher Columbus discovered America, but what did he know about its great lakes, mighty rivers, redwood forests with their towering trees, deep and gorgeous canyons, spectacular mountain ranges and the verdant Mississippi valley? The famous explorer died without knowing much about the land he had discovered. So, too, many of us have discovered something of the love of God, but there are dimensions of it that we do not know. That love is a great ocean. We plunge into it before we really know anything of it! This truth is captured beautifully in the popular Christian hymn, "The Love of God." The final verse of the hymn has a unique way of describing the indescribable:

"Could we with ink the ocean fill,
And were the skies of parchment made,
Were every stalk on earth a quill,
And every man a scribe by trade,
To write the love of God above,
Would drain the ocean dry.
Nor could the scroll contain the whole,
Though stretched from sky to sky.
O Love of God, how rich and pure!
How measureless and strong!
It shall forever more endure,
The saints' and angels' song!"

The cross is a symbol of God's unfailing love. It is said of a Roman Catholic Archbishop of Paris that when he was thrown into prison and condemned to be shot, he saw a window in his cell which was shaped like a cross. Upon the top of the cross he wrote "height," and at the bottom he wrote "depth," and at the end of each arm, "length." When we wish to know the love of God, we should go to Calvary. Can one of us look upon that scene and say "God does not love me?" The cross forever speaks of the love of God! Greater love has never been taught than what the cross of Jesus teaches.

What do you suppose it was that prompted God to give up His one and only Son to suffering and death at the hands of men? What do you suppose it was that prompted Jesus to willingly die upon the cross of Calvary's hill outside the gates of Jerusalem if it were not for love? Jesus Himself had previously told his disciples, **"Greater love has no one than this: to lay down one's life for one's friends** (John 15:13)." Yet, Paul tells the Romans that Jesus did more than lay down his life for his friends. He said, **"But God demonstrates His love for us in this: While we were still sinners, Christ died for us** (Romans 5:8)." Jesus laid down his life for his enemies—even for those who hated him and murdered him! The spirit of the cross and of Calvary is love. When those who crucified him were mocking and deriding him as he suffered excruciating pain, being nailed to the timbers of the cross, what did Jesus say to them? Jesus did not speak one angry word at any of them; instead, he prayed out loud: "**Jesus said, Father, forgive them, for they do not know what they are doing** (Luke 23:34)." That, my friends, is love! Jesus did not call down fire from heaven to consume his tormentors; there was nothing in his heart but love!

The Bible teaches that the love of God is unchangeable. Many who loved you at one time may have grown cold in their affection and perhaps they have even turned away from you. It may be their love has even changed into hatred. This can happen with people. This cannot happen with God! It is recorded of Jesus Christ, when he was parted from his disciples and led away to Calvary's cross, that "**It was before the Passover Festival, Jesus knew that the hour had come for him to leave this world and go to the Father. Having loved his own who were in the world, he loved them to the end** (John 13:1)." Jesus knew that one of his disciples would betray him; yet he loved Judas. He knew another disciple would deny him; yet he loved Peter. It was the love that Christ had for Peter which broke Peter's heart and brought him back in penitence to the feet of the risen Jesus. For three years, Jesus had been with the disciples, teaching them his love, not only by his life and words, but also by his works. And, on the night in which he was betrayed to his captors, Jesus took a basin of water, girded himself with a towel, and taking the role of a servant, he washed the feet of the disciples. Jesus wanted to convince them of his unchanging love!

One of the most beautiful passages of the Bible is chapter 14 of the Gospel of John. Hear what Jesus says as he pours out his heart to his disciples: "**On that day you will realize that I am in my Father, and you are in me, and I am in you. Whoever has my commands and keeps them is the one who loves me. Anyone who loves me will be loved by my Father, and I too will love them and show myself to them** (John 14:20-21)." Just think of the great God Who made the heavens and the earth loving you and me! Jesus went on to say to his disciples, "**Anyone who loves me will obey my teaching. My Father will love them, and we will come to them and make our home with them** (John 14:23)." If only our minds could grasp the wondrous significance of this truth: the Father almighty and His precious Son both so love us that they desire to come and abide with us!

What's more wondrous than this is the fact that God loves us even as He loves His own Son. Notice the thrilling content of Jesus' own words: *"I in them and you in me—so that they may be brought to complete unity. Then the world will know that you sent me and have loved them even as you have loved me* (John 17:23)." This is perhaps one of the most remarkable sayings that ever fell from the lips of our Lord. There is no reason why the Father should not love Jesus. He was obedient unto death itself; He never transgressed the Father's law or turned aside from the perfect path of obedience every hour and every day of his life! But it is quite different with us. Yet, notwithstanding all of our rebellion, selfishness and foolishness, he says that the Father loves us even as he loves his Son. That God could love us as He loves His own sinless Son seems too good to be true. Yet, this is his teaching!

It is hard to make a sinner believe in this unchangeable and matchless love of God. When a man has wandered away from God, he thinks God now hates him. We must make a distinction between the sin and the sinner. The reason why God hates sin is because it mars human life. In fact, it is precisely because God loves the sinner that he hates sin.

God's love is not only unchanging, it is also unfailing. In the Old Testament there is an astounding passage: *"Can a mother forget the baby at her breast and have no compassion on the child she has borne? Though she may forget, I will not forget you! See, I have engraved you on the palms of my hands; your walls are ever before me* (Isaiah 49:15-16)." Think of it! The strongest human love that we know is a mother's love for her child. Many things may separate a man from his wife. A father may even turn his back on his child; brothers and sisters may become terrible enemies. But a mother's love endures through all. In good repute, in bad repute, in the face of the world's condemnation, a mother loves on and hopes her child may turn from errant ways and repent. She remembers the infant smiles, the merry laughter of childhood, the bright promise of youth, and she can never be brought to think her child unworthy. Death cannot quench a mother's love; it is stronger than death.

You may have seen a mother watching over her sick child. How willingly she would take the fever or the disease into her own body if she could by so doing relieve her child's suffering! Week after week, she will keep watch. She will not let another take care of her sick child. I remember hearing the story about a mother whose son was badly influenced by a wayward father. The boy had committed all kinds of crime, and finally he committed murder. The mother sat all through the trial but she did not share the bitterness of the jury and the public. She loved on. After the execution of her son, she craved the body but that was denied her. Soon, the mother herself died, but before doing so, she had made arrangements to be buried by the side of her son in the prison cemetery. She was not ashamed to be known as the mother of a murderer. What made the difference was her love for her son!

Love cannot be confined to thought alone. It cannot be defined as feeling alone, either. Love is thought that gives birth to feeling and feeling that gives birth to action. Love is never complete until it culminates in action. Saying to someone, "I love you," are only words that stir up hopefulness in the person to whom the words are spoken. The veracity of those words can only be determined by the behaviors that substantiate that claim. If a person loves another, they will not ignore them. They will not disrespect them. They will not overlook their obvious needs. They will not purposefully hurt them. They will not be unkind to them. They will not exercise control over them. They will not stifle or smother them and keep them from experiencing their potential to achieve goals that are important to them. I am sure you are able to see where I am going with this description. The all too common fact is that many people use the word "love" erroneously because they do not know how to say other things like, I need you because of what you do for me; I need your companionship, I need your hugs and kisses and the sex you give to me; I need the security you provide because it gives me a standard of living I could not have without you. I need you because you are so attractive that it makes me look good when I can display the fact that you are my girl or my wife! I tell you that I love you because I am afraid you will leave me and find someone else if I do not say I love you. I love you because you make me feel good.

You will notice that all of the examples I have listed have one thing in common: the focus is on the recipient. These expressions define need, not love. Love is giving—even sacrificing, if need be, for the wellbeing of the one loved. If you say to someone, "I love you," you are going on record as being committed to expend whatever it takes to advance the happiness and wellbeing of the other person! The words are then backed up by repeated actions that will convince the person that love is the right word to describe the attitude that drives the lover to love with power and consistency. An example of love in action might be a very busy executive who instructs the secretary to "hold all calls; I do not want to be disturbed unless the caller is my wife or one of my children." It is love for his or her children that will motivate a parent to leave work early or put in for leave time in order to attend an important game in which their child is playing, or to view a performance in which their child is taking part. It is love that translates into duty that spurs a person to leave the house at any hour of the night and drive in a thunderstorm or snowfall in order to find a store that is open where one can get some over-the-counter remedy to help a sick spouse or family member at home. It is love for a friend that will drive a person to get up in the middle of the night and go to the aid of a friend who has called for help. It is not fear that makes these decisions. It is not selfishness that makes these decisions, either; it is love. Love is a power that has no equal! Love is thoughtful. Love is kind. Love is faithful. Love considers. Love commits. Love gives. Love trusts. Love acts!

If you need a model to set a pattern for you as to how to love, you can do no better than to look to Jesus. He, more than any other who ever lived, was the very embodiment of love. Since I have already made a case for love is more than thought and more than feeling— love is action, consider that Jesus loves you and his actions prove it. Only his death could atone for our sins because there was none other who was without sin who could have done the job instead. If ever even a single human being could be saved from sin, it would require a substitute who was without sin to die in his place. This is because, as Paul declared in his epistle to the Romans, "**For the wages of sin is death** (Romans 6:23a)." Therefore, because he loved us, Jesus submitted himself to his captors, endured a mock trial and physical torture, willingly positioned himself on the wooden timbers horizontally laid out on the ground in the form of a cross, stretched out his arms and let the soldiers drive the nails into his palms and through his feet until he was affixed to the cross. He remained committed to his suffering and pain as the cross was lifted up and was dropped with a thud into the hole that was prepared for it, jarring our Lord's bones and stretching his wounds as the blood spurted out and streamed down his body to pool at the foot of his cross! Not for anything he had done nor for anything he deserved, did Jesus submit to this cruel ordeal. He did this for love. It was the love of his Father in Heaven that designed the plan for saving sinners, and it was the love of Jesus—God the Father's Son, who carried out the plan and sacrificed himself to redeem sinners who would believe in him. "**For God so loved the world that he gave his one and only Son, that whoever believes in him shall not perish but have eternal life** (John 3:16)." This, my friends, is the power of love! It is the power of God's love!

The cross for us who live after the fact of Jesus' crucifixion is an amazing example of the power of God's love. Consider those who lived before the fact of Jesus' sacrificial death for sinners. God's chosen people—the nation of Israel—had abundant reason to know the love and the power of the love of almighty God. The Psalms of David are replete with examples of his profound appreciation for the manifest love of God. The love of God so moved David that he often burst forth in song: "**But I will sing of your strength, in the morning I will sing of your love; for you are my fortress, my refuge in times of trouble. You are my strength, I sing praise to you; you, God, are my fortress, my God on whom I can rely** (Psalm 59:16-17)." Again, David declared, "**But I trust in your unfailing love; my heart rejoices in your salvation. I will sing the Lord's praise, for he has been good to me** (Psalm 13:5)." David knew his life depended upon the goodness and the faithfulness of his God. He knew there was great reward for placing trust in God. On one occasion, David wrote: "***Many are the woes of the wicked, but the Lord's unfailing love surrounds those who trust in him*** (Psalm 32:10)." It is a theme David never got tired of sounding. David had an inner joy that could not be extinguished by the miseries and challenges of life. It was as though he were swimming in an ocean of God's love. David said, "***I will sing of the Lord's great love forever; with my mouth I will make your faithfulness known through all generations. I will declare that your love stands firm forever, that you have established your faithfulness in Heaven itself*** (Psalm 89:1-2)."

As you can see, David made no secret of his love for God because God made no secret of his love for David! It is no secret, either, how great a love God has for you and for me. His love is a powerful force. His love transforms lives, turns people around in their tracks; summons them to walk in his ways and to do his will. It is as Paul describes: "***For Christ's love compels us, because we are convinced that one died for all, and therefore all died. And he died for all, that those who live should no longer live for themselves but for him, who died for them and was raised again*** (2 Corinthians 5:14)." Consider that this profound belief in the love of God that David displayed was based upon God's acting in keeping with his promises. It was God's loyalty to David—his steadfast faithfulness and merciful interventions that convinced David that his trust in God was supremely well-placed. David knew nothing of Jesus' life and teachings. He knew nothing of the disciples and the apostles who followed and accompanied Jesus in his earthly ministry. He did not have any concept of the Son of God hanging to die upon a wooden cross as an intervention planned by God the Father to save sinners and make them heirs of God and joint heirs with Jesus in his Divine Kingdom that would have no end. Therefore, if David had so much for which to sing about the matchless love of God, how much more do we have something about which to sing! We can sing of our Redeemer! To Jesus, we who believe and have been washed in his blood can now sing his praises. With John the Apostle we can sing these words: "***To him who loves us and has freed us from our sins by his blood, and has made us to be a kingdom and priests to*** *serve his God and Father—to him be glory and power forever and ever! Amen.* (Revelation 1:5-6)."

There is power in God's love. There is power in man's love, also. That's because love itself is a force; love is power in action. If you question this proposition, open up your mind and open your heart to God. Yield your will to God's will and invite him to be Lord and master of your life. God will love you with an all-encompassing love. When you stray from his love, he will seek you out to bring you back. If you disobey, he will discipline you. He disciplines only because he loves you and wants you to be at your best for him. He corrects you so that he can bestow his blessings upon you. This is the message God gives in his Word: *"Those whom I love I rebuke and discipline. So be earnest and repent. Here I am! I stand at the door and knock. If anyone hears my voice and opens the door, I will come in and eat with them, and they with me* (Revelation 3:20)." I know you will never be the same once you have discovered the love of God in your life. To God be the glory!

Chapter Twelve

LESSONS FROM BETHANY

Two experiences common to all people are birth and death. I suppose it is safe to say that we know quite a bit more about birth than we know about death. Once we are born, it is a matter of time before we die and make our exit from this world. For some, the time of departure from this life is far too soon; for others, it comes quite late in the scheme of things. Depending on a number of things, such as close family ties, quality of life and an array of loving and admiring friends, it becomes very difficult to let go of a person and to accept the reality of their death. When a lot of suffering and unrelenting pain or severe senility constitutes the quality of one's life, death for many can be all too welcomed. In any event, each one of us must face the fact that we are mortals and one day we will breathe our final breath. Not only do we face our own mortality, we must acknowledge the mortality of everyone we love and cherish. Should we live longer than any one of them, we will suffer from the loss of such dear ones. Anyone who loves will know the sting of grief at some time or time, and time again. It is inevitable fact, yet it is never easy to accept nor do we choose to give much time to thinking about it. This very truth leaves us woefully unprepared for facing the experience of losing someone we deeply love.

Such was the case of two sisters about whom we read in the Bible. Their names are Mary and Martha. These women lived in the town of Bethany during the days of Jesus' ministry of teaching and healing in the Middle Eastern land of Palestine. Bethany was west of the Jordan River, which flowed north and south; between Jericho and Jerusalem. Whenever Jesus traveled from the northern area around the Sea of Galilee to Jerusalem in the south, he would stop on the way to visit and lodge with Mary, Martha and their brother, Lazarus. The family was very precious to Jesus because they had a great love for him. The little town of Bethany will forever be remembered as the place where one of the most amazing events in the life of Jesus took place.

The weeks that preceded the death of Christ at Jerusalem were filled with a flurry of activity for our Lord. Jesus had given several indications to his disciples that he needed to go to Jerusalem. On the Mount of Transfiguration, Peter, James and John, who had accompanied Jesus to this remote location, had overheard the prophets Moses and Elijah talking with Jesus about his soon-coming death. The time soon came when Jesus and his disciples were nearing the moment when Jesus would enter Jerusalem where the events of his passion and crucifixion would take place. The unfolding drama is recorded by the Apostle John, chapter eleven, verses one through forty-six.

Jesus was just about at the end of three and one-half years of his public ministry. He had healed the sick, raised the dead and taught with wisdom not of this world. He performed many, many miracles out in the open where the crowds that followed him could witness them. By this point, Jesus had garnered a tremendous following and people were coming to believe that his claim of being the Son of God was absolutely true! The loyalty of the multitudes that believed in Jesus frightened the Jewish Ecclesia and they were convinced he posed a threat to their traditions and their religion. The religious leaders of the day were very angry at Jesus and they could scarcely wait to get their hands on him to destroy him.

The beginning of events took place in the countryside beyond the river Jordan where John the Baptist used to preach and baptize converts. As it happened, Jesus was looking for a place of solitude and safety from the angry Jews who tried to take him by force a few days earlier, when Jesus laid claim to the fact that he was the Son of God. The eleventh chapter of John opens with Jesus receiving the news from a messenger who was sent by Mary and Martha of Bethany—the news that their brother and Jesus' dear friend, Lazarus, was lying very sick and was probably about to die. It was the hope of the two sisters that Jesus would come immediately and would perform one of his miracles; they believed he would heal Lazarus of his illness so that he would not die.

Jesus, however, did not promptly set out for Bethany. After hearing the word of the messengers, Jesus said, "***This sickness will not end in death. No, it is for God's glory so that God's Son may be glorified through it*** (John 11:4)." The text goes on to state, "***Now Jesus loved Martha and her sister and Lazarus. So when he heard that Lazarus was sick, he stayed where he was two more days, and then he said to his disciples, 'Let us go back to Judea*** (John 11:5-7)." Given the intense anger against him on the part of the religious hierarchy at Jerusalem, this impending visit to Bethany was most dangerous both for Jesus and his disciples. The disciples began to protest and reminded Jesus that a short time ago the Jews tried to stone him; it would be too risky to go back to Judea. As a matter of fact, the disciple Thomas was not happy about Jesus taking this risk. When Jesus told the disciples that he was going to Bethany to raise Lazarus from the dead, Thomas jested, "***Let us also go, that we may die with him*** (John 11:16)." Jesus' delay of two days before departing for Bethany was timed by our Lord so that his arrival at Bethany would be after Lazarus had been dead and buried for four days! The sisters and their friends were now in mourning.

There are three very significant statements in John's detailed account that I wish to call to the reader's attention: two statements made by the sisters of Lazarus, and one made by Jesus himself. I believe that by considering these three statements within their context, we may learn some extremely valuable lessons concerning how we might handle the trauma of sickness and death. In understanding the meaning of these three statements, I believe there is a profound message of hope for all of us!

The first statement is that of the sisters, Mary and Martha, as they sent word to Jesus that Lazarus, their brother, was sick. John's text says: "***So the sisters sent word to Jesus, 'Lord, the one you love is sick*** (John 11:30)." The fact that Mary and Martha sent a messenger to find Jesus when Lazarus was so seriously ill is indicative of their belief that no stone should be left unturned to try and help bring healing to the ill. They believed, as many still do today, that where there is life, there is hope. This is good, because many things can be done for the sick. Never was this truer than it is in our day and age. Modern medicine and medical protocols are able to save many lives from diseases and illnesses that people could not have survived just a few generations ago. Here we have, however, in the example of Mary and Martha, a good account of a timeless principle concerning what to do with the ill.

The first thing we can do is to minister to the needs of the ill person. Certainly, from two loving sisters such as were Mary and Martha, Lazarus was lacking in no amount of attention, companionship, moral support and physical nursing. The home of Lazarus was no doubt a veritable beehive of activity as meticulous Martha and matronly Mary lavished their care upon their sick brother. Unfortunately, the best of care may not suffice to save life.

A second thing which can be done when all the care given is not enough to reverse a person's condition is to seek whatever help that is available. This is what we learn from these devoted women. Some will send for the best physicians to attend their beloved ill; they will place the ill person in the care of a top-rate medical clinic or a hospital that is known for their success with their patients. In Lazarus' case, there was no city hospital to which he could be taken—no intensive care units were available. But there was no greater physician in the entire known world, they believed, than Jesus Christ. Therefore, Mary and Martha dispatched a messenger to find Jesus; they asked for nothing less than the best!

A third and most important thing that can be done for the ill is to pray for him or her. By sending for Jesus, Mary and Martha were doing more than seeking the best physician available, they were placing the fate of their beloved brother in the hands of the Lord! The message read, "***Lord, the one you love is sick***." There was a lot implied in this simple message to Jesus. Consider just a few of the most relevant implications. In the first place, there is the implication that the love Jesus has for Lazarus will motivate him to do whatever is needed to save him. The sisters did not ask Jesus to hurry to Bethany. They assumed that simply mentioning the dire need would be enough to say. They were counting on Jesus' love to do the rest. He would do whatever was needed! These women trusted that Jesus loved them and they trusted that he loved Lazarus, also.

In the second place, there is the implication that love will not permit Jesus to let Lazarus die. This is the human perspective on life's tragedies. As far as it is a human perspective, it is the highest form of human rectitude to believe in love doing its duty. It is solid logic—the logic of love! Love will seek to lessen or remove the pain endured by the beloved, with but one exception. That exception, of course, is when a higher good is taken into account than the presence of pain and suffering. Love will permit pain to exist when serving a higher good. In the punishing of children, for example, a loving parent may inflict pain for the higher good of retarding moral decay. The wise parent knows that some suffering on the part of a child may turn the child from practices which later in life would only bring more serious suffering and pain when unrestrained childish folly leads to rebellion and risk. The spared rod leads to the spoiled child. Surely, spoiling the child is not the deed of love! In psychological terminology, failing to correct the erring child is enabling the child to continue along a path that is bound to result in many problematic behaviors that will not easily yield to change.

Another example is the probing of a sterilized needle for an embedded splinter in the flesh of a child's finger is probably going to inflict pain, but the pain is necessary to remove an agent that could create infection and far greater pain than were it not removed. So it is here with Jesus: it is expected that he will act in love. Indeed, he will, but the loving thing Jesus does is far greater than the loving thing Mary and Martha had expected! The women expected that Jesus would heal Lazarus of his sickness unto death. Jesus purposed to meet a greater need: he would deal with the enemy greater than sickness—the enemy of death itself!

In the meeting of this immediate need of a solitary family through the resurrecting of a single corpse, the love of Jesus would extend far beyond the Mary and Martha of little Bethany to the millions of Marys and Marthas, to the Ronalds and Bills, the Joes and the Davids, the Barbaras and the Judys of all time—to you and to me, and in this one decisive miracle, Jesus would speak clearly to the supreme need of each of us, which is the need for hope in the face of death!

It is no wonder that Mary and Martha did what was right and what was best for Lazarus when they sent word to Jesus. And it is no wonder that Jesus did what was right for Mary and Martha to have delayed his coming. The women did what human love would do; Jesus did what Divine love would do—he would wait. Jesus would wait not only until Lazarus had died, but he waited sufficiently long enough that there would be no hope whatsoever. Lazarus would be reckoned to be "deader than a door nail," as the saying goes. In Jesus' way of thinking, there must be no question as to the absolute power of God performing the resurrection of Lazarus. Everyone would know it was a marvelous miracle!

One is reminded of a similar dynamic involving the prophet Elijah in days long before this. In 1 Kings, chapter 18, we find the account of the contest between Elijah and the 450 prophets of Baal. Each built an altar and placed a bull on each altar. The prophets of Baal were challenged to pray to their god to consume the sacrifice on their altar. They prayed, pleaded, shouted, danced and maimed themselves from morning until night time, but failed to receive any response whatsoever from Baal. Elijah, on the other hand, made it as scientifically impossible as he could for the Lord to bring fire down on his altar. He had a trench dug around the altar and he instructed the prophets of Baal to fill four large jugs with water and to pour it on his altar and on the wood. Then he told them to do it the second time and even a third time. The altar and the wood were drenched and the water ran down the altar and filled the trench. Listen to what Elijah did next: "***At the time of the sacrifice, the prophet Elijah stepped forward and prayed: 'Lord, the God of Abraham, Isaac and Israel, let it be known today that you are God in Israel and that I am your servant and have done all these things at your command. Answer me, Lord, answer me, so these people will know that you, Lord, are God, and that you are turning their hearts back again.' Then the fire of the Lord fell and burned up the sacrifice, the wood, the stones and the soil, and also licked up the water in the trench. When all the people saw this, they fell prostrate and cried, 'The Lord—he is God! The Lord—he is***

God! (I Kings 18:36-39)." Elijah wanted to demonstrate beyond the shadow of a doubt that what they were to witness would be the work of almighty God!

So it is with the raising of Lazarus. It must be a miracle that no one could argue against by sighting some explanation from the laws of physical science for the resurrection of Lazarus. This must be clearly to all an act of the omnipotent God; it must say to all that God has the power to raise the dead! Yes, where there is life there is hope. Jesus waits until all hope is gone! Now, please let your mind focus on the scene four days after the death of Lazarus. Jesus now arrives at Bethany. Lazarus is dead and buried. The family is in mourning. Martha first, then Mary some minutes later, both protest to Jesus that he is too late; had he come sooner it would not have meant death for dear Lazarus! Thus, we have the second statement from which we can learn a major lesson: **"*Lord," Martha said to Jesus, "If you had been here, my brother would not have died* (John 11:20)."**

Mary and Martha had done all that was humanly possible to save Lazarus, including sending for Jesus, yet Lazarus dies! We all come to death sooner or later. It does not make it easier to deal with the loss of a loved one even when we believe his or her death is inevitable; it still hurts us so terribly much! Why isn't it easier for us to accept the death of a loved one when we can see it coming? It is never easy to accept a permanent separation from the one we love. It goes against all the grain that is in us—against that which makes us feel important to someone, all that makes us feel secure. It is never easy to accept that loss! We do not grieve so much for the person who dies as we grieve and are in fear of what is to become of us in that loved one's absence. We sorrow for our own sense of loneliness over the vacuum their going leaves behind in our lives!

Mary and Martha acted correctly for ones who dearly loved a brother; they took his death very hard. They took his death hard for more than his being taken from them, however. As hard as it was going to be to reconcile them to the absence of Lazarus, they would in time adjust to it. The sorrowing, in time, can be reconciled to reality. Life does not stop because a dear portion of it is gone. Life must go on; in most cases, grieving ends and people are able to move on. No, Mary and Martha had a greater difficulty to surmount than the loss of their brother. Their greater grief was over the obstacle posed by Jesus' apparent insensitivity to their grief. He had waited. He did not come on time. He could have healed Lazarus and spared them of their broken hearts, thought these women. It is as though they were saying to Jesus, "This is a fine time for you to show up; you are too late! The worse has already happened!"

The grief of these sisters—and a grief to which they could not be reconciled—was in the feeling that their trust in Jesus had been misplaced. Can you imagine the thoughts? "I felt Jesus loved Lazarus; why did he let him die?" Or, "I thought Jesus loved me; why did he let me lose my brother?" Are not these questions valid? Are they not very logical? Are they not questions that you or I may have at the loss of a loved one—at the death of a child, of a family member or of a spouse?

The message I hear in the response of Mary and Martha is, "Does Jesus care? Does he <u>really</u> care?" The answer comes in Jesus' response at this moving scene of Mary weeping at Jesus' feet—her Jewish friends all weeping with her—and Jesus hears her pain-filled words, "***Lord, if you had been here, my brother would not have died*** (John 11:32b)." These words and the circumstances that prompted him were such that Jesus was deeply moved. The response of Jesus is simply astounding: "***When Jesus saw her weeping, and the Jews who had come along with her also weeping, he was deeply moved in spirit and troubled. 'Where have you laid him?' he asked. Come and see, Lord, they replied*** (John 11:33-34)." What comes next is the shortest verse in the entire Bible: "***Jesus wept*** (John 11:35)."

For whom is Jesus weeping? Is he weeping for Lazarus who is wrapped in grave clothes and laid out in a cold, rock-hewn tomb? Is he weeping for the women whose hearts had been put to such a test, whose hopes had been so bitterly crushed and whose trust in him had now been challenged? Or, is Jesus perhaps at that scene weeping for all of us—for the millions upon millions of people down through the ages who have grieved over their dead? Does he now weep over the plight of the whole human race? Does he see in the form of Lazarus, wrapped in linen grave clothes, the form of a little child whose death has broken the hearts of his or her parents? Does he see the form of a young man or woman who has died from an untimely accident or dreadful disease? Does he see the form of a soldier who died on the fields of battle in the fight for freedom? Does he see the form of a beloved mother or father whose children are now alone? Does he see the form of the fire-fighter or the law enforcement officer who died in the line of duty? Who does Jesus see and for whom does he weep? Death is hard to accept. It is so hard to accept, that Jesus wept!

This brings us to the third statement from which we learn a major lesson at Bethany. When Martha confronted Jesus with the consequences of his delayed arrival, Jesus said to her, "**Your brother will rise again** (John 11:23)." Martha was not without faith, even after losing Lazarus. She said to Jesus, "**I know that he will rise again in the resurrection at the last day** (John 11:24)." Now hold on to your seat; listen to these most profound and moving declarations that ever fell from the lips of Jesus: "**Jesus said to her, 'I am the resurrection and the life. Anyone who believes in me will live, even though they die; and whoever lives by believing in me will never die. Do you believe this?** (John 11:25-26)."

Martha had elicited this response from Jesus. He spoke to her need with a profound statement of fact: death is not the end! Those who believe in Jesus will live forever! Yes, and in speaking to Martha, Jesus speaks to us! We need not sorrow as those who have no hope. We have a hope that is anchored to the power and the promises of the Lord of life! Death is a great enemy of us all; Jesus is greater! Martha's expression of grief prompted Jesus' glorious promise that He was more powerful than death and that He will raise from the dead all who believe in Him.

Mary's expression of grief came next. Martha went back to the house and informed Mary that Jesus had come. Mary hurried out to see Jesus and she fell at his feet, weeping. Her expression of grief was the same as Martha's, for she said, "**Lord, if you had been here, my brother would not have died** (John 11:32b)." In response to Martha, Jesus had given a promise. In response to Mary, Jesus asks a question: "**Where have you laid him?** (John 11:34)." The mourners with Mary invited the Lord to come and see where Lazarus was laid. Can you imagine that dreadful scene? The grieving sisters and the weeping Jews were standing there with Jesus before the tomb of Lazarus. Does Jesus care? To get the greatest impact for what comes next, I will cite the words of our text: *"**Jesus, once more deeply moved, came to the tomb. It was a cave with a stone laid across the entrance. 'Take away the stone,' he said. 'But Lord,' said Martha, the sister of the dead man, 'by this time there is a bad odor, for he has been there four days.' Then Jesus said, "Father, I thank you that you have heard me. I knew that you always hear me, but I said this for the benefit of the people standing here, that they may believe that you sent me.' When he had said this, Jesus called in a loud voice, 'Lazarus, come out!' The dead man came out, his hands and feet wrapped with strips of linen, and a cloth around his face. Jesus said to them, 'Take the grave clothes and let him go.**** (John 11:38-44)."*

Does Jesus care? Does Jesus love? Is death the end? Look! Lazarus appears! "Let him go," Jesus commands. Yes, loose him—loose Lazarus from the garments of death for they do not fit one who lives—one who has been raised from the dead! And in letting Lazarus go, Jesus was speaking to yet a broader audience than those who stood at the tomb of Lazarus, saying loose them and let them go! Loose all who mourn for their loved ones from their despair. Loose all the sorrowing from the cords of grief! Loose all who have to face death from their fearfulness and sense of dread. Loose them, and set them free!

Death is not the reward for the believer in Jesus. What awaits all who trust in him is glorious life—eternal life with Jesus in the Heavens. Yes, there were three great statements concerning the events of Bethany: **"Lord, the one you love is sick."** Jesus waited, because he loved. Secondly, **"Lord, if you had been here, my brother would not have died."** Jesus wept because he loved. Thirdly, **"Jesus said I am the resurrection and the life. Anyone who believes in me will live, even though they die; and whoever lives by believing in me will never die. Do you believe this?"** Jesus now wins! He wins because he loves! My friend, the magnificent truth is this: because Jesus wins over death, we win, too!

The words of the Apostle Paul are so very appropriate to quote at this point: *"**Death has been swallowed up in victory. 'Where, O death, is your victory? Where, O death, is your sting?' The sting of death is sin, and the power of sin is the law. But thanks be to God! He gives us the victory through our Lord Jesus Christ. Therefore, my dear brothers and sisters, stand firm. Let nothing move you. Always give yourselves fully to the work of the Lord, because you know that your labor in the Lord is not in vain** (1 Corinthians 15:55-58)."*

Mary—Martha—Lazarus—and Jesus. Thank God for the lessons from Bethany!

CHAPTER THIRTEEN

GOD ALONE MATTERS

Quite often, many of the most profound truths can be expressed by simple statements. When you think on it, many of the deep sayings of the Bible are limited to no more than three words: *"God is love," "Jesus wept," "It is finished," "He is risen."* Take any of these statements by themselves and meditate on the significance embodied in those two or three words and you will be utterly amazed at the world of meaning each phrase delivers! Though centuries have passed and the greatest of thinkers have weighed in on these themes and produced tons of books, these simple statements have never been fully fathomed! If you want to try something very different some day, just take out a note pad and write at the top of the first page any one of those brief phrases referred to above. Then, proceed to think on it without distraction and see what comes to your mind as you begin to write out all the thoughts that might explain the meaning and significance of that brief phrase. It will amaze you, I am sure! What does it mean to you that *"God is love?"* What does it mean to you that Jesus was standing at the grave of his dear friend Lazarus, who had recently died and was buried, and *"Jesus wept?"* How does it touch your soul to think of Jesus suffering a lengthy, agonizing and excruciating death upon the cross of Calvary, offering His own life in your place, dying for your sins and not his own, and hearing him say, *"It is finished?"* What, also does it mean to you that He who died for you and was buried in a borrowed tomb that was sealed and guarded by Roman soldiers was found missing on the third day and the explanation given by angels to the women who came to anoint his body was, He is not here, *"He is risen?"*

I would like to suggest there is a simple statement which every person would do well to grasp and hold on to with great mental tenacity. Although it consists of just three words, it has the potential for revolutionizing one's entire life. These words are packed with power and strike at the most basic of human needs—the need to be free. By this I do not refer to a political freedom, such as when one escapes from a dictatorial, tyrannical regime. Neither do I refer to freedom from a binding contract like an ill-fated marriage, a military enlistment, an automobile or home lease. I do not refer to freedom from a judicial sentence or an incarceration. I do not refer to an outward freedom of any kind, but to one that is far more penetrating and deeper than any of these, no matter how important any of them may be. The freedom to which I refer is an inward release—a liberation of one's spirit and soul from that which has burdened, restricted or confined it. Whether they realize it or not, every person craves an inner freedom, an inward peace that nothing can dislodge or take away. Many study and train to acquire skills and professions which will reward them with feelings of accomplishment and enable them to garner an income that pays the bills, provides for the needs of themselves and their families, believing that taking care of the ones they love will bring peace and contentment to their souls. They are striving for freedom from worry that they might not be adequate for the challenge of doing right by those who are depending on them for survival. People are driven by an inward need to feel adequate and at peace within their innermost being—freedom from failing, from not measuring up to expectations.

The science of psychology is devoted to understanding the tensions, needs and motivations of the inner self. Whether it is the psyche, ego or id, or the self-- call it what you will, the issue is the same: the soul of a person is shielded by layers of defenses that precludes discovery by others. We don't even know this is happening within us because it is going on in our subconscious; an area of our being that we can scarcely get in touch with nor can we understand. The truth is that any person is inwardly bound by any variety of psychological fetters, limiting their freedom to reach their true potential or their ideal self. The fetters may be feelings of inferiority, fears of the unknown, feelings of insecurity, of failure, of guilt, of moral weakness, wrongful longings or desires, need for acceptance or approval from significant others and countless other limiting factors. A person can be all bound up inside oneself, literally barb-wired and mine-fielded with defenses that keep others at bay, preventing them from invading and knowing their innermost self. The desire may be to be free of these restrictions but there is the fear of being wounded and hurt should the attempt to self-reveal be made. Some freedom to be in touch with one's inner self is achieved by intimacy with another whom one trusts and whom one loves. When this happens it is at best tentative and risky because there is the possibility we won't be understood and accepted for who we really are. It is an attempt at becoming free but it is not true freedom of the soul.

In every generation young people are making attempts at breaking the molds of society and are striving to express this innermost freedom. In the 1950's and 60's it was the beatniks and hippies, as they were labeled by society, who were trying to express freedom from conventionalism. They were on a quest for freedom to be the way they wanted to be --- to be liberated from the set patterns of society. They were known as nonconformists. They were on a quest for self expression that would deliver them from pressures of fitting in with the expectations of the general public. By their choice of clothing, styles of fixing their hair or the adornments of their face or bodies, they were sending a message that they are free to be who they want to be—free from pretending, free from being counterfeit. The hippies' search for self-realization is perhaps justified, but sadly misdirected. True liberty does not come with long hair, facial hair and goatees, dark sun-glasses, smoking pot and LSD. Liberty of the soul does not come with spurning responsibilities, shunning labor or casting off societal mores or morality. The drug user on his or her psychedelic trip, the alcoholic in his or her stupor are poor examples indeed of a person finding freedom. They always must come painfully back to the world of reality and face the same problems from which they were seeking escape!

There is a better answer to man's problems than this. What one thinks would bring satisfaction may in the end deliver something less. What one expects to bring happiness may not succeed in delivering happiness. We may think wealth will bring us peace. Perhaps what motivates us may be the need to be popular or to be famous and admired by others. Perhaps what drives us is to earn the respect and trust of others. As worthy as these goals may be, I would suggest something far better. It could be summed up in a simple, three-word statement that can become imbedded in one's thinking. It can be memorized and emblazoned in the mind so that it may never be forgotten. It is the key to peace of mind and the inner-door to self-discovery and the road to inner peace and freedom. This is true liberty, to know that GOD ALONE MATTERS! That's it! That's the statement one must seize and believe: GOD ALONE MATTERS! Think on it!

In saying this simple phrase, I am perfectly aware that many people will be in disagreement. In fact there are two categories of people who would disagree with this statement that GOD ALONE MATTERS. The first categories of people who disagree are PEOPLE TO WHOM NOTHING MATTERS—NOT EVEN GOD. There are hosts of people who are dedicated to nothing. They are not dedicated to family, not to sweetheart, not to their job, not to a solid code of ethics or morality. They are people who are indifferent, riding the moods of each passing day and following the fluctuating inclinations of self-centered pursuits and desires. These people cannot be relied upon. They can't be trusted to do what they say they will do. They demonstrate no loyalty to any person, principle, or code of conduct other than what may suit them and what answers to moods or cravings at any given moment of time.

Usually, these people think of themselves as being free, independent, and possessors of liberty. While they do enjoy a liberty from laws, moral restrictions and the expectations of others, they are slaves to their own desires, servants of their dominating lusts and are shackled to faulty habits which cannot be broken. These people may think they are independent and not committed to anything or anyone but they certainly are not free in soul. They consequently are not happy or contented people. They do not know the true liberty that comes with the conviction that GOD ALONE MATTERS. These people will never really make it in their jobs or careers, won't have successful marriages or the admiration of their children. Because they have also neglected to nurture a faith in God they will end up feeling empty, alone and depressed, totally unprepared for their demise and what awaits them after that.

The second category of people that disagree with the statement that GOD ALONE MATTERS is THEY WHO SAY THAT GOD MATTERS, but will not go so far as to say that He <u>ALONE</u> matters. Many people think they have done God a favor simply to admit they believe there's a God! Such persons do not honor God in the slightest, for recognition is not the same as worship. Recognizing God and serving God are very different responses. The devil recognizes God, but he is his enemy! To concede that God is there—what is this? The trees are there, too, but is not God deserving of more from a person than the trees? To say that one believes there is a God is to say no more than to believe there's a railroad track in Chicago or that there's a Redwood tree in California!

Even if one should get specific and say there is only one God, what more are they saying than there is one Empire State Building, one Golden Gate Bridge, one Theodore Roosevelt or one Elvis Presley? What honor has one brought to God if this is all one could say about him? It is no wonder that so many who attend our churches each Sunday and who call themselves Christians do not know the feeling I am describing here. True liberty does not come by just adding God to one's life like an appendage in the back of a book! Making room for Him among other allegiances is woefully inadequate! God is not satisfied unless He occupies the central part of one's life—when He is asked not to be just a passenger who goes along on the ride but is asked to be the driver who takes one where He would have him go!

Telling God he is important is not enough. One must tell Him he is <u>most</u> important, and then back it up with action!   Doing anything less than this is complete absurdity. One must remember Who God really is! He is the God who created the universe and who made the world in which we live and who supplies the breath that sustains your God-given body. When you bask in sun by the pool, it is God's sun that tans your skin and God's water that refreshes your senses when you splash in to cool off! It is God who sets the wheels of nature into movement to grow the food that is processed in your kitchen, placed on your plate to satisfy your hunger. Even if you eat out in a restaurant and whip out the money or credit card to pay the bill, your part in the process of satisfying your hunger is infinitesimally small. Where did you get the money to pay the bill? You probably got it from your job. Where did you get your job? You probably got it from your abilities. Where did you get your abilities? What do you owe God any way? You owe him everything! What are you giving him? If you are not giving him first place in your affections, the dominant place in determining your attitudes and objectives, you really are not giving him anything!

If you have trouble understanding this, imagine treating your married partner like you treat God. Husbands tell your wife you will see her on Sunday morning for an hour after you have been seeing other women all week. Can you imagine your wife being satisfied with this attention? You may say, "Well, that is ridiculous!" My response is this: it is just as ridiculous as a man who gambles away his life's savings trying to hit it big, drinks like a fish, swears like a trooper, laughs at dirty jokes, shacks up with prostitutes and then comes to church to worship God! In fact, such a man is actually worse than this. He usually feels church is not good enough for him. He feels he can worship God by himself and he doesn't need to go to church to be religious. Rubbish!!

A person who thinks like this—and I am not exaggerating, because there are people like this—is as stupid as a turtle in a horse race. As far as God is concerned, he is not even in the game! The fact is that God has to be given the preeminence or he is being preempted by less important concerns. A Saturday night party that so fatigues a person so that he cannot be in God's house at ten or eleven o'clock on Sunday morning makes partying or boozing more important than God in his life. That is just the way it is, pure and simple! Whatever comes between oneself and one's duty to God is one's God—it is one's idol. God will never bless a life that is lived on such terms! It is not freedom to live like this. It is freedom to have a right relationship with God. When one's life puts God in the center where He belongs, all other things will take their proper perspective. The ways of the world will no longer dominate. Hard times or discouraging circumstances will not bring defeat. When the heart is set upon God, the soul is free of lesser things. This is true liberty: to know that GOD ALONE MATTERS.

It is not enough to say that God matters because it is only giving him a place among a host of other important interests in one's life. Should the creator of your life and the savior of your soul for all eternity have to fight for a little time in your life? God must be lifted up above all other considerations. It must be as the Apostle Paul wrote to the Colossians: "*That in all things He might have the supremacy* (Colossians 3:18)." God alone matters. That means, besides Him, nothing else will do. Nothing else will meet our human need. To know Him is to find that which nothing else can replace. God alone matters. At all costs, one must be right with Him! He holds the keys to my life, my success, my death, my eternal destiny. Nothing else under heaven touches these basics. Therefore, GOD ALONE MATTERS!

Jesus taught that one cannot possibly serve two masters: he cannot please both God and man. A man should, therefore, not be concerned about pleasing man, but God! God alone is our judge, therefore he alone matters. This is what the Apostle Paul was stressing in I Corinthians 4:3-4—"*I care very little if I am judged by you or any human court; indeed I do not even judge myself. My conscience is clear, but that does not make me innocent. It is the Lord that judges me.*" As you can see, Paul was only concerned about answering to God. In being so concerned, Paul enjoyed a wonderful freedom and inner release. Many people live in fear for what others think about them. It is true liberty to know that God alone matters, and if He judges us to be right, we could care less what any man might judge. Criticism cannot harm the individual who believes that GOD ALONE MATTERS.

Think of the vast implications of this concept. We have a reason for living. It is to glorify God. To know that God alone matters narrows our vision and allows us to focus upon a single goal worthy of all our energies. We become determined and purposeful in everything we do. I once had a woman in counseling who was suicidal. What kept her from going through with killing herself, she confided, was her concern for the impact it may have upon her son.

Another woman admitted in counseling that she was suicidal except for one reason—she could not bear the thought of leaving her pet animals to be without her care! People find reasons for carrying on in spite of every impulse to abandon the will to live when some concern transcends their selfish desire to end their life. This is what happens when it is truly believed that GOD ALONE MATTERS.

When a person believes this truth, they are not threatened by losses. Should one lose material possessions, a job or life's savings, it is not enough to sink their ship if they are convinced that GOD ALONE MATTERS. When I served as an Army chaplain with a Field Artillery Battalion that was being deployed to Vietnam in 1968, I can vividly remember what our soldiers were feeling as they separated from their loved ones and prepared to move into fields of battle from which many would never return. Those soldiers who knew that their lives were in God's hands did not worry like those who had no faith in God. They knew that whatever might come, GOD ALONE MATTERS. Even should death come, it would be regarded as gain for I truly believed as did other Christian soldiers that "*We are confident, I say, and would prefer to be away from the body and at home with the Lord* (2 Corinthians 5:8)." It is true liberty to know that GOD ALONE MATTERS!

The matter of setting up priorities in life is solved when God alone matters. This is what Jesus had in mind when he taught, "*But seek first His kingdom and His righteousness, and all these things shall be given to you as well* (Matthew 6:33)." The visit of Jesus to the home of his friend Lazarus is a case in point. Mary was at the feet of Jesus while her sister Martha scurried about tending to chores. Mary knew that chores came with every passing day. She chose, however, to do the more excellent thing—giving devotion and fellowship with Christ. For Mary, GOD ALONE MATTERED.

Then there is the experience of the apostles Paul and Silas as they were incarcerated in a Roman prison. At midnight they were singing joyfully, in spite of their predicament. Although confined in body they were free in spirit because they believed that GOD ALONE MATTERS.

The prophet Daniel was not deterred from his worship of God even though it jeopardized his own life. He would be thrown into a den of lions for holding true to his commitment to God, but that was of no concern to Daniel because he believed GOD ALONE MATTERS!

The most that man can do to a person is put the body to death—he cannot touch the soul. Paul knew this, and so he could say, *"**For me to live is Christ and to die is gain** (Philippians 1:21)."* What does a man who believes like this have to fear? He knows that GOD ALONE MATTERS! Let this inspire you to live up to your true potential as a Christian. Do your level best as unto the Lord in all things you do and take no thought of the possible criticism or abuse you may receive from naysayers and taunters. Know that GOD ALONE MATTERS and you will experience a freedom and a joy and a release from burdens such as you have never dreamed possible!

Failure to come by this attitude will cause you nothing but hardship, frustration, defeat and failure. One can never be truly happy until he is truly free, and true freedom comes when we know that GOD ALONE MATTERS! Circumstances may place one in the cell block of discouragement, but the key which locks one in is one's own rebelling attitude. Bitterness, resentment, frustration, chafing – all of these things are products on one's own attitude. They are the natural fruits of the mind which fails to believe that GOD ALONE MATTERS!

The mission of Christ was to set man free from himself, cleanse him from sin, and bring him into fellowship with God the Father. Christ came to show us that GOD ALONE MATTERS. Listen to the words of Jesus in Luke 4:18:

*"**The Spirit of the Lord is on me because He has anointed me to preach good news to the poor. He has sent me to proclaim freedom for the prisoners and recovery of sight to the blind, to release the oppressed, to proclaim the year of the Lord's favor**."*

True liberty can never come except by Jesus Christ. God anointed Him as His Christ and commissioned Him to *"**Proclaim liberty to the captives and opening of prison to them that are bound**."*

What is your prison? Is it uncontrollable jealousy? Is it a violent temper? Is it incurable indifference? Is it perpetual laziness?

Is your prison family responsibilities and cares? Christ came to open the prison and set you free! It is as Jesus said, **"If the Son shall set you free you shall be free indeed** (John 8:36)." In Romans 8:21 Paul speaks of **"The glorious liberty of the children of God."** To the Corinthians he declared: **"Where the Spirit of the Lord is, there is liberty."** and to the Galatians he urged, **"It is for freedom that Christ has set us free. Stand firm then, and do not let yourselves be burdened again by a yoke of slavery** (Galatians 5:1)."

The Christian knows a release and a freedom from sin, guilt, condemnation and judgment which should be a wellspring of refreshing joy! In Christ there is a release from the old nature and a gift of the new nature. We are now dead to self, but alive to God! He alone counts! He alone matters! That is true liberty, my friends, and there is absolutely nothing in this world that comes close to that feeling!

To feel this is to come alive in the spirit. To breathe this is to draw strength for daily living. To taste this is to find sweetness in living even amidst all of the adversity and pain which life throws in one's path. Nothing matters but God! For the believer in Christ, there is no rat race for popularity, or worry about one's reputation, nor any fretting about material loss or gain. There is freedom from all of this! For this is true liberty, that GOD ALONE MATTERS!

If you have not come to that place in your life where you have made the value choice of what comes first in your priorities, consider these issues. If you would like to have the inner peace of your soul, tranquility and restfulness of your mind, an unmoved dignity and serenity of your spirit no matter what life brings your way, you need to come to the place where you will allow nothing at all —only God—to matter. Believe this one profound truth and act upon it and I am certain you will never be the same again. There is tremendous power in that simple phrase – enough to change lives. This is true liberty, to know that GOD ALONE MATTERS!

ABOUT THE AUTHOR

Roger L. Bradley, formally a Baptist Pastor, Minister of Christian Education, U.S. Army Chaplain, Licensed Marriage and Family Therapist. He holds B.A., M.Div., M.S., and M.A. degrees, Graduate of US Army Chaplain Officer Basic and Advance Courses and the US Army Command and General Staff College. He has had articles published in The Standard Magazine, and The Chaplain Quarterly. Originally from Springfield, MA, Mr. Bradley now resides in Lemoore, CA.

INDEX

A

E

F

S

THE MALE REPRODUCTIVE SYSTEM

The testes are located in the scrotum, which hangs outside the body where the temperature is more suitable for efficient sperm production. The testes are responsible for the production of sperm and the release of the male hormone testosterone. Testosterone controls the development of male secondary sexual characteristics at puberty, such as deepening of the voice, facial hair, changes in the penis and testicles and the production of sperm.

After a boy reaches puberty, his testes create sperm at a rate of approximately 125 million sperm a day. These gather in the testes and then move on to the coiled tubular system known as the epididymis, where they mature. The epididymis drains first into the vas deferens and from there into the ejaculatory ducts. During sexual activity, these ducts contract and push sperm through the urethra during the process of ejaculation.

Sperm are carried in fluid produced by the seminal vesicles and the prostate gland. This fluid, which is known as semen, is rich in nutrients and provides an effective medium within which sperm can stay alive. For about 20 minutes after ejaculation, the sperm hardly move at all, remaining in the gel-like substance. After this, the semen liquefies, and the sperm swim towards their ultimate goal – a female ovum (egg). It is here that fertilization takes place.

Other elements of the male reproductive system are related to the penis and include the urethra, the foreskin and the glans penis. The urethra is the tube through which semen is ejaculated during sexual activity and it is also the tube through which urine passes.

The glans penis is the conical swelling at the tip of the penis. In uncircumcised men, the glans is enclosed by the foreskin, which is attached at the neck of the penis. After about three years of age, the foreskin, or prepuce, usually becomes retractable so that the glans may be exposed; up until this time it sticks to the glans. The inside of the foreskin is covered with sebaceous glands that secrete a substance known as smegma, and this should be removed by regular, careful cleaning of the penis.

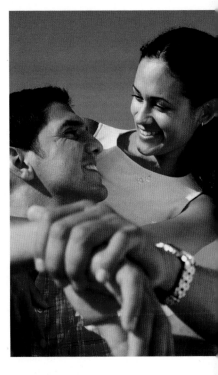

△ It is hormonal changes in the male and female bodies during puberty that prepare them for their ultimate purpose: sexual activity and reproduction.

THE MALE REPRODUCTIVE ORGANS

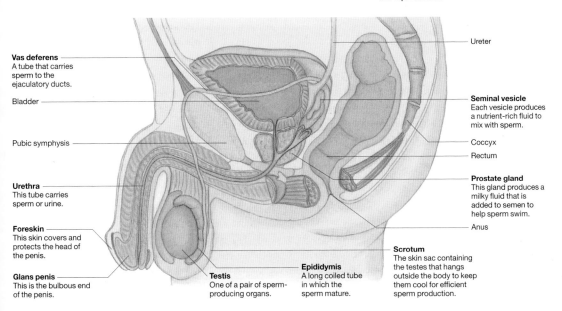

Vas deferens
A tube that carries sperm to the ejaculatory ducts.

Bladder

Pubic symphysis

Urethra
This tube carries sperm or urine.

Foreskin
This skin covers and protects the head of the penis.

Glans penis
This is the bulbous end of the penis.

Testis
One of a pair of sperm-producing organs.

Epididymis
A long coiled tube in which the sperm mature.

Ureter

Seminal vesicle
Each vesicle produces a nutrient-rich fluid to mix with sperm.

Coccyx

Rectum

Prostate gland
This gland produces a milky fluid that is added to semen to help sperm swim.

Anus

Scrotum
The skin sac containing the testes that hangs outside the body to keep them cool for efficient sperm production.

Pregnancy and health

Pregnancy is a time of great excitement and joy for parents-to-be, but the major physical changes experienced by the mother can cause some discomfort and may be stressful. Close contact with your healthcare team is the best way to protect both your own and your baby's well-being. The team will also be able to answer any questions that you have and reassure you that your pregnancy is progressing normally. Although most women feel anxious at some stage, it is important to remember that the vast majority of pregnancies end with a healthy baby.

Once you suspect that you might be pregnant, you should visit your doctor. (Over-the-counter pregnancy testing kits are fairly accurate and will test positive around the time of the first missed period or soon after.) By medical convention, pregnancies are dated from the first day of the last period. Most routine antenatal care will be undertaken by a midwife, who will usually be based at your doctor's surgery.

Your doctor will refer you to a specialist obstetric unit based at a hospital but you will probably only see the consultant once in early pregnancy and a short time before delivery. You will also visit the hospital for ultrasound scans.

Your first antenatal visit will usually involve taking a medical history, followed by an examination. You will have to give a sample of blood and urine for a series of

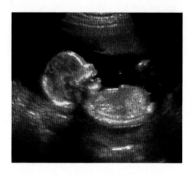

△ An ultrasound scan is vital for checking on the baby's position and development, and is usually carried out at 12 weeks and 20 weeks.

routine tests. At this stage, all tests are designed to pick up any significant risk factors that may complicate the pregnancy as it progresses.

PREGNANCY HEALTH CHECKS

Most women are seen at regular intervals throughout pregnancy. From 20 to 32 weeks, women are checked every 4 weeks. They are then reviewed every 2 weeks until 36 weeks, and at weekly intervals thereafter. At each visit, there is an opportunity for your healthcare team to:
• Carry out routine health checks and answer any questions you have.
• Check the baby's growth and position.
• Listen to the baby's heart.

EATING WELL IN PREGNANCY

A healthy, balanced diet is extremely important during pregnancy in order to maintain your health and nurture your baby. It is usually only in the last couple of

months, when your baby is growing rapidly, that you may need to eat more.

The following foods should be avoided:
• Raw or undercooked eggs.
• Mussels and other shellfish.
• Liver pâté.
• Unpasteurized cheeses, such as brie.

Doctors advise all women trying to conceive, and pregnant women during their first 12 weeks, to take folic acid to prevent spina bifida.

EXERCISE AND PREGNANCY

If you exercised before you were pregnant it is a good idea to continue. If you remain fit, you may experience less backache and your pushes during labour are likely to be stronger. You should avoid situations with a risk of falls – such as horse-riding – and should not push yourself too hard.

As your pregnancy progresses, your increasing weight, size and tiredness will limit the type and amount of exercise you can do. Swimming and yoga may be more appealing than other forms of exercise.

SMOKING AND ALCOHOL

Smoking harms your baby. Smokers should stop while pregnant as they could affect fetal growth, predispose their baby to asthma and increase their baby's chances of cardiovascular disease in later life. If you have trouble stopping, ask your doctor for help. Avoid alcohol for the first 12 weeks (it may be unpleasant to take at this time in any case). After this, try to stick to the occasional tipple only.

▽ There is an increased risk of high blood pressure during pregnancy, so regular health checks are essential to ensure that any changes are picked up as soon as possible.

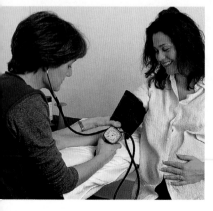

THE MAIN STAGES OF PREGNANCY

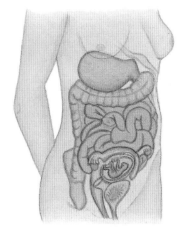

△ **At 12 weeks**
Although still tiny, the fetus is baby-shaped, with fingers, toes, genitalia and facial features.

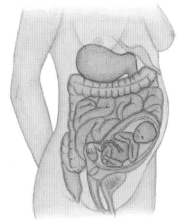

△ **At 18 weeks**
The fetal organs begin to function and bones start to harden at this stage.

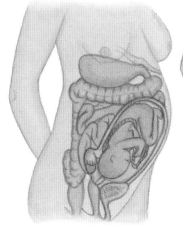

△ **At 24 weeks**
The growth of the fetus begins to place pressure on internal organs.

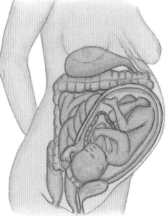

△ **At 36 weeks**
The head sinks down into the pelvis ready for the birth; this is known as "lightening".

AFTER THE BIRTH

It is vital that you continue to look after your health after the birth. Make sure that you eat well and rest as much as possible.

Many women will experience some depression after childbirth, which may be due to the the sudden decline in levels of oestrogen and progesterone once the baby is born. In about 10 per cent of women, this is severe and lasts for months (postnatal depression). Symptoms include persistent low mood, difficulty in relating to the baby, feelings of inadequacy and anxiety and, in some cases, panic attacks. Your healthcare team can provide useful advice, and treatment may not be necessary. However, your doctor may prescribe antidepressants, which help many women.

PREGNANCY PROBLEMS

Fertility problems are very common – as many as one in five women under the age of 35 will fail to become pregnant if they have regular unprotected sex for a year. Infertility may be due to problems such as a failure to ovulate or poor sperm count – or a combination of both.

If you have difficulty conceiving, seek help from your doctor, who can refer you to a clinic for tests. These may include a detailed sperm analysis for the man, or ultrasound and X-ray examinations to check the woman's reproductive organs. Postcoital tests are sometimes carried out, to check if the woman's body is rejecting her partner's sperm.

Treatment will depend on the cause but may include hormonal drugs or microsurgery to clear a blockage. If initial treatment fails, artificial insemination or other conception therapies may be attempted. The success rate for these procedures is low and the couple will be given counselling to help them come to terms with the possibility of failure.

Many women have no difficulty in conceiving but do not carry the baby to term. One in four pregnancies ends in miscarriage – usually in the first three months. Often this is because of an abnormality in the fetus, but infections such as salmonella or a lack of certain hormones are also common causes. Most women who have a miscarriage carry their next baby to full term.

Ectopic pregnancies affect up to one in a hundred women. In this condition the fertilized egg becomes embedded in a Fallopian tube, where it cannot develop normally. As the embryo grows, it may cause the tube to rupture, leading to internal bleeding. Because of this, surgery must be carried out to remove the embryo once an ectopic pregnancy has been diagnosed.

Irregular menstrual periods

SEE ALSO

➤ Diseases of the thyroid gland, p316
➤ Endometriosis, p403
➤ Ovarian cysts, p404
➤ Polycystic ovary syndrome, p404

The average menstrual cycle lasts for 28 days, and a period can last anything between two and seven days. There are, however, considerable variations between individuals: periods may occur as frequently as every 21 days and as infrequently as 35 days. Irregular menstrual periods are not necessarily cause for alarm and can arise for many reasons. However, it is a good idea to seek advice if your menstrual cycle suddenly changes because it may be a symptom of an underlying problem such as stress, or of other more serious conditions.

Menstrual irregularity occurs most frequently just after puberty and in the years leading up to the menopause, due to hormonal fluctuations at these times.

Where an irregular pattern is the result of stress, anxiety or a recent illness, the problem usually corrects itself. Similarly, any irregularities that occur during teenage years also tend to diminish gradually.

If you have a persistently irregular bleeding pattern with no easily identifiable cause, your doctor may investigate. Blood tests and pelvic ultrasound scans are commonly used testing procedures.

For persistent irregularities in younger women, the contraceptive pill may be used to regulate the cycle. Older women nearing the menopause may be offered hormone replacement therapy (HRT).

POSSIBLE CAUSES

Menstrual irregularity may be a symptom of another condition, such as:

➤ Ovarian cysts and polycystic ovary syndrome.

➤ Endometriosis.

➤ Disorders of the thyroid gland.

➤ Unsuspected pregnancy.

➤ Cancer.

Or it may be caused by factors such as:

➤ Stress and anxiety.

➤ Periods of depression or of general physical ill health.

➤ Fluctuating weight.

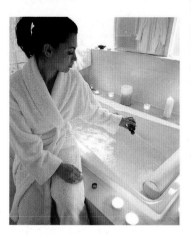

△ Taking time to relax in a warm, soothing environment can help to tackle feelings of stress and anxiety, which may be the underlying cause of menstrual irregularity.

Painful periods (dysmenorrhoea)

SEE ALSO

➤ Endometriosis, p403

Painful periods are extremely common and affect most women at some stage of their lives, to varying degrees. Many women can be quite incapacitated by this problem. Pain is usually most apparent on the day before a period starts and during the first 48 hours of a period.

Painful periods are most common during adolescence and when a woman is in her 20s; the problem often subsides later in life. If you normally have little pain with your periods and suddenly start experiencing unusual levels of discomfort, seek medical advice. Your doctor may want to rule out any gynaecological problems and carry out further investigations.

TREATMENT OPTIONS

Anti-inflammatory drugs are often effective, ideally taken before severe pain takes hold. The combined contraceptive pill can also be taken. This eases painful periods by suppressing ovulation.

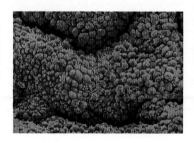

▷ This coloured scan shows the thickening in the endometrium, the lining of the uterus, that occurs during the second half of the menstrual cycle.

Premenstrual syndrome (PMS)

SEE ALSO
➤ Depression, p346
➤ Irregular menstrual periods, p398
➤ Painful periods (dysmenorrhoea), p398

Premenstrual syndrome is a very common problem that affects up to a third of all menstruating women at some point in their lives, and is particularly prevalent in women over 30. Although some people question the existence of PMS, many doctors now believe it is due to an imbalance of sex hormones in the body just before menstruation. The results can be debilitating, even though the problem usually lasts for only one or two days just before or at the beginning of the period. Symptoms range from headaches to severe anger or depression.

SIGNS AND SYMPTOMS

Classic symptoms of PMS are:

➤ Irritability, depression and mood changes.

➤ Tiredness and headache.

➤ Fluid retention and abdominal bloating.

➤ Breast tenderness.

➤ Backache and muscular pains.

If you find that fluid retention is a particularly troublesome symptom then your doctor may prescribe a diuretic to be taken as needed. You might be able to relieve muscular aches and headaches using simple painkillers and anti-inflammatory drugs. Mood changes and depression may respond to antidepressants, which are taken during the second half of the menstrual cycle or on a regular basis. A variety of progesterone preparations have also been tried with varying degrees of success.

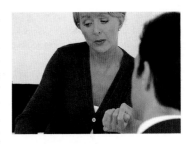

△ Your doctor may prescribe antidepressants to alleviate depression and control the mood swings that can occur in premenstrual syndrome.

Menopausal complaints

SEE ALSO
➤ Osteoporosis, p356

The menopause is the time in a woman's life, typically between 45 and 55, when her periods gradually stop. Hormone replacement therapy can help treat the symptoms associated with the menopause, although it should be discussed carefully with your doctor.

SIGNS AND SYMPTOMS

Many women have only mild symptoms attributable to the menopause. Some, however, experience a range of problems, including:

➤ Hot flushes and excessive sweating.

➤ Mood changes that may include anxiety and depression.

➤ Tiredness and loss of libido.

➤ Vaginal dryness.

➤ An increased susceptibility to urinary tract infection.

Almost all menopause-related symptoms can be treated with hormone replacement therapy (HRT). Here, small amounts of oestrogen and progesterone are given – just enough to minimize the natural oestrogen withdrawal of the menopause. HRT is usually taken for a few years in pill or skin patch form, but may also be given as under-the-skin implants. Women on HRT are periodically assessed for weight, blood pressure and general state of health.

THE LONG-TERM OUTLOOK

There are some advantages in taking HRT on a long-term basis, principally that oestrogen tends to protect bones from osteoporosis. There may also be a small reduction of heart disease among women on HRT. There are also certain health risks associated with HRT, including a slight increase in the risk of breast cancer in women who have taken HRT for more than seven years.

POSTMENOPAUSAL RISKS

Oestrogen protects against heart disease so after the menopause, the risk of cardiovascular problems rises. The decline in oestrogen levels also means you may be more prone to osteoporosis.

Breast pain and lumpiness

SEE ALSO

➤ Pregnancy and
   health, p396
➤ Premenstrual
   syndrome, p399
➤ Menopausal
   complaints, p399

Many women notice a generalized lumpiness and pain that occurs in their breasts at particular stages of their menstrual cycle. This is most apparent in the days immediately before a period, and during puberty and pregnancy. Breast tissue changes as it is affected by female sex hormone fluctuations that occur throughout menstrual life. There are several methods that can help reduce breast pain, but you should always seek advice from your doctor if symptoms persist or you are concerned about any unusual lumps or pain.

Lumps in the breast may often be accompanied by cyclical occurrences of breast pain. Postmenopausal woman often experience this less, although it may be more persistent in women on hormone replacement therapy.

Some simple self-help measures may be helpful for painful and lumpy breasts:
• Taking daily oil of evening primrose.
• Relaxation exercises.

WHAT MIGHT YOUR DOCTOR DO?

Lumpy breasts that are not painful do not usually require any specific treatment. However, your doctor may refer you to a breast specialist for further investigation if:

• Lumpiness is persistent and not affected by your menstrual cycle.
• There is a specific area of lumpy tissue.
• A definite lump can be felt, which may turn out to be either a fibroadenoma or a cancerous tumour.

THE STRUCTURE OF THE BREAST

▷ The breasts are made of fatty tissue, milk-producing lobules and a system of ducts designed to carry milk to the nipple. Breast tissue is subject to constant hormonal stimulation, allowing it to prepare for pregnancy and lactation (milk production) whenever the need arises. As a result, the tissues of the breast are undergoing continual change.

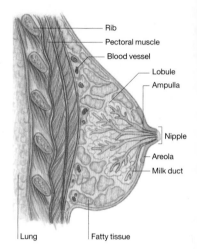

- Rib
- Pectoral muscle
- Blood vessel
- Lobule
- Ampulla
- Nipple
- Areola
- Milk duct
- Lung
- Fatty tissue

Fibroadenoma

SEE ALSO

➤ Breast cysts, p401

This non-cancerous (benign) breast lump tends to develop in women aged between 20 and 30. Doctors believe that fibroadenomas may arise because of the effects of oestrogen on breast tissue. They may develop at a number of different sites within the breast.

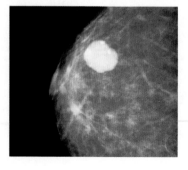

Fibroadenomas are the most common reason for lumps in the breast. They grow very slowly, sometimes over a number of years, and are generally harmless. However, they can be difficult to distinguish from cancerous lumps so you should always seek

◁ Mammographs are X-rays that clearly reveal the soft tissue of the breast. A fibroadenoma (seen here as a white mass) is a small tumour of fibrous tissue; although usually benign, these can become malignant if left untreated.

medical advice if you find an unusual lump. Your doctor will refer you to a breast unit where specialist staff will scan the breast, using ultrasound, and perform a biopsy – taking a sample of tissue from the lump that can be tested to confirm the diagnosis.

Small fibroadenomas can be safely left untreated. They often diminish in size and may disappear completely in time. If the lump is large or growing, it may be appropriate to remove it surgically.

Breast cysts

SEE ALSO
➤ Fibroadenoma, p400
➤ Breast cancer, below
➤ Ovarian cysts, p404

Breast cysts are small, fluid-filled lumps that can develop in the breasts, most commonly in women between the ages of 30 and 50. These lumps are simply lobules that have filled with fluid and they are generally harmless. Occasionally, however, a cyst may contain cancerous cells, so your doctor should investigate any breast cyst to make absolutely sure that it is not malignant. Half of the women affected by cysts find that they have more than one, or that they affect both breasts; recurrence of breast cysts is also not uncommon.

Although breast cysts are usually harmless, as with any lump in the breast it should be checked out to rule out the possibility of breast cancer. Your doctor will normally refer you to a breast unit for specialized scanning and to get the cyst drained (aspiration). A sample of the fluid from the cyst is sent for laboratory analysis to check for signs of cancer.

Aspiration may be the only treatment that is required. Women who suffer from recurrent cysts may need to have them removed surgically.

BREAST ASPIRATION

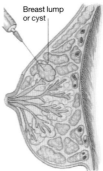

Breast lump or cyst

▷ A breast cyst can be treated by aspiration, where a doctor uses a needle syringe to draw fluid from the lump.

SCREENING AND SCANNING
Although breast cysts are usually harmless, in rare cases they may contain cancerous cells. Specialized scanning can identify the nature of the lump and catch the disease at an earlier, more treatable, stage. Many countries now have screening programmes for older women, between the ages of 50 and 65, who are more susceptible to breast cancer and HRT is thought to be a causative factor.

Breast cancer

SEE ALSO
➤ Lymphomas, p458

Breast cancer is the most common female cancer. Most often seen in women over 50, it also occurs in younger women. Particular factors put women at higher risk of breast cancer and these include aging, a family history of the condition, obesity and being on HRT.

SIGNS AND SYMPTOMS
Breast cancer may not produce any symptoms in the early stages but when signs do appear they include:

➤ A painless lump in the breast.

➤ Blood-stained discharge from the nipple.

➤ "Orange-peel" dimpling of the skin around the lump.

➤ Inversion of the nipple.

If your doctor suspects breast cancer you may be referred to a specialist breast unit. Your breast will be scanned and a sample of the lump will be taken and its fluid drained; cells will be sent for analysis. Only about one in twenty breast lumps turns out to be cancerous. If cancer is confirmed, you may have other scans to determine whether it has spread to other parts of the body.

TREATMENT OPTIONS
Breast cancer is treated with varying combinations of surgery, radiotherapy, chemotherapy and hormone treatment.

• Small tumours are surgically removed (lumpectomy) while large tumours usually involve removing a greater amount of breast tissue. Sometimes the whole breast is removed (mastectomy). Some lymph nodes are removed from the area to check if the cancer has spread.

• Radiotherapy is now used routinely for six weeks after the removal of all lumps.

• Where the cancer has already spread to other organs, chemotherapy is used in conjunction with other treatment.

• Oestrogen-blocking drugs shrink some tumours or impede their growth.

Fibroids

SEE ALSO

➤ Pregnancy and health, p396
➤ Painful periods (dysmenorrhoea), p398
➤ Fibroadenoma, p400

Fibroids are non-cancerous growths that develop within the walls of the uterus (womb). They are very common and may be found in up to a third of all women during their childbearing years. Fibroids occur most frequently in women between the ages of 35 and 55. It is believed that they arise from stimulation of uterine tissue by the female sex hormones, resulting in some pain and unusually heavy menstrual periods. Although these tumours are non-cancerous, they can cause infertility. Treatments vary according to the size and severity of the fibroids.

SIGNS AND SYMPTOMS

A bigger fibroid tends to produce a range of symptoms, including:

➤ Prolonged and heavy menstrual bleeding.

➤ Severe pain during menstruation.

➤ Infertility.

➤ An increased risk of miscarriage.

Fibroids are non-malignant tumours, formed from muscular tissue, which develop in the uterine wall. Fibroids vary in both size and the symptoms that they produce. Some fibroids are very small and produce no symptoms whatsoever, while others grow to the size of a grapefruit. Sometimes fibroids occur in multiples.

They can cause heavy periods and some pain. If they grow to a substantial size, they may even cause infertility or miscarriage.

DIAGNOSING FIBROIDS

Fibroids can sometimes be diagnosed during a pelvic examination. Once your doctor suspects fibroids you may be referred for a pelvic ultrasound scan, which will confirm the diagnosis.

TREATMENT OPTIONS

Smaller fibroids that display no symptoms can safely be left untreated. For larger growths that are causing problems, drugs may be used to try to reduce them in size, but if this is not successful they may need to be removed. This can be done in a number of ways:

• Hysteroscopy – Small fibroids growing on the inner uterine wall may be removed

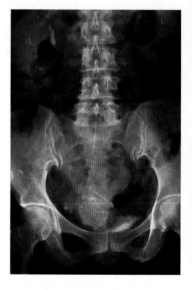

△ On this X-ray of a uterus, a fibroid shows up as an orange lump in the centre of the image. Fibroids are benign tumours formed from fibrous and muscular tissue.

during this procedure, in which a small telescopic instrument is passed into the uterus so that your doctor can see inside your abdomen to locate and then remove the fibroids.

• Abdominal surgery – Larger fibroids can be removed using an abdominal incision in order to gain access to the uterus.

• Hysterectomy – If fibroids are causing a number of serious problems and their size and location means they are difficult to remove, a hysterectomy may be considered. However, this procedure is only used in cases where the fibroids are causing severe pain or discomfort.

WHERE FIBROIDS ARE FOUND

▷ Fibroids are formed from muscular tissue that builds up in the wall of the uterus. There may be just one, which is relatively unusual, or several may develop at the same time.

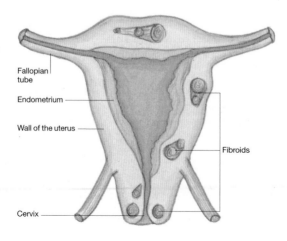

Fallopian tube

Endometrium

Wall of the uterus

Fibroids

Cervix

Endometriosis

SEE ALSO
▶ UTIs, p390
▶ Irregular menstrual periods, p398
▶ Ovarian cysts, p404
▶ Female genital infections, p407

The endometrium is the lining of the uterus. This lining is shed once a month during menstruation, and then regrows. The condition known as endometriosis occurs when endometrial tissue starts to develop in other organs within the pelvis (such as the ovaries or Fallopian tubes), usually because it has been affected by hormones released during the menstrual cycle. Endometriosis may also develop outside the pelvis – the intestines are sometimes affected and the condition can reach as far as the abdominal cavity or even the lungs.

SIGNS AND SYMPTOMS
Typical symptoms of pelvic endometriosis include the following:

➤ Painful, heavy and irregular periods.

➤ Deep pain during sexual intercourse.

➤ Urinary discomfort.

➤ Infertility.

Doctors do not know what causes this condition but it is common in women who have their first child over the age of 30 and in those who remain childless.

When endometriosis develops outside the pelvis, the symptoms depend on which organs are affected. Intestinal endometriosis, for example, tends to cause a change in bowel habit, abdominal pain and sometimes rectal bleeding.

TREATING ENDOMETRIOSIS
Hormone therapy may be used to suppress the menstrual cycle in order to reduce production of the oestrogen on which endometrial tissue depends. Such treatment may be used for up to one year, after which the condition may subside.

Doctors can destroy small areas of endometriosis during a laparoscopy – a minimally invasive procedure where rigid viewing devices are inserted through the abdomen to illuminate, examine and treat organs. If the patient is an older women, or the condition is extremely severe, a total hysterectomy may be considered.

Endometriosis sometimes resolves with pregnancy but may recur afterwards.

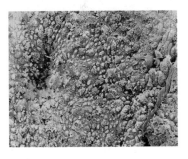

▽ This shows the surface of an endometriotic cyst. It has formed where fragments of uterine lining have attached to an ovary.

Uterine cancer

SEE ALSO
▶ Ovarian cancer, p405

Cancer of the uterus is most common in women between the ages of 55 and 65. It occurs more frequently in women that have had no children and in those who have had a late menopause. The specific cause of the cancer is not known, but early diagnosis and treatment is essential.

SIGNS AND SYMPTOMS
Common symptoms include:

➤ Heavy menstrual bleeding.

➤ Bleeding after sexual intercourse.

➤ Vaginal "spotting" after the menopause.

Uterine cancer usually causes unusual patterns of vaginal bleeding. If your doctor suspects cancer from your symptoms you may be urgently referred to a gynaecologist, who will take tissue samples from your uterus. This can be done easily using a procedure known as a hysteroscopy. If a cancer is diagnosed, a range of other tests are carried out to determine whether or not the cancer has spread to any other organs.

HOW IS IT TREATED?
This cancer is usually treated by removing all the pelvic organs by means of a total hysterectomy. Cancer that has spread beyond the uterus is usually treated with chemotherapy and hormonal treatment.

After treatment, the outlook is good if the tumour has been diagnosed at an early stage, with at least 80 per cent of women surviving for five years or longer.

Ovarian cysts

SEE ALSO

➤ Irregular menstrual periods, p398

➤ Fibroids, p402

➤ Endometriosis, p403

➤ Female genital infections, p407

Ovarian cysts – fluid-filled sacs that develop within the ovary – are very common during a woman's reproductive years. These cysts may be very small or grow to considerable size and there may be just one or several (the latter is called polycystic ovary syndrome). Ovarian cysts are usually non-cancerous but some have cancerous potential. For this reason your doctor will normally refer you to a specialist for further investigation. It can be difficult to diagnose ovarian cysts as they do not necessarily present symptoms, and the symptoms can come and go.

SIGNS AND SYMPTOMS

Most cysts do not cause symptoms, and many will develop and disappear spontaneously without a woman being aware of their existence. Larger, persistent cysts may produce symptoms, and these include:

➤ Abdominal pain, which may be felt on the same side as the affected ovary.

➤ Abdominal distension or bloating.

➤ Deep pain during sexual intercourse.

➤ Menstrual irregularities.

The presence of a cyst might be obvious from your symptoms, and your doctor may be able to feel the cyst during a pelvic examination. For confirmation, your doctor may refer you for an ultrasound examination. A blood test may also be done to check for the presence of tumour markers, which are proteins produced by tumours that can be measured in the blood. Where a cyst is large, persistent or problematic, a gynaecologist will assess the situation by monitoring the cyst for a while.

This is to determine whether it is growing or starting to regress naturally. Large cysts require draining or removal. A cyst is removed surgically if there are cancerous changes within it, but as much of the ovary is conserved as possible.

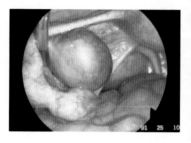

▷ This inside view of a woman's abdomen has been taken with a device called a laparoscope. The round, fluid-filled swelling seen left of centre is an ovarian cyst.

Polycystic ovary syndrome

SEE ALSO

➤ Diabetes, p314

This common syndrome, caused by a relative excess of luteinizing hormone and testosterone, is characterized by multiple fluid-filled ovarian cysts. Women with this condition are at greater risk of developing diabetes and high blood pressure, and of suffering ovulatory failure.

SIGNS AND SYMPTOMS

➤ Irregular, scanty or absent periods.

➤ Excess body hair.

➤ Ovulatory failure.

This condition may result in infertility, so a correct diagnosis and prompt treatment is very important. If your doctor suspects this condition from your symptoms, you may be referred for a pelvic ultrasound to identify the multiple ovarian cysts that form part of this syndrome. Blood tests carried out to measure levels of luteinizing hormone and testosterone may reveal a hormonal imbalance.

Treatment depends on the severity of the condition and whether you want to have children. Fertility drugs may be given to stimulate ovulation, and irregular menstrual patterns may be controlled by prescribing the combined contraceptive pill.

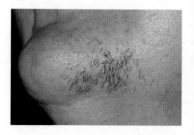

△ Excessive body hair (this shows a woman's chin) may indicate polycystic ovary syndrome, caused by an excess of particular hormones.

Ovarian cancer

SEE ALSO
➤ Uterine cancer,
  p403
➤ Ovarian cysts,
  p404
➤ Cancer of the cervix,
  p406

Cancer of the ovary causes many thousands of deaths worldwide each year. This cancer is often difficult to diagnose because many patients show no symptoms until a relatively late stage of the disease. By the time any symptoms become apparent, the tumour may have already spread beyond the ovary. For this reason it is essential to seek advice if you are demonstrating any of the symptoms listed below, especially if you fall into any of the high-risk groups for this disease. At present, there is no effective way of screening for this form of cancer.

SIGNS AND SYMPTOMS

The possible symptoms of ovarian cancer include:

➤ Abdominal pain and distension.

➤ Frequent urination.

➤ Abnormal menstrual patterns.

➤ General malaise and weight loss.

Certain groups of women have been identified as more likely to develop ovarian cancer. These at-risk groups include:
• Childless women.
• Women who have a late menopause.
• Women who have family members affected by the disease.

SURGICAL TREATMENT

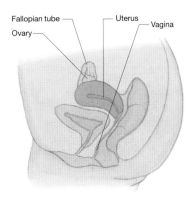

Fallopian tube — Uterus
Ovary — Vagina

△ If the cancerous tumour has spread beyond the ovary a hysterectomy may be necessary. This surgery involves the removal of the uterus, Fallopian tubes and ovaries, the top part of the vagina and the lymph nodes.

Ovarian cancer can affect women of any age, although there are more cases diagnosed between the ages of 50 and 60 than any other age-group. Also, women who have taken oral contraceptives appear to be less likely to develop the disease.

HOW IS IT DIAGNOSED?

If there is any question about the possibility of cancer, you will be urgently referred to a gynaecologist for further investigation. Tests include a pelvic ultrasound scan, blood tests to look for tumour markers and keyhole surgery (diagnostic laparoscopy) to inspect the ovary and take a sample of tissue for analysis. If cancer is confirmed, you may need to undergo a series of other scans to determine whether or not the cancer has spread to other internal organs, such as the liver or lungs.

TREATMENT OPTIONS

If the cancer is limited to one ovary and the woman still wants to have children, every effort will be made to avoid performing a full hysterectomy. In these cases, surgery will be limited to the removal of the affected ovary and Fallopian tube.

Where the tumour has spread from the ovary to other parts of the pelvis, or in cases where child-bearing is not an issue, a total hysterectomy is recommended as the safest method of removing all cancerous material from the area. During the hysterectomy operation, the uterus, both ovaries and both Fallopian tubes will be removed, along with some other tissue. In most cases, this surgical treatment is followed by a course of chemotherapy and possibly radiotherapy.

The best prognosis for ovarian cancer occurs when the cancer has been diagnosed in its earliest stages, preferably when it is confined to just one ovary. However, the greatest difficulty in diagnosing this cancer lies in the fact that it can be "silent" (not show any symptoms) until the more advanced stages of the disease, and may then continue to present no symptoms until the tumour has already spread to other parts of the pelvis. Currently, three-quarters of women are diagnosed with ovarian cancer after the disease has already spread to other parts of the body.

There is currently considerable research being undertaken to develop an effective screening test for this disease, although no widespread programmes are in use at the present time. Until screening is available, any symptoms should be taken seriously and investigated without delay.

▽ A viewing device called a laparoscope may be used to diagnose ovarian cancer. During this procedure, several small incisions are made in the abdomen to insert a fibre-optic video camera, along with tools that are used to carry out an examination of the ovaries.

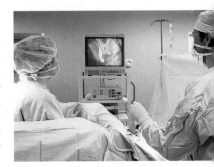

Cervical dysplasia

SEE ALSO

➤ Smoking and your health, p268

➤ Cancer of the cervix, below

➤ Sexually transmitted infections, p411

The cells of the cervix may change from normal to cancerous over a period of many years. Between the extremes of normal and cancerous cells are a range of cellular abnormalities commonly referred to as cervical dysplasia. Doctors can detect cervical dysplasia by taking a cervical smear, which all women should have at least every three years. During an internal examination, cells from the cervix are collected using a spatula or brush. These cells can then be examined microscopically for any evidence of significant cellular change.

The exact cause of this condition is not known but it is associated with the sexually transmitted papilloma virus. Therefore, one risk factor is unprotected sex, and a greater number of sexual partners increases the risk of coming into contact with this virus. People who smoke are more likely to develop cervical dysplasia and cancer, as are people who take immunosuppressant drugs.

TREATMENT OPTIONS

Mild cervical dysplasia requires no specific treatment but you will usually be asked to go for a repeat smear six months after the initial diagnosis. If mild dysplasia persists, or if there is moderate or severe dysplasia, preventative treatment identifies and removes the abnormal cervical cells. During a painless procedure called a colposcopy, a magnifying instrument is used to examine your cervix closely and so identify any abnormalities. Areas of dysplasia (abnormal tissue) can be removed with laser treatment.

After a colposcopy, smears are taken at intervals to ensure that there are no further signs of dysplasia. As the cervical tissue returns to normal, the intervals between smears are lengthened.

TYPES OF CERVICAL DYSPLASIA

There are three grades of dysplasia – mild, moderate and severe. Mild dysplasia may disappear without treatment, whereas moderate and severe types may develop slowly, sometimes over several years, in to cancer if not treated. The chance of a good outcome is improved if abnormalities are caught early and any cancer is treated before it starts spreading through the pelvis.

Cancer of the cervix

SEE ALSO

➤ Uterine cancer, p403

Cervical cancer is a common female cancer. Fortunately, it is one of the few cancers that can be prevented by regular screening. Most developed countries have national screening programmes that detect precancerous changes in the cervix years before cancer develops.

Once cancerous cells have been detected in the cervix, further tests will be carried out to discover how far the tumour has spread. If the tumour is confined to the cervix, doctors may be able to remove the affected area without harming a woman's ability to conceive and bear children.

Where child-bearing is not an issue, a hysterectomy may be considered to remove the cervix and uterus, but the ovaries will usually be conserved. If the cancer has already spread to the uterus, a total hysterectomy will be necessary. If the cancer has spread to other parts of the body, chemotherapy and/or radiotherapy is used to try to contain the disease.

SIGNS AND SYMPTOMS

Cervical cancer may cause few symptoms initially. Symptoms that may develop include:

➤ Vaginal bleeding.

➤ Deep pain during sexual intercourse.

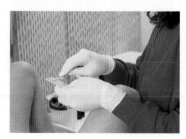

▷ Regular screening by cervical smear tests is widely available in developed countries. This test involves cells being scraped from the cervix (the neck of the womb). The cells are then checked for abnormalities so that cancer can be detected in the very early stages.

Female genital infections

SEE ALSO
➤ Diabetes, p314
➤ The urinary organs, p386
➤ UTIs, p390
➤ Sexually transmitted infections, p411

Most women will experience inflammation and itching in the vaginal area at some point in their lives. This may simply be a reaction to using perfumed soaps or bath products. However, this condition also commonly arises from infection by the *Candida albicans* fungus (thrush), or by sexually transmitted micro-organisms such as *Trichomoniasis vaginalis* (trichomoniasis). Most genital infections clear up quickly when treated, but some may spread up into the pelvis, causing pelvic inflammatory disease. This is a major cause of infertility among women.

SIGNS AND SYMPTOMS OF VAGINAL INFECTION

See your doctor if you experience any of the following symptoms:

➤ Itchiness, irritation or soreness in or around the vagina.

➤ An abnormal vaginal discharge, which may or may not have a strong odour.

➤ A burning sensation experienced on passing urine.

➤ Discomfort during sexual intercourse.

Many women feel embarrassed about visiting their doctor with vaginal irritation (known medically as vaginitis). However, vaginitis has many different causes, including serious infection, so it is essential that you have the condition investigated.

If your doctor suspects that you have an infection, vaginal swabs of any discharge may be taken and sent for testing. In most cases, the problem clears up once the infecting micro-organism is identified and the correct treatment given. You should usually abstain from sexual intercourse until the inflammation and irritation has gone. In many cases, your sexual partner should also be treated.

THRUSH

Thrush causes severe itching and a thick white discharge. Many women suffer repeated bouts of thrush, and the infection often seems to be related to general stress and fatigue. Pregnant women, those suffering from diabetes and people on a course of antibiotics or immunosuppressive drugs are particularly prone to thrush.

Antifungal pessaries and creams normally relieve symptoms and clear up the infection. Single doses of oral antifungal drugs are also available, and are safe and effective to use.

If you suffer from recurrent thrush, your doctor may suggest further tests to ensure that the diagnosis is correct. You may find it helpful to lower your intake of dietary sugars and eat *acidophilus* bacteria in the form of live natural yoghurt or acidophilus tablets. Male partners should also be treated as they may carry fungal infection and re-infect you after treatment.

BACTERIAL VAGINOSIS

Bacterial vaginosis causes an off-white vaginal discharge with a fishy odour. It occurs when normally harmless bacteria living in the vagina start to multiply excessively. The usual causes are *Gardnerella vaginalis* or *Mycoplasma hominis*. The condition can be effectively treated with a course of antibiotics.

TRICHOMONIASIS

Trichomoniasis is a sexually transmitted infection, causing severe itching, pain on passing urine and an unpleasant-smelling yellow discharge. The condition clears up quickly if the correct antibiotics are taken.

Men can carry the disease without having symptoms, but they may develop non-specific urethritis (inflammation of the urethra). If a woman has trichomoniasis, her sexual partner should be treated, too.

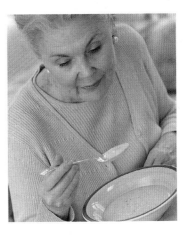

△ A simple self-help option for thrush is eating live natural yoghurt which contains helpful *acidophilus* bacteria.

PELVIC INFLAMMATORY DISEASE (PID)

PID is the largest single cause of female infertility. It starts as an infection in the vagina – usually chlamydia or gonorrhoea, which are sexually transmitted. The infection spreads up from the vagina to infect the Fallopian tubes and other pelvic organs.

Pelvic pain, pain during sex and fever can all be signs of PID, but it often causes no symptoms, with the result that many women are unaware that they have the condition. If PID is treated promptly with antibiotics, most women recover completely. However, if it is untreated, the Fallopian tubes may become damaged, which will affect fertility.

Enlarged prostate gland

Prostate gland enlargement occurs naturally with age and becomes more apparent from the age of 50 onwards, but it can also arise as a result of bacterial infection. Doctors refer to the condition as prostatism (benign prostatic hypertrophy). Whether or not symptoms occur depends on the degree of enlargement. As the gland enlarges, it squeezes the urethra and starts to prevent adequate emptying of the bladder, and so one of the key symptoms is a frequent desire to urinate. Avoiding consumption of certain fluids can help control the symptoms.

SIGNS AND SYMPTOMS

Typical symptoms are:

➤ A frequent need to urinate.

➤ A sensation that the bladder is not completely empty after urination.

➤ Dribbling after urine has been passed.

➤ A need to get up at night to pass urine.

➤ A poor stream of urine.

If untreated, urine can collect in the bladder and cause urinary tract infection.

Inflammation of the prostate gland is commonly caused by bacterial infection. It causes pain when passing urine, the need to urinate frequently (causing disruption to sleep patterns because of the need to get up during the night), pain on ejaculation, blood in semen, pain at the base of the penis and in the testes, fever and general malaise. Sometimes the prostate gland may become inflamed (prostatitis) during episodes of infection and is prone to cancerous change in middle-aged and older men. The symptoms of prostate cancer are similar to those experienced by someone suffering from an enlarged prostate gland but there may be some back or hip pain as well.

Your doctor will base diagnosis on your medical history and an examination. The prostate can be felt and its size assessed by a finger inserted into the rectum. An ultrasound can be done to assess to what degree bladder emptying has been impaired.

THE POSITION OF THE PROSTATE GLAND

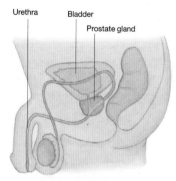

Urethra

Bladder

Prostate gland

△ The prostate gland is a chestnut-sized organ located at the base of a man's bladder. It is wrapped around the urethra as it exits the bladder. The prostate gland produces secretions that are added to semen during the process of ejaculation.

DRUG TREATMENT

When your condition starts to affect your quality of life, it can be treated. It may be possible to control the condition using drugs – alpha-blockers (which make it easier to pass urine), antiandrogens (which shrink the prostate over time) and oral antibiotics (to treat an infection).

SURGICAL MANAGEMENT

If symptoms become progressively worse and drugs have failed to control the condition, there are a number of surgical options and these include:

• Partial transurethral prostatectomy – This is the most common procedure, during which an operating telescope is passed along the urethra to reach the prostate gland. A heated wire is then introduced and used to cut away some prostate tissue. As the operation removes only part of the prostate it may need to be repeated. Some men become impotent following this operation.

• Total prostatectomy – If the prostate gland is extremely large, it may be removed completely. This operation may result in infertility and impotence.

Research into new treatments is ongoing and new procedures that are currently being evaluated include prostate laser surgery.

MONITORING FLUID CONSUMPTION

Mild symptoms may not significantly interfere with lifestyle. It may be possible to control symptoms of an enlarged prostate by ensuring that you do not drink too much fluid during the evening and by avoiding fluids that stimulate the desire to pass urine, such as caffeine-containing drinks and alcohol.

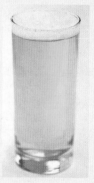

◁ Alcoholic drinks tend to over-stimulate the need to pass urine.

Prostate cancer

SEE ALSO

➤ Routine health checks, p272

➤ Enlarged prostate gland, p408

➤ Testicular problems, p410

Cancer of the prostate gland is most common in men over 50, and especially in those over 65. This tumour generally grows slowly and may not cause significant symptoms for many years. When the tumour is confined to the prostate gland, 90 per cent of men survive for at least five years after diagnosis and many live much longer. As with all cancers, early diagnosis and the right treatment is essential for recovery. Treatments vary according to the size and spread of the cancer. Screening can pre-empt development of the disease, but is not widespread at present.

SIGNS AND SYMPTOMS

Prostate cancer often produces no symptoms at all. If symptoms do become apparent, they include:

➤ A poor stream of urine.

➤ A need to pass urine frequently.

➤ Rarely, blood in the urine.

If prostate cancer is suspected, your doctor will perform a rectal examination to assess the size and regularity of the prostate gland. At the same time, a blood sample will be taken to check the level of prostate-specific antigen (PSA), which may give an indication of cancerous change.

▽ Blood samples are sent away for testing but this only shows changes in the blood that might indicate cancer, and other tests will be needed.

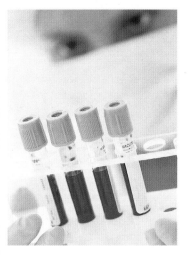

Your doctor will refer you to a specialist (urologist). Further tests include a prostate scan, in which some samples of prostate tissue are removed for microscopic analysis. Other scans to determine cancer spread will be done if cancer is diagnosed. PSA readings can be used to monitor cancer.

HOW IS IT TREATED?

If the cancer is confined to the prostate gland, the general approach is:
• Regular check-ups.
• Hormone therapy to reduce testosterone which can stimulate prostate cancer.
• A radical prostatectomy.
• Radiotherapy.

In elderly men with localized prostate cancer and no symptoms, the best approach is usually to monitor the condition as it is likely that the disease will not progress.

When prostate cancer develops in a younger man, however, there is a greater chance that the cancer may spread. In many cases, the cancer will be treated surgically, although radiotherapy may be offered as an alternative option. Possible treatment options include:
• Surgery – A radical prostatectomy removes the whole prostate gland. This operation, however, results in high levels of postoperative impotence and some urinary incontinence.
• Radiotherapy – The delivery of radiotherapy is now more sophisticated so it is possible to implant radioactive seeds into the prostate gland. This allows a lower total dose of radiation to be delivered more accurately.

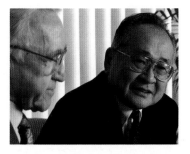

△ Prostate cancer usually occurs in men over the age of 50. In many cases, the cancer remains in the prostate and does not spread. The appearance of this cancer in a younger man indicates that it is particularly malignant and may spread more quickly, so surgery is often the best form of treatment.

SCREENING FOR PROSTATE CANCER

There is much scientific debate regarding prostate cancer screening. A blood test can measure prostate-specific antigen (PSA), which is secreted by the prostate. The levels of PSA can rise during infection, gland enlargement, trauma and cancer. A raised PSA level can indicate cancerous change requiring investigation but is not indicative of cancer. Similarly, a normal reading does not exclude cancer.

Although used routinely in the United States, screening for prostate cancer is not carried out worldwide. This is because the test is not foolproof. Also, there is debate as to which treatements are effective and all the treatments available have the potential to cause serious side effects.

Testicular problems

SEE ALSO
➤ Routine health checks, p272
➤ The reproductive organs, p394

Several testicular-related problems can occur in men, from harmless cysts to cancer. Regular self-examination is key to identifying changes in the testicular region, and medical advice should be sought promptly if any inexplicable symptoms are found. Like many harmless tumours and cysts, conditions such as epididymal cysts may be very worrying when first discovered as they can be mistaken for cancerous growths. Although testicular cancer is relatively rare, any abnormality should be investigated by a doctor, if only to set your mind at rest.

EPIDIDYMAL CYSTS

Small, harmless cysts commonly form in the epididymis – the coiled tubules that conduct semen from the testes. These cysts are very common in men over 40.

DIAGNOSIS AND TREATMENT

Your doctor can identify a cyst by simple manual examination and may confirm the diagnosis by ultrasound examination. Treatment depends on the size of the cyst – small cysts may be safely left alone but larger cysts must be surgically removed, as they may cause considerable discomfort.

TESTICULAR CANCER

Cancer of the testis is rare but is one of the most common cancers in young men between the ages of 20 and 40. This cancer is relatively easy to pick up by regular self-examination and is one of the few completely curable cancers.

WHEN TO SEE YOUR DOCTOR

It is advisable that you report any lump in a testicle to your doctor immediately. Many lumps turn out to be harmless cysts, but if there is any doubt your doctor will refer you to a specialist. Further investigations may include an ultrasound scan and a biopsy where a sample of tissue is taken for testing. If cancer is diagnosed, further scans are done to determine whether or not the tumour has spread to other organs.

HOW IS IT TREATED?

If the tumour is confined to one testicle, the testicle can be removed and it is likely that there will be no need for further treatment.

SIGNS AND SYMPTOMS OF TESTICULAR CANCER
➤ A hard, pea-sized lump, which is usually painless, in a testicle.
➤ Changes in the skin of the scrotum and a dull ache.

If the cancer has already spread, treatment involving a combination of surgery and sessions of chemotherapy or radiotherapy may still be successful.

VARICOCELE

A varicocele is a collection of varicose veins in the scrotum. This condition is not uncommon and is due to faulty valves within the testicular venous system.

WHAT MIGHT YOUR DOCTOR DO?

Your doctor will be able to feel the varicocele – it feels rather like a bag of worms. The treatment given will then depend on the degree of discomfort that the condition is causing. Very mild cases can usually be left alone quite safely as they may not progress any further. More advanced cases, however, will require surgical intervention in which the affected veins are carefully dissected and removed.

SIGNS AND SYMPTOMS OF VARICOCELE
➤ Pain in the testicle or scrotum.
➤ A dragging sensation on the affected side of the scrotum.

HYDROCELE

A hydrocele is a collection of fluid that gathers between the two-layered membrane that surrounds the testicles. It results in a soft swelling in the scrotum and is common in infants and older men. There is usually no apparent cause, although a hydrocele may develop in response to testicular infection or injury.

The classic test to confirm the diagnosis is to shine a light from behind the swelling. In a hydrocele the light shines through the fluid.

Some cases subside without treatment. If it becomes painful, your doctor can treat it either by draining the fluid or by removing the membranous sac that contains the fluid.

A HYDROCELE

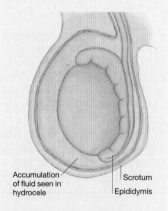

Accumulation of fluid seen in hydrocele

Scrotum

Epididymis

△ A hydrocele literally means a "water hollow". It is a collection of fluid that gathers and causes a swelling in the tissue capsule around the testicle.

Sexually transmitted infections

SEE ALSO
➤ Urinary tract infections, p390
➤ Female genital infections, p407
➤ HIV and AIDS, p468

Sexually transmitted infections (STIs) are passed from one person to another during sexual activity. They are usually transmitted during vaginal and anal intercourse, but some infections may also be transmitted by oral sex. STIs affect both sexes, and can occur in any person that is sexually active, whether young or old. Inevitably, the risk of infection rises among sexually active people who change their partners frequently. Consistent use of an appropriate protective contraception will dramatically reduce the spread of these diseases.

NON-SPECIFIC URETHRITIS (NSU)

A common infection in men.

Symptoms A burning pain when urinating; soreness at tip of penis; penile discharge.

Diagnosis A urethral swab and a urine culture may identify the causative organism.

Treatment One-week course of oral antibiotics. Where chlamydia (see below) is suspected or diagnosed as the cause, it is important that sexual partners are screened.

CHLAMYDIA

A common bacterial infection in sexually active men and women.

Symptoms May show no symptoms. Women may suffer vaginal discharge, urinary frequency, pelvic pain or pain during intercourse. It can cause infertility, pelvic inflammatory disease and ectopic pregnancy.

Diagnosis Chlamydia may be diagnosed by taking a swab from the cervix or urethra.

Treatment Oral antibiotics. Sexual partners should also be treated.

GONNORHOEA

An infection that affects sexually active men and women of any age, and that may be transmitted by oral sex.

Symptoms There may be no symptoms. Pain may develop on passing urine, and there may be penile or vaginal discharge. Women may also have vaginal bleeding.

Diagnosis By taking appropriate swabs. Diagnosis is difficult because a large number of infections have no symptoms.

Treatment Usually responds to oral antibiotics but should be treated early on. If not treated, chronic inflammation in the prostate gland, urethra and epididymis may result. Women risk chronic infection, scarring in the Fallopian tubes, recurrent pelvic inflammatory disease and infertility.

SYPHILIS

A long-term bacterial infection that results in acute genital symptoms. It can spread to other organs if it is not treated early.

Symptoms It has three stages of infection:
- Primary syphilis – Development of a painless ulcer on the penis or vulva and enlarged lymph glands in the groin. The ulcer heals on its own, but secondary syphilis will develop if the condition is not treated at this stage.
- Secondary syphilis – A rash over the whole body. Fever, tiredness and malaise. This may resolve over several weeks. No further symptoms may ever develop but some cases progress (20 or 30 years later).
- Tertiary syphilis – Progressive dementia with confusion, memory disturbance and disorientation. Destruction of the spinal cord resulting in paralysis of the legs.

Diagnosis By taking swabs from the urethra, anus and mouth, and blood tests.

Treatment Primary and secondary syphilis can be treated with injections of penicillin.

GENITAL HERPES

Recurring viral infection that affects both sexes, and can affect a baby during labour and a Caesarean section must be performed.

Symptoms Includes painful, fluid-filled blisters on genitals; tingling and burning sensations in the genitals; fever, aches and pains, tiredness. Symptoms usually subside over a period of two to three weeks.

Diagnosis Usually made from history and examination; can be confirmed by swabs.

Treatment Responds well to antiviral drugs, which reduce the life of infection and degree of infectiousness, but will not eliminate the virus. For recurrent attacks, regular preventative antiviral drugs are advised until the predisposition to recurrent attacks has diminished. The disease often burns itself out over several years.

HEPATITIS

Both hepatitis B and C are viral infections. Hepatitis B virus is transmitted by blood contact and penetrative sex. Hepatitis C virus is transmitted by the blood-borne route, although some cases are believed to be sexually transmitted.

Symptoms These viruses mainly affect the liver. Initial infection is followed by many years of asymptomatic infection and the liver functions normally. Some hepatitis B-positive individuals, and a larger number of hepatitis C-positive individuals, may develop a slowly progressive inflammation of the liver. This may result in liver failure and risk of developing liver cancer.

Diagnosis Blood tests can identify the nature of the virus.

Treatment Increasingly effective antiviral drugs, often used together over a course of about six months. Hepatitis B can be prevented by practising safe sex. People at risk can be immunized against hepatitis B. At-risk groups are gay men, intravenous drug-users, partners of known cases, healthcare workers and workers in long-stay residential units. As yet there is no immunization to prevent hepatitis C.

Impotence

The inability to achieve or sustain an erection is common and affects most men at some time in their lives. The incidence of impotence rises with age and occurs much more frequently among the middle-aged and elderly, although it can affect any man at any age. Occasional impotence is normal and can be caused by a number of factors, including depression or stress. If the problem persists, visit your doctor for further investigation, as more serious diseases may be the root of the problem, including vascular problems or diabetes.

The causes of impotence may be physical, psychological or a combination of the two. Psychological factors often underlie the problem as sexual performance is so closely related to emotional wellbeing. Any man struggling to deal with depression, anxiety, tiredness, relationship problems or a host of other interrelated factors may develop impotence as one physical expression of the stress in his life.

The condition often has physical causes, the most common of which are:
• Vascular disease.
• Drugs (including several used to treat high blood pressure and depression).
• Diabetes.
• Damaged nerves during prostate surgery.
• Liver disease.
• Multiple sclerosis.

Cigarette smoking is known to promote atherosclerosis, which may affect the blood supply to the penis, eventually causing impotence. Heavy and prolonged alcohol consumption may damage the liver and thereby interfere with testosterone production, which affects sex drive and erectile function.

WHAT MIGHT YOUR DOCTOR DO?
Your doctor will want to discuss more easily reversible factors, such as:
• Reducing levels of stress and anxiety.
• Stopping smoking.
• Cutting down alcohol consumption.
• Reviewing regularly taken medication.

To ensure there is no unidentified physical reason, your doctor may examine you and take blood for testing.

PSYCHOLOGICAL COUNSELLING
Psychological factors need to be explored and may require referral to a counsellor. It is very important to have a supportive partner during this process and it is often helpful to agree not to have sexual intercourse for an agreed period of time; this removes pressure of performance and the fear of failure. Attention can then be focused on addressing relevant emotional issues within a relationship.

DRUG THERAPY
The advent of sildenafil, better known as Viagra, has revolutionized the drug treatment of impotence. It works by dilating the small arteries that supply the penis, allowing more blood to flow into the organ and resulting in an erection. Viagra starts to work about one hour after it is swallowed. Some medications used for certain heart disorders may prohibit the use

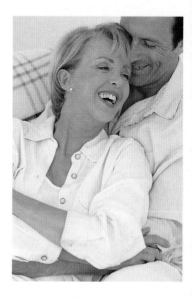

△ Impotence is extremely common and affects most men at some point in their lives. A supportive partner plays a vital role in dealing with the possible causes.

of Viagra, so it is very important that you only obtain such drugs from your doctor.

A number of alternative drugs have been or are in the process of being developed. These include:
• Apomorphine hydrochloride (Uprima), which has recently become available, stimulates the brain into activating the genital areas. It works more quickly than Viagra and achieves erection within 20 minutes of being taken.
• Alprostadil is a drug that is inserted into the penis using a small applicator. It works by acting on the blood supply to produce an erection.

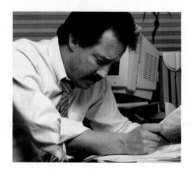

▽ Impotence can be caused by stress, anxiety and overwork. Addressing these psychological factors may well alleviate the problem.

10

THE EARS, NOSE AND THROAT

The ears, nose and throat are exposed to the air, and are therefore vulnerable to attack by harmful micro-organisms and foreign bodies. However, these potential invaders have to get past the body's defensive devices. The nose is lined with tiny hairs which serve to trap foreign bodies and prevent them from entering the airway. Protective immune tissue lies at the top of the throat, stopping infection from spreading into the lungs. The outer part of the ears contains cells that produce wax, which traps and expels foreign bodies. When these front-line defences fail, infection, inflammation and blockage may follow.

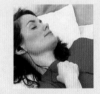

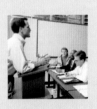

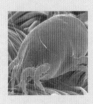

The function of the ears, nose and throat

In medicine, the ears, nose and throat are treated as one speciality, which is known as ENT. This is because all are located within the head and neck, and are directly linked by a passageway called the Eustachian tube. The body has a range of ways to repel infection and protect these vulnerable organs, and to prevent micro-organisms from spreading into internal organs such as the lungs. However, because infection can pass easily from one hollow organ to another, sore throats, sinusitis and ear infections are very common.

The ears, nose and throat are vital to our senses of smell, taste and hearing as well as our ability to balance and to breathe.

THE EARS

Organs in the ear are responsible for our hearing and balance. The three parts of the ear – the outer ear, middle ear and inner ear – all play a part in processing sound and transmitting it as nerve impulses to the brain. Our hearing provides the brain with information about our surroundings, and helps us to communicate through the medium of language.

THE NOSE

The nose is part of the respiratory system and is also responsible for smell. Receptors in the nose are stimulated by odours and these then send nerve impulses to the brain.

HOW WE CAN HEAR

Sounds are heard in the ears as a series of air pressure waves. The outer ear acts like an ear trumpet, collecting and focusing sound on to the eardrum, causing it to vibrate. These vibrations then pass to the middle ear, where three connected bones – the malleus, incus and stapes – transmit the sounds to the inner ear, amplifying the sounds as they do so. Sounds enter the inner ear at a junction called the oval window and travel to a specialized hearing organ called the cochlea. The spiral cochlea converts sound waves into nervous impulses, which it then transmits to the brain via the cochlear nerve.

HOW WE BALANCE

Your sense of balance is vital to your ability to remain upright and to move without falling over. The inner ear contains a structure called the vestibular apparatus, which helps with balance by detecting the position of the head and which way it is moving. The vestibular apparatus comprises three semicircular canals, which move when the head rotates, and the vestibule, which senses the head's position. Once the brain knows where the head is in space and how it is moving, it can use information from the joints to work out the positions of other parts of the body, and adjust them as necessary.

The human sense of smell is not as acute and well used as that of animals, but we can distinguish more than 10,000 odours.

Our sense of smell is responsible for most of our sense of taste. Your tongue detects only the tastes of salt, sweet, sour and bitter, and the aromas from the foods you eat help to build on these four basic variants. The role of the nose in tasting food becomes obvious if your nose is blocked, when your sense of taste diminishes.

The lining of your nose is packed with small blood vessels, which warm the air as you inhale. Tiny hairs lining the nose help to trap foreign bodies, preventing them from entering the lungs. You breathe with one nostril at a time – the nostrils shut down in rotation to allow the lining to recover from the drying effects of air passing in and out during breathing.

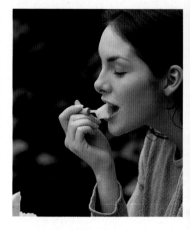

△ Our sense of smell is crucial to our sense of taste – helping us to distinguish tiny differences in flavours.

THE THROAT

A ring of immune system tissue sits at the back of the nose and throat, which helps prevent infection moving into the lungs. This ring – known as Waldeyer's ring – is formed by the tonsils, adenoids and lymph nodes at the back of the tongue. The airway and oesophagus meet in the throat (pharynx), so food and drink, and air, pass through it. During swallowing, a flap of cartilage known as the epiglottis closes over the airway, so that food does not enter the respiratory system.

The larynx ("voice box") acts as a valve, to divert food from the airway, and has the role of producing speech and other sounds. Vocal cords within the larynx vibrate to produce sounds, which are modified by the tongue and the lips to produce the elements of comprehensible speech.

THE STRUCTURE OF THE EARS, NOSE AND THROAT

▷ The structures of the ears, nose and throat are closely linked, which is why medicine groups them together. A problem in one of these three areas often affects the others.

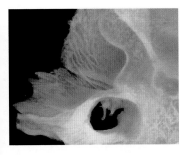

△ The middle ear bones transmit sound waves from the eardrum towards the inner ear, where vibrations are turned into nerve impulses.

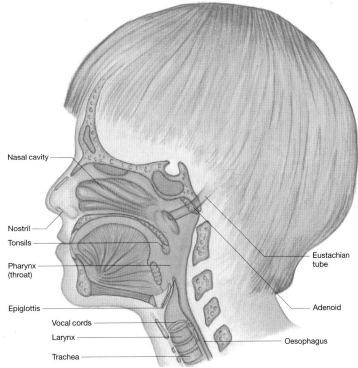

Nasal cavity

Nostril

Tonsils

Pharynx (throat)

Epiglottis

Vocal cords

Larynx

Trachea

Eustachian tube

Adenoid

Oesophagus

These artworks have been designed to show the location of different parts of the ear, nose and throat clearly, and are therefore not to scale.

INSIDE THE EAR

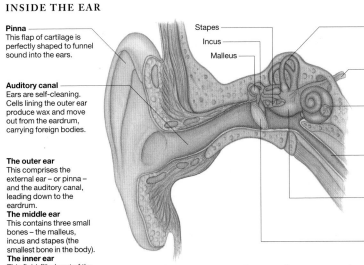

Pinna
This flap of cartilage is perfectly shaped to funnel sound into the ears.

Auditory canal
Ears are self-cleaning. Cells lining the outer ear produce wax and move out from the eardrum, carrying foreign bodies.

The outer ear
This comprises the external ear – or pinna – and the auditory canal, leading down to the eardrum.
The middle ear
This contains three small bones – the malleus, incus and stapes (the smallest bone in the body).
The inner ear
This fluid-filled part of the ear contains the cochlea, the semicircular canals and the vestibule.

Stapes

Incus

Malleus

The outer ear

The middle ear

The inner ear

Semicircular canals
These fluid-filled canals, at right angles to each other, are responsible for balance and detect rotational movements of the head.

Cochlear and vestibular nerves
These nerves take data on sound (from the cochlea) and balance (from the vestibule) to the brain.

Cochlea
This spiral organ is full of sensitive hair cells, each tuned to a different frequency of sound. Movement in the hairs triggers nervous signals to the brain.

Eustachian tube
This links the middle ear to the back of the nose and aids the equalizing of air pressure on either side of the eardrum.

Vestibule
Two devices in this part of the inner ear send information about linear movement – travelling up or down – and static position – which way is up.

Eardrum
This vibrating membrane, known as the tympanic membrane, separates the outer and middle ears.

Earache

Pain in the ear can be distressing, particularly for young children. It is often due to an infection in the middle or outer ear, but can also be caused by an injury or the build-up of wax. Diseases of the ear, jaw or anywhere within the head and neck can also cause pain in the ear. It is advisable to consult your doctor if you have an earache that lasts longer than 24 hours, since an untreated infection could damage your hearing. Antibiotics are usually necessary if there is a bacterial infection, and most causes of earache can be sorted out within days or weeks.

Earache can be painful and debilitating but it usually has a straightforward cause, and usual causes include:

• Inflammation or infection in the ear canal – also known as otitis externa. The skin becomes red and inflamed, and there may be pus discharge from the ear.

• Inflammation or infection in the middle ear – otitis media. In this condition, the middle ear can fill with fluid or pus, leading to partial hearing loss.

• Pressure changes causing damage or pain in the middle ear – barotrauma. This is usually the result of scuba diving or travelling by air. It should correct itself without treatment, but see your doctor if it persists for more than a few hours.

• Jaw or teeth-related problems such as temporomandibular joint disorder. The temporomandibular joint is just in front of your ears. It can become inflamed, often as a result of poor or loosely fitting teeth or dentures, causing severe pain near your ears.

WHAT MIGHT YOUR DOCTOR DO?

If you have pain in your ear, your doctor will look into the outer ear canal using an instrument called an otoscope. Any ruptures of the eardrum, wax blockages or pus collections will be visible. The treatment depends on the cause.

• Otitis externa – Ear drops or sprays with a steroid antifungal agent and antibiotics usually settle the problem in a few days.

• Otitis media – Most cases are caused by a viral infection and usually clear up without treatment. However, if the cause

△ A doctor examines his patient using an otoscope, which comprises lenses, a light and a funnel-shaped tip which is inserted into the ear.

is bacterial, antibiotics are usually given.

• Temporomandibular joint disorder is often eased by dental treatment. Stress can play a part in some cases, so relaxation techniques may be advised.

Noises in the ear (tinnitus)

Tinnitus can be alarming. It results from sounds generated within the ear itself and affects up to 15 per cent of us at some time in our lives. The noises are usually high-pitched and vary from ringing to hissing or whistling. People notice it most when it is quiet, so it disturbs sleep.

Tinnitus can affect people on and off, as brief episodes, or almost non-stop. Some of those affected hear noises only when they concentrate on them, while for others it is persistently intrusive and disruptive.

Many cases of tinnitus relate to the aging process while others are related to conditions such as anaemia and an overactive thyroid gland. Symptoms similar to tinnitus may be experienced if the ears are blocked with wax. Both ears tend to be affected and noises that occur in one ear only could be due to other causes.

COPING WITH TINNITUS

After an examination to exclude any other cause, your doctor may discuss strategies for managing tinnitus. These include:

• Using a masker – This is a device, similar to a hearing aid, which produces sounds in order to mask the tinnitus. Some people find having a radio under their pillow at night can be helpful.

• Drug therapy – Occasionally, if tinnitus is causing severe disruption and upset, your doctor may prescribe sedatives and antidepressants.

Hearing loss and deafness

SEE ALSO
➤ Routine health checks, p272
➤ The function of the ears, nose and throat, p414

About one in five adults has some form of hearing impairment, ranging from mild hearing loss to complete deafness. The first thing people notice is difficulty listening to conversations, which may be particularly troublesome if there is background noise. There are different types of deafness and your doctor will be able to diagnose the exact type by an examination of your ears and eardrums, together with a series of tests with tuning forks. If hearing loss is permanent, hearing aids can usually enable you to participate in normal daily life.

Doctors categorize hearing loss into types:
- Conductive – This is where there is a problem conveying sound often caused by a blockage or an infection. As the nerves are intact, treatment is usually successful.
- Sensorineural – The most common type, where the sound-detecting hair cells of the inner ear, or the nerves taking messages to the brain, are damaged.
- Combined sensorineural and conductive.

CONDUCTIVE LOSS
Hearing is usually restored once the cause is treated, and causes include:
- Wax – This common cause can treated with wax softening ear drops which can

THE STRUCTURE OF A COCHLEAR IMPLANT

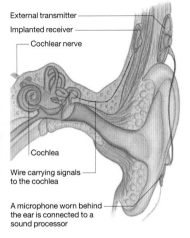

External transmitter
Implanted receiver
Cochlear nerve

Cochlea
Wire carrying signals to the cochlea
A microphone worn behind the ear is connected to a sound processor

△ In a cochlear implant (hearing aid), sound impulses are picked up by a receiver under the skin, then sent along a wire to tiny electrodes implanted in the cochlea.

HEARING AIDS
Initially, wearing a hearing aid can be disappointing since all noise, including background noise, is amplified. With perseverance, however, hearing usually improves. Hearing can be better if both ears are fitted with an aid. There are several types:

➤ Behind-the-ear-aids are widely used. A battery, microphone, amplifier and speaker are housed in a case worn behind the ear, and a transmission tube is passed into the ear canal.

➤ In-the-ear aids are smaller. All the components are contained in a case, which fits neatly into the ear canal.

➤ Newer hearing aids can be anchored directly in to the bones of the skull.

➤ Cochlear implants can be used for profoundly deaf people. They create an impression of sound which, combined with lip-reading, can help profoundly deaf people to understand speech.

be purchased in pharmacies, or in severe cases by gently syringing your ears.
- Otitis externa – In which the ear canal is filled with skin debris. A spray or drops containing antibiotic and an antifungal agent usually clears up the problem.
- Otitis media (glue ear) – In which pus and fluid prevent the three bones of the middle ear vibrating. The condition may respond to antibiotics but if not it needs draining surgically via grommets.
- Perforated eardrum – It often follows an infection and can heal without treatment in a few weeks, but can require surgery.
- Otosclerosis – In which the bones of the middle ear fuse. It usually affects older people and does not respond to drugs. Possible treatments are surgery to replace the stapes bone or a hearing aid.

SENSORINEURAL LOSS
This is hard to treat, but a hearing aid can help. Some causes include:
- Noise trauma – Regular exposure to loud noise, or exposure to one very loud noise, can destroy the hair cells of the inner ear.
- Exposure to very high air pressure.
- Increasing age – Inner ear function declines as you get older.
- Drugs – Inform your doctor of any drugs being taken because this can be a factor.
- Skull fracture.
- Viral infections such as mumps.
- Labyrinthitis – An inner ear infection.

▽ Listening to loud music on a personal stereo can put you at risk of hearing loss.

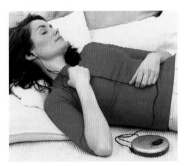

Vertigo

SEE ALSO

➤ High blood pressure, p278

➤ Stroke, p328

➤ Cervical spondylosis, p360

Vertigo is the unpleasant sensation of spinning: the person feels that either they or their surroundings are moving when in fact they are still. This distressing feeling develops suddenly and may last from a few minutes to several days. It is commonly due to problems in the ear and is often associated with nausea and vomiting. Occasionally there is a more serious underlying cause, so if you experience any such symptoms you should see your doctor urgently. Vertigo usually clears up by itself or once the underlying cause has been treated.

Vertigo is often the result of a problem in the inner ear, which contains the organs that control balance. The causes include:

• Acute labyrinthitis – This is an inflammation of the labyrinth, part of the vestibule in the inner ear. The condition can be extremely unpleasant and there may be associated nausea and vomiting. A simple viral infection is the most common cause. The problem usually settles in a few days and antiemetic drugs can help control the sickness.

• Chronic labyrinthitis – In this condition vertigo lasts for a few minutes, but recurs over weeks and months. It can be due to a long-term bacterial infection in the middle ear (otitis media) or to deposits of crystal in the balance mechanisms, which cause dizziness when the head moves.

• Ménière's disease – This is a rare disorder of the inner ear, in which the balance

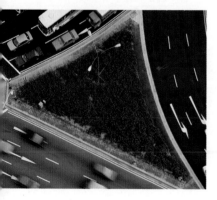

▽ Medically, vertigo does not mean the fear of heights and the sensation of dizziness that you feel when looking down from a high place. This condition is known as acrophobia.

mechanism becomes filled with fluid. The symptoms can be severe and include recurrent bouts of vertigo, deafness, tinnitus and pain in the ears.

• Acoustic neuroma – This rare tumour affects the nerve connecting the inner ear to the brain. It is non-cancerous but can press on the nerve or part of the brain, causing dizziness and balance problems.

Non-ear-related problems such as a stroke can also cause vertigo. In these cases, the person affected may have difficulty in speaking or seeing and may experience weakness in the limbs, and medical treatment should be sought as a matter of urgency. Some people develop vertigo as a result of high blood pressure or arthritis in the neck (cervical spondylosis). Older people are most likely to be affected but either condition can occur at any age.

WHAT SHOULD I DO?

A bout of vertigo is usually relieved if you lie down and keep the head still for a few minutes. However, if the vertigo persists or if you suffer from repeated attacks, you should see your doctor to rule out any serious underlying cause.

INVESTIGATING VERTIGO

Your doctor will examine your eyes, ears and neck, and check your blood pressure. Antiemetic drugs may be prescribed to relieve symptoms. Vertigo can often clear up on its own, but you may need treatment for the underlying cause. For example, antibiotics will be necessary if you have a bacterial infection in the middle ear.

MOTION SICKNESS

Also called travel sickness, this condition causes the same spinning sensation as vertigo. It affects almost everyone at some point in their lives and most often occurs during travel. The problem arises when the brain receives conflicting messages from the balance organs in the inner ear and the eyes. For example, your ears will register the motion of the car even though your body is not actually moving. If you suffer from motion sickness, there are a number of self-help options to try the next time you travel.

➤ Eat only a light meal before you set off on a journey. Fatty foods can aggravate feelings of nausea.

➤ Avoid reading while travelling and keep your eyes on the horizon.

➤ Take an antihistamine drug before the journey, but if you are driving be aware that some cause drowsiness.

➤ Suck ginger-based sweets – ginger can help to soothe nausea.

▽ Many people develop motion sickness on a boat, and the spinning sensation can persist for a few hours afterwards.

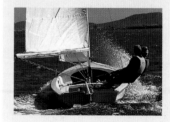

Nosebleeds

SEE ALSO
► Endoscopy, p295
► Asthma, p378
► Hayfever and perennial rhinitis, p420
► Haemophilia, p453

The lining of the nose has a plentiful blood supply, with many small blood vessels just beneath the surface. These serve to warm the air as it passes through the nose on its way to the lungs. Unfortunately, they mean that the nose is prone to bleeding. Nosebleeds are particularly common in children. The cause is usually straightforward – for example, damage to the lining caused by a blow or by nose-picking. Occasionally, however, nosebleeds can be a symptom of a serious disorder, so you should consult a doctor if bleeding is persistent.

The commonest cause of a nosebleed is nose-picking, which can damage the fragile blood vessels in the nose lining. Children and some adults habitually pick their nose, some even in their sleep.

Forceful nose-blowing, or inserting a foreign body into the nostril, can also result in a nosebleed. Very rarely, nosebleeds may be a sign of a serious disorder, such as cancer of the nasopharynx (the passage that connects the nose and throat) or a bleeding disorder. It is therefore very important that you seek medical advice for persistent or recurrent bleeding.

The cause of persistent nosebleeds can also be investigated by means of an endoscopy. In this procedure, a flexible narrow tube is passed into each nostril to look for the presence of a tumour or damage to the blood vessels. A sample of tissue can be taken at the same time.

TREATING NOSEBLEEDS

Seek medical advice if a nosebleed lasts longer than 30 minutes but these steps will usually stop a nosebleed in minutes:

► Gently squeeze the soft end of the nose. Apply this pressure to the nose for at least ten minutes, breathing through your mouth.

► If bleeding persists, apply the pressure for a further ten minutes.

► Do not dab, wipe or blow your nose – this just prolongs the nosebleed.

▽ Avoid blowing the nose for three hours after a nosebleed, since this can interrupt clotting and cause further bleeding.

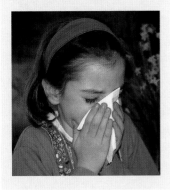

THE SOURCE OF A NOSEBLEED

In almost all cases, the bleeding comes from a patch just inside the nose called Little's area. Applying pressure to the end of the nose (see treating nosebleeds box) usually stops the bleeding.

Bleeding from the back of the nose is less common but may have a more serious cause. It is harder to treat since it is difficult to apply direct pressure, and may therefore lead to significant blood loss.

Anyone with a bleeding disorder (such as haemophilia), or those taking blood-thinning drugs (anticoagulants), tends to bleed for longer.

PERSISTENT NOSEBLEEDS

You should seek urgent medical treatment if a nosebleeds lasts longer than half an hour, or if so much blood is lost that the person feels dizzy or turns pale.

The bleeding may be stemmed either by packing the nose tight with ribbon gauze or by using a urinary catheter (hollow tube). The balloon that normally holds a urinary catheter in the bladder can be blown up inside the nose to apply pressure to the bleeding spot. Another form of treatment is to destroy some tissue just inside the nose using heat or by freezing. You may need such cauterization again if nosebleeds recur.

NASAL POLYPS

Many people develop nasal polyps, non-cancerous fleshy growths that arise from the sinuses. Their cause is unknown, but they are more common in people who suffer from asthma and hayfever. The severity of the symptoms depends on the number of polyps and their size. Symptoms often include:

► A blocked nose.

► A decreased sense of smell.

► A runny nose, in some cases.

Nasal polyps can be shrunk by using a steroid spray, or removed via endoscopic surgery, in which a fine, flexible telescope device is guided up your nose.

▽ A nasal polyp may disappear without treatment, but will usually be removed under general or local anaesthetic.

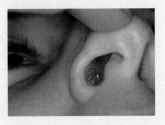

Hayfever and perennial rhinitis

SEE ALSO

➤ Asthma, p378

➤ The function of the ears, nose and throat, p414

➤ Sinusitis, p421

Hayfever is an acute allergic reaction that causes inflammation of the membranes lining the nose and throat and also affects the eyes. It is usually caused by sensitivity to pollens – of grasses, trees, flowers and weeds. Hayfever is a seasonal condition, with symptoms usually occurring in spring and summer. Some people suffer from hayfever-like symptoms all year round, a condition known as perennial rhinitis which is triggered by additional allergens. Symptoms can usually be brought under control by avoiding known triggers (allergens) and using medication.

SIGNS AND SYMPTOMS

The same symptoms occur in both hayfever and perennial rhinitis, but may be more severe in hayfever sufferers. The signs and symptoms include:

➤ A runny nose.

➤ Watery, red and itchy eyes.

➤ A dry and uncomfortable throat.

➤ Frequent sneezing.

➤ A general feeling of irritability and being unwell.

Hayfever or perennial rhinitis can affect anyone but will occur most commonly in people who have other forms of allergic disorder such as asthma. The trigger for hayfever is usually pollen, so symptoms occur in spring and summer when pollen counts are high. Perennial rhinitis can be triggered not only by pollen but by other allergens, such as house-dust mites,

▷ Tiny dust mites (shown magnified in this picture) are common triggers for perennial rhinitis and other allergic disorders.

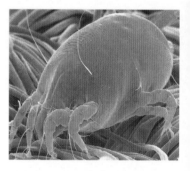

feathers, animal fur and mould. Symptoms may occur all year, but are often exacerbated during the hayfever season.

TREATMENT OPTIONS

The main treatment for hayfever and perennial rhinitis is the management of symptoms and can include:

• Antihistamines – These drugs are taken orally to treat the acute symptoms of hayfever and allergy. They may be taken as needed for intermittent symptoms or on a regular preventative basis when symptoms are persistent. They are usually taken once a day and have few or no side-effects.

• Nasal sprays and eye drops – These act on a preventative basis and need to be taken at least twice a day to have a beneficial effect. Inhaled steroid sprays often provide good control for individuals with troublesome nasal symptoms.

PREVENTING HAYFEVER AND PERENNIAL RHINITIS

The following can help to reduce the effects of pollen in spring and summer:

➤ Avoid areas with long grass or where grass is being cut.

➤ Stay indoors in late morning and early evening, when pollen counts are high, and keep windows and doors closed.

➤ Wear sunglasses outside to reduce eye irritation.

If you suffer from perennial rhinitis, the following may help to reduce symptoms:

➤ Avoid the provoking allergen where possible. For example, do not keep cats if you are allergic to them.

➤ Keep house dust to a minimum. Have wooden floors rather than carpets, blinds rather than curtains.

➤ Regular vacuuming of the mattress and bedding removes skin scales, which form a dust mite's food.

▽ Swollen eyes are a common symptom of hayfever, and are caused by an allergic response to airborne allergens such as pollen.

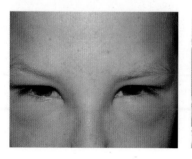

▽ Feather-filled pillows and duvets can trigger allergic disorders such as perennial rhinitis, so foam-filled bedding helps to reduce attacks.

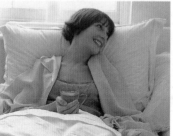

Sinusitis

SEE ALSO
- Colds and flu, p376
- Hayfever and perennial rhinitis, p420

The sinuses are air-filled cavities around the eyes and nose, within the bones of the skull. Doctors do not know the precise function of our sinuses but it is thought that they may serve to modify the quality of the voice. Inflammation of the sinuses – or sinusitis – is often associated with an infection in the upper respiratory tract, such as a cold or hayfever, and the condition can be both painful and distressing. It often clears up without treatment but may recur with more severe symptoms. In severe cases, bouts of sinusitis can last for several months.

SIGNS AND SYMPTOMS

The usual symptoms of sinusitis include:

- Headache.
- Fever.
- Blocked nose and discoloured nasal discharge.
- Pain and tenderness over the affected sinus.
- Sometimes, redness around an eye.

THE LOCATION OF THE SINUSES

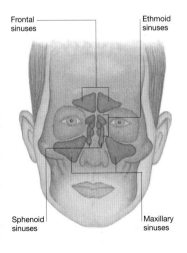

Frontal sinuses

Ethmoid sinuses

Sphenoid sinuses

Maxillary sinuses

△ The different sinuses are named after the bones in which they are found. The maxillary sinuses are located in the cheekbones, the frontal sinuses are in the spaces above the eyebrows, and the ethmoid and sphenoid sinuses lie deep within the skull.

Many people suffer from pain in the sinuses, but some individuals are more prone to regular episodes of sinusitis. Young children rarely suffer from the condition because the sinuses do not develop fully until they are four or five years old.

WHAT CAUSES SINUSITIS?

An attack of sinusitis is usually the result of infection by common cold viruses. The sinuses can block, fill with fluid and cause facial pain. Most symptoms occur between three and ten days after a cold. Simple painkillers and steam inhalation to loosen the discharge are the best treatments, along with rest if you have a fever and feel unwell.

Consult your doctor if your symptoms last longer than three days. You should also seek medical advice if symptoms suddenly recur along with more pain and a fever. This so-called "secondary sickening" is due to an infection by bacteria.

MAKING A DIAGNOSIS

Your doctor will press on your cheeks and forehead to check for tenderness, and may shine a light through your skin to see if your sinuses are clear. If a secondary bacterial infection is likely, you will be prescribed a short course of antibiotics, which usually clears up the problem. Your doctor may also arrange for X-rays of the sinuses if chronic sinusitis is suspected.

SIMPLE SELF-HELP

- Take decongestant tablets which are available from pharmacies.
- Avoid smoky atmospheres and prolonged exposure to dust and irritants.

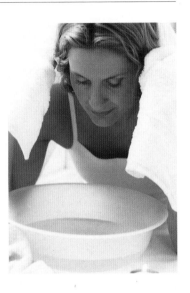

△ Inhaling steam from a bowl of boiling water, for a few minutes at a time, loosens discharge and helps it to drain away more easily.

- Do not blow your nose too forcefully during a cold since this can push the infection up into the sinuses.

CHRONIC SINUSITIS

If short-lived infections occur frequently in the sinuses, they may never seem to clear up. This form of the condition is known as chronic sinusitis. The cause is not known, but smoking and industrial pollution appear to make the condition worse. Symptoms usually improve with steroid nasal sprays, although in some very severe cases the problem may be referred to an ENT specialist, who will wash out and drain the sinuses.

Snoring

SEE ALSO

➤ Weight control, p264

➤ Smoking and your health, p268

➤ Sensible drinking, p270

Breathing noisily during sleep is a common and usually harmless condition. However, it can disturb the snorer's sleep and can also be disturbing to those sleeping near them. The noise is due to vibration of the soft palate (the back of the roof of the mouth) because people often breathe through their mouths when they are asleep. Snoring is common in children, and in adults between 30 and 50 – men are more likely to be affected than women. Loud snoring may be a symptom of a more serious condition called obstructive sleep apnoea.

Snoring can affect anyone, but certain factors are more likely to make you breathe noisily when you are asleep. These include:
• Smoking.
• Drinking alcohol or taking sedatives.
• Being overweight or obese.
• Having a cold or nasal congestion.

Most snoring problems in children are not caused by adenoidal disease, but enlarged adenoids can sometimes cause snoring.

WHAT CAN I DO?

Sleeping on your back promotes snoring so try another sleeping position – sewing a bumpy object into the back of your night clothing can help. You should also give up smoking, lose weight if you are overweight and refrain from drinking alcohol or taking sedatives before bedtime.

Consult your doctor if you have other symptoms, such as daytime drowsiness, as this may suggest sleep apnoea.

HOW SNORING OCCURS

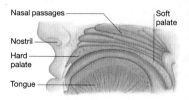

△ Air passes the soft palate on its way to the nasopharynx. If the airway is blocked, the soft palate tissues vibrate, causing snoring.

Obstructive sleep apnoea

SEE ALSO

➤ Heart disease, p282

In obstructive sleep apnoea, the airway is sucked closed, causing you to stop breathing briefly. This interruption in breathing means that less oxygen reaches your lungs and the oxygen level in your blood falls. Low oxygen levels prompt you to wake up and take a deep breath.

SIGNS AND SYMPTOMS

The typical pattern in obstructive sleep apnoea is for a person to snore more and more loudly and then stop breathing for ten seconds or more. Breathing begins with a choke or splutter as the airway reopens. This pattern continues during the night. Other symptoms include:

➤ Daytime sleepiness.

➤ Morning headache.

➤ Reduced libido (sex drive).

➤ Feeling drunk in the morning.

➤ Ankle swelling.

Sleep apnoea usually occurs in middle-aged men but can affect anyone, including children. It is often the result of an obstruction in the airway but may have other causes. It is important to have the sleep apnoea diagnosed since it can contribute to serious disorders such as heart disease or high blood pressure.

WHAT MIGHT A DOCTOR DO?

Your doctor will examine your nose and throat for signs of obstructions, and may arrange for you to have an endoscopy, where a narrow tube is passed through the nostrils to allow a more detailed examination. Sleep tests, in which oxygen levels in the blood and heart rate are measured, can confirm the diagnosis. Treatment is aimed at removing the causes of sleep apnoea. If this fails, a positive pressure device may be used, which involves air being pumped from a compressor to keep the airway open.

CAUSES OF SLEEP APNOEA

Sleep apnoea is usually the result of an obstructed airway, caused by:

➤ Obesity.

➤ Enlarged tonsils or nasal abnormality.

➤ Drugs that decrease breathing or relax the airway, such as alcohol, sedatives and opiate painkillers.

Sore throat and tonsillitis

SEE ALSO
➤ Colds and flu, p376
➤ The roles of blood and lymph, p448
➤ Glandular fever, p467
➤ Colds, sore throats and earache, p474

The tonsils are large lymph nodes that are situated either side of the back of the tongue. They are part of the ring of immune tissue around the mouth and nose which serves to intercept any invading viruses or bacteria. Infections and inflammation of the throat and tonsils are common and the vast majority are viral infections that last a few days. Most can be treated at home with simple self-help measures, but you should seek medical advice if your symptoms are particularly severe, if you have any difficulty in breathing, or if symptoms persist.

SIGNS AND SYMPTOMS

A sore throat or tonsillitis causes similar symptoms, such as:

➤ Pain and inflammation in the throat.

➤ Swollen lymph nodes in the neck.

➤ Difficulty in swallowing.

➤ A high temperature.

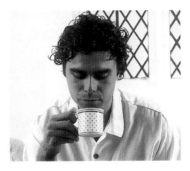

△ Most sore throats clear up quickly with plenty of fluids, painkillers and rest.

Most sore throats are caused by a viral infection and usually clear up in a few days. The only treatments needed are:
• Rest.
• Plenty of fluids.
• Simple painkillers. (Gargling with soluble aspirin can be helpful for a sore throat but you should be very careful that you do not exceed the safe dosage levels for painkillers.)

If symptoms persist, consult your doctor. Glandular fever may have similar symptoms to a sore throat but tends to last

▽ Tonsillitis is usually easy to spot: the tonsils become red and inflamed, with a white coating.

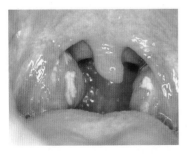

for weeks rather than days. Glandular fever can be easily diagnosed by a blood test.

STREP THROAT

An extremely sore throat can be the result of infection by *Streptococcus* bacteria. This requires treatment with antibiotics.

Distinguishing a viral sore throat from a bacterial infection can be very difficult, and doctors now try to avoid unnecessary use of antibiotics as this contributes to bacteria becoming resistant to antibiotics. In general, a bacterial sore throat will make you feel more unwell than a viral one. You may also have pus and ulcers on your tonsils and throat. To aid diagnosis, a swab may be taken and sent to the laboratory for testing.

RECURRENT TONSILLITIS

Tonsillitis is an infection that is confined to the tonsils. The tonsils are larger in children than adults, which is why so many more children are prone to tonsil infections. In the past, thousands of children had their tonsils surgically removed (tonsillectomy) to prevent recurrent infections. Nowadays, doctors are reluctant to remove the tonsils because they perform a useful function as part of the body's defences, and because there is always a danger that the operation, like any other, can lead to complications.

However, those affected by recurrent tonsillitis – that is, those suffering more than three bouts a year for two years or more – are usually referred to an ear, nose and throat specialist so that surgical treatment can be considered.

PERITONSILLAR ABSCESS

Rarely, the infection causing tonsillitis causes an abscess or a collection of pus to form behind the tonsil – this is called a peritonsillar abscess. This is very painful and can cause severe malaise. An operation to drain the abscess is required as well as a course of antibiotics.

▽ Hot or very cold drinks will help to ease the irritation of a sore throat, and drinking different fruit juices will increase your vitamin intake at the same time.

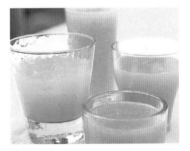

Hoarseness of the voice

SEE ALSO

➤ Smoking and your health, p268

➤ Sensible drinking, p270

➤ Sore throat and tonsillitis, p423

The most common cause of a hoarse voice is a viral infection of the larynx that has led to inflammation. People who put a lot of strain on their voices, such as actors or singers, and people who smoke and drink excessively, may also suffer from temporary hoarseness. It can also be caused by air-conditioned atmospheres, pollution or high pollen levels. In most cases, the hoarseness will settle without treatment if the voice is rested and you refrain from smoking. However, hoarseness can be a sign of serious illness so if it persists it is advisable to seek medical advice.

If you notice a change in your voice that is persistent, it is advisable to visit your doctor. Most causes are relatively simple, and do not result in long-term damage. However, persistent hoarseness can be a symptom of more serious conditions such as cancer.

Any vocal changes lasting over three weeks will be referred to a ear, nose and throat specialist. In this case, your throat will be inspected by means of an angled mirror and a light, or by an endoscope – a flexible telescopic device that is passed through the nostril into the throat. A local anaesthetic may be given. To help with diagnosis, a small sample of tissue may be taken. This procedure is called a biopsy.

WHAT THE LARYNX DOES

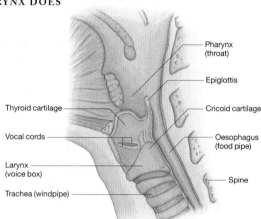

▷ The larynx, or voice box, is situated at the back of the tongue, at the start of the airway that leads down into the lungs. The larynx acts as a valve to close off the airway during swallowing, but it also contains the vocal cords, which produce sounds and speech.

Pharynx (throat)

Epiglottis

Thyroid cartilage

Cricoid cartilage

Vocal cords

Oesophagus (food pipe)

Larynx (voice box)

Spine

Trachea (windpipe)

CAUSES OF HOARSENESS

• Chronic laryngitis – This is a long-standing inflammation of the larynx. It is usually the result of smoking or the persistent overuse of the voice. There is no specific treatment but it usually improves if the voice is rested. If you smoke, you should give up, and you should also reduce alcohol consumption.

• Vocal polyps – These are fleshy, non-cancerous growths on the vocal cords. They are quite common and can easily be removed by a minor surgical procedure.

• Vocal nodules – These thickenings on the vocal cords are caused by overusing the voice. They are most often seen in people such as singers and teachers, but sometimes affect persistently noisy children. In most cases, the nodules disappear if the voice is rested, but they may have to be removed surgically.

• Cancer of the larynx and the pharynx – Cancers of the larynx and of the lower pharynx are more common in smokers and people who regularly drink alcohol to excess, and are also more likely to affect men than women. If caught in the early stages when the tumour is small, radiotherapy can often effect a cure. Larger tumours of the larynx require surgery and these operations can make it difficult or impossible for a person to speak and they may end up with a permanent opening to their airway in the neck (tracheostomy). As with most cancers, the smaller the tumour, the better the prognosis.

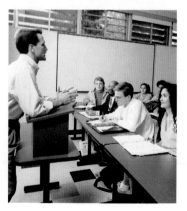

▽ Teachers and lecturers may suffer from vocal nodules as they regularly strain their voices.

PERSISTENT HOARSENESS

Persistent hoarseness can be caused by cancer of the larynx and the pharynx, so seek medical advice if hoarseness persists for over three weeks. Other symptoms might include difficulty in swallowing or a feeling of a lump in the throat. Treatment has a high success rate if the cancer is caught early.

11

THE EYES

It is easy to take sight for granted, but this is one of the most intricate and miraculous senses a human being enjoys. Light bouncing off objects around us enters the eyes and forms images on the retina. These images are translated into electrical impulses which are sent along the optic nerve to the brain, where the information is interpreted. The structure of the eyes and how they function is impressive, and an investigation of the range of disorders and infections that can threaten your sight highlights the importance of protecting the health of these incredible and fragile organs.

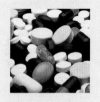

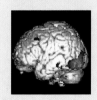

CONTENTS

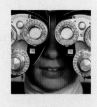

How the eyes function

The human eye is a truly impressive organ and human beings have the most sophisticated light-detection system of any animal on Earth. Of all the senses, sight is perhaps the most important, supplying vast quantities of information about the world in which we live. Our sight allows us to interact with other people, judge speeds and distances, work in bright sunlight or semi-darkness, discern colours and work up close in tiny detail. The eyes are well protected by the skull and the eyelids, and produce tears to keep them lubricated, clean and free of infection.

The eyes perform one of the most important functions in the human body. In conjunction with the brain, they allow you to see, recognize, remember and react to objects and people around you.

THE EYE AS A CAMERA

The eye is similar to a video camera in that visual information from your surroundings streams in continuously. Cameras, in fact, mimic the features of the eye. A series of lenses bends and focuses light rays on to a light-sensitive layer (the film) at the back of the camera. Even the aperture, in SLR cameras, reflects the actions of the pupil of the eye – it expands to let more light in or gets smaller to restrict the amount of light.

In a video camera, the end product is the series of images captured on the film or disk. But in humans, the light rays hitting the back of the eye are registered as images and then are converted to nerve impulses that travel to the brain, where the information is interpreted.

▽ As light hits the eyes, impulses are sent from the retina to the brain, which analyses and interprets this information to form a rounded, colour image of the object you have seen.

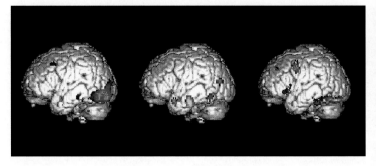

△ These coloured scans of the left side of the human brain show which areas are active while images are processed. The far left scan shows the brain responding as an object is seen, while the middle scan shows part of the temporal lobe lighting up as the object is recognized. The far right scan shows which areas are active when a person speaks to name the object.

The layers (cornea and lens) that bend light in the eye are of a much poorer quality than those in the average camera. However, the human eye compensates for this by having a much more sensitive light-detection system and a truly immense computer (the brain) to analyse and enhance the images. Each eye views objects in a slightly different way, so healthy eyes produce very detailed information for the brain to interpret and use.

HOW THE BRAIN SEES

The visual centres at the back of the brain do much more than receive simple signals from the retina. Most of the processes that produce a sharp, full-colour image in three dimensions occur within the brain. Visual signals are integrated with many other kinds of information in different parts of the brain. The brain also stores detailed information, about people and objects, provided by the eyes.

CONDITIONS AFFECTING THE EYES

Despite being fairly well protected, some outer parts of the eye can become infected, causing styes or conjunctivitis. Most of these conditions are easily treated and, while uncomfortable, do not cause lasting damage. More serious eye conditions occur when the complex inner workings of the eye are affected.

Many people suffer from myopia (short sight) or hypermetropia (long sight, usually in later life). These can be corrected by special lenses (glasses or contact lenses). These days more people are opting for laser

PROTECTING THE EYE

The eye is served by two kinds of protection: eyelids help to keep harmful particles out of the eye, while tears prevent infection, wash away dangerous material and even contain an antiseptic.

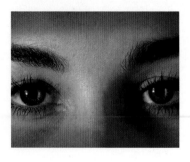

THE STRUCTURE OF THE EYE

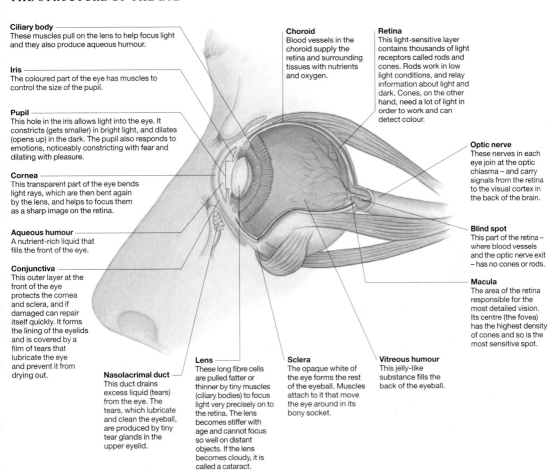

Ciliary body
These muscles pull on the lens to help focus light and they also produce aqueous humour.

Iris
The coloured part of the eye has muscles to control the size of the pupil.

Pupil
This hole in the iris allows light into the eye. It constricts (gets smaller) in bright light, and dilates (opens up) in the dark. The pupil also responds to emotions, noticeably constricting with fear and dilating with pleasure.

Cornea
This transparent part of the eye bends light rays, which are then bent again by the lens, and helps to focus them as a sharp image on the retina.

Aqueous humour
A nutrient-rich liquid that fills the front of the eye.

Conjunctiva
This outer layer at the front of the eye protects the cornea and sclera, and if damaged can repair itself quickly. It forms the lining of the eyelids and is covered by a film of tears that lubricate the eye and prevent it from drying out.

Choroid
Blood vessels in the choroid supply the retina and surrounding tissues with nutrients and oxygen.

Retina
This light-sensitive layer contains thousands of light receptors called rods and cones. Rods work in low light conditions, and relay information about light and dark. Cones, on the other hand, need a lot of light in order to work and can detect colour.

Optic nerve
These nerves in each eye join at the optic chiasma – and carry signals from the retina to the visual cortex in the back of the brain.

Blind spot
This part of the retina – where blood vessels and the optic nerve exit – has no cones or rods.

Macula
The area of the retina responsible for the most detailed vision. Its centre (the fovea) has the highest density of cones and so is the most sensitive spot.

Nasolacrimal duct
This duct drains excess liquid (tears) from the eye. The tears, which lubricate and clean the eyeball, are produced by tiny tear glands in the upper eyelid.

Lens
These long fibre cells are pulled fatter or thinner by tiny muscles (ciliary bodies) to focus light very precisely on to the retina. The lens becomes stiffer with age and cannot focus so well on distant objects. If the lens becomes cloudy, it is called a cataract.

Sclera
The opaque white of the eye forms the rest of the eyeball. Muscles attach to it that move the eye around in its bony socket.

Vitreous humour
This jelly-like substance fills the back of the eyeball.

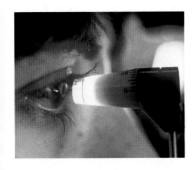

△ This test is used by an ophthalmologist to check for glaucoma. The instrument is an applanation tonometer, it gently presses the eye to give an indication of its internal pressure.

surgery to correct impaired vision caused by these conditions.

Glaucoma can be treated if caught early on, but damage is often irreversible, and treatment focuses on trying to prevent any further deterioration.

OPHTHALMOLOGY

An ophthalmologist should check all parts of the eye: the eyelids and the skin around the eyes, as well as using ophthalmic instruments, such as a slit-lamp microscope, to check for internal disorders. The movement of the eye, the vision fields and the pressure within the eye should also be

checked. A regular check-up will probably involve a vision acuity test to detect signs of long or short sight in either or both eyes.

FIND YOUR BLIND SPOT

With your left eye shut, look at the cross with your right eye and move closer to the page. The dot disappears when its image falls on to your blind spot.

Conjunctivitis

SEE ALSO
➤ Hayfever and
  perennial rhinitis,
  p420
➤ Autoimmune
  diseases, p459
➤ Causes of infectious
  disease, p462

Conjunctivitis is the name given to an inflammation of the conjunctiva – the thin layer of cells that lines the front of the eye and the inside of the eyelids. This condition can cause a lot of discomfort but is rarely serious and often looks worse than it actually is. Conjunctivitis is usually caused by an infection; other causes include allergies, most notably hayfever, which can produce serious swelling of the conjunctiva. Like any viral infection, viral conjunctivitis does not respond to antibiotic treatment but usually clears up naturally in a few days.

SIGNS AND SYMPTOMS

The first time you notice conjunctivitis symptoms is likely to be when you wake up in the morning. It is usual for both eyes to be affected, with any of the following symptoms:

➤ The whites of the eyes become red and inflamed.

➤ Stinging, itchy or watering eyes.

➤ A gritty or uncomfortable sensation in the eyes.

➤ The eyelids may become stuck together with discharge.

The commonest causes of conjunctivitis are:
• Infection – Bacteria, and more commonly viruses, can cause conjunctivitis.
• Allergy – There are a number of factors that can cause allergic conjunctivitis, the most common being pollen.
• Irritants – Irritant chemicals in make-up, contact lens solution and some eye-drops can inflame the conjunctiva. Other irritants include dust, smoke, pollution and ultraviolet light.

DRY EYE SYNDROME

If your eyes feel dry and gritty, it may be due to decreased tear production. The most common cause is old age, but it can occur in people with autoimmune conditions such as rheumatoid arthritis or SLE. You can restore moisture levels with drops called "artificial tears".

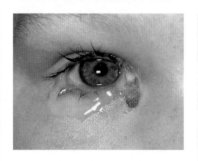

△ Severe bacterial conjunctivitis can cause great discomfort and a heavy discharge of water or pus, as seen here. Bacterial conjunctivitis usually responds well to antibiotic treatment.

The conjunctiva heals quickly, so most problems settle down with treatment or if the causative factor is removed.

MAKING A DIAGNOSIS

Your doctor will examine your eyes and try to establish a cause. If infection is suspected, antibiotic ointment or eye-drops are prescribed; if the likely cause is an allergy, anti-allergy eye-drops will help. Other types usually clear up in 5 to 7 days.

SIMPLE SELF-HELP MEASURES

An infection such as conjunctivitis is easily spread from hand to eye so it is important to pay close attention to hygiene to ensure you do not spread infection or pass it on to someone else:
• Use separate face cloths or towels; do not share them.
• Wash your hands after bathing your eyes or touching them.
• Bathe your eyes with warm water or with artificial tear eye-drops.

CORNEAL ULCERS

The most common cause of this condition is when a foreign body, such as a tiny piece of grit, gets into the eye and scratches the conjunctiva, exposing the underlying cornea. It can be extremely painful but once the foreign body has been removed, the conjunctiva heals itself within a few days. Other possible causes include:

➤ Viral infections, such as herpes simplex or shingles.

➤ Severe blepharitis.

➤ Acids and alkalis can cause large corneal ulcers if accidentally splashed into the eye. The eye must be washed with copious amounts of saline, water or eyewash to minimize damage. Medical help must be sought as a matter of urgency.

People who wear contact lenses are susceptible to these ulcers and should take great care with eye hygiene.

▽ Corneal ulcers affect the outer layer of the cornea. Doctors can identify the affected area by introducing a coloured dye to the eye. A corneal ulcer can be seen, stained green, in the picture below.

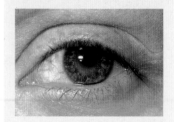

Styes

SEE ALSO
➤ Diabetes, p314
➤ How the eyes function, p426
➤ Blepharitis, below

Common styes are pus-filled swellings (abscesses) of the eyelash hair follicles. They can cause the eyelid to become inflamed and painful, usually because the small head of pus stretches the follicle and the surrounding skin. Most styes are caused by infection with *Staphylococcus aureus* bacteria and can be spread easily to other eyelash follicles. Antibiotic cream usually cures the infection, but recurrent styes can be a sign of general ill-health and occasionally of even more serious conditions such as diabetes, so medical advice should be sought if the problem persists.

SIGNS AND SYMPTOMS
You may first notice a stye as a slight red lump on the edge of your eyelid, but it will then swell up, become very painful and the eyelid will grow red and inflamed.

A stye will usually rupture, drain and heal within a few days. If it persists or becomes worse, then visit your doctor, because some antibiotic eye ointment may be necessary.

SIMPLE SELF-HELP MEASURES
Whether you have a stye or are suffering from blepharitis, there are ways to ease the discomfort and speed up recovery. Doctors offer the following advice:
• Place a clean, warm, damp washcloth on your eye and leave for about 20 minutes. Repeat this cleansing and soothing treatment three or four times a day.
• Avoid spreading infection by not sharing towels or cloths with others, and washing your hands after touching your eyes.

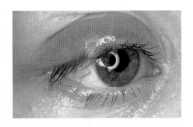

△ Styes are caused by a swelling in the gland at the base of an eyelash hair. A pus-filled abscess develops at the centre of the stye and the whole eyelid is affected.

Blepharitis

SEE ALSO
➤ Styes, above

In this condition, which may affect one or both eyes, the edges of the eyelids become inflamed and sore, and scaly skin may develop at the base of the eyelashes. Blepharitis may be caused by an allergic reaction to make-up, dust or smoke, or by a bacterial infection.

This condition is not easy to get rid of and even with the right treatment it may take many days to show an improvement. The best approach is regular, gentle cleaning of the edges of the eyelid with warm water, to remove the caked-on crusts. Once you have had blepharitis it is likely to recur, so take great care with eye hygiene. People who

SIGNS AND SYMPTOMS
Your eye may be sticky and crusts may appear on the lashes. Your eyelids will be swollen, red and itchy, and sometimes a stye may develop at the same time.

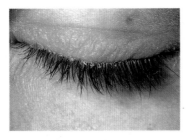

△ Blepharitis is characterized by inflammation of the upper eyelid along with scaly skin at the edges of the lid.

have dandruff and eczema seem to be prone to blepharitis, perhaps because they have dry, sensitive skin.

EYELID DISORDERS
In entropion, the eyelid turns in so that lashes rub the cornea and conjunctiva, causing irritation and, in severe cases, corneal ulceration. It can be present at birth (but usually clears up after a few months) and it affects older people.

In ectropion, the lower lid turns out and exposes its inner surface, which becomes dry and sore. This condition is most common in older people.

Both conditions risk damaging the cornea and may require minor surgery, to realign the eyelids.

Short sight (myopia)

SEE ALSO

➤ Routine health checks, p272

➤ Glaucoma, p433

➤ Macular degeneration, p434

Myopia sufferers can focus on nearby objects clearly but have difficulty focusing on objects in the distance, so their vision is blurred and fuzzy. The condition is caused by variations in the structure of the eyeball – such as the distance from the cornea to the retina, or the focusing power of the cornea. Short sight can be corrected by wearing concave lenses (see diagram below), in the form of either glasses or contact lenses. It is also – increasingly – corrected by laser surgery, which flattens the curve of the cornea to solve the problem.

Short sight is rare in children under the age of six, but vision will often change very rapidly during the teenage years. It seems to be that the earlier a person develops short sight, the more severe it becomes with age. In cases where sight deteriorates rapidly, the eyes will be tested and glasses may need to be changed every six months.

If you wear glasses, it is essential that you visit an ophthalmologist so your eyes can be checked for symptoms of other conditions. People with myopia are more prone to retinal detachment, glaucoma and macular degeneration, so it is important to tackle these problems as soon as they arise.

RETINAL DETACHMENT

Short-sighted people are more susceptible to this condition which is where the photoreceptor layer of the retina peels away from its blood supply. It can result in partial or complete blindness. If your retina detaches you might notice flashes of light or new "floaters" (tiny marks in your field of vision which everyone experiences to a certain degree).

If you have the impression of a dark curtain or shadow in one eye you should see a doctor as soon as possible.

▽ This is a refractor – a complex piece of equipment used by opticians to measure eye function very precisely and so determine the right lenses to correct any defects.

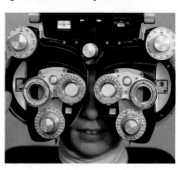

NORMAL FOCUSING

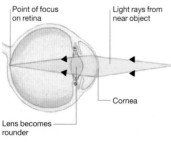

Point of focus on retina

Light rays from near object

Cornea

Lens becomes rounder

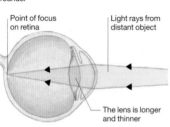

Point of focus on retina

Light rays from distant object

The lens is longer and thinner

△ The cornea bends light on to the lens. The lens changes shape to bend light to a greater or lesser degree, depending on the distance of the object, so that a sharp image is formed on the retina.

HOW THE EYE FOCUSES

Light rays are directed on to the retina via the cornea and lens, through a process called accommodation. This is the process by which the ciliary muscles push and pull the lens into different shapes to change the angle of the light rays entering the eye. To focus on distant objects, the lens needs to be long and thin in order to bend light accurately on to the retina; to focus on closer objects, the lens becomes rounder. Focusing depends on the focusing power of the cornea and lens as well as the distance from the cornea to the retina – the length of the eyeball.

LASER EYE SURGERY

Surgery can be carried out to remove a small piece of the cornea, making it flatter, and so can restore vision in people with mild short sight. Laser-assisted in-situ keratomileusis (LASIK) is the most widely used method, but is not suitable for everyone with short sight.

MYOPIC FOCUSING

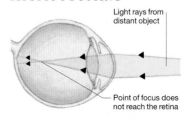

Light rays from distant object

Point of focus does not reach the retina

△ If the distance from cornea to retina is longer than normal, the lens focuses distant objects just short of the retina, causing a blurred image.

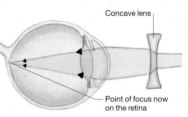

Concave lens

Point of focus now on the retina

△ Concave lenses are used to correct myopia. These lenses bend light outwards and so help to focus the image on the retina, not in front of it.

Long sight (hypermetropia)

SEE ALSO
➤ Routine health
checks, p272
➤ High blood pressure,
p278
➤ Diabetes, p314

People with long sight, or hypermetropia, are able to focus on distant objects but struggle to focus on those closer to them. Reading can be particularly problematic. The condition is more common in older people, because the elasticity of the lens declines naturally with age.

Hypermetropia can be caused by the shape of a person's eyeball, where the focal length of the eye is too short, or by the ability of the cornea and lens to focus light on to the retina. Convex lenses (see diagram below) are normally used to correct this focusing error.

PRESBYOPIA

This form of long sight is caused by the lens becoming stiffer and less able to focus on near objects. Presbyopia is particularly associated with aging – it affects everyone to some extent as they get older, which is why so many people start to wear reading glasses from around their mid-40s.

▽ The focusing ability of the eyes changes with age, but lenses are able to correct even very severe sight problems.

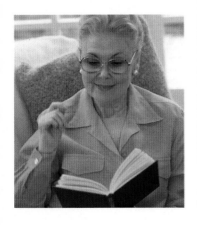

EYE TESTS

Regular eye tests, carried out by a qualified ophthalmic optician or optometrist, are vital for people who already wear glasses, as an incorrect prescription may cause blurred vision, headaches and/or migraines. However, even if you do not wear glasses, it is advisable to have an eye test every couple of years because eyesight deteriorates so gradually. Good vision is especially vital for people who drive regularly.

As well as assessing your sight, your optician checks the general health of your eyes to assess any ongoing conditions.

➤ Sight check – To test how well the eyes work together (sometimes using a Snellen chart and phoropter).

➤ Ocular examination – Using an instrument called an ophthalmoscope, to inspect the optic nerve, retina and lens. Early signs of diabetic retinopathy, damage from high blood pressure or macular degeneration can be picked up during this examination.

➤ Pressure check – Using a tonometer to measure the pressure within the eyeball. Raised pressure can indicate glaucoma, which needs to be treated promptly to avoid further damage to the optic nerve and loss of sight.

➤ Examination of the eyelids, lashes and cornea, using a slit lamp.

➤ Visual field test – To check there are no areas of missing vision.

People with diabetes should have an eye test at least once a year and may need more regular checks and treatments if diabetic changes occur in their eyes. This test usually includes dilating the pupils with a special chemical, so that the optometrist can examine the back of their eyes.

Many problems affecting the eyes can be treated as long as they are detected promptly, so it is a good idea to visit a doctor or optician as soon as you notice any problem with your eyes.

ASTIGMATISM

A normal cornea is curved like the surface of a ball, but sometimes the cornea is not perfectly round and has flat areas. This condition is known as astigmatism, and the abnormal shape of the cornea means that the eyes can focus on either vertical lines or horizontal ones, but not both at the same time. The problem can be corrected totally by wearing the right kind of lenses.

HYPERMETROPIC FOCUSING

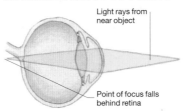

Light rays from near object

Point of focus falls behind retina

△ For someone with long sight (hypermetropia), images of close objects appear blurred. This is because their eyeball is shorter than normal or the cornea is weak.

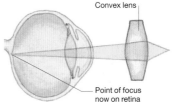

Convex lens

Point of focus now on retina

△ A convex lens can be used to correct long sight. This lens bends light more before it reaches the eye, so that a sharp image is focused on the retina.

Cataracts

Cataract is the term used when a lens becomes cloudy or opaque, causing blurred vision. In the West, the most common cause of cataracts is aging, as the fibres that make up the lens deteriorate naturally over time. Cataracts are found in 75 per cent of people over 65. It is usual for both eyes to be affected, but one eye will tend to have more severe vision problems than the other. The changes to the lens fibres are irreversible, but cataracts rarely cause total blindness; even in severe cases, sufferers can usually distinguish light from darkness.

SIGNS AND SYMPTOMS

Typical symptoms include the following:

➤ Blurring and gradual loss of vision.

➤ Objects have blurred edges as light is "scattered" by the opaque lens.

➤ Deterioration in colour vision so that dimmer colours are seen.

If you have a cataract in just one eye, you may have difficulty judging distances. Also, cataract-sufferers who wear glasses may find that their prescription keeps changing.

The lens of the eye consists of elongated fibre cells. In a cataract, changes in these cells' proteins cause the normally transparent lens to become cloudy or opaque. The transparency of the lens is crucial in allowing light through it and into the eye. Any cloudiness restricts and scatters light entering the eye and therefore affects how well a person can see.

CAUSES OF CATARACTS

The majority of cataracts are simply a sign of aging, and most sufferers from the condition are over the age of 65. However, there can be other causes for cataracts. These include:

• Diabetes – Diabetes mellitus can cause complications in the eyes and anyone with cataracts will have blood or urine tests to check sugar levels.
• Rubella – If a pregnant woman has rubella (German measles) it can cause cataracts in her baby.
• Eye injury.
• Prolonged exposure to sunlight.
• Ionizing radiation, including X-rays.
• Long-term steroid drug therapy.
• Smoking.

DIAGNOSING CATARACTS

A cataract can affect just one eye, in which case the sufferer may well be aware of a difference between the vision in each of the eyes. If your doctor or optometrist suspects that a variation in vision is caused by a cataract, your eyes will be examined with an ophthalmoscope. An optometrist may also use a slit-lamp microscope and dilate your pupils with eye-drops to allow a more thorough examination.

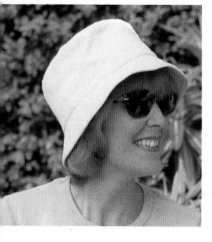

◁ Prolonged exposure to harmful ultraviolet rays in sunlight is one of the causes of cataracts. Wearing sunglasses and a hat will help to protect your eyes.

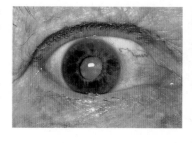

△ Cataracts are usually easy to diagnose – the normally transparent lens of the eye appears clouded or "milky".

HOW ARE CATARACTS TREATED?

Your cataracts may only be treated when the loss of vision seriously disrupts your life, and this obviously varies from person to person. For example, a 50-year-old lorry driver with only minor cloudiness of the lens will need treatment but an 80-year-old who doesn't read much may be relatively unaffected by fairly advanced cataracts.

Currently, no treatment exists for restoring the transparency of the lens once cataracts have appeared. The only treatment available to cure cataracts is an operation to remove the affected lens and replace it with an artificial one. In the most advanced technique – called phako-emulsification – a small incision is made in the cornea and the lens sac. The lens is broken up, using an ultrasound probe, and is sucked out. A replacement soft lens is then positioned within the lens sac. For most people, this operation is done under local anaesthetic as a day-case procedure. You may need to wear glasses for driving or watching television after this operation.

Glaucoma

SEE ALSO
➤ Diabetes, p314
➤ Diseases of the thyroid gland, p316
➤ Parkinson's disease, p340
➤ Short sight, p430

Glaucoma is the name given to conditions in which the optic nerve is damaged at the point where it leaves the retina at the back of the eye. The cause of the damage is usually raised pressure from the fluids within the eyeball. Glaucoma can occur suddenly (acute glaucoma), but it is more usual for the condition to develop gradually over a period of years (chronic glaucoma). Untreated glaucoma is a major cause of blindness, but regular check-ups can detect the condition in its early stages, when it can easily be treated.

SIGNS AND SYMPTOMS

Obvious symptoms tend not to appear until glaucoma is well developed, so regular check-ups are vital. For example, testing may reveal patterns in a person's field of vision that suggest glaucoma, even in the early stages. The individual would not notice this themselves because, initially, areas of visual loss are filled in by the two eyes' overlapping visual fields.

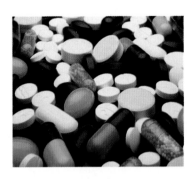

△ Some drugs such as antidepressants or those prescribed for Parkinson's disease may exacerbate an existing glaucoma.

Glaucoma usually affects both eyes, although one eye tends to be worse than the other, and it slowly destroys vision. If glaucoma is left untreated, it causes blindness. In the West, glaucoma affects 1 in 50 people over 40. Chronic glaucoma accounts for 90 per cent of glaucoma cases in the developed world.

HOW PRESSURE BUILDS UP

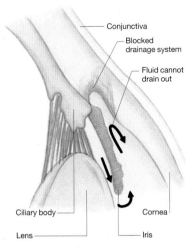

Conjunctiva
Blocked drainage system
Fluid cannot drain out
Ciliary body
Cornea
Lens
Iris

△ In a healthy eye, fluid known as aqueous humour circulates between the cornea and the iris. If a blockage occurs, the fluid cannot circulate. This creates a build-up of pressure, resulting in glaucoma.

CAUSES OF GLAUCOMA

Glaucoma may be due to high pressure in the eye affecting the blood supply to the optic nerves, causing damage to nerve fibres as they leave the eyes. Pressure within the eye is created by the level of a liquid called aqueous humour, which maintains the shape of the eye. This liquid is produced and drained at a certain rate in order to maintain the right pressure. Abnormally high pressure in the eye is caused by blockages or faulty draining of the eye via the trabecular meshwork (drainage system).

WHO IS MOST AT RISK?

Groups that are at risk of developing glaucoma include:
• People with a family history of glaucoma.
• People over 80 years old – One in ten suffer from the condition.
• Short-sighted people.
• Diabetics.
• Thyroid eye disease sufferers.

At-risk groups need to have regular eye checks to monitor their intraocular pressures, the appearance of their optic nerves and visual fields.

TREATMENT OPTIONS

Treatment aims to control the condition by reducing pressure in the eye, which can usually be done simply by using eye-drops. These drops ease the pressure by either improving the circulation of the fluid within the eye or decreasing its rate of production. If these treatments fail, there are surgical or laser options to increase the circulation of the fluid within the eye. There is, however, no cure for the optic nerve damage, which is permanent.

ACUTE GLAUCOMA

This rare form of glaucoma needs urgent treatment to prevent loss of vision. It occurs because of a sudden blockage to the drainage of fluid within the eye. It usually occurs in one eye, which becomes red and painful; the iris may also bulge forwards. Your vision becomes blurred, your pupils may be fixed and dilated, and you may feel sick and see coloured halos around lights. Acute glaucoma tends to occur in middle-aged people with long sight and it affects four times as many women as men.

Macular degeneration

This condition is generally age-related and commonly affects older people, although there is a juvenile form. It is due to degeneration of the light-sensitive cone cells in the macular area of the retina. The macula is the site of your most sensitive vision in terms of detail and colour. In macular degeneration there is a gradual loss of visual details and of the central field of vision (in contrast to glaucoma, where sight at the outer edges of the visual field is lost). It can affect both eyes, but usually one eye is affected a few weeks before the other.

SIGNS AND SYMPTOMS

Macular degeneration may cause:

➤ Difficulty in focusing on the text in a book.

➤ Inability to recognize faces easily.

➤ Problems making out details when watching television.

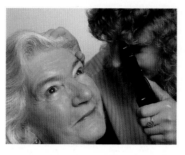

◁ Macular degeneration often occurs as part of the aging process. An ophthalmologist will test for the condition by examining the interior of the eye to check for changes in the macula.

Sandwiched between the choroid and the retina of the eye lies a protective insulating layer. With age, this layer may develop defects that allow some of the eye's fluid to escape into the retina itself. This fluid can then cause progressive damage to the sensitive rods and cones that are key to producing clear, recognizable images – a disorder known as macular degeneration.

WHAT IS THE MACULA?

The macula is a very small but highly sensitive area in the centre of the retina. Its function is specifically to allow you to focus on objects in the centre of your field of vision. Macular degeneration results in increasing loss of sight in this central area, but the outer edges of the field of vision will be relatively unaffected.

SPOTTING THE CONDITION

It is not always easy to spot the signs of macular degeneration, because the deterioration can happen very slowly and gradually over a period of several years. However, if you notice a gap or distortion in your central field of vision you should seek immediate medical advice.

WHAT MIGHT YOUR DOCTOR DO?

Your doctor or optometrist may be able to identify changes in the macular region of the retina when inspecting your eye with an ophthalmoscope. Further tests are sometimes done to assess the extent of the damage and include a procedure called fluorescein angiography, in which pictures of the blood vessels in the eye are taken.

Laser eye treatment can be helpful in some cases, although it can only halt the progress of the disorder, rather than reversing damage that has already been done. For most people, however, this condition is untreatable.

THE STRUCTURE OF THE RETINA

At the centre of eye function is the light-sensitive layer at the back of the eye called the retina. The retina is made up of specialized cells – called rods and cones – that produce electrical signals when exposed to light. These signals then travel along the optic nerve to the brain, where they are processed.

Rods

These cells are sensitive to light, and several share one connection to the brain. They work in low light conditions and relay information only in black and white. Rods are sensitive to movement, but do not give a very sharp image. They are concentrated at the edges of the retina, hence the ability to see movement out of the corner of your eye.

▷ This picture shows the microscopic light-sensitive cells of the retina – rods (blue) and cones (blue-green).

Cones

These cells respond to colours – red, blue and green – and each cell has its own connection to the brain. They produce sharp colour images but only work well in high light intensities. Cones cluster in the centre of the retina, especially at the point where the lens focuses an image – the macula.

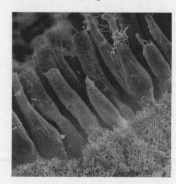

THE SKIN

The skin is the largest organ in the human body. Able to heal and renew itself continuously, it also provides an essential heat-regulation system for the body, as well as providing it with a covering and protection from infection. This front-line exposure, however, means that your skin is vulnerable to damage from various outside elements, particularly the sun. Human skin is exceptionally sensitive to both internal and external changes and stimuli. This sensitivity is a wonderful quality in many ways, but any disruption to it can lead to many different kinds of problems, from irritant or allergic reactions to stress-related rashes.

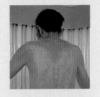

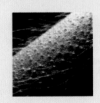

CONTENTS

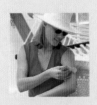

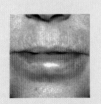

The functions of the skin

SEE ALSO

➤ Travel health and safety, p274

➤ Skin cancers, p442

The skin is the body's largest organ because, on average, it measures an impressive 2 m² (21½ ft²). Your skin cells are constantly growing, dying and replacing themselves so that this organ can keep doing its main job efficiently – keeping out potentially harmful micro-organisms such as bacteria. Kept waterproof and supple by an oily substance called sebum, your skin helps to control body temperature and to shield you from the harmful effects of the sun. Its receptors also give you all kinds of sensory information about the world around you.

The skin is composed of two layers – the epidermis and the dermis.

• Epidermis – This upper layer of your skin is made of sheets of dead cells. Cells at the base of the epidermis continually grow, divide and migrate to the surface. As they travel upwards, they fill with a tough, fibrous protein called keratin, which gives skin its strength and suppleness. (Your hair and nails are also made principally of keratin, and so are considered to be closely allied to skin.) By the time they reach the surface, the skin cells are dead and are then shed as flakes of skin, making way for new skin. The epidermis also contains cells called melanocytes. These make the pigment melanin, which is responsible for filtering ultraviolet (UV) light from the sun (see below) and also gives your skin its colour.

• Dermis – This lower layer is made of strong elastic tissue. The dermis contains all the blood vessels, nerves, lymph vessels, sweat glands, sebaceous glands, hair follicles, muscle fibres and receptors

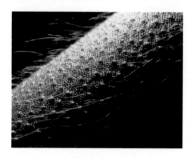

△ This close-up image of the epidermis on the arm shows "goosebumps" and erectile hairs. These hairs trap warm air – part of the skin's way of controlling body temperature.

(sensitive organs that detect touch, pressure, heat and cold) that supply and support the epidermis. The cells that repair any damage are also found here.

CONTROLLING BODY TEMPERATURE

As well as protecting the body's internal organs from the outside world, the skin has another vitally important function – helping to control body temperature. If your body becomes too hot, then the blood vessels in the dermis widen to disperse the heat, and sweat glands release perspiration to cool you down. If the body starts to get too cold, the blood vessels become narrower to hold on to the warm blood, and hairs all over your skin stand on end to trap a layer of warm air around your body.

THE SUN AND YOUR SKIN

Most of us love to be out in the sunshine and the sun does have beneficial effects, but its ultraviolet radiation can also do great damage to the skin. The skin's pigment, melanin, reduces the amount of UV that can reach the dermis, but this is often not enough. Even the indigenous populations of very hot climates, whose dark skin means that they have high levels of filtering melanin, can still suffer from sunburn if over-exposed to the sun. As its name suggests, sunburn can be a serious burn and, apart from being very painful, can cause scarring and premature aging of the skin.

Regularly exposing your skin to the sun with no or insufficient protection can quickly lead to damage that may go much deeper into the skin's layers than you might expect. UV light can trigger a cancer of your skin's pigment-producing cells – called a

▽ Prolonged exposure to the sun can have long-term effects on the skin. It is essential to use sunscreens to protect it from damage – especially if you are fair-skinned.

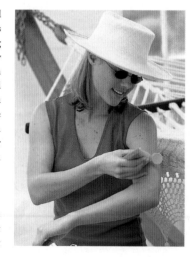

BE SAFE IN THE SUN

It is wise during the summer months to stay out of direct sunlight between the hours of 10 am and 4 pm. If you are out in the sun there are three main ways to avoid damage to your skin:

➤ Wear a T-shirt.

➤ Put on a wide-brimmed hat.

➤ Apply sunscreen regularly.

THE STRUCTURE OF THE SKIN

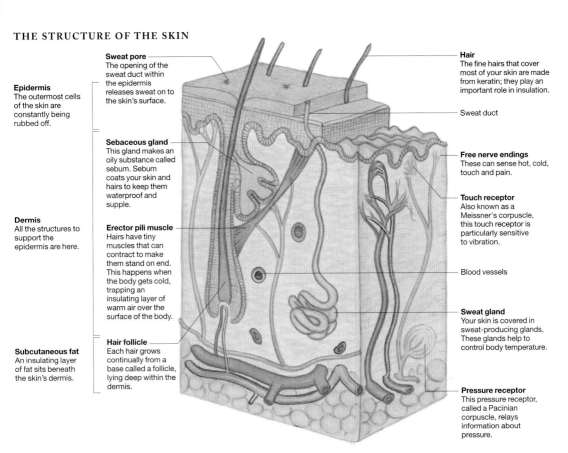

Sweat pore
The opening of the sweat duct within the epidermis releases sweat on to the skin's surface.

Epidermis
The outermost cells of the skin are constantly being rubbed off.

Sebaceous gland
This gland makes an oily substance called sebum. Sebum coats your skin and hairs to keep them waterproof and supple.

Dermis
All the structures to support the epidermis are here.

Erector pili muscle
Hairs have tiny muscles that can contract to make them stand on end. This happens when the body gets cold, trapping an insulating layer of warm air over the surface of the body.

Subcutaneous fat
An insulating layer of fat sits beneath the skin's dermis.

Hair follicle
Each hair grows continually from a base called a follicle, lying deep within the dermis.

Hair
The fine hairs that cover most of your skin are made from keratin; they play an important role in insulation.

Sweat duct

Free nerve endings
These can sense hot, cold, touch and pain.

Touch receptor
Also known as a Meissner's corpuscle, this touch receptor is particularly sensitive to vibration.

Blood vessels

Sweat gland
Your skin is covered in sweat-producing glands. These glands help to control body temperature.

Pressure receptor
This pressure receptor, called a Pacinian corpuscle, relays information about pressure.

---

malignant melanoma. This cancer is responsible for a large number of deaths worldwide each year. However, it can be cured if it is caught early enough – prompt detection is the key.

The message is simple: Always cover up properly with creams, hats and other clothing in strong or prolonged sun – especially if you are fair. Research has shown that several episodes of serious sunburn in childhood can lead to cancer later in life, so keep babies and children well protected.

UV BENEFITS

UV light does, however, bring some good news. A certain amount of UV is vital to body processes and the UV light that does penetrate the skin is crucial to production of Vitamin D, which is in turn essential for strong bones.

TACKLING SKIN COMPLAINTS

The skin's role as protector of the body from infection and injury means that it is exposed to a wide range of dangers, including viral and bacterial infection and various allergens and irritants. Many skin conditions manifest themselves as rashes or raised red marks and typical symptoms include itchiness and sore or broken skin.

While skin diseases are often distressing and uncomfortable, they are rarely fatal. Most, including the many rashes whose cause is never discovered, can be relieved by topical steroid or antibiotic creams, and sometimes with tablets. The psychological impact of some skin diseases should never be underestimated when devising treatment – an unsightly rash on the face or some other visible part of the body can cause the sufferer great anxiety.

DIAGNOSING SKIN CONDITIONS

Your doctor will ask you about your symptoms and then examine the affected area of skin. A magnifying glass may be used for a detailed examination, and a swab may be taken if there is any weepiness or fluid. The samples will be sent to a laboratory for analysis to try to establish the underlying cause.

Many skin conditions will disappear without treatment over a period of time. It is advisable, however, to seek medical advice if a problem is persistent or is particularly troublesome or painful, as some skin conditions can develop into more serious complaints and are sometimes indicative of more general underlying problems and ill-health.

Eczema (dermatitis)

SEE ALSO

➤ Asthma, p378

➤ Hayfever and
perennial rhinitis,
p420

Eczema, or dermatitis, refers to a family of diseases that usually inflame the skin, making it dry and itchy; there may also be small blisters. The cause often remains a mystery, although an allergy may be to blame. Infection is common because the skin easily becomes very dry, scaly and cracked, allowing micro-organisms to enter. Eczema can affect any part of the body, but is most commonly found on the hands, legs and feet. Treatment focuses on soothing the itching and preventing scratching – using ointment and perhaps dressings or wearing cotton gloves.

SIGNS AND SYMPTOMS

➤ Dry, scaly and cracked skin.

➤ Red and inflamed skin.

➤ Itchiness and irritation.

➤ Fluid-filled blisters, also known as vesicles, which can burst, causing "weeping".

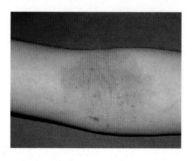

△ Atopic eczema (pictured) can occur without any identifiable cause and often develops in skin creases at joints. It is usually treated with emollient or antibiotic ointments.

There are several different types of eczema:

• Atopic eczema – This usually starts in childhood and is related to other diseases such as hayfever and asthma. It tends to improve as the child gets older, and can usually be managed using emollients (hydrating creams), but persistent cases may need short courses of steroid cream.

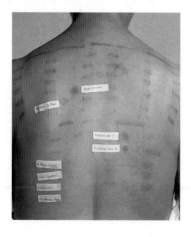

▽ An allergy patch test. Small amounts of common allergy-producing substances are applied to light scratches on the skin, to find out which ones, if any, are causing reactions.

• Irritant-induced eczema – This tends to affect the hands, which can become red, sore and cracked. Detergents, soaps, oils, acids, alkalis and solvents are common causes. If contact with the irritant cannot be avoided, wearing gloves or applying emollient cream will help.

• Allergic contact eczema – With this form, the reaction to an irritant lasts longer and can be triggered by minimum exposure. Common culprits are dyes, nickel (in gold and zips), chromium (in leather), lanolin (in cosmetics), resins and certain plants (such as ragweed). Often, the reaction is restricted to the area in contact with the irritant, for example in a band around a finger under a nickel-containing ring. Patch-testing of the skin may be able to uncover the cause. Avoidance of the irritant is the best solution, although topical steroid creams also work well.

• Seborrhoeic eczema – This affects areas of skin rich in sebaceous glands, such as the face, scalp and joint creases. Steroid creams are useful, but should not be used on the face. Coconut oil is helpful for soothing itchy scalps.

PATCH TESTING

To find out what is triggering your allergic reaction, a dermatologist applies small strips or discs containing allergy-provoking substances to your skin. Two days later, results are assessed. Red, inflamed patches indicate the cause of your eczema.

TREATMENT OPTIONS

The mainstays of treatment are:

➤ Emollients – These help to keep moisture locked into the skin; creams can be used, or special products can be added to the bath.

➤ Corticosteroid (steroid) creams – These are effective in reducing inflammation. However, if used in excess or for too long, they can make the skin thin and fragile. They must be used very sparingly on the face and only if prescribed by a doctor.

➤ Steroid ointments – These moisture-retaining, water-repelling ointments are useful in treating eczema.

➤ Antibiotic creams – These creams may be helpful where there is evidence of infection, particularly if combined with steroid creams.

➤ Steroid drugs – These are needed very rarely and only in the most severe cases of eczema.

Psoriasis

SEE ALSO
➤ Anxiety, p342
➤ Psoriatic arthritis, p359
➤ The functions of the skin, p436

This is a common skin complaint, found all over the world. Psoriasis can strike at any age and the cause remains unknown. The condition produces areas of red, thickened skin known as plaques, which may have a covering of silvery scales and are often itchy and painful. These plaques can occur anywhere, but are most commonly found on the backs of the elbows, on the knees and in the scalp; they may also develop on scar tissue. In affected areas, the epidermis layer of the skin produces new cells at a much faster rate than normal – hence the thickening.

SIGNS AND SYMPTOMS

➤ Areas of red, inflamed, thickened skin.

➤ Flaky skin – often silvery in colour.

➤ Pitted or discoloured nails.

➤ Pain in the joints.

➤ Occasionally the infected area will produce a sterile pus.

Stress, physical injury, infection and some drugs, such as lithium and beta-blockers, can trigger psoriasis, although the precise cause of this skin problem is unknown. Many psoriasis sufferers have a family history of the condition. In some rare cases, the condition can be associated with an arthritis, similar to rheumatoid arthritis, known as psoriatic arthritis.

Although it can be distressing and cause great discomfort, only the most severe cases of psoriasis are life-threatening. If the thickened plaques appear across large areas of skin, then the condition may interfere with the body's all-important heat regulation mechanisms and a potentially dangerous rise in body temperature could occur. Such patients need specialist treatment in hospital, so medical advice should be sought as early as possible if psoriasis seems to be spreading.

As with many skin conditions, cases where the problem is widespread may cause the sufferer a great deal of embarrassment and anxiety – especially if the face is affected in any way. In these instances, the sufferer may well be referred for psychological counselling.

▶ TREATING PSORIASIS

There is no cure, so the various treatments are aimed at controlling the condition:

• Steroid creams rapidly improve psoriasis; unfortunately psoriasis quickly returns once treatment is stopped.

• Coal tar preparations and dithranol (originally from the Indian Goa tree) have formed the backbone of psoriasis treatment for decades and are very effective. The strength of the cream is slowly increased until an effective dose for an individual's psoriasis is found. These preparations can be unpleasant to use and they stain clothing or bedding.

• Vitamin D derivatives have been developed as alternatives to coal tar and are now generally preferred because they do not smell or stain skin or clothes and are usually effective.

▽ This picture shows an area of skin affected by psoriasis. Typical cases cause red, inflamed skin that may also be scaly and itchy. There may be stiffness in joints – knees or elbows are commonly affected by the condition.

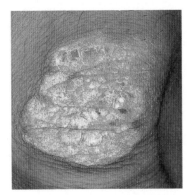

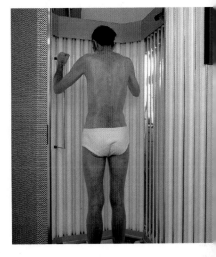

△ Ultraviolet radiation therapy may be used for chronic cases of psoriasis. However, this treatment can prematurely age the skin and studies suggest that it increases the risk of skin cancer, so it is prescribed with caution.

• Ultraviolet (UV) light treatment can be very effective when psoriasis is affecting large areas of the body. However, UV light ages the skin and may increase the risk of skin cancer so this treatment is usually only recommended for people suffering from very severe psoriasis.

• Powerful drugs, such as the anticancer drug methotrexate or the immuno-suppressant cyclosporin, are sometimes prescribed for severe cases of psoriasis. Like UV treatment, however, these drugs can produce various problematic side effects and so patients taking them should always be very closely monitored by their doctor.

Urticaria

SEE ALSO

➤ Learn to manage stress, p260

➤ Eczema (dermatitis), p438

Urticaria, also known as hives or nettle rash, produces itchy red weals, usually caused by an allergic reaction. It may also be provoked by infections and physical stimuli such as cold, pressure, heat or stress. In most cases, no definite cause can be pinpointed. Urticaria tends to develop fast – sometimes within just a few minutes – and can occur anywhere on the body. It can vary in severity, appearing as a small patch or covering the entire surface of the body, and lasting from a few minutes to a few hours. It usually clears up without treatment.

Conditions associated with this skin complaint include dermographism (see below) and angioedema. Angioedema is a sudden and severe swelling of the mouth, eyes and tongue. It may sometimes affect the throat, which in turn can give rise to breathing difficulties that need emergency care, so always seek medical advice urgently. Urticaria is an extension of the allergic response and may occur at the same time as anaphylactic shock (a life-threatening allergic reaction).

WHAT YOUR DOCTOR MIGHT DO

It is often difficult to pinpoint the exact cause of urticaria. Your doctor may arrange a skin-prick test, using potentially allergenic substances, to see if any of these might be the culprit. This is a common diagnostic step for many skin complaints. It should be remembered, however, that this form of testing may yield no positive results.

Urticaria usually disappears on its own within the space of a few hours. Recurrent

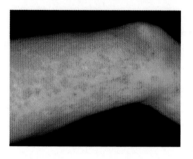

△ The hundreds of small, raised weals on the skin that indicate urticaria are often caused by stress but can also be the result of a severe allergic reaction.

sufferers often find the condition distressing and may be prescribed antihistamine tablets (which can produce side effects such as drowsiness). Prolonged attacks of urticaria may respond well to steroid drugs.

▽ Swelling of the mouth's soft tissue is a typical symptom of angioedema. This condition is similar to urticaria and is usually caused by an allergic reaction to foods or insect bites. It can cause difficulty in breathing, so seek medical help urgently (this usually involves treatment with anti-inflammatory drugs or antihistamines).

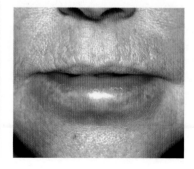

CHRONIC URTICARIA

In some cases, urticaria persists for weeks or months. Such chronic urticaria is very common and it can be impossible to find the cause – to the frustration of the patient and doctor alike. Possible causes include:

➤ Food allergies – fish, eggs, dairy products, chocolate, nuts.

➤ Food additives – tartrazine dyes.

➤ Inhalants – house dust.

LUMPS AND BUMPS

The skin is prone to a whole family of minor skin lumps that tend not to cause problems. You can, however, have some removed, if they become large or develop in an awkward spot.

➤ Lipomas – These are mobile fatty lumps that sit just beneath the skin's surface.

➤ Sebaceous cysts – These blocked sebaceous glands can feel hard and smooth to the touch. They may grow to quite a size and are often susceptible to infection.

➤ Skin tags – These harmless flaps of skin most often occur on the neck, trunk, groin and/or armpit.

DERMOGRAPHISM

Literally meaning "drawing on the skin", dermographism is a highly over-sensitive reaction to pressure. It sometimes develops in people suffering from urticaria. A raised red rash appears on the skin when it is stroked firmly, with the end of a pencil or a finger nail for example; the rash follows the line of pressure. (However, similar reactions may occur in other skin disorders and on exposure to heat, cold or water.)

This extreme sensitivity can be a long-term problem. Doctors are still unsure of the exact cause, although it is thought to be related to a high level of immunoglobin E. It also seems to be particularly prevalent in fair-skinned people and those who suffer from other allergic skin conditions.

Teenage acne (acne vulgaris)

SEE ALSO

➤ Blepharitis, p429
➤ The functions of skin, p436
➤ Bacterial skin infections, p444

This is a common condition that affects 90 per cent of adolescents to some degree. It follows the onset of puberty, and typically affects the face and trunk. These areas are particularly rich in sebaceous glands, which produce the oily sebum that keeps our skin moist. Adolescent acne is more common in boys than girls and can be very upsetting, because it appears at a time when people are especially self-conscious about their appearance. Acne also occurs in adults (acne rosacea), and in contrast to the teenage type affects women more commonly than men.

The root cause of acne is an overproduction of sebum by the sebaceous glands, so sufferers' skin often looks obviously greasy. Instead of flowing on to the skin and hair, the excess sebum blocks the hair follicles and sebaceous glands, giving rise to tiny blackheads. If a plug of keratin forms over the top, bacteria (*Proprionibacterium acnes*) can colonize the area, causing inflammation and pustules of acne. In severe cases, or when spots are picked, prominent scars (keloids) may be left behind when the skin heals.

The overproduction of sebum may be triggered by hormonal changes at puberty. There is no significant evidence that eating fatty foods, chocolate and sweets causes or aggravates acne.

HOW IS IT TREATED?

There is no quick fix for acne, and treatment may last from six to twelve weeks. It is also likely that you will need

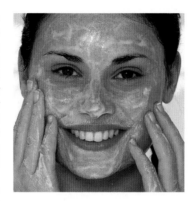

△ Careful cleansing of affected areas can help keep acne at bay and moderate exposure to sunlight can also be beneficial.

repeat treatment in the future. Cases occasionally respond to treatment within two to three weeks, although it normally takes longer than this. Possible treatments include the following:

• To begin with, you may be given creams or gels containing benzoyl peroxide – to combat the acne bacteria.
• If benzoyl peroxide proves ineffective, the next line of attack involves antibiotic creams, or courses of oral antibiotics if the cream alone fails to work.
• For women, certain types of contraceptive pill can be helpful in preventing the occurrence of acne.
• If your acne is particularly severe, you will be seen by a hospital specialist, who may prescribe retinoid drugs. Once you start taking these drugs, you have to be monitored closely as they can cause side effects, including birth defects if given to pregnant women.

ACNE ROSACEA

Also known as adult acne, this tends to affect the face only and usually develops between the ages of 30 and 55. It more commonly affects women, often runs in families, and is possibly caused by overuse of corticosteroid creams. Acne rosacea usually affects the nose, cheeks and forehead. The white- and yellow-headed pimples often itch or sting, and the sebaceous glands may become inflamed and scarred. If the skin of the nose is involved, particularly in cases affecting men, it can become enlarged, red and scarred – a condition known as rhinophyma. Occasionally, an eye condition called blepharitis also develops. There is no known cure, so treatment is aimed at reducing symptoms, and includes antibiotics in the form of creams and capsules.

▽ The skin on this 16-year-old's forehead is affected by acne. In this skin disorder, overactive sebaceous glands lead to the infection and blockage of hair follicles, causing blackheads and spots.

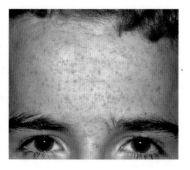

▽ This 36-year-old woman has acne rosacea, a chronic skin disease. It can start as temporary flushing of the skin, and then permanent redness usually develops, often followed by the appearance of large yellow pustules.

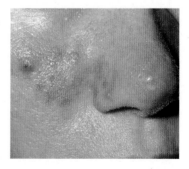

Skin cancers

There are several different types of skin cancer. Most are associated with prolonged exposure to the damaging ultraviolet radiation in sunlight and fair-skinned people are most at risk. Skin cancer is very common, affects millions of people around the world and causes a large number of deaths every year. However, most types can be treated successfully if they are detected at an early stage. Most skin cancers grow slowly, confine themselves to the skin and do not spread to other parts of the body. The exception, however, is malignant melanoma.

Skin cancer is one of the most treatable forms of the disease, but like most cancers, it is essential to seek advice if you have any symptoms at all, to make sure that you catch the problem in its earliest stages.

Skin cancer may have no apparent cause, or it may develop as the result of external factors – as in exposure to strong sun. Cancer of the skin can also arise because cancer has spread there from other parts of the body, such as the breast, kidney or lung. This latter type usually forms hard skin nodules, most frequently on the scalp.

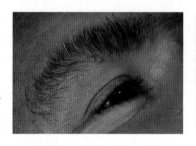

△ This raised lump on the eyebrow is known as a rodent ulcer – one of the most common forms of skin cancer.

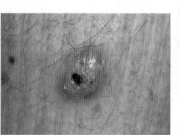

△ Squamous cell carcinomas produce wart-like swellings on the skin. They are most often seen in the fair-skinned and the elderly.

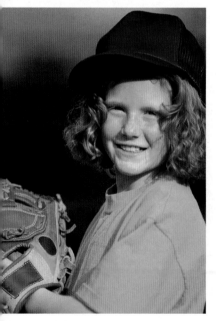

▽ People who are fair-skinned are among potential risk-groups for skin cancer, as they are more likely to suffer from sunburn.

MOLES

The ordinary moles that you have on your skin are also known as non-cancerous melanomas. Most moles are perfectly harmless, but some may develop into malignant melanoma. Moles are typically flat and brown, of differing size, and sometimes hairy. Usually present from birth, more may develop during a person's lifetime. Although cancerous moles are rare, it is wise to keep an eye on them, as changes can indicate malignancy (see signs and symptoms of malignant melanoma box). Remember that hairy moles will very rarely become cancerous.

BASAL CELL CARCINOMAS

Also known as rodent ulcers, these carcinomas look like small pearls with open sores (ulcers) in the centre. Rodent ulcers mainly affect skin that is exposed to the sun, especially around the nose and eyes. They grow slowly and do not spread to other organs (metastasize). However, if not treated, a basal cell carcinoma can spread, causing tissue damage to other parts of the body local to the skin cancer.

This skin cancer is more common later in life. If your doctor suspects you have a rodent ulcer, the diagnosis can be confirmed by taking a biopsy, where small samples of the tissue are removed and sent to a laboratory for testing. The ulcer can be removed surgically or treated with a course of radiotherapy, or a combination of both, to ensure complete removal of the cancerous cells. Superficial ulcers may be frozen off using a process called cryotherapy. Treatment is likely to be effective – 90 per cent of people with basal cell carcinomas are treated successfully.

SQUAMOUS CELL CARCINOMAS

These cancers look like small nodules with raised hard edges. They occur:
• On sun-exposed areas of the skin.
• In chronic leg ulcers.
• On the lips of smokers.

SIGNS AND SYMPTOMS OF MALIGNANT MELANOMA

Any of the following changes to a mole could indicate development of a malignant melanoma. It is advisable to see your doctor as soon as possible if you develop a new skin growth, or if a pre-existing mole changes in any way. The changes to look for include:

➤ Any rapid change in size.

➤ Changes in shape or an irregular border (normal moles have a smooth, regular shape).

➤ Change in colour, especially darkening to blue-black.

➤ Bleeding.

➤ Pain or itching.

➤ A softening of the mole.

➤ Crumbling, or the breaking away of pieces of the mole.

➤ The appearance of new moles around the original one.

Squamous cell carcinomas are similar to rodent ulcers. They start out as small, firm lumps in certain parts of the body and, although they are painless, they can grow quite rapidly. It is rare for them to spread to other parts of the body, but this does happen in some cases. They can also occur

▽ Solar keratosis is a red skin-growth caused by too much exposure to the sun over a number of years. Although not cancerous to begin with, it may develop into skin cancer, so your doctor will always recommend its removal.

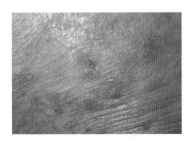

at multiple sites in the body. Squamous cell carcinomas can be very destructive, especially when they occur on the face and if left untreated. They are cured by radiotherapy or are removed surgically.

MALIGNANT MELANOMAS

Malignant melanoma is the most serious form of skin cancer. It affects the melanocytes – the skin's melanin-producing cells – and can strike any part of the body. In women, malignant melanomas are often found on the legs; in men, the back is a common site. Rarely seen in children, these cancers are more usually found in adults of middle age and older, although there have been occurrences in young adolescents.

This cancer is connected with excessive exposure to the sun and so is especially common in fair-skinned people and in countries such as Australia. Incidence has risen because people travel more widely and like having a tan.

About 50 per cent of these cancers develop from moles. They grow quickly and if untreated can spread rapidly to other parts of the body. Melanomas can be cured by surgical removal, but only if caught while small. A first step in treatment is analysing a sample of the cancer. Radiotherapy and/or chemotherapy may be used.

POTENTIALLY CANCEROUS CONDITIONS

There are certain conditions that can change, in rare cases, into skin cancers and these include:

• Bowen's disease – This produces slow-growing, red, scaly patches on the skin. Rarely, these turn into squamous cell carcinomas. Your doctor can diagnose the patches under a microscope and can cure the condition using a drug called 5-FU, surgery or radiotherapy.

• Acitinic (or solar) keratoses – These pinkish red crusts appear on sun-exposed areas of skin and can develop into squamous cell carcinomas. They can be cut out or treated with 5-FU paint.

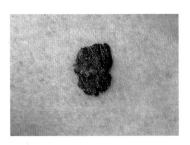

△ This picture shows a malignant melanoma on the skin of the lower leg. Malignant melanomas are more common in people with pale skin because their skin contains less of the pigment melanin, which provides protection against the harmful effects of the sun.

Although most forms of skin cancer are eminently treatable, with a survival rate much higher than most other types of cancer, the signs of skin cancers should be taken seriously. Prevention is better than cure, and taking care in the sun will often stop cancer from developing.

SKIN CANCER AWARENESS

At risk groups include:

➤ People who work outdoors.

➤ People over 50 years old.

➤ People who have had radiation treatment or who are exposed to radiation as part of their job.

➤ People who had severe sunburn regularly in childhood.

It is a good idea to examine yourself every few months for any skin changes, and to check existing moles and the appearance of new ones. Ask a friend or partner to inspect areas you cannot see. If you are familiar with marks on your skin you will notice any change and can bring it to the attention of your doctor.

Changes to look out for include:

➤ New growths or sores that do not heal within four weeks.

➤ Spots or sores that itch, hurt, scab or bleed persistently.

Fungal skin infections

SEE ALSO

➤ Diabetes, p314
➤ Female genital infections, p407
➤ Causes of infectious disease, p462

Millions of fungi, including yeasts, live naturally on your skin. Normally, there is healthy competition in the body between bacteria and fungi. However, if the bacteria are wiped out by a course of antibiotics, the fungi can be free to colonize and infect certain areas. Some people are more prone to fungal infections than others, although there is no known medical reason for this. If fungal infections recur, this can be an indication of diabetes or of other more general disorders, so it is a good idea to contact your doctor as a precautionary measure.

RINGWORM

This is caused by a fungus and not, despite its name, by a worm. The infected skin develops well-defined, scaly patches, which are usually itchy. Ringworm commonly affects the scalp and groin. It disappears quickly with antifungal cream treatment.

ATHLETE'S FOOT

The fungi that cause this itchy rash between the toes thrive in warm, humid conditions. They can also affect the nails, making them brittle and deformed. Wearing certain types of footwear, such as trainers, makes the feet sweat and more likely to develop this infection. The skin rash settles rapidly with antifungal creams, but the nail infection can need extended treatment with antifungal tablets or nail paints.

▽ This picture shows ringworm on the skin of a farmworker. The condition may have been picked up from an infected sheep.

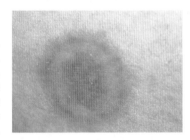

ORAL THRUSH

The yeast *Candida albicans*, which lives normally on the skin, can easily infect the mouth and/or vagina (vaginal thrush). With oral thrush, the mouth and tongue become red and sore, with white patches. The condition often occurs after a course of antibiotics, when the bacteria that normally control levels of *Candida* in the body have been killed. While oral thrush is easily treated and usually clears within a matter of days, recurrent infections can occur in people with diabetes or any long-term illness. Anticandidal creams and tablets can be used to treat oral thrush, and pessaries are available for vaginal thrush.

Bacterial skin infections

SEE ALSO

➤ Bacterial infections, p464

Bacteria are just one of the many groups of micro-organisms that can affect the skin. There are two main types of bacteria – *Streptococcus* and *Staphylococcus*. Bacteria can live on the skin without symptoms but if the skin's protective barrier is breached, infection can result.

CELLULITIS

This infection tends to be found in the feet and calves and can be quite extensive. Many patients need antibiotic injections in the first three to five days in order to control the infection. Once it is under control, this is usually followed by a few weeks of oral antibiotics to clear up the infection.

A type of infective cellulitis that affects only the face – called erysipelas – is caused by a particular *Streptococcus* and clears up with penicillin treatment.

IMPETIGO

This usually affects children. A moist rash develops, often around the mouth or nose, with yellow crusts. Treatment involves antibiotic creams and a course of antibiotics.

FOLLICULITIS

This is usually a mild inflammation of the hair follicles due to infection and requires little, if any, treatment. Antibiotic cream can be used in extensive infections. It usually clears up in a week.

ERYTHEMA NODOSUM

This firm, tender, dark-red rash occurs on the legs and resembles bruising as it settles down. It commonly affects young adults, particularly women, and is caused by:
• Bacteria or fungi.
• Drugs, such as the contraceptive pill or sulphonamide drugs.
• Inflammatory bowel disease, such as Crohn's disease and ulcerative colitis.
Treatment involves bed-rest and non-steroidal anti-inflammatory drugs.

Viral skin infections

SEE ALSO
➤ Sexually transmitted infections, p411
➤ The roles of blood and lymph, p448
➤ Causes of infectious disease, p462

A whole host of viruses give rise to various different skin rashes. These viral rashes include cold sores, warts and molluscum contagiosum. Treatments usually include antiviral creams, although some conditions clear up untreated, given time (in the case of infections such as warts, however, this can be several years). Once you have had certain viral infections, such as the herpes simplex virus that causes cold sores, symptoms are likely to recur. These infections are often contagious and should be treated early to avoid any spread.

COLD SORES

These sores form around the mouth and are caused by the herpes simplex virus. This occurs naturally in most human bodies, but usually it is controlled by the immune system. If the immune system is actively fighting off other viral infections, even those as mild as the common cold, the herpes simplex virus can take hold. The eruption of cold sores is preceded by an itching sensation. This usually develops into groups of small blisters where the skin and the lip membrane meet. Sores can also occur around the nose. They are best treated as soon as the itching develops, with an antiviral cream – a choice of these is available over the counter at your local pharmacy. Cold sores tend to recur.

WARTS AND VERRUCAS

These flat, scaly skin growths are caused by the human papilloma virus. Most people develop immunity to the virus with time and the warts may disappear within three to six months. Most warts will disappear without any treatment.

Verrucas are flat warts on the sole of the foot and require no treatment unless they are painful. However, like other types of wart, they are highly infectious and can be spread easily around the infected area or from person to person. It is recommended that verruca sufferers should wear protective socks – when swimming, for example, or around the house.

Warts that persist or cause discomfort can be removed. Ways of doing this include destroying the tissue with heat, freezing or laser treatment. Such treatments can usually be performed by your doctor, although several sessions may be needed to clear the warts completely. The best method, however, is applying caustic paints containing salicylic acid.

Warts that affect the genitals need specialist treatment in a genitourinary clinic. Informing/tracing of sexual partners must be carried out.

▽ Cold sores are a common affliction. They usually begin as an itch and develop into small, fluid-filled blisters. As with other viral skin infections, cold sores are highly contagious and can be spread to other areas of the body.

▽ Verrucas are flat warts which appear on the soles of the feet and the toes. The infection is usually contracted from contaminated floors and can be spread easily in public places such as swimming pools.

ERYTHEMA MULTIFORME

In this condition the skin becomes covered with raised red patches. This inflammation is caused by the dilation (opening up) of underlying blood vessels. The centre of each red patch may appear blue, giving the rash a characteristic "target" appearance. The rash has a tendency to affect both sides of the body and in severe cases can cause ulcers on the mouth and genitalia.

The rash is caused by:

➤ Viruses, such as herpes simplex, Epstein-Barr virus, HIV and the weakened virus of BCG vaccination.

➤ Chronic autoimmune diseases, such as systemic lupus erythematosus and sarcoidosis.

➤ Drugs, such as penicillins and barbiturates.

➤ Some cancers, including myeloma, Hodgkin's lymphoma and carcinomas.

The rash settles quickly if treated with steroid creams but tends to recur.

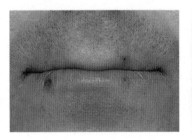

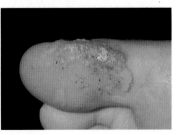

MOLLUSCUM CONTAGIOSUM

These pearl-like lumps, caused by viral infection, are common in children and may occur in multiple clusters around the body. The condition can be caught during contact with an infected person. It usually disappears in six to twelve months, once the child develops immunity to the virus.

Leg ulcers

SEE ALSO

➤ High blood pressure,
  p278
➤ Peripheral vascular
  disease, p280
➤ Angina, p284
➤ Diabetes, p314

These open sores can cause the skin around the ankle or foot to break down. They are common in the West and mainly affect people later in life, when they often cause a long-term problem. About 1 per cent of people over the age of 70 suffer from leg ulcers. People who are bedridden or have reduced mobility are especially at risk. There are different types of leg ulcer: some can be painless but others cause a great deal of discomfort, usually as a result of poor circulation. Treatment ranges from bandaging to amputation in severe cases.

There are several types of leg ulcer, each with its own symptoms and characteristics. Each of these types also responds to different levels of treatment. All ulcers can become unpleasant and problematic if left untreated, so they should be brought to the attention of a medical expert:

- Venous ulcers – These painless ulcers are the most common and are associated with varicose veins that cause the skin around the ankle to become thin and fragile. Early changes to the skin include a brown rash and/or a form of eczema.
- Ischaemic ulcers – These painful ulcers are caused by poor blood supply to the leg (peripheral vascular disease). They are common in smokers and people with a history of high blood pressure, angina and claudication (crampy pain in the legs). This silting up of arteries taking blood to the legs is also a common problem in people with diabetes.

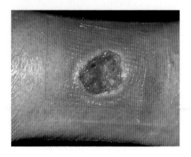

▽ This picture shows an example of a leg ulcer. It formed after a blow to the leg caused severe skin damage. Treatment depends on the type of ulcer, but ulcers like this one would be cleaned, dressed and left to heal. Antibiotics might also be taken to clear up any infection.

- Diabetic ulcers – People with diabetes are prone to losing the sensation of pain in their feet and so can easily damage the skin without knowing it. Huge infected ulcers can occur and these may be impossible to heal.

WHEN TO SEE YOUR DOCTOR

If you notice unusual skin changes on your legs you should bring them to the attention of your doctor. If your doctor suspects a leg ulcer, you may be referred to a specialist for a Doppler scan – a type of ultrasound scanning – to assess the blood flow in the affected leg.

TREATMENT OPTIONS

Most ulcers are slow to heal and have a tendency to recur. Treatments vary and include the following:

- Venous ulcers – Your doctor will treat your varicose veins in order to prevent ulcers from forming. Once an ulcer has formed, it can take weeks or months of regular high-compression bandaging and leg elevation to ease or heal it. Skin grafts may occasionally be used as a way of healing the ulcer.
- Ischaemic ulcers – An operation to bypass a blockage to the leg arteries may improve the circulation, but these ulcers heal poorly, are prone to infection and can be very painful. To prevent large ulcers developing further the affected leg may be amputated below the knee.
- Diabetic ulcers – If ulcers on the feet are severe, amputation may be the only cure, although this treatment will only be considered as a last resort.

CORNS AND CALLUSES

These patches of thick, hardened skin occur at points of abnormal pressure on the skin and the commonest cause is ill-fitting shoes. Once a corn or callus is formed it is unlikely to settle without treatment, and will probably need to be removed by a chiropodist.

Maintaining good leg and foot health (keeping skin soft and supple, and gentle exercise to improve circulation) is likely to be beneficial for people with diabetes and circulatory disease, in order to prevent the formation of ulcers.

▽ Taking care of your legs and feet can help prevent leg sores and ulcers, and problems such as corns and calluses, especially if you suffer from diabetes or circulatory diseases.

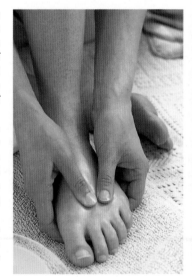

13

BLOOD AND THE IMMUNE SYSTEM

Your blood contains red and white blood cells, plasma and platelets, creating a very efficient system for supplying oxygen and nutrients, getting rid of waste products, fighting infection and healing wounds. The latter two functions mean that the blood is a major component of our immune system – how the body protects itself from illness. Another component of our immunity "machinery" is the network of nodes, vessels and organs that make up the lymphatic system. This system defends the body and also returns our watery tissue fluid to the blood. Closely linked, the blood and lymphatic systems work together to promote optimum health. Problems range from anaemia caused by low red cell counts to cancers of the lymph nodes.

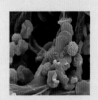

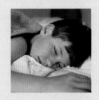

CONTENTS

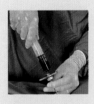

The roles of blood and lymph

Blood is the body's internal transport system. It flows constantly around the body, supplying oxygen and nutrients to the tissues and removing carbon dioxide and waste products. Important signalling chemicals – such as hormones – and dissolved minerals travel in the bloodstream and help to keep the body's internal environment in perfect balance. Vitally important to the circulation is the lymphatic system, which removes excess fluid, or lymph, from the tissues and plays a crucial role in the immune system – the body's defence against foreign invaders.

The average person has 5–6 litres (8½–10½ pints) of blood in their bodies and in a drop of blood the size of a pinhead there are several million red blood cells.

WHAT IS BLOOD?

Blood is a mixture of cells floating in a straw-coloured fluid called plasma. Most blood cells are made in the bone marrow and some white blood cells are made in the spleen and thymus gland.

Plasma is 90 per cent water. Water-soluble substances dissolve in it and are transported to their destination. Substances dissolved in the plasma include:

• Food – Products of digestion such as glucose and fats are taken round the body for use as fuel.

• Waste products – These include carbon dioxide and urea.

• Hormones – These chemical messengers are secreted into the blood and travel to their site of action.

• Proteins – These include the vital clotting factors and antibodies.

• Minerals – Such as sodium, calcium and potassium, vital to body function.

Water-insoluble substances travel around by being bound to a protein called albumin.

FIGHTING FOREIGN INVADERS

Your body is constantly under attack by microbes – potentially harmful invaders. The blood, lymphatic system, specialized cells, antibodies and various organs all work together as an immune system to deal with threats each second of every day.

The lymphatic system includes lymphatic vessels, lymph nodes and lymph fluid. As well as removing excess fluid from the tissues, lymph filters out microbes and triggers the immune response in the lymph nodes – home to disease-fighting white cells called lymphocytes.

RECOGNIZING INVADERS

Special cells and chemicals within the immune system are able to recognize invading microbes:

• You are constantly exposed to infectious agents such as bacteria and viruses. Your immune system deals with the attack, but also remembers the attacker so that it can fight back even more effectively next time.

• Cell division and growth is not infallible and thousands of abnormal, potentially cancerous cells are made every day. The immune system usually recognizes and destroys these cells.

HOW BLOOD CLOTS TO HEAL A WOUND

▽ Your body has an elaborate clotting system that plugs any leaks in the blood vessels. Small leaks are plugged by clumps of platelets. For leaks that are too large to plug, the platelets initiate a cascade of chemical reactions so that a clot is formed to seal the injury. Sometimes the clotting system fails (as in haemophilia), or it may work too well, blocking healthy blood vessels and causing possible heart attacks.

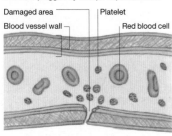

Damaged area | Platelet
Blood vessel wall | Red blood cell

1 As soon as a blood vessel is damaged, it narrows to reduce blood flow. Platelets nearby are activated to become sticky and clump together to plug the damaged area.

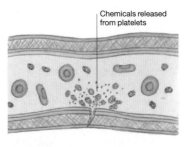

Chemicals released from platelets

2 Chemicals are released from damaged tissue and clumped platelets. These set off a chain reaction involving the blood's clotting factors, each one setting off the next.

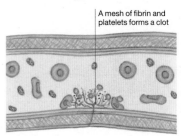

A mesh of fibrin and platelets forms a clot

3 Plasma contains a dissolved protein called fibrinogen. Clotting factors cause fibrinogen to form strands of fibrin, which mesh and trap blood cells to form a clot.

THE LYMPHATIC SYSTEM

▷ This system comprises a network of nodes connected by vessels, plus other organs and tissues. One role of the system is to fight infection, via white blood cells. The other is to return any of the watery fluid (lymph) that has drained into the lymphatic vessels back to the bloodstream. The nodes contain concentrations of white cells, and the major collections of nodes lie at the neck, armpits and groin.

Axillary (armpit) nodes
All the nodes filtering lymph from the arms and breast are concentrated here.

Heart

Liver
This organ plays a crucial role by acting as a "sieve" for toxins entering the body via the digestive tract, which it then destroys. It also produces many of the blood-borne chemicals controlling the destruction of foreign particles.

Inguinal (groin) nodes
This large collection of nodes filters lymph from the legs and pelvis.

Bone marrow
Antibodies made here by white cells stick to foreign proteins (antigens) on the surface of invading organisms and label them for destruction. (Note that red blood cells are also made in the bone marrow.)

Lymph vessels
Lymph circulates through a network of vessels. It passes from the body's tissues into small lymphatic capillaries and from there into larger vessels called lymphatics.

This artwork has been designed to show the different elements of the lymphatic system clearly, and it is therefore not to scale.

Cervical (neck) nodes
These lymph nodes can often be felt as they enlarge to fight infection. A protective ring of lymph nodes around the throat comprises the tonsils and adenoids.

Subclavian veins
Lymph from the whole body drains into the heart via these veins, and so returns to the bloodstream.

Thymus gland
This produces mature T-cell lymphocytes, which fight viruses and parasites.

Spleen
This large, fragile organ produces all types of lymphocytes and nestles under the lower ribs on the left. It is home to many white cells that produce antibodies. People who have had their spleen removed need particular vaccines and antibiotics to protect them from infections.

Intestines
This collection of lymph tissue is in an area exposed to the outside world – the digestive tract – and so is more prone to attack by bacteria.

BLOOD CELLS

Red blood cells
These doughnut-shaped cells are full of the chemical haemoglobin, which carries oxygen to cells around the body. Haemoglobin gives cells their red colour.

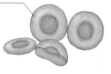

Lymphocytes

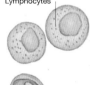

White blood cells
These cells play a vital role in your immune system. Some – the lymphocytes – produce antibodies to alert your body to foreign invaders while others – the phagocytes – destroy debris and bacteria.

Platelets
These tiny blood cells are vital for blood-clotting and for repairing injuries.

Phagocytes

PROBLEMS WITH THE SYSTEM

Sometimes, the immune system over-reacts, producing allergies. "Immunodeficiency" diseases arise when the immune system fails in some way. The system may also attack the body's tissues, such as joints, giving rise to "autoimmune" diseases. Problems can often arise with organ transplantation, as the immune system may see the organ as an "invader" and attack it.

ENLARGED LYMPH NODES

You may notice your glands (especially in the neck) are enlarged, this may be due to:
• Most commonly, a response to infection.
• Invasion by cancerous cells; as part of the body's drainage system, lymph nodes receive fluid from all parts of the body and are a common place for cancers.
• Development of cancers of the lymphatic system (lymphoma).

BOOSTING IMMUNITY

Vaccination is a way of protecting people against infectious diseases. Vaccines, which are usually given by injection, are weakened or dead micro-organisms that prompt the immune system to produce antibodies to fight a disease. People may also be given ready-made antibodies.

Anaemia

SEE ALSO

➤ Haemolytic anaemia, below

➤ Macrocytic and Microcytic anaemia, p451

➤ Sickle cell anaemia, p452

Anaemia describes a group of conditions in which there is a lower-than-normal count of red blood cells (and so less of the oxygen-carrying pigment haemoglobin) in the blood. Anaemia is classified by the size and appearance of the red blood cells. The common types of anaemia are haemolytic, macrocytic and microcytic, and they share similar symptoms, including fatigue and weakness. People suffering from illnesses such as angina may find they are more likely to have attacks if they are also anaemic. A good supply of oxygen in the blood is essential to good health.

SIGNS AND SYMPTOMS

Symptoms include the following:

➤ Tiredness.

➤ Headaches.

➤ Faintness.

➤ Pale skin.

➤ Breathlessness following exercise.

➤ Palpitations (patients with anaemia often have high heart rates).

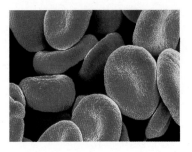

△ Red blood cells get their colour from haemoglobin, an oxygen-carrying protein. Anaemic people have a shortage of these cells.

INVESTIGATING ANAEMIA

Several routine investigations are used to diagnose anaemia:

➤ Full blood count check, which gives numbers of all the cell types.

➤ A blood film test, which examines the red blood cells' colour and shape.

➤ A test to check for low levels of vitamin B_{12} and folic acid.

➤ A test to estimate the body's stores of iron.

➤ A reticulocyte count to measure how many young cells the bone marrow is producing.

There are three main causes of anaemia:
1 Not enough red blood cells being made.
2 Red blood cells being lost from the body at an abnormal rate by slow, chronic bleeding, as with heavy menstrual periods or gastrointestinal bleeding.
3 Red blood cells being destroyed faster than they can be produced.

Haemolytic anaemia

SEE ALSO

➤ Anaemia, p450

The normal lifespan of a red blood cell is 120 days. In haemolytic anaemia, this lifespan is severely shortened as red blood cells are destroyed faster than normal. There are several reasons for this, and the condition can be inherited.

SIGNS AND SYMPTOMS

As well as the common symptoms of anaemia, the patient may be jaundiced, due to abnormally high levels of bilirubin, the breakdown product of haemoglobin. The spleen may enlarge as it is the main site of red cell destruction and in this condition is working harder than usual.

CAUSES OF HAEMOLYTIC ANAEMIA

• Inherited disorders of the cell surface membrane; and disorders of cell contents e.g haemoglobin in sickle cell disease.
• Other inherited disease (see box, right).
• Reactions to blood transfusions.
• Drugs, for example antimalarial drugs.
• Burns.
• Infections such as malaria.
• Mechanical heart valves.

SPHEROCYTOSIS

Hereditary spherocytosis is the commonest inherited haemolytic anaemia. A defect in the red blood cell membrane means that, as the cells pass through the spleen, part of the cell membrane is lost and they become spherical rather than doughnut-shaped. The cells can no longer travel through the spleen and so die.

Macrocytic anaemia

SEE ALSO

➤ Eat healthily, p262
➤ Anaemia and Haemolytic anaemia, p450
➤ Microcytic anaemia, below

In macrocytic anaemia, the red blood cells are larger and paler than normal. These defective red cells are known as macrocytes and they most commonly arise because of a vitamin deficiency – of either vitamin B_{12} or folic acid. Both of these vitamins are essential for the efficient formation of red blood cells in the bone marrow. There may be number of reasons for these deficiencies and these include a poorly balanced diet, too much alcohol, or intestinal problems that mean nutrients are not absorbed properly by the body.

SIGNS AND SYMPTOMS

As well as general anaemia symptoms, this may produce signs such as nervous system dysfunction (B_{12} deficiency) or a sore tongue (folic acid deficiency).

VITAMIN B_{12} DEFICIENCY

The main cause of vitamin B_{12} deficiency is a disease known as pernicious anaemia, in which the cells of the stomach, where B_{12} is absorbed, are destroyed (an autoimmune disease). Pernicious anaemia is more commonly found in people over 60, and in women. It is important that it is treated because it can result in irreversible degeneration of the brain and the spinal cord. B_{12} deficiency can also occur in patients who have undergone a gastrectomy (removal of part or all of the stomach).

FOLIC ACID DEFICIENCY

A lack of folic acid (also known as folate) can result in macrocytic anaemia. Folate deficiency can be caused by:

• A diet low in fresh vegetables.
• Alcohol abuse, because it interferes with folic acid absorption.
• Pregnancy, because larger quantities are needed for the healthy development of the fetus.
• Drugs, such as anticancer and anti-convulsant drugs.

TREATMENT OPTIONS

If anaemia is due to B_{12} deficiency, injections of B_{12} are given. Folic acid deficiency is treated with folic acid tablets.

Microcytic anaemia

SEE ALSO

➤ Anaemia, p450

This form of anaemia is characterized by small, pale red cells. The most common cause is a deficiency of iron, an essential component of haemoglobin. Unfortunately, diets are often deficient in iron. Certain foodstuffs can also interfere with absorption.

SIGNS AND SYMPTOMS

As well as the general symptoms of anaemia, microcytic anaemia can cause brittle, spoon-shaped nails, a smooth, painful tongue and brittle hair.

CAUSES OF IRON DEFICIENCY

• Blood loss – In women this is commonly due to heavy menstrual periods, made worse by the fact that iron-rich red meat is now less popular. Iron deficiency in men is also due to blood loss, usually caused by diseases in the gut or kidney.

• Increased demand for iron – this occurs most commonly while the body is still growing and developing, and during pregnancy.
• Eating iron-poor foods; a problem with some vegetarians and vegans.
• Decreased iron absorption from the intestine.

WHAT MIGHT YOUR DOCTOR DO?

Test results confirm microcytic anaemia when they reveal red cells that are small and pale, and levels of iron that are lower than normal. Your doctor will investigate causes of blood loss and ask about your diet.

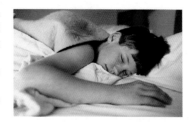

△ In most forms of anaemia, tiredness can be one of the symptoms.

Most people with anaemia can correct the condition by taking an iron supplement, although in very severe cases a blood transfusion may be required.

Sickle cell anaemia

SEE ALSO
➤ Anaemia, p450
➤ Bone marrow
   transplant, p454

Normal haemoglobin – the substance that carries oxygen around the body inside red blood cells – comprises a haem unit within four globin chains (two alpha and two beta). If the globin structure is abnormal, it can affect the oxygen-carrying capacity of the blood and cause this serious form of anaemia. An inherited condition, sickle cell may first appear very early in life and occurs most commonly in the populations of Africa, India, southern Europe and the Middle East. Sufferers have episodic "crises", where even a simple infection can bring on a life-threatening illness.

THE GENETICS OF SICKLE CELL ANAEMIA

Hb A is the gene responsible for normal haemoglobin; the abnormal haemoglobin gene is Hb S. All is well if an individual inherits an Hb A gene from both parents. Someone inheriting two Hb S genes, one from each parent, will have sickle cell anaemia. Inheriting an Hb S gene from one parent and an Hb A from the other means that you are a carrier of sickle cell trait but do not have the full-blown condition.

Sickle cell anaemia sufferers may feel fine most of the time, but are prone to serious health "crises". In general, these episodes start suddenly and last from a few hours to several days. They may come on seemingly for no reason or be prompted by a variety of factors, such as:

SICKLE CELL ANAEMIA AND MALARIA

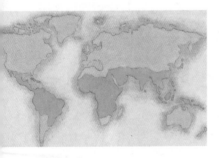

△ The sickle cell condition has one advantage: it protects against the malaria parasite. This means that it is much more common where malaria is endemic (red on the map above).

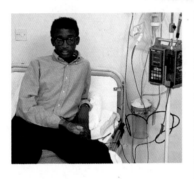

△ In severe sickle cell anaemia, regular blood transfusions are carried out to boost the levels of normal haemoglobin in the blood.

• Cold.
• Dehydration.
• Lack of oxygen (e.g. if at high altitudes).
• Infections.

These factors can cause red blood cells to change from their normal doughnut shape to a sickle shape and clump up, causing a range of severe symptoms (see box, right).

DIAGNOSIS AND TREATMENT

To confirm a diagnosis, you may have blood tests – a full blood count, a blood smear analysis and haemoglobin electrophoresis.

Avoiding the triggering factors is the main method of preventing a sickle cell crisis. A blood transfusion may be given to correct anaemia and may be carried out before major surgery so that the level of abnormal Hb S is reduced. Drugs to boost levels of Hb F, another form of haemoglobin that resists sickling, can be useful, although these are not yet widely available. Transplants of normal red cell-producing cells from the bone marrow of close relatives are another alternative. In the future, gene therapy may be possible, to replace the abnormal haemoglobin gene.

SIGNS AND SYMPTOMS

The abnormal red blood cells are destroyed by the spleen, and this can lead to the development of anaemia – causing fatigue, pale skin and shortness of breath on exertion. Sickle-shaped cells are inflexible and may block small blood vessels. This leads to symptoms including the following:

➤ Bone pain – the most common symptom.

➤ Breathing difficulties.

➤ Priapism in men, a painful persistent erection of the penis that can destroy the penis if left untreated.

➤ Abdominal pain, due to spleen and liver damage.

➤ Strokes and fits if vessels in the brain are blocked.

➤ Blood in the urine, due to kidney damage.

THE OUTLOOK

In the long term, people with sickle cell anaemia can suffer from recurrent infections, leg ulcers, gallstones, bone destruction (particularly of the femur) and blindness. Sufferers and carriers are also advised to seek counselling if they are thinking about having children.

Thalassaemias

SEE ALSO
➤ Anaemia, p450
➤ Sickle cell anaemia, p452

In this condition, production of the globin element of haemoglobin is abnormal. Instead of producing alpha and beta globin chains in equal amounts, someone with thalassaemia fails to make enough of one of these chains. Too few alpha chains causes alpha-thalassaemia, but the most common form is beta-thalassaemia, in which there are few or no beta chains. As with sickle cell anaemia, the signs and symptoms may be evident from childhood. Some forms need little or no treatment, but others may require blood transfusions.

SIGNS AND SYMPTOMS

In mild forms of the disease there may be few symptoms. In more severe cases, signs appear from the age of four to six months. Symptoms may include:

➤ Severe anaemia, causing pale skin, shortness of breath and abdominal swelling due to an enlarged spleen and liver.

➤ Susceptibility to infections.

➤ Bony deformities, particularly of the face, develop as the bone marrow expands to try to produce enough haemoglobin.

TREATMENT OPTIONS

Mild forms need no treatment. Severe cases require lifelong regular blood transfusions, which unfortunately overload sufferers' bodies with iron. To get rid of this excess, drugs are given that bind to the iron, so that it passes out in the urine and doesn't damage the liver, pancreas and heart.

THE STRUCTURE OF HAEMOGLOBIN

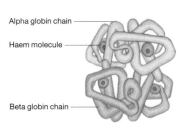

Alpha globin chain

Haem molecule

Beta globin chain

△ Normal haemoglobin has two alpha and two beta globin chains around a haem molecule.

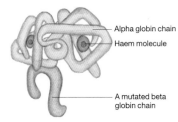

Alpha globin chain

Haem molecule

A mutated beta globin chain

△ Beta-thalassaemia haemoglobin looks very different and causes symptoms of this disease.

Haemophilia

SEE ALSO
➤ How blood clots, p448

Someone with this condition lacks an essential clotting factor in their blood. There is usually a family history of this rare disease. Abnormally severe bleeding can occur after injury or surgery, or spontaneous bleeding may even occur during ordinary daily activities.

SIGNS AND SYMPTOMS

Symptoms depend on the individual and the severity of the condition, but include:

➤ High susceptibility to bruising.

➤ Painful swelling of muscles and joints, due to internal bleeding.

➤ Prolonged bleeding after minor injury.

➤ Blood in the urine.

Haemophilia is a bleeding disorder caused by a deficiency in clotting factor VIII. The condition most commonly affects men, and women are carriers of the condition.

In order to confirm a diagnosis of haemophilia, your doctor will take a sample of blood to send to a laboratory for tests which will include a full blood count, blood film and blood clotting tests.

People with haemophilia are treated with injections of factor VIII. This used to be obtained from donated blood plasma but is now produced using genetically modified yeasts and is known as recombinant factor VIII. Those with mild haemophilia can have levels of their own factor VIII boosted using a drug called DDAVP.

Other rare bleeding disorders include Christmas disease, that is caused by a lack of factor IX, and von Willebrand's disease, in which a factor, that carries clotting factor VIII, called von Willebrand's is missing.

Acute leukaemias

SEE ALSO
➤ The roles of blood and lymph, p448
➤ Bone marrow biopsy, p457

These rare cancers of the white blood cells fall into two types. Acute lymphoblastic leukaemia (ALL) involves lymphocytes and tends to affect children. Acute myelogenous leukaemia (AML) affects a white blood cell called a myeloblast and occurs more often in adults. Acute leukaemia generally develops quickly, whereas chronic leukaemia tends to progress fairly slowly. People suffering from acute leukaemias may find they need regular blood and platelet transfusions. A bone marrow transplant will be considered if chemotherapy alone is unlikely to lead to cure.

SIGNS AND SYMPTOMS

The symptoms of leukaemia are caused by bone marrow failure, where normal marrow is infiltrated and replaced by cancerous cells, and include:

➤ Symptoms of anaemia – pale skin, shortness of breath, fatigue.

➤ Repeated infections.

➤ Bruising or bleeding.

➤ Occasionally, lymph node, liver and/or spleen enlargement.

In leukaemia, blood test results show low numbers of normal red blood cells, white blood cells and platelets, and may also show the presence of characteristic cancerous white blood cells. The blood tests carried out will include:
• A full blood count.

▽ Leukaemia treatment reduces the effectiveness of the immune system; here, a mother wears a mask to protect her child against infection.

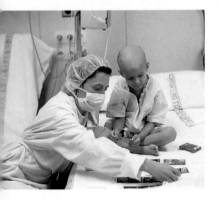

• Bone marrow biopsy (taking a sample of bone marrow tissue).

TREATING ACUTE LEUKAEMIAS

The treatment of these conditions is divided into general treatments and treatment specific to the type of leukaemia. General treatments include:
• Blood and platelet transfusions.
• Rapid treatment of any infection with intravenous antibiotics.

Specific treatments for each form of leukaemia are evolving and improving all the time. The mainstay approaches are chemotherapy (drug treatment to kill the cancerous cells) and bone marrow transplantation. Specific treatments for each form include:
• Acute myelogenous leukemia (AML) – This potentially curable disease can be treated with multidrug chemotherapy. Recurrences of the disease are also managed with chemotherapy, but usually with less success.
• Acute lymphoblastic leukaemia (ALL) – This most commonly affects children. It is also potentially curable through the use of a variety of chemotherapy drugs. Ninety per cent of patients respond to this treatment and 50 to 60 per cent are cured by it. Treatment is usually continued for two to three years. If ALL recurs, it tends to do so in the bone marrow, in which case a bone marrow transplant can be life-saving. Particular drugs can be injected into the spinal fluid to reduce the effects on the nervous system.

BONE MARROW TRANSPLANT

First, the patient's cancerous bone marrow is destroyed using high doses of radiation or chemotherapy and is then replaced by bone marrow from either a close relative or a matched donor. The patient receives bone marrow as an infusion into the bloodstream. Destroying the bone marrow leaves patients vulnerable to infection, bleeding and anaemia, so they are isolated until they start to produce new bone marrow. After the transplant, the patient has to take powerful immunosuppressant drugs, to control rejection of the bone marrow and also to prevent graft-versus-host disease, in which the new bone marrow attacks the recipient's body tissues.

▼ A bone marrow transplant may be the best treatment for a leukaemia sufferer. Here, a doctor harvests genetically compatible bone marrow from a donor; the bone marrow will then be filtered and infused into the recipient's bloodstream.

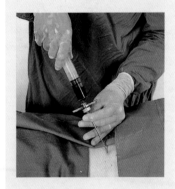

Chronic leukaemias

SEE ALSO
➤ Anaemia, p450
➤ Acute leukaemias, p454
➤ Myeloma, p456

These white blood cell cancers usually affect adults and, as with acute leukaemias, there are two types – chronic lymphocytic leukaemia (CLL) and chronic myeloid leukaemia (CML). CLL is the most common leukaemia in the world. Chronic leukaemias can be slow to show any symptoms, beginning only with fatigue but gradually showing more definite signs. The exact cause of the chronic types of leukaemia is not yet known, although radiation, some viruses and industrial chemicals have all been connected with the disease.

SIGNS AND SYMPTOMS
Most people with chronic leukaemias have no symptoms, and this may be the case for several decades with CLL. Symptoms can include:

➤ Signs of anaemia – pale skin, shortness of breath, fatigue.

➤ Recurrent infections.

➤ Bleeding.

➤ Enlarged lymph nodes.

➤ Abdominal swelling, due to an enlarged liver and spleen.

➤ Fever and night sweats.

In chronic leukaemia, too many white blood cells are made in the bone marrow. The two different forms of chronic leukaemia reflect the different types of white cell that are affected. In CLL, too many lymphocytes are produced; in CML, it is granulocyte cells.

The first sign for many sufferers is simply feeling tired. However, over a period of time, the spleen gradually enlarges and eventually begins to cause pain in the abdomen. The patient may notice that they have lost weight and begin suffering from nose bleeds or aching in the bones. They may also find they sweat a great deal and are more sensitive to hot conditions than usual.

MAKING THE DIAGNOSIS
All types of leukaemia are progressive, and chronic leukaemias show signs only very gradually. Elderly people – who form the majority of those affected – should seek medical advice as soon as symptoms are apparent. As with acute leukaemias, your doctor will diagnose the condition by undertaking a full blood count to check the levels of red and white cells in the blood.

TREATMENT OPTIONS
There are several treatments, depending on the type of chronic leukaemia, including:
• Chronic lymphocytic leukaemia (CLL) – Most patients are asymptomatic for many years and only require treatment if they develop symptoms. Many patients are treated with supportive measures, such as blood transfusions, and may survive for over ten years after diagnosis. Infection is the commonest eventual cause of death.
• Chronic myeloid leukaemia (CML) – The disease often starts in a mild form that produces few symptoms for three or four years. It may develop into an acute

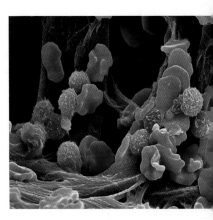

△ These are blood cells taken from a patient with chronic lymphocytic leukaemia. In this condition, too many white blood cells known as lymphocytes (shown here in purple) build up in the body. No one understands why this occurs.

leukaemia, which can be difficult to treat. Life expectancy used to be approximately five years but advances in drug therapy have increased survival times for this disease, and bone marrow transplants may be curative in younger patients.

▽ Chronic leukaemias are most common in elderly people.

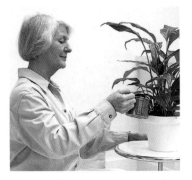

HAIRY CELL LEUKAEMIA
Occurring most often in middle age, this rare leukaemia causes bone marrow failure. Its name relates to the appearance of the cells on a blood film. Symptoms include those of anaemia, recurrent infection and abdominal pain (due to an enlarged spleen). Hairy cell leukaemia responds well to, and is often cured by, a drug called 2-CDA.

Myeloma

This bone-marrow cancer involves a type of antibody producing white blood cell known as a plasma cell. In this condition, these cells produce large amounts of an abnormal antibody known as paraprotein, some of which (Bence-Jones protein) may be excreted in the urine.

Myeloma is a disease that affects elderly people; the average age of sufferers is about 60. The disease can systematically destroy the bone marrow and bones. Treatment options vary but they are aimed at minimizing symptoms rather than effecting a cure and survival rates are poor.

SIGNS AND SYMPTOMS

Common symptoms include:

➤ Bone pain – most commonly backache.

➤ Anaemia – pale skin, fatigue and shortness of breath.

➤ Kidney failure – feeling unwell, infrequent urination and jaundice.

➤ Bleeding – due to low platelet levels.

Myeloma has several characteristics:

• Bone destruction – The bones of the spine are often affected, leading to collapse and fractures. This may compress the spinal cord and so trap nerves, causing weakness of various parts

▽ As myeloma systematically destroys the bones, one of its most common symptoms is bone pain, often in the form of backache.

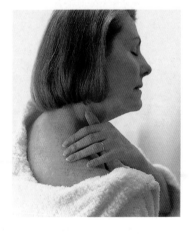

of the body, depending on which nerves are compressed.

• Raised blood calcium levels – The destruction of the bone releases calcium into the bloodstream (hypercalcaemia).

• Bone-marrow destruction – This leads to anaemia and low levels of platelets and white blood cells.

• Kidney damage – This is due partly to excretion of excess antibodies, and partly due to hypercalcaemia.

Patients with myeloma are also susceptible to recurrent infections.

WHAT MIGHT YOUR DOCTOR DO?

Your doctor will arrange a series of tests to confirm the diagnosis and help decide on suitable treatment. Tests include:

• Full blood count – Myeloma is suggested if the results reveal anaemia, low white blood cell count or low levels of platelets.

• Kidney function tests – The results may be abnormal and may show high blood calcium or uric acid levels.

• Electrophoresis – The Bence-Jones protein can be detected through a process called electrophoresis, which is where blood proteins are separated in a gel by using electricity.

• X-rays – Various X-rays may show bony deposits that point to myeloma; these are most easily detected in the skull.

• Urine tests – These are often able to detect the fragments of antibody called Bence-Jones protein.

• Bone marrow biopsy – The tissue sample taken in a biopsy may show infiltration by cancerous cells.

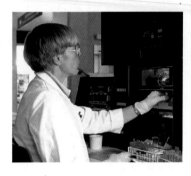

△ A full blood count test is one of the ways of diagnosing myeloma. Here, a technician uses a Coulter counter to measure the sizes of red, white and platelet cells in a blood sample.

TREATMENT OPTIONS

All symptoms are treated appropriately. For example, bone pain usually responds well to radiotherapy, and research shows that raised calcium levels can be reduced using drugs called bisphosphonates. Steroid drugs are also used to relieve the symptoms of bone deposits. Kidney dialysis may be the only treatment option for patients who suffer from kidney failure.

Certain chemotherapy agents have increased the long-term survival of myeloma patients, and new drug regimens show signs of further improvements.

WHAT IS THE OUTLOOK?

Until recently, few people diagnosed with myeloma lived much longer than six or seven months, and for a shorter time if they had complications such as anaemia and kidney failure. Now, myeloma sufferers without complications may survive up to two to three years and possibly longer.

Bone marrow disorders

SEE ALSO

➤ Heart disease, p282
➤ Anaemia, p450
➤ Acute leukaemias, p454
➤ Chronic leukaemias, p455

Bone marrow fills the inside of many of the bones of the body – those of the arms and legs, sternum (breastbone), shoulderblades, pelvis and ribs. Bone marrow produces stem cells that become red blood cells, white blood cells and platelets. When the bone marrow fails to perform this essential task, severe problems may arise, as the correct balance of these cells is vital for efficient functioning of the blood system. The bone marrow disorders covered here include: aplastic anaemia, polycythaemia, myelofibrosis and myelodysplasia.

APLASTIC ANAEMIA

This causes symptoms of anaemia, recurrent infections and bleeding. All cells made by the bone marrow are reduced in number. In half the cases no cause is found, but other common causes include:

- Chemotherapy drugs and occasionally sulphonamide drugs.
- Radiotherapy.
- Pregnancy.
- Chemicals such as benzene.
- Infections, such as measles, tuberculosis and hepatitis.

The outlook for aplastic anaemia is poor. Some patients' bone marrow will recover over time, but recurrent infections can prove life-threatening. Blood transfusions and antibiotics may be used to prevent and treat anaemia and infection. When the bone marrow fails to recover, a bone marrow transplant may correct the problem.

POLYCYTHAEMIA

In this condition there are too many red cells in the blood. The blood becomes significantly thicker, which may cause

BONE MARROW BIOPSY

Bone marrow diseases can be confirmed by taking a sample of bone marrow tissue (biopsy) and analysing it under a microscope. A sample is usually taken from the posterior iliac crest of the pelvis or the sternum (breastbone). Biopsies are carried out to diagnose leukaemias and are swift, safe procedures.

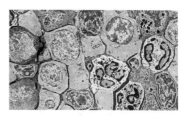

▷ This coloured micrograph shows the three different types of blood cell that are produced in the bone marrow: red blood cells, platelets and some white blood cells.

blood clots and thus strokes, and so some patients have blood removed from their circulation every week until red cell levels return to normal.

NATURAL ADAPTATIONS

Polycythaemia occurs naturally in people who live at high altitudes, in order to compensate for lower levels of oxygen in the air. It can also arise in people with chronic lung or heart diseases, as their bodies try to increase the amount of oxygen in their blood. Smoking is a common cause.

Symptoms of polycythaemia include:
- Ruddy complexion and bloodshot eyes.
- Headache.
- Ringing in the ears.
- Blurred vision.

MYELOFIBROSIS

Here, the bone marrow is replaced by scar tissue. Anaemia and bleeding disorders may develop, as the marrow fails to make enough red cells and platelets. Tiredness and weakness are common symptoms. The cause is unknown, and blood transfusions and drugs are used to control the symptoms.

MYELODYSPLASIA

This failure of the stem cells that produce red cells causes severe anaemia. About 30 per cent of sufferers eventually develop acute myelogenous leukaemia. Myelodysplasia usually affects the elderly and is treated with blood transfusions and/or chemotherapy. In young patients, a bone marrow transplant can be a successful treatment.

BONE MARROW LOCATIONS

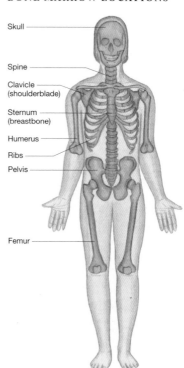

Skull

Spine

Clavicle (shoulderblade)

Sternum (breastbone)

Humerus

Ribs

Pelvis

Femur

Lymphomas

SEE ALSO

➤ Heart disease, p282

➤ Disorders of the liver, p302

➤ The roles of blood and lymph, p448

This general term refers to any cancer of the immune system's lymphoid tissues – principally the lymph nodes and spleen. These tissues produce the white cells that help protect our bodies against invading organisms. There are two main kinds of lymphoma. The type that displays classic abnormalities is called Hodgkin's lymphoma. All other kinds are grouped together under the term "non-Hodgkin's lymphoma". Most lymphomas cause enlargement of the lymph nodes. Rarely, cancer may develop in an organ, such as the thyroid gland, testis or breast.

SIGNS AND SYMPTOMS OF HODGKIN'S LYMPHOMA

➤ Pain-free swelling of lymph nodes in the neck or armpits.

➤ General malaise, fever, night sweats, poor appetite and weight loss.

➤ General itchiness.

➤ Pain after drinking alcohol (rare).

Lymphomas are divided into low- and high-grade, according to how fast they divide and grow. Paradoxically, the aggressive high-grade lymphomas are all potentially curable while the low-grade diseases often resist treatment.

INVESTIGATING LYMPHOMAS

You may undergo the following tests:

• Full blood count – The results may show anaemia, high white blood cell counts and low platelet levels.

• Kidney and liver function tests – Affected lymph tissue within these organs can affect their function.

• Chest or abdominal X-rays or CT scans – Abnormal masses may be seen.

▽ A surgeon carries out a lymph-node biopsy. The sample is then tested for cancerous cells.

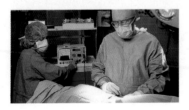

• Lymph node biopsy – This can detect cancerous cells in a sample of tissue.

• Uric acid test to reveal significantly raised levels in the blood.

HODGKIN'S LYMPHOMA (HODGKIN'S DISEASE)

This is a rare condition, affecting men more than women. Usually seen between the ages of 15 and 30 and 55 and 75, it is especially common in later life. Modern treatment has made this condition curable in most cases. The cause is unknown, though the Epstein-Barr virus is a possible link.

TREATMENT OPTIONS

Treatment consists of radiotherapy and/or chemotherapy, repeated over several sessions. The therapy will depend on the distribution and extent of the disease.

NON-HODGKIN'S LYMPHOMAS

This refers to a family of lymphomas – basically any lymphoma that is not Hodgkin's disease. These cancers usually affect those over 50. Each lymphoma in this family represents a cancer of one particular type of B- or T-type white blood cell.

BURKITT'S LYMPHOMA

First identified in West African children, this non-Hodgkin's lymphoma usually affects the jaw. The vast majority of people affected by this lymphoma, particularly children, can be treated successfully with chemotherapy.

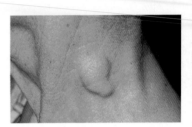

△ This swelling in a patient's neck is caused by an enlarged cancerous lymph node – in this case from a non-Hodgkin's lymphoma.

Again, the exact cause of these conditions has not yet been established, although it is possibly the result of a malfunctioning immune system, and various viruses, including the Epstein-Barr virus, have also been implicated.

TREATMENT OPTIONS

Lymphomas may be slowed by radiotherapy. Powerful anti-cancer drugs are used – chemotherapy – if the cancer has spread. A bone marrow transplant may be necessary.

SIGNS AND SYMPTOMS OF NON-HODGKIN'S LYMPHOMAS

➤ Pain-free swelling of lymph nodes in the neck or groin.

➤ Fever, night sweats, fatigue, weight loss, poor appetite.

➤ Abdominal swelling, enlarged spleen, or enlarged liver.

There may be different symptoms, if the cancer spreads to other organs.

Autoimmune diseases

SEE ALSO

➤ Raynaud's disease,
p289

➤ Diabetes, p314

➤ Rheumatoid arthritis,
p362

Rheumatoid arthritis and diabetes are common examples of autoimmune diseases, in which the body's immune system attacks normal body tissue for reasons as yet unknown. Autoimmune conditions are often seen in young adults and it seems that women are more commonly affected than men. Symptoms for the different types of autoimmune disease can vary, but any and all should be investigated as early as possible. The severity of the symptoms and the outlook also varies greatly depending on which parts of the body are affected.

The term autoimmune disease covers a range of conditions in which areas of tissue become inflamed, causing a variety of problems. The inflammation arises when autoantibodies attack the tissue, seeing it as "foreign" matter that must be destroyed.

LUPUS ERYTHEMATOSUS

This condition, often called simply lupus, causes inflammation in various parts of the body. One form, discoid lupus, usually attacks the skin only. A more severe type – systemic lupus erythematosus, or SLE – may strike just about any part of the body, from the skin and joints to internal organs and membranes ("systemic" conditions are those that affect the whole body). In most sufferers, a few organs are affected at the same time.

Lupus is characterised by the production of autoantibodies that target genetic material, but why this occurs is unknown. The general outlook for sufferers is good

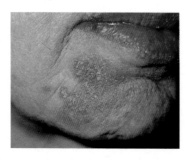

△ The skin rash associated with lupus erythematosus often appears on the face and neck and consists typically of red patches with grey-brown scales.

and symptoms can be controlled by taking corticosteroid drugs for joint inflammation and painkillers. Symptom-free periods do occur. There is usually a family history of the disease and it is rarely found in people outside the 12 to 55 age bracket.

SYSTEMIC SCLEROSIS

Also known as scleroderma, which means "hard skin", systemic sclerosis affects the body's connective tissue (any type of tissue that helps to hold together the body's form and organs). Affected tissues become inflamed, thickened and hardened, and also tighten up. Symptoms may be confined to the skin and joints but the condition can also affect internal organs. Signs of systemic sclerosis may be mistaken for other conditions – for example the joint discomfort is often thought to be rheumatoid arthritis. The disease is most commonly found in people between the ages of 20 and 50, and affects four times more women than men.

SIGNS AND SYMPTOMS OF SYSTEMIC SCLEROSIS

Symptoms depend on the severity and spread of the condition and include:

➤ Fingers that are particularly sensitive to the cold (as in Raynaud's phenomenon).

➤ Small areas of hardened skin on the fingers.

➤ Swollen, painful joints.

➤ Muscle weakness.

➤ Difficulty swallowing, due to stiffening of the oesophagus.

There is as yet no cure. The outlook can be good if the skin alone is affected, but is harder to tackle if organs such as the heart, lungs or kidneys are implicated. However, in many people – thankfully – the disease progresses very slowly.

▽ In systemic sclerosis, the immune system turns against the body, causing a hardening of connective tissue. It may affect just one or several parts of the body.

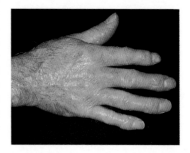

SIGNS AND SYMPTOMS OF SYSTEMIC LUPUS ERYTHEMATOSUS

Symptoms vary greatly from one person to another, and depend on which organs are affected, but they may include:

➤ Joint pain.

➤ Fever.

➤ Fatigue.

➤ Skin rashes, often a butterfly-shaped rash on the face.

POLYMYOSITIS

This is a rare condition where the skeletal muscles become inflamed and painful. Other characteristics can include a red rash on the skin (usually on the face, chest and the backs of the hands), and if this occurs it is known as dermatomyositis.

Polymyositis usually settles down well following treatment with steroid drugs, but unfortunately it can be associated with certain cancers, including those of the lung, ovary, breast and stomach.

The outlook is much more hopeful for children with this disease than it is for adults, with 70 per cent of children recovering in around two years.

SIGNS AND SYMPTOMS OF POLYMYOSITIS

➤ Weak muscles.

➤ Fatigue.

➤ Difficulty swallowing and speaking, due to the oesophagus being affected.

➤ Shortness of breath, as the chest muscles become affected.

POLYMYALGIA RHEUMATICA

Another relatively rare condition, this inflammation of tissues causes aching and stiffness in the neck, shoulders, hips and lumbar spine. Symptoms of polymyalgia rheumatica tend to be worst first thing in the morning but usually wear off after a few

SIGNS AND SYMPTOMS OF POLYMYALGIA RHEUMATICA

➤ Aching and morning stiffness in the muscles of the neck, shoulders and hips. The torso and lower back can sometimes be affected too.

➤ Fatigue.

---

hours. There may also be tiredness, fever and weight loss. It almost always affects people over 50.

Diagnosis can be fairly straightforward because a blood test will show signs of inflammation. The condition often occurs together with temporal arteritis. Steroid treatment is usually successful in reducing inflammation, although steroids may need to be taken for several months. The condition tends to recur.

TEMPORAL ARTERITIS

This condition most commonly affects elderly people and causes an inflammation of the arteries in the temples at the sides of the head. It often develops in association with polymyalgia rheumatica.

As with polymyalgia rheumatica, diagnosis will usually be confirmed with a simple blood test, and sometimes by testing a sample taken from one of the temporal arteries. Treatment usually involves high-dose steroid drugs in the first instance; once the symptoms start to subside, the dose is gradually reduced over a period of months. However, this condition does have a tendency to recur.

▽ Many autoimmune disorders, such as polymyalgia rheumatica and temporal arteritis, are common in elderly people. They generally affect more women than men.

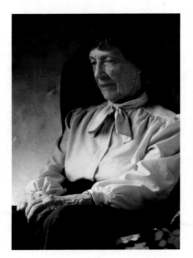

SJÖGREN'S SYNDROME

This chronic condition damages the glands that produce tears and saliva, causing dry eyes and a dry mouth. Nine times more women suffer from this condition than men and it affects people in the 40–60 age group. It is very commonly associated with rheumatoid arthritis. There is no cure but people with this condition use artificial tears, and drinking plenty of fluids can be helpful. A dry mouth may lead to dental problems, so regular check-ups are recommended.

▽ In Sjögren's syndrome, the salivary glands are unable to produce saliva, causing a dry tongue.

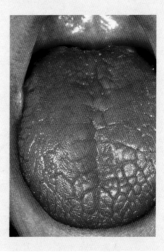

SIGNS AND SYMPTOMS OF TEMPORAL ARTERITIS

➤ Localized headache usually over the temple, which may be very tender to the touch.

➤ Fatigue.

Any visual disturbance, whether temporary or permanent, should be reported to your doctor as a matter of urgency because if this condition is left untreated, it can cause blindness.

14

INFECTIOUS DISEASES

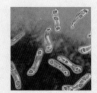

Humans pick up, incubate and pass on infectious diseases every day. Many infections are caught from droplets in the air produced by coughing and sneezing and so are difficult to avoid – just think how many people suffer from the common cold every year. However, your immune system is designed to deal effectively with infections – viral or bacterial – and they often pass with little more than a cough, sneezing, a runny nose and general malaise. Some infectious diseases, however, can be highly dangerous, particularly for very young children or the elderly, so an understanding of the different types and the issues involved can prove invaluable.

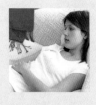

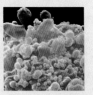

Causes of infectious disease

SEE ALSO

➤ Travel health, p274

➤ CJD, p339

➤ The roles of blood and lymph, p448

➤ Protection against infection, p472

A vast range of tiny pathogens – disease-causing micro-organisms – are able to infect your body and cause all kinds of problems, from a mild cold to life-threatening malaria. An infection may be localized, where it affects only one part of your body, or systemic, which means that it affects the whole body. Infections can be spread in water or food, through touch or sexual contact, in the air and by insects. These micro-organisms also have the ability to change and adapt in order to outwit medication, so controlling them is a constant battle.

Invading micro-organisms, commonly called "germs", can be classified broadly into several distinct groups – bacteria, viruses, protozoa, and fungi and yeasts. Your body can also be invaded by larger, more complex organisms, such as worms and lice; these are often referred to as "infestations" rather than infections.

BACTERIA

Bacteria are microscopic organisms consisting of one cell. They are able to multiply (by division) very rapidly and are found everywhere – all around us and inside our bodies. There are, in fact, more bacterial cells inside us than body cells. Most bacteria are harmless and many are beneficial – bacteria in our large intestine help us to

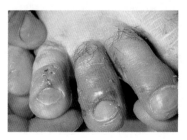

△ Athlete's foot is a fungal infection that causes irritation and inflammation of skin on the feet – typically between and on the toes.

digest and absorb certain food substances, for example. Of the thousands of different types of bacteria that exist, only a handful cause disease in humans. In some cases bacteria disrupt the normal working of cells themselves, while in others they release toxins that do the damage. Bacteria come in various shapes, which can be broadly grouped as:
• Cocci (spheres).
• Bacilli (rods).
• Spirochaetes (curved or twisted forms).

Common bacterial infections can include tuberculosis, pneumonia, meningitis and urinary tract infections.

FUNGI AND YEASTS

Fungi that cause disease tend to fall into two groups – filamentous fungi and single-celled yeasts. Yeasts resemble human cells (which is why they are used in genetic engineering, to produce copies of human substances such as insulin). They tend to cause only mild diseases such as skin infections but they can prove deadly in people with a reduced immune system, such as people suffering from AIDS or those receiving a transplant.

Fungal infections include thrush (candidiasis), which can be vaginal or oral and can be treated with antifungal medication.

VIRUSES

These powerful organisms are made up of simple protein packets containing a few strands of genetic material. They are so tiny that millions of viruses could fit inside one human cell. Viruses bind to animal and plant cells and use these cells' own machinery to replicate themselves. In this process the host cell is destroyed, resulting in disease. Because viruses interfere with the

▽ The common cold is the most frequent, and usually one of the mildest, viral infections. Avoid spreading the virus through the air by covering your mouth as you cough or sneeze.

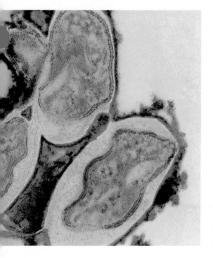

▽ *Mycobacterium tuberculosis* is the rod-shaped bacteria that causes tuberculosis in humans. It has become resistant to many drugs.

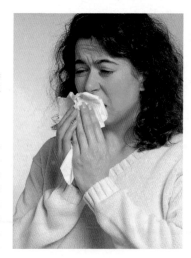

genetic structure of cells, many viruses have been implicated as factors that may lead to cancer. They have a great ability to dodge the defences of the immune system and can lie dormant for years.

Viruses cause diseases that range from relatively mild problems – the common cold or an upset stomach – to very severe and often fatal conditions, which include ebola, rabies and HIV.

PROTOZOA

A protozoan is a single-celled organism that scavenges food from other micro-organisms. They live mainly in moist environments such as soil and water but some can live inside creatures, such as the parasitic protozoan that causes malaria, which is found inside mosquitoes.

Common protozoal infections include malaria, sleeping sickness and toxoplasmosis.

PARASITIC WORMS, MITES AND LICE

These creatures live in close contact with one another and cannot live without their hosts. This is why the most advanced parasites do not kill their host.

Common parasitic worm and lice infestations are tapeworm, pinworm, scabies and head lice.

▽ Head lice are a common problem in schools as they are easily spread when an infested child is in close contact with other children.

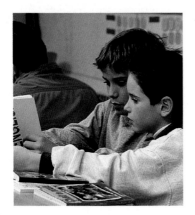

CONTROLLING INFECTION

Until the last 60 or so years, infectious diseases killed huge numbers of people all over the world; the very young and the elderly being particularly vulnerable. The spread of infectious diseases has been greatly controlled in recent times, thanks to better hygiene, cleaner water and pest control. Other vital factors that have made a significant difference to fighting infectious disease are widespread vaccination programmes and the use of drugs – antibiotics, antivirals and antifungals.

➤ Immunization – For many infectious diseases, especially viral ones, this is the only treatment available. Vaccines work by prompting and boosting the immune system to deal with a specific pathogen so that, next time around, it can deal with the infection more effectively.

➤ Antibiotics – The treatment of bacterial infections was revolutionized by the discovery of penicillin. This antibiotic was first made generally available to allied troops in the Second World War. Other antibiotics quickly followed and their ability to deal with infectious disease was dramatic – formerly fatal diseases were cured in a few days. Unfortunately, some bacteria have developed resistance to certain antibiotics. New drugs continue to be developed, but doctors are concerned that they won't always be able to keep a step ahead in the battle against bacteria, and many are now more cautious in prescribing antibiotics for routine illnesses.

➤ Antiviral drugs – A few viral infections, such as herpes or HIV, can be controlled by drugs, but on the whole there is no treatment for viral illness other than trying to support the patient as they fight off the infection. Vaccines are still the best weapons against viral disease.

➤ Other drugs – These are used against pathogens such as parasites, fungi and yeasts. Unlike an antibiotic, which may defeat a range of bacteria, each of these drugs is usually efffective against just one particular pathogen.

▽ Immunization is one of the most effective ways to prevent infection, by boosting the immune system to fight specific pathogens.

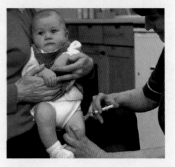

PRIONS

These unusual pathogens are protein particles without any DNA or RNA (genetic material). For reasons that are presently unknown, prions are able to replicate themselves rapidly, damaging surrounding body cells in the process. The term prion stands for proteinaceous infectious particle, and was suggested by Stanley Prusiner – who isolated the particle – to demonstrate that this was not a virus.

Prions are responsible for many diseases of the brain. The most notable being the new variant Creutzfeldt-Jakob disease (vCJD) in humans, which is the equivalent of bovine spongiform encephalopathy (BSE) in cows.

Other diseases assigned to prions include fatal familial insomnia, which usually starts to affect people in middle age and causes worsening insomnia, memory loss, speech defects, muscle spasms and general physical and mental deterioration.

Prions are resistant to heat and all forms of sterilization and so can be passed around in contaminated food. Currently, there is no treatment available for diseases caused by prions.

Bacterial infections

SEE ALSO
➤ Meningitis, p332
➤ Urinary tract infections, p390
➤ Bacterial skin infections, p444

In the past, bacterial infections were a major cause of death all over the world. Since the advent of antibiotics, however, even the most serious bacterial infections can often be dealt with quickly and effectively. There are numerous bacterial infections that can attack the body, including tetanus, diphtheria and tuberculosis, most of which are now rare in developed countries because of long-standing and effective vaccination programmes. If a bacterium causes disease by releasing a powerful toxin, specific antitoxins can be prescribed.

PERTUSSIS

Also known as whooping cough, pertussis is caused by the bacterium *Bordetella pertussis*. It is highly contagious and is spread through the air in droplets formed by coughing and sneezing. It tends to occur in epidemics every few years, although most children under two are now vaccinated and so cases are rare.

Pertussis can occur at any age, although it is mainly found in children under the age of five. As with many bacterial and viral infections, its occurrence in adulthood can be much more severe.

The incubation period for the infection is seven to ten days, and in the initial catarrhal stage the patient is highly infectious. The early symptoms are tiredness, lack of appetite, a runny nose and

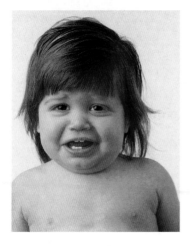

▽ Pertussis, or whooping cough, most commonly affects young children. It is highly contagious and can be very distressing.

streaming eyes – symptoms very similar to those of the common cold.

As the infection progresses, however, it reaches a paroxysmal stage, so-called because of the paroxysms (bouts) of coughing that characterize this disease. A run of coughing as the child breathes out is followed by a large intake of breath, often causing the typical whooping sound. Vomiting may follow. This distressing stage can last for two weeks and may lead to serious complications as it affects the ability to breathe properly.

If caught in the first stage, an antibiotic can abort or reduce the severity of the disease. There is no effective treatment, however, once the cough starts, and often the only thing to do is wait for the infection to run its course.

TETANUS

In this disease, a powerful neurotoxin made by the bacterium *Clostridium tetani* attacks the nerves and causes muscle spasm. It occurs when these bacteria (which live in soil and in the intestines of humans and animals) contaminate a wound. In

SIGNS AND SYMPTOMS OF PERTUSSIS

➤ Tiredness and loss of appetite.

➤ Symptoms as for the common cold.

➤ Severe and prolonged coughing, followed by a sharp intake of breath.

➤ Vomiting.

DIPHTHERIA

A toxin made by the bacterium *Corynebacterium diphtheriae* causes diphtheria. Typical symptoms are:

➤ A sore throat.

➤ Fever.

➤ Swelling of the throat and larynx, which can block the airway.

Diphtheria may also affect the heart, causing inflammation of the heart muscle (myocarditis), and the brain, again causing inflammation (encephalitis).

Most people recover completely if treated promptly with antibiotics and antitoxin injections. Prevention is the best approach, however, via vaccination.

It is thanks to vaccination that diphtheria is now uncommon in developed countries, although it is on the increase in Eastern Europe and Russia. It is vital to keep vaccination levels up to prevent recurrence of this serious disease.

▽ The bacteria *Corynebacterium diphtheriae* – the cause of the dangerous condition diphtheria. Fortunately it is now uncommon in the developed world.

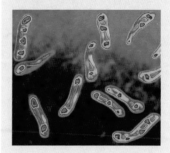

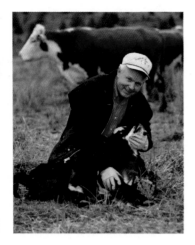

△ Tetanus bacteria thrive in soil and animal intestines, so farmers are particularly at risk – these bacteria are easily passed to humans.

developed countries, tetanus often occurs in elderly people who have injured themselves while gardening.

The toxin causes muscle spasm, particularly of the jaw muscles, hence tetanus's familiar name of "lockjaw". Other symptoms of the disease may include a high fever and headache, along with a characteristic grinning facial expression called *risus sardonicus*. The muscle spasm can also affect the muscles of the larynx, bladder and chest, which can be extremely dangerous because it affects the efficient functioning of these organs.

Occurrences of the disease used to be far more common than they are now, and 60 per cent of cases were fatal. This has been massively reduced to 20 per cent with the

widespread use of antibiotics, antitoxins and, most importantly, good nursing care.

Immunization is the key to preventing cases of tetanus. All children in developed countries now have a course of three tetanus injections followed by regular boosters. Adults need a booster at least every ten years, but those most at risk, such as farmers, should have boosters every five years.

TUBERCULOSIS

This disease is caused by *Mycobacterium tuberculosis*, which is a slow-growing bacterium that causes a chronic infection. Tuberculosis is often rife among people who live in substandard social conditions in poorer parts of the world. In the world's richer countries, improvements in food, sanitation and housing over the past 50 years or so have led to significant reductions of tuberculosis cases. However, since 1985 there has been an increase in cases of tuberculosis worldwide, and this is possibly because the disease is becoming resistant to antibiotics, and may also be due to the rising prevalence of HIV and AIDS because so many more people are vulnerable to this type of infection.

Infection with *Mycobacterium tuberculosis* often causes only a mild illness with fever and cough, although this may persist for many weeks and produce a greenish-yellow sputum, but more severe cases can be dangerous. Tuberculosis bacteria are spread from person to person in airborne droplets in coughs and sneezes. Once a case has been detected, it is vital to trace and screen any contacts the patient may have had, in order to prevent the start of an epidemic. The infection can lie dormant for many years and reactivate itself long after the initial illness.

Fortunately, tuberculosis is readily treated nowadays, although it often needs treatment with multiple antibiotics for many months. It is also partially prevented with the BCG vaccine, which many people receive during adolescence. The efficiency of this vaccine depends on latitude – with 94 per cent protection in higher latitudes of

SCARLET FEVER

Scarlet fever bacteria (*Streptococcus pyogenes*) are spread by airborne droplets in coughs and sneezes. The red rash, which often develops after a throat infection, mainly affects the face and hands. It spreads rapidly and skin layers may peel away. The tongue may have a white coating with red spots (strawberry tongue). One week of antibiotic treatment usually clears it up.

▽ Scarlet fever rash is caused by toxins produced by the offending bacteria. The rash may spread all over the body.

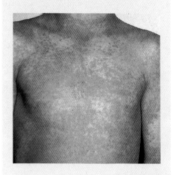

the globe to 0–20 per cent of the population near the equator.

Tuberculosis usually focuses on the lungs but it can spread to affect many different parts of the body, including the brain, the bones, the digestive tract and the skin.

Doctors use a chest X-ray to diagnose the disease but may also take a sputum sample to culture the bacterium.

SIGNS AND SYMPTOMS OF TETANUS

➤ Fever.

➤ Headache.

➤ Muscle spasms, particularly in the jaw.

➤ A grinning facial expression.

➤ Stiffness of the limbs.

SIGNS AND SYMPTOMS OF TUBERCULOSIS

➤ Fever.

➤ Persistent cough.

➤ Greenish-yellow sputum, or sputum streaked with blood.

➤ Night sweats.

➤ Weight loss.

Viral infections

SEE ALSO

➤ Viral encephalitis, p333
➤ Hepatitis, p411
➤ Sore throat and tonsillitis, p423
➤ Viral skin infections, p445

Most of the everyday infections you pick up will be viral – from a cough and cold to bouts of diarrhoea. Treatment for such conditions is usually supportive, which means it is aimed at managing the symptoms while your immune system conquers the viral attackers. Supportive treatment involves painkillers, bedrest and plenty of fluids. Sometimes, an antiviral drug is available to kill a particular virus, but on the whole your body's immune system does all the work. Common viral infections include chickenpox and measles.

CHICKENPOX

The virus *Varicella zoster* causes chickenpox. It is spread through the air and by contact with the characteristic skin blisters. The infection usually occurs in childhood and confers lifelong immunity. The disease is much more severe in adults who did not have it as children, and so it is important to

∇ A chickenpox rash is made up of small, itchy red spots which turn into fluid-filled blisters. Calamine lotion can be used to soothe irritation.

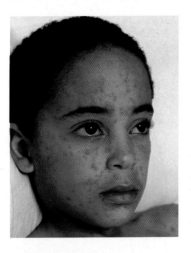

SHINGLES

Shingles is caused by the chickenpox virus. Most people have chickenpox in childhold, and then the virus usually lies dormant in the nerves of the spinal cord. Sometimes it reactivates to produce shingles – pain along a nerve and a skin rash following the line of the nerve. There may be fever, headache and malaise too.

keep infected children away from public places. Pregnant women are vulnerable to chickenpox, which could damage the fetus, and so should seek medical help if they may have been exposed to the virus.

The course of the disease takes two to three weeks from incubation to recovery. It often begins with fever, malaise and headache. A red blistering rash develops all over, even inside the mouth in many cases, and the red spots quickly fill with fluid and crust over. Children must be kept isolated until all the blisters have dried up.

Rarely, chickenpox can cause a severe form of pneumonia and viral encephalitis. Children usually require no specific treatment, but in people over 16 and in those with a reduced immune system, antiviral drugs may be used.

RUBELLA

Also known as German measles, this viral infection produces a mild illness in children. In adults, the disease can be more serious.

SIGNS AND SYMPTOMS OF CHICKENPOX

➤ Headache.

➤ Fever.

➤ Malaise.

➤ Itchy red rash all over the body, which develops into fluid-filled spots.

SIGNS AND SYMPTOMS OF RUBELLA

➤ Fever.

➤ Mild malaise.

➤ A fine red rash all over the body.

There are rarely any complications in children but unimmunized pregnant women are particularly vulnerable to this infection. Rubella can cause congenital rubella syndrome in a woman's developing baby, resulting in various complications including heart malformations, cataracts, mental retardation and deafness. There is no treatment for these malformations once the infection has developed, so it is vital to prevent outbreaks of this disease via vaccination. Rubella vaccine is now combined with those for measles and mumps in the MMR vaccine.

It can be spread through airborne droplets produced while sneezing or coughing. The incubation period (the time after infection before symptoms develop) of the rubella virus is two to three weeks.

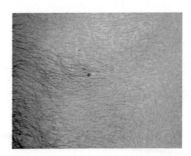

▷ A rubella rash consists of tiny red spots. Rubella is most dangerous if it affects pregnant women in the first four months of pregnancy.

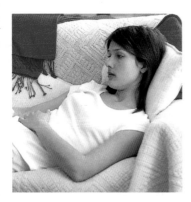

△ Listlessness and fatigue are often the longest lasting symptoms of glandular fever.

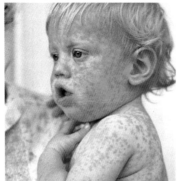

△ A measles rash appears first on the face and then spreads over the body.

GLANDULAR FEVER

Also known as infectious mononucleosis, this disease is common worldwide among adolescents and young adults. It is caused by the Epstein-Barr virus and is transmitted by saliva (hence its nickname, "kissing disease") and via small droplets in the air.

Infection causes swollen lymph nodes (commonly known as glands) and a sore throat (making it difficult to swallow), along with fever, headache and malaise. These symptoms appear weeks after the initial infection and develop over several days. Once established, symptoms last for a few weeks.

Glandular fever may produce a rash and an enlarged spleen. Furthermore, the person may have a poor appetite and lose weight. Some people can be debilitated for months and become depressed. To confirm the disease, your doctor tests a blood sample for the presence of antibodies against the virus.

There is no specific treatment for glandular fever and supportive treatments are usually all that is required. Almost everyone makes a full recovery and one attack provides lifelong protection. However, a lengthy illness can prove disastrous for some, especially young athletes and those about to sit examinations.

MEASLES

The measles virus causes a serious infection in children. One child in 500 with the disease will die. In developed countries, occurrence is rare due to vaccination, but the number of cases rises when parents stop getting their children vaccinated after scares about the vaccine leading to various illnesses.

The virus passes from person to person in the air, carried in droplets of water, and is contagious from four days before until two days after the rash develops. In the initial phase the symptoms include fever, malaise and a cough. Characteristic grey patches with a red base (known as Koplick's spots) may appear in the mouth. A widespread, non-itchy red rash then develops, initially on the face but spreading to other parts of the body.

In healthy children there are usually no complications, but serious complications can occur in those with other diseases, including pneumonia, infection of the heart muscle (myocarditis) and inflammation of the brain (encephalitis). The measles virus does not cause fetal malformations but it can cause premature labour and abortion.

There is no specific treatment for measles. The best way is to avoid it altogether via vaccination.

MUMPS

This viral infection is now rarer, due to vaccination. The mumps virus is spread by sneezing and coughing and by skin contact, and affects mainly schoolchildren and young adults. Early symptoms of fever, malaise and headache are followed by painful swelling of one or both parotid salivary glands in the cheeks, causing a hamster-like appearance. Symptoms usually subside after two or three weeks. Mumps can have serious complications, including inflammation of the brain (encephalitis) and painful swelling of the testicles (epididymo-orchitis), which can cause sterility.

▽ The mumps virus causes swelling of the parotid glands in the angle of the jaws, resulting in red, swollen cheeks.

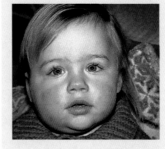

SIGNS AND SYMPTOMS OF GLANDULAR FEVER

➤ Swollen lymph nodes.

➤ Listlessness and fatigue.

➤ Headache.

➤ Fever.

➤ Rash.

➤ Sore throat.

SIGNS AND SYMPTOMS OF MEASLES

➤ Cold and fever.

➤ An angry red rash.

➤ Malaise.

➤ A cough.

➤ Conjunctivitis.

➤ Sneezing.

HIV and AIDS

The first cases of human immunodeficiency virus (HIV) infection were identified on the west coast of the US in 1981. The World Health Organization now estimates that there are about 40 million people worldwide infected with HIV. The parts of the globe that have been particularly affected are sub-Saharan Africa and the Indian subcontinent. The source of the virus is still not fully understood but, like many tropical viral illnesses, it is believed to have developed first in apes and then to have been transmitted to humans.

It took some years after the first cases of this new and aggressive disease before the virus was identified and medical experts began working on treatments and possible cures. In that time, before many people were even aware of it, the number of cases rose dramatically. Today, awareness of the disease and how it is contracted is so widespread that the incidence should have dropped, but this appears not to be the case. Precautions should always be taken when having sexual intercourse with any partner who has not been tested for HIV or AIDS.

In the US, Canada and the UK, HIV is most commonly transmitted during sex between homosexual men and via shared needles in intravenous drug-users. There are, however, increasing reports of new cases among heterosexual men and women, which may be due to changes in the virus and to increases in sexual promiscuity amongst younger people. In sub-Saharan Africa and India, where HIV has reached epidemic proportions, the patterns of transmission are different and it is most commonly transmitted via heterosexual sex.

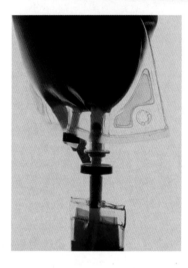

△ Blood that is used for transfusions is screened for HIV, among other things, to ensure there is no danger of the virus being transmitted.

HOW IS HIV TRANSMITTED?

The HIV virus can be found in blood, semen, vaginal secretions and breast milk. The known modes of transmission for the HIV virus are:

• Sexual intercourse (vaginal, anal and oral) – The most common mode of transmission worldwide is vaginal intercourse but in the US, Canada and the UK, HIV is more commonly spread among gay men.

• Contaminated blood and blood products – Before compulsory screening was introduced for donated blood, after the virus had been identified in 1981, thousands of people with haemophilia became infected with HIV. Routine screening in many countries has made this much rarer.

• From mother to child – Transmission can occur either in the womb via the placenta, during birth or through breastfeeding.

• Contaminated needles – Intravenous drug-users often share needles; this route to infection is a common one in the US and Europe.

• Needlestick injuries – Healthcare workers can become infected with HIV if they accidentally injure themselves on a needle contaminated with HIV-positive blood from a patient.

There are a number of less common ways of becoming infected. For example, some cases are believed to have been contracted when a tattooist used the same needle for several customers.

SIGNS AND SYMPTOMS OF THE ONSET OF AIDS

Deterioration of the immune system causes symptoms that vary in each case and which may signal AIDS:

➤ Oral thrush.

➤ Recurrent vaginal thrush.

➤ Recurrent herpes infections.

➤ Intermittent fever.

➤ Weight loss.

➤ Diarrhoea.

➤ Muscular aches and pains.

SIGNS AND SYMPTOMS OF HIV

Initial infection may cause minor illness or none at all. These early symptoms can typically include:

➤ Flu-like symptoms.

➤ Generalized lymph node enlargement.

➤ Fatigue and dizziness.

WHAT HIV DOES TO THE BODY

HIV infects and eventually destroys particular white blood cells, which reduces the efficiency of the body's immune system. Once the virus starts to destroy these white blood cells, then the door to illness opens.

HIV infection typically progresses through three stages. In the first stage, when a person has just been infected, the virus starts to reproduce rapidly. Some people experience flu-like symptoms for a week or two at this time; others have no symptoms at all. During this early phase, blood tests may well not reveal the presence of antibodies to HIV – which is how doctors can tell whether someone is HIV-positive. It usually takes some weeks (in a few cases, up to a year) after infection before the antibodies reach a detectable

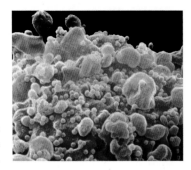

△ This electron micrograph shows white blood cells that have been infected with the HIV virus – the virus is shown in green.

level. At this stage, the immune system is still generally effective but there may be an increasing susceptibility to infections.

In stage two of the HIV cycle, there is an asymptomatic (showing no symptoms) period. This may last for around ten years. Further deterioration in the immune system generally follows, due to falling levels of white blood cells. This increases the chance of developing more serious and potentially life-threatening illnesses, often called "AIDS-defining conditions". An HIV-positive person who develops any of these conditions has reached the third stage – full-blown AIDS (acquired immunodeficiency syndrome). At present, most HIV-positive people go on to develop AIDS, but a few do not, and they may provide clues as to how the disease can be beaten in the future.

MANAGEMENT OF HIV AND AIDS

Although there is no cure for HIV infection or AIDS, treatment has been transformed over the past ten years by the development of a number of antiviral drugs capable of significantly delaying the progression of this condition. Anyone who is diagnosed with the HIV virus will usually be prescribed these HIV-protease inhibitor drugs. They reduce the ability of the virus to replicate itself in human cells and slow down the process of deterioration. Several have been proven to work and others are currently being investigated and tested.

PREVENTING HIV INFECTION AND AIDS

As there is no vaccine available for HIV at present, prevention is currently based on education and changing behaviour patterns to take on board the following:

➤ Using condoms during sexual intercourse.

➤ Treating other sexually transmitted infections to reduce genital ulceration.

➤ Always using clean needles and syringes for intravenous injections.

➤ Screening blood and blood products. (This has been in place in the West since 1985.)

➤ Taking part in confidential HIV screening followed by specialist advice on how to limit transmission of the infection to others.

These drugs are usually administered in combinations of three drugs on an indefinite basis. A number of other medications may also be taken – in order to prevent various bacterial, fungal and viral infections from taking hold and causing complications. Someone suffering from HIV will probably need to take these drugs for the rest of their life, but we have seen that life-expectancy can be greatly extended through their use.

Drug treatment and public health programmes have decreased the number of HIV-related deaths in the US, Canada and parts of Europe, but in countries that are unable to afford such treatments, the number of deaths continues to rise rapidly.

Awareness and understanding of HIV and AIDS has grown as people realize that it cannot be transmitted through the air or via normal contact with infected people. However, many still seem unaware of the real dangers of this disease and do not take preventative measures seriously. Educating people is key to preventing the worldwide spread of this virus.

COMMON AIDS-DEFINING CONDITIONS

Infections:

➤ Pulmonary tuberculosis.

➤ *Pneumocystis carinii* pneumonia.

➤ Systemic toxoplasmosis.

➤ Systemic cytomegalovirus.

Tumours:

➤ Kaposi's sarcoma.

➤ Non-Hodgkin's lymphoma.

Neurological disease:

➤ Dementia.

▽ Skin lesions such as this – known medically as Kaposi's sarcoma – are a common symptom of AIDS.

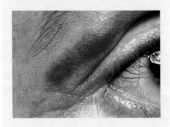

Malaria

Malaria is a disease that is widespread throughout the tropics, and it is caused by a group of parasites that colonize the red blood cells and the liver. These parasites (protozoa) belong to the *plasmodium* group and there are four subtypes that infect humans – *p. falciparum,* *p. malariae, p. ovale* and *p. vivax.* Each causes a slightly different illness and needs particular treatment. The most serious form of the disease is *falciparum* malaria. The parasites are carried by mosquitoes, which pass them on to humans when they bite them to suck their blood.

SIGNS AND SYMPTOMS

The symptoms are caused by the parasite multiplying inside red blood cells, often destroying them in the process. Symptoms usually start ten days to six weeks after being bitten and infected. The symptoms include:

➤ Intermittent high fever.

➤ Anaemia – with fatigue, pale skin and headache.

➤ An enlarged liver or spleen, with abdominal pain.

Malaria is a common disease in tropical countries and cases are increasingly found amongst travellers. It currently affects 250 million people and is fatal in around 1 per cent of cases. It is endemic in India, parts of Africa and Central and South America.

▽ This magnified image shows a red blood cell infected with the malaria parasite, which will eventually destroy it.

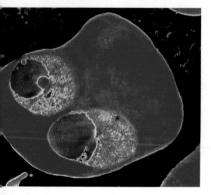

MALARIAL FEVER

The fever characteristically goes through three phases:

1 The "cold stage" – The patient feels cold and shivery despite having a high fever.

2 The "hot stage" – The patient feels very hot and may be delirious.

3 The "sweating stage" – The bedclothes may be drenched, but the patient feels better, although they will be very tired and may sleep for large parts of the day.

In most forms of malaria, the fever occurs every other day, can last for several weeks and has a tendency to recur.

In the most serious form – *falciparum* – the malarial fever is more severe and is usually continuous. During this time, the parasite kills large numbers of red blood cells. This form of the disease can be fatal within 48 hours. It can also damage the kidneys, liver, brain and gut, and may leave the patient permanently debilitated if they survive at all. In addition, it causes two unique complications:

• Cerebral (brain) malaria – This causes convulsions, coma and death.

• Blackwater fever – The large number of dead red blood cells causes the urine to become dark brown-black and can lead to kidney failure.

WHEN TO SEE YOUR DOCTOR

If you have recently visited a malarial zone and develop a fever shortly after returning home, see your doctor immediately.

Your doctor may suspect malaria if you have recently returned from a tropical country and have a fever. The diagnosis can be confirmed by laboratory examination of a blood sample, which will identify the presence of the malarial parasite.

The mainstay of treatment of this very serious illness is antimalarial drugs. Painkillers and drugs to reduce fever are also helpful. In severe cases, urgent hospitalization may be needed in order to treat the disease effectively.

PREVENTING MALARIA

One of the most effective ways to prevent malaria is antimalarial drugs. Seek medical advice on the most up-to-date recommendations for the country you intend to visit. It is also important to avoid being bitten (remember that mosquitoes are more active at night):

➤ Apply insect repellents at dusk.

➤ Sleep under a mosquito net.

➤ Wear light-coloured long-sleeved shirts and trousers in the evening.

▽ When travelling to countries where malaria is endemic, it is advisable to sleep under a protective net to avoid being bitten by mosquitoes.

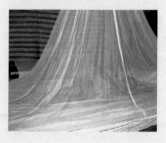

15

CHILDREN'S HEALTH

Children are vulnerable to infections and certain illnesses because their immune systems, along with all their other body systems, are still developing. They are also more likely than adults to suffer complications from diseases such as pneumonia. It is therefore important that parents monitor their child's illness, and consult a doctor if there are any unusual, severe or persistent symptoms. However, most children have an ability to bounce back to health with enviable speed, and many recurrent childhood problems – such as eczema and asthma – improve as a child gets older.

CONTENTS

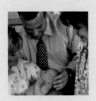

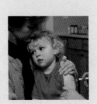

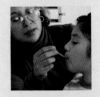

Protection against infection

SEE ALSO

➤ The roles of blood and lymph, p448

➤ Bacterial infections, p464

➤ Viral infections, p466

Infectious diseases used to be the most common cause of death in children and young adults. However, since doctors started using immunization – injecting vaccines, for example – to help our immune systems fight harmful invaders, infections such as meningitis, measles and tetanus are no longer widespread killers. A range of methods have been developed to boost the immune system, and if immunized early in life a child can be protected even before they are at risk from infection. Most immunizations are very safe and produce few side effects.

"Immunization" is a general term for the ways in which medicine can help the body prepare in advance to fight disease. Immunization is achieved by giving vaccines, typically by injection. These may be dead or weakened forms of disease-causing micro-organisms (bacteria or viruses), which stimulate the body to produce disease-fighting antibodies against that illness. In this way, the immune system is primed to recognize and defeat the micro-organism if the child encounters it at a later date. This method is also known as vaccination. (The other immunization method involves giving people actual antibodies, which provides shorter-term protection.) Vaccination can give your child

WHAT VACCINATIONS ARE CURRENTLY AVAILABLE?

National vaccination programmes may vary slightly but they tend to follow the schedule outlined below. Your doctor will advise you on the best specific schedule for your child.

Age	Vaccination
2 months	DTP, Hib, polio, meningitis C
3 months	DTP, Hib, polio, meningitis C
4 months	DTP, Hib, polio, meningitis C
12–15 months	MMR
4–5 years	DT, MMR
10–13 years	BCG

Key: D = Diphtheria; T = Tetanus; P = Pertussis; Hib = *Haemophilus influenzae* B; MMR = Measles, mumps and rubella; BCG = bacillus Calmette-Guérin for tuberculosis.

HOW ANTIBODIES FIGHT INFECTION

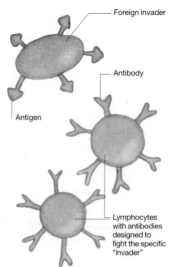

- Foreign invader
- Antibody
- Antigen
- Lymphocytes with antibodies designed to fight the specific "invader"

◁ ▽ Lymphocytes (a type of white blood cell) produce antibodies that fight infection. Specific antibodies "recognize" specific antigens (substances that form part of disease-causing micro-organisms) and so can destroy invaders.

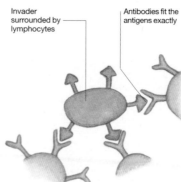

- Invader surrounded by lymphocytes
- Antibodies fit the antigens exactly

long-term protection from a range of infectious diseases that either cannot be treated or that spread so rapidly that treatment is inadequate.

A different vaccine is given for each disease, because the immune system produces specific antibodies to kill each invader. For most infections, several vaccinations are needed so that the immune system builds up and maintains a protective level of antibodies.

WHY VACCINATE?

Vaccination gives a significant level of protection against potentially fatal diseases. Many of these diseases still do not have an effective treatment, so vaccination may be the only way to protect your child.

Immunization can also help to eradicate the virus or bacterium from circulation. This is because, when the majority of

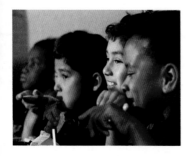

△ Immunization effectively protects your child against disease-causing micro-organisms, even if they come into close contact with a child who has already been infected.

children in a population are fully immunized, there are fewer potential carriers – if the virus or bacterium cannot spread it will gradually die out.

Smallpox, the first disease for which there was a vaccine, has been eradicated worldwide, and vaccination is no longer necessary. By contrast, cases of measles are becoming more common, because concerns over possible side effects cause some parents to decide against vaccinating their children.

SIDE EFFECTS OF VACCINATION

Most vaccines produce few side effects – the polio, diphtheria and tetanus vaccines are all extremely safe. Others – notably the MMR vaccine – are capable of causing very mild forms of the diseases they are designed to fight. Common side effects for all forms of immunization include the following:

• A mild fever for 24–48 hours after the immunization. This may be relieved by giving the child paracetomol syrup.
• A localized allergic reaction, causing redness, swelling and pain at the site of the injection. This usually subsides within days and has no lasting effect.

The MMR vaccine may cause the following side effects:

• A fever and a measles-like rash, which may occur one week after the vaccination.
• Swelling in salivary glands (the parotid glands which are just in front of the ears) up to three weeks after vaccination.

• Sore joints two to three weeks following the vaccination.

If a child falls ill after receiving a vaccination, it is worth remembering that the two events are not necessarily linked. Babies and children succumb to a large number of minor infections in the first years of life, and it is inevitable that some of these will coincide with a vaccination.

WHAT IS THE RISK OF SERIOUS SIDE EFFECTS?

Serious side effects are rare and are thought to occur in about one out of every 100,000 vaccinations. Severe reactions can take several different forms:

• A local allergic reaction may occur, in which an extensive area of redness and swelling spreads out from the site of the original injection.
• General reactions may include a high fever (39.5°C/103°F or above) that develops within 48 hours of the vaccination, severe irritability and/or convulsions.
• Rarely, a child may suffer a severe allergic reaction that can lead to anaphylactic shock. This can be fatal if emergency medical treatment is not provided.

The pertussis (whooping cough) vaccine carries a minimal risk of brain damage. However, the disease is more likely to

▽ This two-year-old girl is receiving her MMR vaccination, which will protect her against measles, mumps and rubella.

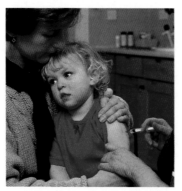

SAFE VACCINATION
Your child should not receive a vaccination if he or she:

➤ Is suffering from a severe illness with fever. Minor coughs and colds that are not accompanied by fever are not a problem.

➤ Has previously suffered a severe local or generalized reaction to a vaccination. Specialist medical advice should be sought in these cases.

The following factors should not stop your child having a vaccination (but you always discuss concerns with your doctor or health visitor):

➤ A family history of allergies or adverse reactions following vaccinations.

➤ A family history of convulsions.

➤ A family history of inflammatory bowel disease, such as ulcerative colitis or Crohn's disease.

➤ If a baby has been born prematurely.

➤ Neurological conditions such as cerebral palsy.

cause damage than the vaccine. Some people have suggested a link between MMR and autism, but this is not proven. Generally it is safer for a child to be vaccinated than not, and most people decide that the advantages of vaccination outweigh the risks. However, if you are worried, you should discuss your concerns with your health visitor or doctor. If your child develops any serious side effects after a vaccination, you should seek medical help immediately.

IS THERE AN ALTERNATIVE?

There are no proven and effective alternatives to the vaccination programme available now. Homeopathic medicines have been developed but there is no evidence that they provide children with significant levels of protection.

Colds and sore throats

SEE ALSO
➤ Colds and flu, p376
➤ The function of the ears, nose and throat, p414
➤ Hayfever, p420
➤ Sinusitis, p421

All children suffer from frequent colds and sore throats. A normal, healthy child may have at least five or six colds in a year, and more if he or she attends a nursery or has older brothers and sisters. Most colds and sore throats are caused by viruses and result in a relatively short episode of illness from which your child quickly recovers. Usually all that is needed is simple treatment to reduce fever and relieve other symptoms. Only if the child has a very high fever, symptoms such as a rash on the skin, or a headache is there usually any cause for concern.

SIGNS AND SYMPTOMS
A child with a cold or sore throat may feel reasonably well or they may have:

➤ Fever.

➤ Tired, heavy, aching feeling.

➤ Runny nose.

➤ Earache.

Colds and sore throats generally get better with supportive treatment such as:
- Painkilling syrup, such as paracetamol, to help to bring down a fever.
- Simple decongestants in the form of liquid drops for the pillow or a rub for the chest to relieve a blocked nose.
- Plenty of fluids to prevent the child from becoming dehydrated.

▷ Sponging with tepid water is a possible way to reduce a fever.

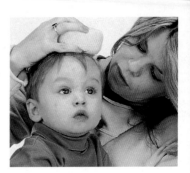

Earache in children

SEE ALSO
➤ Earache, p416

One of the most common childhood health problems is earache, which is usually the result of teething or an infection. Most earaches get better by themselves, but painkilling syrup can relieve discomfort. If the cause is a bacterial infection, antibiotics may be necessary.

Ear infections can damage hearing, so it is important that you take your child to the doctor if they have a persistent earache.

Most ear infections start in the throat and then travel via the Eustachian tube to the middle ear chamber. This condition, known as otitis media, is the most common ear infection suffered by children.

TYPES OF OTITIS MEDIA
In acute otitis media, the middle ear can become filled with infected secretions. The eardrum turns red and bulges out. It may rupture, which is a defensive reaction to allow the infection to drain, and there may a small amount of blood too. The earache often improves once the eardrum has burst and any perforation usually heals very quickly. Painkilling syrup relieves the pain.

Otitis media with effusion (glue ear) is a common cause of earache, but many children with this condition have no pain. The ear becomes filled with a thick, sticky secretion or "glue", often as a result of repeated viral infections. This fluid fails to drain via the Eustachian tube, which leads to temporary deafness. Repeated bouts of deafness can affect a child's speech.

Most cases of glue ear settle on their own, but an operation to drain the glue may be required. This operation consists of making a small hole in the eardrum and inserting a plastic tube – which is known as a grommet – to keep the hole open.

If a child suffers recurrent and severe earache, antibiotics are usually advised.

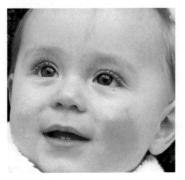

◁ Babies often develop earache when teething. Fever and vomiting may be the only symptoms.

Bronchiolitis

SEE ALSO
➤ Smoking and your health, p268
➤ The breathing process, p374
➤ Viral infections, p466

Bronchiolitis is an infection of the tiny airways (the bronchioles) in the lungs. It is usually caused by the respiratory syncytial virus (RSV), which is spread via coughing and sneezing. Bronchiolitis most commonly affects children during the first year of their lives, and may occur in epidemics during winter. Children living in overcrowded conditions or whose parents smoke are at greater risk. The condition can be serious: the airways may become inflamed, restricting breathing. If your child has difficulty breathing, urgent hospital treatment is required.

SIGNS AND SYMPTOMS

The typical symptoms of bronchiolitis include:

➤ An initial cold or sore throat.

➤ A dry cough.

➤ Wheezing.

➤ Rapid breathing.

➤ Difficulty in breathing.

➤ Difficulty in feeding.

You should consult a doctor if your child develops the symptoms of bronchiolitis. Mild cases can be managed at home with regular doses of painkilling syrup to control fever; sitting your child in a steamy bathroom can help to ease breathing. More serious cases need to be admitted to hospital for intravenous fluids, inhaled bronchodilator drugs and oxygen.

Many infants are prone to recurrent episodes of wheezing for a year or two after developing bronchiolitis. These usually occur when they have a cough or cold.

CROUP

This viral infection of the windpipe most often affects children of six months to three years. Typical symptoms are:

➤ A barking cough.

➤ Rapid, harsh and noisy breathing.

➤ Fever.

Sitting the child in a steam-filled bathroom often helps to relieve symptoms, but severe attacks require hospital treatment.

Pneumonia

SEE ALSO
➤ The breathing process, p374

Pneumonia is an inflammation of the air sacs (alveoli) within the lungs. It is caused by a viral or bacterial infection. The alveoli become inflamed and fill with white blood cells, which makes it harder for oxygen to cross into the blood vessels and circulation.

SIGNS AND SYMPTOMS

Pneumonia is a serious condition which causes the child to:

➤ Feel severely unwell.

➤ Look flushed and have a high fever.

➤ Have a persistent cough.

➤ Wheeze.

➤ Breathe rapidly.

➤ Breathe in so strongly that the spaces between the ribs are sucked in.

Young children are at greater risk of developing pneumonia than adults because their immune systems are not fully developed. They are also more likely to suffer life-threatening complications.

You should take a child with the symptoms of pneumonia to see a doctor immediately. Most children with pneumonia require hospital admission to treat the infection. They will usually start to improve rapidly once treatment with oxygen, intravenous antibiotics and fluids has been started.

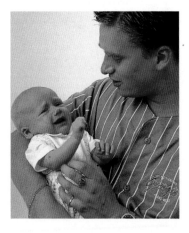

▷ A baby or child with pneumonia will usually appear flushed and will develop a fever.

Diarrhoea, vomiting and constipation

Children frequently suffer from bouts of diarrhoea and vomiting (often caused by gastroenteritis), and may also suffer from constipation. Most cases are straightforward and clear up in a matter of days. However, children suffering from vomiting or diarrhoea are at risk of dehydration because it is difficult for them to replace lost fluids quickly enough. It is therefore important that you encourage a child to drink during an illness. You should take your child to visit a doctor if the symptoms are particularly severe or last longer than a few days.

In general terms, the number and consistency of bowel motions passed by children is variable, especially during infancy. Breastfed babies often pass yellow, very loose stools several times a day while bottle-fed babies usually pass firmer stools less frequently. Many older children continue to have three or four bowel motions a day. This is not usually a cause for concern, unless a child is also failing to gain weight normally. Children of any age may also be prone to occasional episodes of constipation.

DIARRHOEA

Bouts of diarrhoea may have a simple cause such as the introduction of a new food into a baby's diet, or excitement or anxiety in a child. However, they can also be due to conditions such as:

• Infection of the gastrointestinal tract by a virus or, less commonly, a bacterium. This condition, known as gastroenteritis, is the most common cause of diarrhoea in

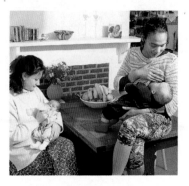

▽ The bowel habits of babies can vary widely, and may depend on whether they are fed from a bottle or the breast.

children and infants. It can also cause bouts of vomiting.

• Difficulty in absorbing certain foods. This can be due to coeliac disease, in which there is a sensitivity to gluten in wheat and other foods.

• An allergy to cow's milk, which occurs in 1 in 25 babies. It is caused by sensitivity to proteins in cow's milk or ordinary formula milks.

VOMITING

Vomiting is a distressing symptom. It is an unpleasant experience for a child and can also be very upsetting for the parents. The causes of vomiting are many and varied, and they include:

• Infection – gastroenteritis is a common cause of vomiting, but almost every childhood infection – including ear, urinary and respiratory infections – can make a child sick.

VOMITING WARNING

If your child is suffering from any of the following symptoms in addition to vomiting, you should seek urgent medical attention.

➤ Bloody or black stools.

➤ Purple spots on the skin that do not fade after being pressed with the side of a glass.

➤ Prolonged abdominal pain.

➤ Unusual drowsiness.

➤ Signs of dehydration (see box).

• Difficulty in absorbing certain substances – for example, a sensitivity to gluten.

• An allergy to cow's milk.

• Emotional problems. Stress or anxiety can lead to vomiting in children.

• Digestive disorders such as a weakness in the muscles around the entrance to the stomach (gastro-oesophageal reflux), or an abnormality in the outlet of the stomach (pyloric stenosis).

• Rarely, vomiting can be the result of a head injury.

WHAT SHOULD I DO?

Vomiting is commonly the result of gastroenteritis, which clears up by itself. The main supportive treatment is to ensure that your child drinks plenty of fluids (see the entry on gastroenteritis).

You should always seek medical help if a child seems particularly unwell, if they have had abdominal pain for longer than four hours, or if the vomiting is persistent.

DEHYDRATION WARNING

If a child becomes dehydrated, they may develop the following symptoms:

➤ Drowsiness and listlessness.

➤ Dry tongue and lips.

➤ Sunken eyes.

➤ Passing a small amount of dark urine.

➤ In infants, a sunken fontanelle (the soft spot on the crown of the head).

Seek immediate medical help if your child develops any of these symptoms.

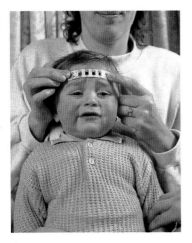

△ A high fever can indicate gastroenteritis. When checking a temperature, bear in mind that strip thermometers such as this one are easier to use on small children, but are not epecially accurate or reliable – you may want to double-check with a conventional thermometer.

Unexplained vomiting in babies or small children requires medical assessment.

GASTROENTERITIS

Most cases of gastroenteritis are mild. They usually clear up by themselves after a few days or perhaps a week. The focus of treatment should be to ensure that your child remains well hydrated.

Doctors usually tell you to give a child plenty of clear liquids and to avoid giving

SIGNS AND SYMPTOMS OF GASTROENTERITIS

The symptoms of gastroenteritis often develop quite quickly over the course of one or two days. Your child may have any combination of the following symptoms:

➤ Vomiting.

➤ Abdominal pain.

➤ Diarrhoea.

➤ High temperature.

➤ A cough and/or runny nose.

milk unless you are breastfeeding. Milk and the lactose it contains are difficult to digest effectively during such an infection, and it may cause more diarrhoea. Antidiarrhoeal drugs are too toxic for small children and should never be given.

HOW TO AID RECOVERY

• Encourage your child to drink small amounts of fluid at frequent intervals. This should be a glucose and electrolyte mixture for small children or clear fluids for older children (water, diluted fruit juice or lemonade).

• Breastfed babies should continue to breastfeed throughout their illness, even though this may provoke more diarrhoea.

• Infants on bottled formulas should be given clear fluids to drink. They can also be given half-strength milk (milk that is made up with half the normal number of scoops of milk powder).

• Once your child has started to recover, reintroduce a very light diet and upgrade to full-strength milk where appropriate.

CONSTIPATION

Many children have difficulty in passing hard faeces at some point. Constipation in childhood is usually a temporary complaint and rarely indicates a more serious problem.

Constipation is often related to diet. It may occur when an infant changes from breast to bottle milk, or if an older child is not eating enough fibre. A healthy, varied diet – that contains plenty of fruit and vegetables and does not rely on convenience and fast foods – will help both to prevent and ease constipation. It is also important that your child drinks plenty of clear fluids such as water or diluted juice. Regular exercise and sport will also be helpful.

Constipation may indicate that a child is distressed. For example, a small child can become constipated if their parents are going through a stressful time at home. If this is the case, more attention to a child's

▷ Children usually make a quick recovery from stomach upsets, but persistent abdominal pain or vomiting should be investigated.

COLIC

Colic is a common problem in small babies. It usually starts at two or three weeks of age and may last until the child is about four months old. The usual symptoms, which are often worse in the evening, may include:

➤ Prolonged crying at roughly the same time each day, with the baby proving to be inconsolable.

➤ Drawing the legs up.

Colic can be distressing but is harmless and not an indication of any serious condition. The cause is not known, but doctors no longer think that it is connected with wind or abdominal pain. There are some over-the-counter preparations that may help and painkilling syrups will help to make a child more comfortable.

emotional needs may be necessary. Some toddlers develop constipation when they are being toilet-trained. The problem usually resolves itself, given time and patience.

Consult a doctor if a child's constipation persists for longer than a week. The doctor may examine the child's rectum by inserting a gloved finger into it. Mild laxatives may be prescribed in persistent cases or if straining to pass hard faeces has caused a tear in the anal tissue.

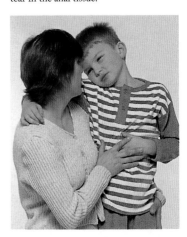

Migraines in children

A migraine can be a very distressing and debilitating condition, and it can affect children as well as adults. The symptoms of childhood migraine may be different to the adult form – the main symptom is usually abdominal pain, although headaches and other adult symptoms may occur as the child gets older. Migraines can affect children as young as two and will usually recur. The cause is not fully understood, and there will often be a history of migraines in the family. Statistically, more girls than boys suffer from migraines.

SIGNS AND SYMPTOMS

A young child with a migraine may demonstrate quite different symptoms to those experienced by adults. They may suffer from:

➤ Abdominal pain.

➤ Nausea and vomiting.

➤ Dizzy spells.

➤ Pale skin.

Older children usually develop more typical adult symptoms:

➤ One-sided headache.

➤ Nausea and vomiting.

➤ Visual disturbance, such as seeing flashing or shimmering lights.

➤ Aversion to bright lights.

➤ Occasionally, weakness in an arm or a leg.

There may be a warning period during which the child feels unwell and in time they may be able to recognize that a migraine is about to start.

About 1 in every 20 children has suffered a migraine by the age of 15, and children as young as 2 have been affected. The exact cause of migraines is not fully understood but may be connected to changes in blood flow inside the skull. Temporary alterations in brain chemicals may also be a factor, causing symptoms elsewhere in the body.

Migraine attacks may be triggered by stress and anxiety, or by particular food

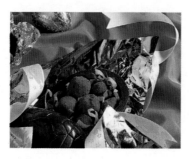

△ If your child suffers from migraines, it is often worth looking at their diet. Chocolate is one of the common food triggers.

substances – some of the most common food triggers are bananas, chocolate, citrus fruits and cheese. Perfume, petrol, tobacco smoke and other inhaled substances may also trigger an attack.

As with adult migraines, the symptoms usually develop gradually over several hours, and an attack can last for several days. In most cases, the child will suffer from recurrent attacks.

WHAT MIGHT YOUR DOCTOR DO?

Doctors can usually diagnose migraine from the child's symptoms, and further hospital investigations are rarely necessary. Occasionally, a CT scan or an MRI of the head may be arranged to discount other possible causes. Young children may be sent for ultrasound scanning of the abdomen.

If the attacks are short-lived, simple painkillers may be all that is needed to relieve symptoms. These are best given during the very early stages of an attack. It can also be helpful for the child to lie down in a darkened, quiet room.

For children who suffer from frequent attacks, your doctor will be able to recommend a number of effective antimigraine drugs that can be used on a regular preventative basis.

Since dietary factors may be significant in approximately 10 per cent of cases, your doctor may arrange for the child and parents to see a dietician. This is often helpful because it can pinpoint any dietary triggers for the attacks, and these foods can then simply be avoided.

The migraines often disappear once a child reaches adulthood, however, in some cases migraine episodes will continue throughout life.

▽ A simple painkilling syrup can help to relieve the symptoms, and is most effective if given in the early stages of a migraine.

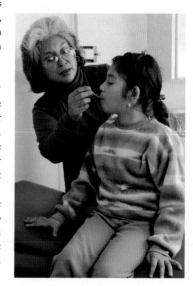

Febrile convulsions

SEE ALSO
➤ The breathing process, p374
➤ Protection against infection, p472

A febrile convulsion is a fit that has been induced by a high fever. This fairly common condition affects about 5 per cent of children between the ages of six months and five years, and is more likely to affect boys than girls. Febrile convulsions often run in families, and about one-third of children that have had one fit are likely to have another. Although frightening to witness, febrile convulsions are rarely serious. They are usually due to an infection in the body, and do not indicate a brain disorder or epilepsy, as is often feared by parents.

SIGNS AND SYMPTOMS

Febrile convulsions often occur in association with an upper respiratory tract infection, such as a runny nose or sore throat. The symptoms include:

➤ Loss of consciousness.

➤ Stiffness of limbs.

➤ Jerking of limbs.

➤ Abnormal eye movements such as the eyes rolling upwards.

A febrile convulsion normally lasts for between two and four minutes. The basic first-aid procedure is as follows:

• Lie your child on his or her side.
• Make sure the child is safe by placing cushions all around him or her, and by clearing the area of any objects that could cause injury. Do not try to restrain the child in any way.
• If this is the first time that your child has had a fit, call the emergency services immediately.
• Sponge your child down with tepid water to bring the fever down.
• Give painkilling syrup once your child comes round, to help to reduce the fever.

AFTER A FIT

The child usually falls asleep after a fit. Contact your doctor if you have not already done so. Where minor infection is diagnosed, keeping the child cool and giving painkilling syrup to bring down the fever are all that is needed. Where there is uncertainty about the cause, the child will usually be admitted to hospital for further investigations, such as antibody tests, tests on blood and urine, and a lumbar puncture.

Balanitis

SEE ALSO
➤ Causes of infectious disease, p462

Balanitis is an infection of the tip of the penis and the foreskin. It is a common childhood infection and may be caused by a bacterium or, more rarely, by a fungus. This type of infection is less likely by the age of five when in ninety per cent of boys the foreskin can be retracted.

In balanitis, the tip of the boy's penis and his foreskin become sore and itchy. There may also be some discharge or a rash.

As soon as you notice any symptoms take the child to your doctor who will examine the area and may take a swab to check for infection. The problem may clear up on its own, but antibiotics may be given. Some doctors use steroid ointment which has been shown to be effective in some studies. Further treatment is not usually necessary unless the child has phimosis, in which case balanitis may recur. Surgery may be recommended in some severe cases.

PHIMOSIS

Phimosis is a contraction of the foreskin. It occurs when the foreskin is too tight or the opening too narrow. It may:

➤ Make a child more vulnerable to balanitis.

➤ Cause difficulty passing urine.

➤ Result in ballooning of the foreskin when urine is passed.

➤ Cause recurrent infections.

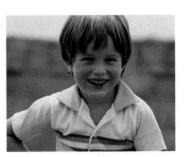

▽ Until they are about five, boys are prone to balanitis because cleaning under the foreskin is difficult as it does not always retract (pull back).

Nappy rash

SEE ALSO

➤ Causes of infectious disease, p462

➤ Bacterial infections p464

Nappy rash is an almost inevitable consequence of wearing nappies. A nappy allows urine and faeces, which have irritant effects, to come into contact with the skin. Eventually the skin becomes red and sore, sometimes causing the baby distress. Nappy rash usually clears up in a matter of days if soothing cream is applied and air is allowed to reach the area. If the problem remains after a few days and the rash seems especially sore, contact your doctor for advice. The baby may have a fungal or bacterial infection that needs medical attention.

Nappy rash is more likely to occur if the baby's nappy is not changed regularly or if the area is not cleaned thoroughly. However, almost every baby will develop it at some point. Simple nappy rash can easily be treated at home. Emollients such as aqueous cream are usually sufficient to clear up the problem in less than a week.

WHEN TO VISIT THE DOCTOR

Take the baby to the doctor if the rash is severe, if it persists longer than a week or if you are worried. The doctor will check for signs of fungal infection and may prescribe antifungal creams or oral drops, to reduce the amount of the *Candida* fungus in the digestive tract. Oral antibiotics may be necessary if a bacterial infection is suspected.

◁ Changing your baby's nappy regularly will reduce the risk of nappy rash.

HELPING TO PREVENT NAPPY RASH

➤ Change your baby's nappies frequently.

➤ Wash the nappy area at each change and allow the skin to dry thoroughly.

➤ Use a simple barrier cream at the earliest sign of irritation.

➤ Avoid perfumed skin products.

➤ Have nappy-free periods during each day.

Eczema in children

SEE ALSO

➤ Asthma, p378

This common skin condition affects as many as 20 per cent of children under the age of five. The cause is not well understood but there may be a genetic link as the condition often runs in families. Diet, such as sensitivity to cow's milk, is a possible causative factor.

SIGNS AND SYMPTOMS

➤ Intense itching and inflammation of the skin.

➤ In infants, a red, scaly rash on the face, neck, elbows and knees.

➤ In older children, a red, scaly rash in creases of the skin.

Children with eczema may also suffer from asthma and hayfever.

Childhood eczema can last several years, but it may clear up as the child gets older. Scratching the skin can cause it to become infected and make the problem worse.

MANAGING ECZEMA

If your child has eczema, they should avoid perfumed skin products, and should use skin moisturizers and moisturizing soaps. A doctor may prescribe corticosteroid creams for persistent rashes, and steroid-antibiotic creams for up to two weeks at a time to clear infected eczema.

OTHER ITCHING CONDITIONS

Scabies – Caused by a mite burrowing into the skin. Typical symptoms include intense itching, raised pink spots and brown lines between fingers and toes. Anti-parasitic lotion clears the condition.

Head lice – Tiny insects infest the scalp, causing intense itching. Spread by close contact and sharing combs and hats, poor hygiene is not a cause. Wet combing and special shampoo cures the problem.

Urinary tract infection in children

SEE ALSO

➤ The urinary organs, p386

➤ Urinary tract infections, p390

➤ Febrile convulsions, p479

Infections of the urinary tract often occur when bacteria around the anus find their way up the urethra, which empties the bladder. An abnormality in the tube (ureter) that connects the bladder to the kidneys can also make infection more likely. A urinary infection is not always easy to spot, especially in young children. However, prompt treatment is vital. If the infection is missed, it could damage the kidneys. This may make the child more prone to further infections and will also increase the likelihood of kidney disease in later life.

SIGNS AND SYMPTOMS

In babies or young children, the symptoms of urinary infection can be hard to distinguish from those of other conditions. They may include:

➤ Fever.

➤ Vomiting.

➤ General ill-health.

➤ Failure to thrive.

➤ Febrile convulsions.

In older children, symptoms may be similar to those experienced by an adult.

➤ A frequent need to pass urine.

➤ A painful, burning sensation when urine is passed.

➤ Discomfort or pain in the side or the lower abdomen.

➤ Wetting during the day or night after a period of being dry.

Urinary infections are easily treatable with antibiotics, as long as they are caught at an early stage. If you suspect that your child has a urinary infection, you should visit your doctor immediately.

WHAT MIGHT A DOCTOR DO?

The child will need to provide a urine sample, and the doctor will test this for the presence of any protein and/or red and white blood cells, which indicate infection. If infection is shown, a course of antibiotics will be prescribed. A sample of urine should also be sent to a laboratory so that the specific bacteria responsible can be identified. Once the doctor knows the cause of the infection, the antibiotic treatment may be changed.

If the infection has reached the kidneys – a condition known as pyelonephritis – the child may need to be treated in hospital with intravenous antibiotics. Babies and very young children may also be referred to hospital for treatment. Most children make a full recovery from an infection in the urinary tract. However, the infection may recur, so you should ensure that they always drink plenty of fluids.

FURTHER INVESTIGATION

Your child may need to undergo further investigation in hospital in order to identify abnormalities in the urinary tract or to check for kidney damage.

DMSA scanning is carried out to look for scarring in the kidneys. In this procedure, a dye is injected into the child's arm. A photograph of the kidneys is then taken using a special camera (a gamma

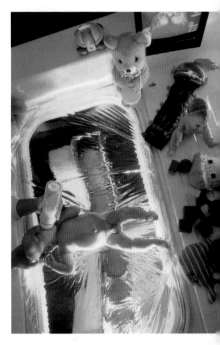

△ This infant is having his kidneys scanned on a special "water bed" scanner. A clear ultrasound image is recorded on the nearby screen.

camera). Ultrasound scanning of the kidneys may also be performed.

Other tests include a special X-ray to examine the urinary tract. This involves a dye being introduced into the bladder, and then X-rays being taken as the child passes urine. This test will identify whether the child has urinary reflux, in which urine flows back towards the kidneys rather than being passed out of the body. In this case, the child may be given low-dose antibiotics until the risk of infection has diminished.

▽ A simple test using a dipstick can determine whether or not your child has a urinary infection.

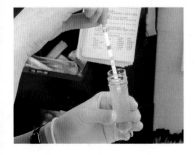

Cystic fibrosis

SEE ALSO
➤ The process of
digestion, p292
➤ The breathing
process, p374

Cystic fibrosis is the most common inherited condition in the Western world, affecting about 1 in every 1000 babies. This disease affects the mucus-producing glands in the pancreas and in the lungs, causing extra-thick secretions to be produced. As a result, children with the condition experience recurrent chest infections and have problems absorbing nutrients from their food. Current treatments have extended the life expectancy of those affected well into adulthood, and researchers hope that gene therapy will soon be used to treat the disease.

Cystic fibrosis is caused by an abnormal gene carried by both parents. The parents may be "carriers" of the gene and need not necessarily have the disease themselves.

The symptoms usually appear within the first few weeks of life. The baby is fretful and fails to thrive, has a swollen abdomen and passes greasy stools (faeces) that float and have an offensive smell.

WHAT MIGHT YOUR DOCTOR DO?

The earlier the diagnosis, the better the outcome. A diagnosis can be confirmed by a sweat test – high levels of salt in the sweat indicate cystic fibrosis. Treatment involves daily physiotherapy to clear excess mucus from the lungs. The baby is given pancreatic enzyme granules before food, along with a high-calorie diet, to maximize digestion and nutrition. Antibiotic treatment is necessary if a chest infection occurs.

Heart problems

SEE ALSO
➤ The cardiovascular
system, p276

A congenital heart disease is one that is present from birth. They affect about 1 in every 100 babies and are usually diagnosed during the very early stages of life. Most problems are mild and disappear as the baby grows, although some can be life-threatening.

Many heart problems cause no symptoms, and are picked up only during routine examinations. A doctor may hear a heart murmur – caused by turbulent blood flow – when listening to the heart with a stethoscope. If a congenital heart defect is suspected the child is referred to a specialist for tests, such as an electrocardiogram (ECG) and an echocardiogram (ultrasound). In approximately two-thirds of cases, the problem clears up by itself, but one in three children may need surgery.

COMMON CONGENITAL HEART PROBLEMS

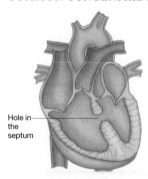

Hole in the septum

△ A septal defect, also known as a hole in the heart, is where there is a hole in the septum (the part of the heart that divides it in two).

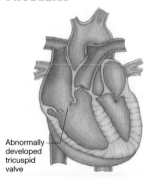

Abnormally developed tricuspid valve

△ A valve defect is when a heart valve develops abnormally, and any of the heart's four valves can be affected in this way.

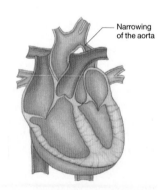

Narrowing of the aorta

△ Coarctation of the aorta is a narrowing of the main artery. This restricts blood flow to the lower body, which places strain on the heart muscle.

Congenital hip dysplasia

SEE ALSO
➤ The musculoskeletal system, p354
➤ Osteoarthritis, p360

This condition affects newborn babies and is much more common in girls than in boys. It often affects babies who are born by breech delivery, which puts excessive strain on their hip joints. In mild cases, there is a looseness of the ligaments around the hip joint, which results in excessive flexibility. In very severe cases, the hip joint is permanently dislocated. Hip dysplasia may correct itself within weeks of the baby's birth, but a plaster cast might need to be worn for up to six months. Corrective surgery may be necessary in some cases.

SIGNS AND SYMPTOMS

Mild cases may show no symptoms at all, but babies with severe hip dysplasia often have the following:

➤ Asymmetrical skin creases on the backs of the legs.

➤ Shortening of the affected leg.

An older child may have a limp if congenital hip dysplasia has not been picked up by doctors during development tests. This condition is most effectively treated early on, and if treatment is delayed, a child is at risk of developing osteoarthritis at a young age, and may also suffer permanent damage to the hip joint.

Congenital hip dysplasia may be due to weakness of the hip joint ligaments or, in more severe cases, to an abnormality in the hip socket.

If the problem does not right itself within the first few weeks, it is vital that the

▽ Babies are examined in the first weeks of life to check the stability and range of movement of their hips. Any problem is then fully investigated.

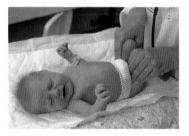

ROUTINE HIP EXAMINATION

All babies are examined during the first day or two of life by a paediatrician or family doctor, and this examination is repeated at the age of six weeks. If there is any suspicion of hip looseness or dislocation, the baby will be referred immediately to a paediatric orthopaedic specialist. An ultrasound scan can be done to confirm or refute the diagnosis.

affected head of the femur is correctly positioned in the hip socket, so that the hip can develop normally. The orthopaedic specialist will use a harness or a plaster cast to keep the hip in correct alignment, and this may need to be worn for six months.

Perthes' disease

SEE ALSO
➤ Osteoarthritis, p360

Perthes' disease is a rare condition in which the head of the femur (thigh bone) breaks down and gradually reforms over about two years. The condition tends to occur in boys between the ages of four and eight. Typical symptoms are limping and pain in the hip or knee.

Doctors do not know why children develop Perthes' disease, but it may be due to disrupted blood supply to the femur. If your child has an unexplained limp, you should arrange to see your doctor about it.

WHAT A DOCTOR MIGHT DO

X-rays or MRI scans of the affected hip will be done to confirm the diagnosis. The condition usually responds to bed-rest but sometimes a child's legs may need to be put in plaster to relieve pressure on the bone. In severe cases, surgery may be needed. Most children make a full recovery, but some may develop osteoarthritis in later life.

▷ This is a broomstick plaster, which may be used to treat Perthes' disease. It holds the child's legs apart, reducing friction on the bone.

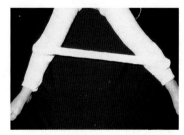

Sudden infant death syndrome

SEE ALSO

➤ Smoking and your health, p268

➤ Addictive behaviours, p350

➤ The grieving process, p490

The death of a child is a tragic event and one of the most distressing aspects of sudden infant death syndrome (SIDS) is that it happens without warning, usually in the place where a baby should be safest – at home. We still do not know what causes SIDS, but doctors have identified certain risk factors. Since new advice based on this research has been made known to parents, the incidence of SIDS has fallen and there are a number of measures that you can take to minimize the risk. Babies between one and six months old are most at risk from SIDS.

Despite much research, the causes of sudden infant death syndrome are still not fully known. However, doctors believe that it may be related to unusual breathing patterns. SIDS is more common in premature babies who were born before 37 weeks gestation. Statistically, siblings of children who have died of SIDS are slightly more at risk.

KNOW THE RISK FACTORS

The risk factors that increase the likelihood of SIDS include:

- Parental smoking.
- Parental drug abuse.
- Recent upper respiratory tract infection such as a cold.
- Putting babies to sleep on their fronts.
- Putting babies to sleep in an overheated room or overwrapping them, particularly during illness, so that they overheat.
- Bottle-feeding rather than breastfeeding your baby.

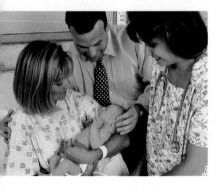

▽ Health visitors will advise parents on ways to protect their baby from SIDS and provide the best possible chance of good health.

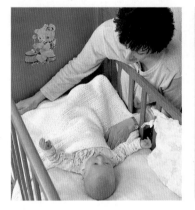

△ Placing your baby on his or her back to sleep is one of the most important steps that you can take to reduce the risk of SIDS.

PREVENTING SIDS

Research has identified many risk factors for SIDS. There are a number of ways in which you can reduce the risk, and these include the following:

- Putting your baby down to sleep on his or her back at the foot of the cot.
- Using a firm mattress in the cot.
- Not using a pillow until your baby has reached the age of one year.
- Not using too many blankets, as there is a danger that your baby may overheat.
- Not smoking at home, or allowing visitors to smoke in your house. Avoiding taking your baby anywhere where people are smoking.
- Breastfeeding for the first few months of your baby's life, because this can boost his or her immune system and may help to make SIDS less likely.

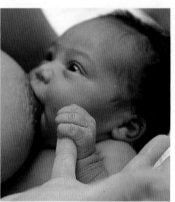

△ Research suggests that babies who are breastfed have a slightly lower risk of SIDS than those who are bottle-fed.

Although many parents use baby monitors to check on their baby's breathing, there is no research to suggest that these devices reduce the likelihood of a baby being affected by SIDS. Often they can heighten the parents' anxiety rather than alleviate it.

Some parents learn cardiopulmonary resuscitation so that they feel able to deal with the situation more confidently. In the unlikely event that SIDS affects your baby, ring the emergency services – or send a helper to do so – and start resuscitation while you wait for them to arrive. Doctors will try to resuscitate a baby on its arrival at hospital, but this is rarely successful.

If a baby dies from SIDS, parents will need support and help. Specialist counselling can be helpful in coming to terms with such a loss and support groups can provide valuable long-term help.

16

CARING FOR THE TERMINALLY ILL

Coping with an advanced disease can be traumatic for both the patient and for family, friends and carers. Under these circumstances it is important that everyone knows and understands the patient's wishes and that they in turn have someone they trust who can make decisions on their behalf if they find themselves unable to do so. There is a confusing range of decisions to be made when it comes to making choices about caring for the terminally ill, and an understanding of the practical issues will help family and friends deal with the situation as well as facing the emotional repercussions and, eventually, the grieving process.

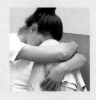

CONTENTS

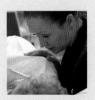

Coping with terminal illness

SEE ALSO
➤ The grieving process, p490
➤ Acupuncture, p493

During the more advanced stages of a terminal illness, the focus of medical treatment often shifts. Although treatments will continue for as long as possible, an increasing emphasis may be placed on quality of life. To this end, your doctor or carers will increasingly involve the patient and/or his or her family in decisions about how to manage the illness. It is important that everyone concerned starts to think through the many issues associated with an impending death, both emotionally and practically, and how they want to deal with them.

Treatment of terminal illness involves weighing up a huge number of medical, physical, psychological and emotional issues. These issues are often difficult to tackle and are often best resolved if the patient, their family and doctors or health workers discuss them carefully together.

MAKING CHOICES

Some people may need, or want, to stay in a hospital, while for others hospice care is the better option. If there is a strong family network to provide care, the patient may even be able to go home.

If particular medicines are unlikely to prolong life, or if they are doing so at considerable personal cost, for example by causing unpleasant side effects, it may be appropriate to stop them. This may apply

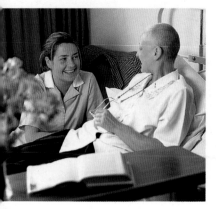

▽ Open and honest discussion with family members may not be possible, so relationships with carers can often provide invaluable understanding and advice, and the chance to talk in-depth about feelings and anxieties.

WHAT IS A LIVING WILL?

A "living will" (also called an advance statement) outlines your beliefs, wishes and values specifically related to medical treatment during the course of a terminal illness. If you or someone you know wishes to write a living will, it may be helpful to do so with your doctor. Such documents usually include some of the following issues:

➤ Nominating a person who understands what you would like to happen in different situations and who will be able to make decisions for you if you are unable to do so.

➤ Setting out clear guidelines about whether you would like a specific treatment up until a particular time or whether you want to refuse certain treatments, such as tube feeding, up until the time of death.

➤ Deciding that you do not want to receive life-sustaining or reviving treatment, such as resuscitation, if it becomes necessary.

➤ Making it clear whether or not you would like to donate any of your body organs to be used after your death.

to medicines that have previously been taken to prevent or delay disease progression. This is inevitably a difficult decision to make and should ideally be taken by the affected person in close consultation with those most involved in his or her care, and with the full support of relevant healthcare professionals.

It may also be appropriate to plan ahead and consider what to do in the event of further deterioration. A terminally ill person is often prone to acute episodes of infection, and much thought needs to be given to whether this should be actively treated or whether it is preferable to refrain from treating these further diseases or infections.

The situation, which places an incredible strain on family and friends, becomes more difficult if the dying person is confused or not fully conscious. Some time may be needed for appropriate courses of action to become clearer to all concerned. Some

patients will have already discussed these issues and may have made a "living will" (see box) that explains what they would like to happen under such circumstances.

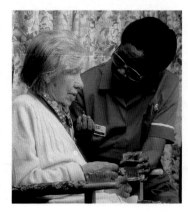

▽ Healthcare professionals are trained to provide care and support for patients who are confused and anxious about their situation.

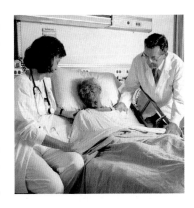

△ Doctors should consult with the patient at every stage about pain relief and life-sustaining treatments, and about what to do if the patient becomes unable to make such decisions.

Where someone chooses to spend their last days or weeks is very important. Many people choose to die at home if they are asked but some choose hospice care instead if it is offered. This wish should be honoured wherever possible, although practical considerations may sometimes make this difficult.

AN EMOTIONAL TIME

For a patient, the process of acknowledging and accepting terminal illness involves a very complex mix of emotions, and will often result in severe mood swings. The range of feelings may include:
• Shock, disbelief and denial.
• Anger and frustration.
• Fear, anxiety and depression.
• Resignation and acceptance.

It is important to remember that a similar range of emotions will also be experienced by those closest to the dying person.

Generally, it is more common to be honest and open about the reality of the situation and prognosis. Many terminally ill patients find that they experience less depression and anxiety once they have had the opportunity to discuss all their fears with both loved ones and healthcare professionals. However, each case should be considered individually, and openness and honesty are not always appropriate. Each person should be offered understanding and support to enable them to cope with the

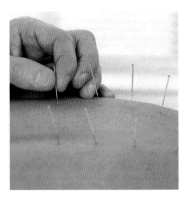

△ Acupuncture is thought to stimulate endorphins, the body's natural painkillers. It is offered to some terminally ill patients as an alternative to drugs that have unpleasant side effects such as nausea or constipation.

situation in their own way. Carers and friends and family may well need to be perceptive and intuitive in order to gauge accurately how a patient feels, because in many cases they are simply not able to make their wishes clear, and do not want to face the reality of their situation.

CONTROLLING PAIN

Pain can be an important factor in advanced and terminal illness, and fear of pain can cause great anxiety and agitation for many patients. Most physical pain can be effectively relieved by the use of strong painkilling drugs. Opiates such as morphine can be administered orally or via a subcutaneously sited infusion (which delivers drugs into the fatty tissue below the skin to disperse slowly) if it is too difficult to swallow. Opiate drugs tend to have an anxiety-reducing effect but also induce constipation and a degree of nausea, particularly for a few days after they have been started. Fentanyl (similar in potency to morphine) can be administered via a patch applied to the skin every 72 hours and is a useful alternative.

Many patients find acupuncture is effective for relieving pain and this treatment is available in some hospices as an alternative to prescribed drugs.

HOSPICE CARE

Hospices provide a range of nursing and medical services. Nurses, carers and doctors provide specialized palliative care for patients with advanced diseases such as cancer, neurological disease and cardiorespiratory disease. Palliative care is designed to provide appropriate treatments and support for patients in the weeks and months following a terminal diagnosis, and generally focuses on dealing with symptoms, and controlling pain and anxiety throughout the course of a terminal illness.

Hospices also offer respite care, which provides a break for patients and carers. Individuals are often admitted to a hospice for two or three weeks at a time.

A range of other services is often available, for example physiotherapy, occupational therapy, various complementary therapies and access to counsellors and spiritual care.

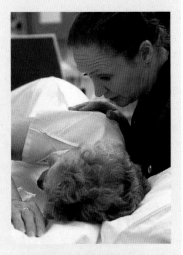

△ A hospice can offer specialized care for terminally ill patients, focusing on quality of life and offering respite to relatives.

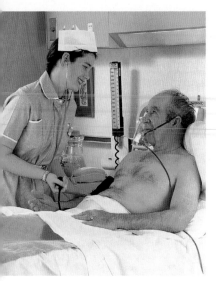

△ Regular blood pressure checks and sessions with an oxygen mask may be vital for a patient's care, but relying on others in this way can cause feelings of powerlessness and frustration.

CONTROLLING NAUSEA AND VOMITING

Nausea and vomiting are common symptoms of terminal illness and can be distressing. This may be a result of disease or a side effect of certain drugs, notably those used to control pain. Antisickness or antiemetic drugs are usually effective and may be administered orally, by suppository or by subcutaneous infusion.

RELIEVING CONSTIPATION AND DIARRHOEA

Constipation is a common symptom in people who are confined to bed and whose movements are limited. It may be caused by lack of fluid (dehydration) and food, and it can be aggravated by deteriorating health and the use of strong opiates. Constipation usually responds to extra fluids where this is possible and to the use of simple laxatives.

Diarrhoea is more common in people dying from advanced HIV infection and usually responds to a range of antidiarrhoeal medicines, including opiate painkillers.

Both diarrhoea and constipation can be distressing for the patient, who may also feel humiliated if they are unable to relieve themselves without assistance. Drugs can alleviate these symptoms, but it is important that carers understand the feelings of frustration that this dependence can cause, and help the patient to feel as normal and capable as possible.

TREATING SHORTNESS OF BREATH

Difficulty with breathing sometimes affects terminally ill patients, especially those with advanced heart or lung disease, and can be very distressing – both for sufferers and for onlookers. It may trigger panic attacks and serious anxiety, which makes breathlessness even worse. Morphine is often an effective treatment, but if the underlying cause is a lung infection, the breathlessness may be relieved by antibiotics, which can help to clear any infection. A person may receive oxygen therapy if it helps to improve symptoms of breathlessness, and this can be particularly useful for those dying from progressive cardiorespiratory disease. Oxygen tents are sometimes used, but in most cases an oxygen mask over the nose and mouth, or oxygen tubes fitted into the nostrils, is more appropriate.

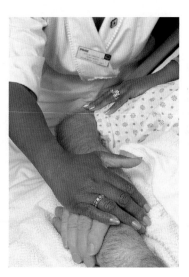

CALMING ANXIETY AND AGITATION

Terminally ill patients are often anxious and agitated. It may be helpful to talk things through to make sure that they are as fully informed as they want to be. This will hopefully reduce feelings of powerlessness and frustration by making the patient feel more in control.

Opiate drugs tend to have an anxiety-reducing effect. There are also a number of other anxiety-reducing and mildly sedating drugs that can be used orally or via an infusion if necessary.

Certain complementary therapies, such as massage and aromatherapy, and the use of touch in general, may be invaluable in relieving anxiety. Simply holding someone's hand can be soothing and comforting, helping the patient to feel less alone and alleviating feelings of panic and agitation.

For many people, dying with dignity is very important and one of their greatest fears is of becoming increasingly dependent on others and being unable to make their own decisions. This can cause anxiety and frustration and it is usually helpful for

▽ Patients who are confined to bed and are more or less immobile require special nursing care to keep their skin clean and healthy, and free from pressure sores.

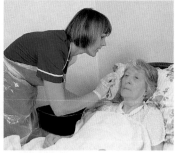

◁ The prospect of dying can be terrifying, and this can cause more anxiety than the pain or symptoms of the terminal disease itself. Talking things through and offering a comforting touch can help people to work through their fears. Touch can be remarkably calming and makes the patient feel less alone.

someone close to the patient – whether family or carer – to calm these fears by talking through every eventuality and making it clear that their wishes have been understood and will be followed.

Another cause of anxiety is being in a strange environment. Many people do not want to die in a hospital and may feel the need to be in their own homes, surrounded by their possessions and loved ones. If possible, this desire should be respected and the patient allowed to return home. However, this is often not practical and indeed many people choose to remain in hospital, or to move to a hospice, where they can be given the best medical treatment and specialized care and support.

INTAKE OF FOOD AND FLUID

People naturally tend to eat less and less as they become more ill. This can be very distressing for those closest to the dying person. Emphasis should always be placed on the needs of the patient and they should not be forced to eat if they do not want to – it may be uncomfortable for them to do so. Usually a lack of appetite and calories in the last stages of an illness does not cause any specific problems.

As the dying person's condition deteriorates, there comes a point when he or she cannot drink much fluid, if any at all. Once again, in the later stages of terminal illness this will not cause specific problems. The sensation of thirst can be prevented by keeping the mouth, lips and gums moist and clean. Tiny sips of water may suffice for this process.

Fluids will often be taken for some time after food has been rejected, but eventually even fluids cannot be tolerated. Again, this is a natural progression and is not usually a specific problem. As long as care is taken to maintain oral hygiene, and the mouth is kept moist, the sensation of thirst is often not apparent. This rejection of food and drink comes towards the end of a terminal illness and, although it is upsetting for family and friends, it is a normal process and should not be a cause of concern.

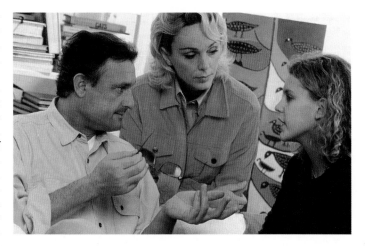

PREVENTING PRESSURE SORES

When a person is in bed all day or is for the most part immobile, he or she can develop aches, pains and sores on the skin. Special beds and mattresses are available that cushion the body and enable carers to wash and move patients more easily and so prevent the development of pressure sores. Specialized nursing care is essential for all-round patient comfort and skin health.

MAKING PLANS

Although many terminal patients can make a "living will", giving directions about their treatment (see earlier box), planning what will happen after death can be too distressing for many to contemplate and this should be respected. In some cases, sufferers may turn to their religion or beliefs to help them, and representatives of their faith can help to make plans and will be the most comforting figures at the end.

The question of whether or not healthy organs should be removed for donation after the patient has died is an issue that many people do not want to discuss with the dying, but the idea of helping someone else live after their death can be a comforting thought. Many people carry donor cards or they may broach the subject themselves. Some patients feel they need to discuss how organ donation works with a medical expert before they make a decision.

△ Discussing funeral plans or organ donation as a family is very important. It is often difficult to make these decisions alone, and sharing the responsibility is usually helpful.

As with many other aspects of dealing with the terminally ill, making plans about matters such as these may help them feel they are still in control.

Another matter that family and friends often avoid when dealing with terminal illness is the arrangement of the funeral. Once again, many patients may not want to discuss this, but others may welcome the opportunity to make some of these decisions for themselves. Planning the funeral, or at least making certain stipulations, can help the patient come to terms with the situation. It can also relieve some of the pressure on family and friends, who are often too grief-stricken after the death of a loved one to think through what they might have wanted. Many people, for example, request that there should be no flowers at their funeral and that the money should be donated to a charity. They may also have a preference for certain music or readings, or feel strongly about whether people should be dressed in black.

It is often a comfort to all concerned that the wishes of the patient in such matters are respected, and making these plans can help the dying person and their friends and family.

The grieving process

SEE ALSO
➤ Learn to manage
   stress, p260
➤ Depression, p346

Coming to terms with the death of someone close to you is a difficult and traumatic issue, and it can be particularly difficult if you have been taking care of someone during a prolonged illness. The situation is emotionally exhausting and life-changing, and most people find that they seriously reconsider their own lives as a result. Grief manifests itself in many different ways and the grieving process is unique to each individual. It may, however, be both possible and helpful to identify certain stages during the grieving process.

FACING LOSS

Anticipating grief may be helpful before an inevitable loss. Where a loved one is dying from a terminal illness, this can at least give relatives and friends the opportunity to take stock of the situation and to start dealing with the loss before it actually happens. This may result in a greater feeling of strength and acceptance when death actually occurs. The chance to say goodbye to a loved one can help enormously.

▽ Initially, in the first hours or days after the death of a loved one, the overpowering emotions are those of shock, confusion and numbness.

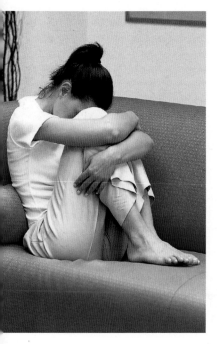

INITIAL REACTIONS

Feelings of numbness and detachment are common after death has occurred, and the emotions one may have anticipated may not arrive for some time. There is usually shock and an overwhelming sense of loss, along with feelings of emptiness, despair and helplessness. Your pattern of life will probably be disrupted for some time, and you may experience a lack of appetite and difficulty in sleeping.

DEPRESSION AND SADNESS

Initial numbness will at some point give way to a range of emotions that tends to include depression and sadness. There may be a feeling of isolation and incredible loneliness. There may also be frustration and anger. Anger might be directed at other people or at yourself. There may be terrible guilt and self-reproach for not having been more available, or for failing to say enough before it was too late. Helplessness and frustration are two key emotions that people feel after someone they know has died.

These are all natural reactions and most will be present to greater or lesser degrees and for different lengths of time in everyone experiencing grief. It is often helpful to know that during this confusing and difficult time others will be going through similar emotions to you. They too will be reproaching themselves and feeling lonely. Often talking to other people who knew the loved one can help. As with most types of trauma or grief, bottling it up can make it worse, and talking can often be a relief and a comfort.

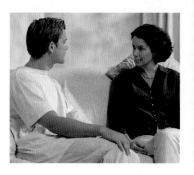

△ At first, most people simply feel numb when someone close dies. This usually develops into a wide range of emotions that can be difficult to deal with. Specialist grief counsellors can help you through this difficult time.

While it may be a comfort to talk thoughts and feelings through with your family and friends, it may also be helpful to seek specialist advice from your doctor or from a counsellor.

RESOLUTION

At some point, life starts to return to some semblance of normality. The timing of the recovery process is different for everyone – it can take from six months to several years. You will find that you start to have more energy and are able to reorganize your life and adjust to your loss. There will often be feelings of guilt for having moved on; the process of recovery may be slow and all the emotions can come flooding back at any time. Birthdays and anniversaries are difficult and you will often relive many of the feelings of initial grief. Eventually, however, you will feel able to start making plans and decisions about your future.

COMPLEMENTARY THERAPIES

17

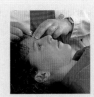

Therapies such as acupuncture and aromatherapy were first used by some of the most ancient civilizations in the world, many thousands of years ago. Until recently, they have been regarded with suspicion by many practitioners of Western medicine. Nowadays, however, increasing numbers of people are turning to these less invasive and more natural forms of treatment for a wide variety of conditions. More doctors accept the effectiveness of various complementary therapies and many incorporate them into their treatment programmes or suggest them as alternative methods of diagnosis and relief.

CONTENTS

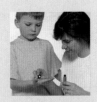

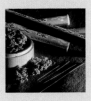

Complementary therapies and their uses

SEE ALSO
➤ Headaches and migraine, p324
➤ Colds and flu, p376
➤ Asthma, p370
➤ Eczema, p438

There has been a considerable growth of interest in complementary therapies in recent years – it is not that long ago that such therapies were viewed with suspicion and hostility in the West. This trend has been accompanied by a shift in attitude by some members of the medical and allied professions. Over the last few decades, there have been attempts to integrate some therapies into mainstream medical settings. It is now not uncommon, for example, to find massage and aromatherapy available on some hospital wards.

Many complementary therapies have evolved from ancient traditions and represent systems of medicine that were first practised many thousands of years ago. All complementary therapies take a holistic approach to health rather than simply treating physical symptoms.

General practitioners regularly refer patients to osteopaths, and a small but growing number of doctors are undertaking some training in homeopathy and acupuncture for example.

CHOOSING A THERAPY

Complementary medicine covers a wide range of therapies and the therapy that you choose will depend upon a number of factors. You may already have had experience of one or more therapies. Sometimes it may be necessary to try a range of approaches before deciding on the right one for you.

Evidence of the effectiveness and safety of any therapy is also important. Osteopathy and chiropractic and traditional Chinese medicines such as acupuncture all have a growing evidence base that testifies to the effectiveness of treatment in a variety of situations. There is a wide range of other specialities, for example reflexology and shiatsu, that have been less vigorously and objectively examined. This does not mean, however, that a less researched therapy is not effective. There are usually many people who are prepared to testify that these therapies have worked for them.

FINDING A THERAPIST

Most complementary therapists practise alone or in one of a growing number of complementary medicine or natural health centres. A fee is usually charged at the end of each session. People with private healthcare insurance may be covered for a

BE WISE, BE SAFE

It is advisable to consult your doctor before trying out any complementary therapy, especially if you have a particular medical condition. Your doctor may advise against therapies that interfere with prescription medicines you are taking on a regular basis. Chinese herbalism, for example, often uses powerful ingredients that could interact with certain drugs and cause serious side-effects. Aromatherapy oils must also be used carefully, as many are very potent and are not advised if you have certain conditions, and especially if you are pregnant. Most oils should be diluted in carrier oil before being applied to the skin. If you are regularly having any type of complementary therapy, tell your doctor when you next visit.

limited number of treatments by a specified range of therapists (most commonly osteopaths and acupuncturists).

The best way to find a therapist is via personal recommendation – from a friend, relative or doctor – and it is a good idea to check that any therapist that you consult is well qualified and a member of the appropriate professional body (remember that anyone can set themselves up in practice as a complementary therapist, so tread carefully). Contact details for the Institute of Complementary Medicine are in the Useful Addresses listing at the back of this book. The Internet is another valuable source of information about professional bodies.

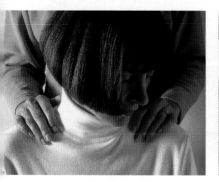
▽ Many complementary therapies use the concept of the soothing and comforting power of healing hands.

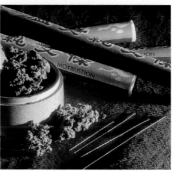
▽ Acupuncture points are also stimulated by "moxibustion": burning of herbs over the skin, using acupuncture needles or special sticks.

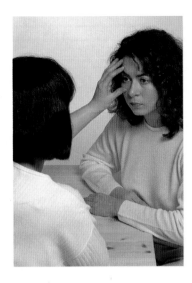

△ As with any treatment, your practitioner will begin by taking a full history of your symptoms and medical problems.

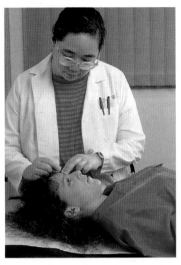

△ An acupuncturist inserts fine needles into the skin in order to correct imbalances in the flow of energy around the body.

effect is the result of stimulating the production of endorphins (the body's natural painkillers, produced in the brain).

AROMATHERAPY

The therapeutic properties of aromatic oils have been understood for thousands of years and ancient records describe their widespread use. The use of essential oils which became known as aromatherapy was developed in Europe during the early 20th century by doctors in France.

During treatment, an essential oil is either applied to the skin in a diluted form or inhaled. Each oil has certain properties and is used alone or in combination for a specific condition or ailment. Aromatherapy can treat a wide range of physical and emotional problems. There is a growing interest in administering essential oils orally (medical aromatherapy) – never do this unsupervised as it can be very dangerous.

WHAT TO EXPECT

Most therapists, like other medical practitioners, will start by taking a formal history. This is followed in most therapies by a physical examination. The therapist will explain the treatment to be used and give you your first session. The length of treatment depends on the nature of your problem. An acute back problem may require one or two sessions with an osteopath, whereas a chronic condition may require a much longer course of treatment.

ACUPUNCTURE

Acupuncture originated about 5000 years ago as one component of traditional Chinese medicine. The system is based upon the belief that there is an energy system within the body and that imbalances within this system result in different forms of illness. The ancient Chinese identified 14 "meridians" in the body, through which they believed a strong energy flowed. The meridians link a series of points where energy and blood flow converge. There are 365 of these acupuncture points. Each point or group of points is believed to be

associated with a specific organ or bodily system. An acupuncturist tries to diagnose such energy imbalances by taking a history, examining the tongue and feeling the range of pulses (six at each wrist). Once the imbalances have been identified, fine, sterile needles are inserted at various points to restore the body's equilibrium.

Western medicine does not generally accept the system of Chinese medicine, although there is some acknowledgement that acupuncture is an effective treatment for certain conditions, notably pain relief. Western medicine explains the effects of acupuncture by asserting that any detectable

▽ In aromatherapy, essential oils (usually diluted in carrier oil) are placed on the skin, or a few drops are placed on a tissue and inhaled.

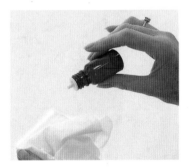

ACUPUNCTURE/MAIN USES
➤ Arthritis.

➤ Digestive disorders.

➤ Hayfever.

➤ High blood pressure.

➤ Migraines.

➤ Pain relief.

AROMATHERAPY/MAIN USES
➤ Colds.

➤ Asthma.

➤ Skin disorders, e.g. acne and ezcema.

➤ Stress-related illnesses.

➤ Urinary tract infections.

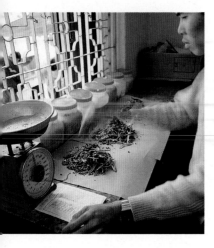

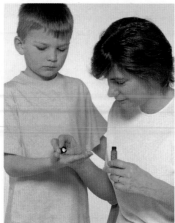

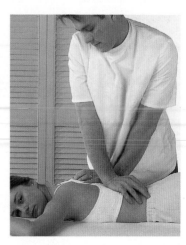

△ This herbalist is using scales to weigh out remedies. This must be done with the utmost precision, according to stringent rules.

△ Homeopathic remedies can be given in the form of ointments, powders, tinctures or pills, to treat a variety of ailments.

△ This chiropractor is manipulating the spine to ease pain and correct faulty alignment caused by an injury.

HERBALISM

Herbalism is an ancient therapy which makes use of the medicinal properties of plants. Most cultures throughout the world have a history of using plants to heal and to maintain health.

The majority of herbal therapies use a holistic approach based on the idea that an emotional and physical balance is required for overall health and wellbeing.

Herbal remedies are usually taken in the form of infusions, powders, tinctures, ointments and capsules. Some nausea or diarrhoea may be experienced when starting to take these remedies, and it is always advisable to consult both your doctor and a recognized herbalist about your treatment.

HOMEOPATHY

In homeopathy, a practitioner works on the principle of treating "like with like". Homeopathy stimulates the body's self-healing abilities by exposing it to tiny amounts of a substance that produces similar symptoms to those of the illness.

In the 5th century BC, the Greek physician Hippocrates was the first person to recognize that like cures like. However, it was not until the late 18th century that the German physician Samuel Hahnemann started to develop homeopathy.

Homeopathy can be used to treat most complaints, although some people respond better than others. A wide variety of homeopathic preparations are available

from health food shops and pharmacies, but it is advisable to consult a homeopath for a full and thorough assessment before taking any remedy.

OSTEOPATHY AND CHIROPRACTIC

These therapies evolved during the 19th century and have much in common, although each has its own system of learning and accreditation. Both disciplines aim to prevent and treat health problems, often musculoskeletal pain, by restoring structural balance and function with a combination of counselling, nutritional advice, manipulation of the spine and other joints, and massage of soft tissues.

HERBALISM/MAIN USES
➤ Digestive disorders, such as irritable bowel syndrome.

➤ Eczema, psoriasis and other skin disorders.

➤ Fatigue.

➤ Migraines.

HOMEOPATHY/MAIN USES
➤ Allergies.

➤ Anxiety.

➤ Asthma.

➤ Eczema.

➤ Menstrual and menopausal problems.

OSTEOPATHY AND CHIROPRACTIC/MAIN USES
➤ Asthma.

➤ Back and neck pain and sciatica.

➤ Digestive disorders.

➤ Headaches.

➤ Insomnia.

REFLEXOLOGY

The practice of reflexology is based on the principle that it is possible to influence and affect the functioning of the body by stimulating specific points on the feet and hands. Each area of the foot and hand relates to a different body system.

This belief system is related to that of ancient Chinese medicine, following the idea that energy flows in certain ways around the body. When this energy is disrupted or out of balance, then illness or pain can result.

By stimulating the hands and feet it is possible to interpret energy patterns and redirect the flow of energy. Reflexology is therefore both diagnostic and therapeutic.

REFLEXOLOGY PRESSURE POINTS

▽ The art of reflexology is based on the belief that stimulating different parts of the feet and hands can relieve symptoms or identify problems in related areas of the body. This diagram shows the pressure points on the bottom of the foot.

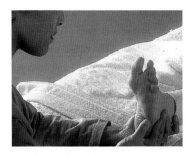

△ A reflexologist manipulates the foot to work out how your body's energy is flowing. If there is blockage, the skin will feel tender or tight, and this can be unblocked using massage.

REFLEXOLOGY/MAIN USES
➤ Anxiety.

➤ Back and neck pain.

➤ Circulation.

➤ Diagnosing other illnesses.

➤ Headaches.

SHIATSU

Shiatsu massage developed in Japan in the early 20th century but has its roots in ancient Chinese medicine. Shiatsu means finger pressure. It follows the principles of meridians and energy flow as in acupuncture. The meridians run through all the body organs and channel energy flow. All meridians, or energy channels, start or end in the fingers and toes. The energy flow maintains your physical body and affects your mind and spirit too. Massage and exercises can stimulate the meridians to maintain wellbeing.

SHIATSU/MAIN USES
➤ Arthritis.

➤ Circulatory problems.

➤ Headache and migraine.

➤ Insomnia.

➤ Stress.

▽ Shiatsu therapy applies pressure to certain points along meridian lines (energy channels in the body) using massage, stretches, holds and supportive touch. This seated position is used by the shiatsu therapist to treat the large intestine and the gall bladder meridians, which cross in the shoulder.

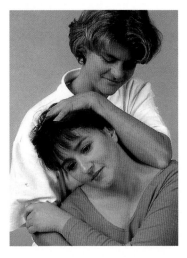

Lymph nodes and lymph drainage

Top of head
Back of head
Pituitary gland
Thyroid gland
Eyes
Ear
Shoulder
Trachea
Spine
Lung
Liver
Stomach
Pancreas
Adrenal glands
Duodenum
Gallbladder
Kidneys
Ascending colon
Small intestine
Appendix
Rectum/anus
Bladder
Sciatic nerve

Ear
Shoulder
Lung
Heart
Spleen
Transverse colon
Descending colon
Sigmoid colon

Glossary

Note: this glossary also includes useful terms that are not used in the book itself.

Abdominal thrust Technique used to expel an obstruction from the airway of a conscious person who is choking.

Abrasion Superficial wound caused by either a blunt object of some kind or by falling on a rough surface.

ACE inhibitors Drugs that block the action of angiotensin, a hormone involved in blood pressure; used in heart failure.

Acute Term used to describe an illness of short duration.

Adrenaline Naturally occurring hormone produced synthetically as a drug for the treatment of cardiac arrest, anaphylactic shock and asthma.

AIDS See HIV.

Airway Passage from the nose and mouth through the windpipe to the lungs; it must be unobstructed to allow breathing.

Allergen Substance that induces an abnormal hypersensitive reaction (allergy).

Anaesthetic Any drug used to numb a certain area of the body (local anaesthetic) or induce unconsciousness (general anaesthetic).

Analgesics Collective term for a diverse range of drugs used to relieve pain.

Anaphylaxis, anaphylactic shock Immediate hypersensitive reaction to an allergen, leading to severe symptoms of circulatory shock and potentially fatal respiratory distress.

Aneurysm Weakness in an artery, which may leak or burst at that point.

Angina pectoris Pain in the chest caused by temporary blockage of coronary arteries.

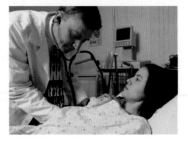

Antacids Substances that neutralize stomach acids and ease indigestion.

Antibiotics Drugs that kill disease-causing bacteria. Different antibiotics are needed for different bacteria.

Antiemetics Drugs that work on organs of balance in the ear to reduce nausea.

Antihistamines Drugs that block histamine, a chemical released by cells during allergic reactions.

Antihypertensives Drugs that reduce blood pressure.

Antioxidants Compounds that mop up harmful molecules in the bloodstream. (See Free radicals.)

Antivirals Drugs that fight viruses. Very few effective antivirals have been developed.

Arrhythmia Abnormal heart rate.

Artery Blood vessel carrying oxygenated blood away from the heart. Arterial blood is bright red and spurts rapidly and rhythmically from a wound; the resulting severe blood loss can quickly lead to shock.

Artificial respiration Mouth-to-mouth resuscitation or "the kiss of life".

Asymptomatic Term used to describe a condition that causes no obvious symptoms.

Atherosclerosis Accumulation of fatty plaques on the inner arterial wall, which impairs blood flow and may eventually block an artery, leading to heart attack.

AVPU code Checklist (Alert, Verbal, Painful, Unresponsive) used by medical practitioners to assess a casualty's level of responsiveness in an emergency.

Beta-blockers Drugs used to control high blood pressure by slowing the heart rate or by reducing the contraction of the arteries.

Biopsy Removal and examination of a tissue sample in order to aid diagnosis.

Blood film Test in which blood smeared on a slide is examined under a microscope.

Blood sugar test Test that measures the concentration of glucose in the blood; a high level may indicate diabetes.

Blunt trauma Internal injury caused by impact with a blunt object that does not penetrate the skin.

Breaking of the waters Rupture of the membrane filled with amniotic fluid that surrounds the baby in the uterus, normally at the onset of labour.

Bronchodilators Drugs that widen the airways. They are used in the treatment of asthma and bronchitis.

Bronchoscopy An examination of the airways in which a small, flexible viewing tube is passed through the nose or mouth and into the lungs.

Cardiac arrest Cessation of heartbeat and circulation of the blood, most often caused by heart attack.

Cardiac compressions Rhythmic compressions of the chest used in a case of cardiac arrest to keep blood circulating until medical help arrives. Also known as chest compressions or heart massage, the technique is combined with rescue breaths in cardiopulmonary resuscitation.

Cardiology Specialist branch of medicine that deals with the heart.

Cardiopulmonary resuscitation (CPR) Provision of basic life support using chest compressions and artificial respiration.

Cardiovascular system Heart and blood vessels.

Catheter Thin tube that is inserted into a cavity or organ to allow fluid to drain. A catheter may be used, for example, to drain urine from the bladder.

Cellulitis Spreading of bacterial infection (from a wound) under the skin.

Chemotherapy Treatment that uses drugs to kill cancerous tissue or harmful micro-organisms. These drugs also destroy some normal cells, so rest periods are needed between treatments.

Chest thrust Technique used to expel an obstruction from the airway of an unconscious person who is choking.

Chronic Term used to describe an illness of long duration.

Clinical Term used to describe anything that relates to the observation of ill people.

Clinical trial Evaluation of a medicine by studying its effects on a group of patients

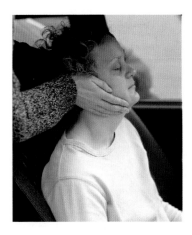

and comparing them with those of a placebo (inactive substance) given to another group.

Colonoscopy Examination of the colon using a flexible tube that is passed through the anus.

Complementary medicine Therapies that can be used alongside orthodox medical techniques. Osteopathy and acupuncture are forms of complementary medicine that are gaining wider acceptance by doctors.

Compress Pad of cloth, soaked in cold or hot water, applied to the skin using pressure to reduce pain, swelling or bleeding.

Contraindication Condition that makes a particular form of treatment undesirable. For example, high blood pressure is a contraindication for certain drugs.

Croup Viral infection of the larynx and vocal chords.

CT scan Computed tomography scan: an X-ray-based imaging technique in which a computer builds up images of "slices" of the body. CT scanning is routinely used to examine the brain and abdominal organs.

Cystoscopy Examination of the urethra and bladder using a flexible viewing device.

Defibrillation Application of electric shock to the chest wall in an attempt to restart the heart after cardiac arrest.

Dermatology Specialist branch of medicine dealing with problems of the skin.

Dialysis Treatment to filter impurities from the blood and remove excess fluid from the body. In healthy people, these processes are carried out by the kidneys; dialysis is needed by people whose kidneys have failed.

Dislocation Injury in which the end of a bone is pulled or pushed out of a joint.

Diuretic Substance that increases the excretion of urine. Diuretics are used to treat high blood pressure and heart failure.

DVT Deep vein thrombosis: the formation of a blood clot in a deep-lying vein, usually in the leg. It can cause pain and swelling, and part of the clot may become a potentially fatal obstruction if it breaks free and travels to the heart and lungs.

Echocardiogram Ultrasound examination that presents a moving image of the structure and function of the heart.

Ectopic pregnancy Unviable pregnancy in which the fertilized egg implants outside the uterus, usually in the Fallopian tube. It causes serious internal bleeding and constitutes a medical emergency.

Electrocardiogram (ECG) Recording of the electrical activity of the heart using electrodes attached to the skin, used to measure heart rate and function.

Electroencephalogram (EEG) Test that measures electrical activity within the brain by means of electrodes attached to the skin.

Embolism Blockage of an artery caused by an embolus, an obstruction such as a blood clot, air bubble or piece of tissue. A pulmonary embolism is a blockage of an artery supplying blood to the lungs and is a likely cause of sudden, unexpected death.

Emphysema Breathing disorder that causes shortness of breath and can lead to respiratory failure or heart failure.

Endemic Used to describe a disease that is established in a region or group of people.

Endocrine glands Organs that produce hormones and secrete them into the blood or lymph. The pancreas, ovaries, testicles, adrenal glands and thyroid are all examples of endocrine glands.

Endorphins Natural painkilling substances produced by the body.

Endoscopy Examination of an internal area of the body by means of a small camera mounted on a flexible viewing tube.

ENT Specialist branch of medicine that deals with the ear, nose and throat, plus other organs in the neck.

Epidemic Outbreak of an infectious disease that spreads rapidly through an entire group of people, commonly as a result of a viral mutation leading to a new strain.

Expectoration The coughing up of mucus from the airways.

Flail chest Multiple rib fractures causing unusual movement of the chest.

Fracture Break in a bone. In an open (compound) fracture the broken ends emerge through the skin; in a closed (simple) fracture they do not.

Free radicals Unstable molecules that have the potential to harm body cells. They are produced by normal bodily processes such as breathing, and increased by smoking or environmental damage. (See Antioxidants.)

Full blood count Blood test to count the number of different blood cells per litre of blood. Cell size and concentration of haemaglobin are also checked. The test is used to diagnose anaemia and leukaemia.

Full-thickness burn Burn that extends through all layers of the skin and beyond, requiring skin grafts.

Gastroenterology Specialist branch of medicine dealing with the digestive system.

Geriatrics Specialist branch of medicine dealing with the health of older people.

Greenstick fracture In children, a fracture in which only one side of the bone breaks, while the other side bends.

Gynaecology Branch of medicine dealing with the female reproductive system.

Haematology Branch of medicine specializing in the blood and blood-producing tissues.

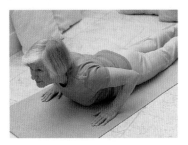

Haematoma Accumulation of blood within tissue from a ruptured blood vessel.

Haemorrhage Medical term for bleeding, which may be visible or internal.

Hepatitis Inflammation of the liver, most commonly by viral infection. Of five named viruses (A, B, C, D and E), A and E are mainly picked up from contaminated drinking water and faeces while B and C are transmitted sexually or through blood and blood products.

History Combination of underlying state of health and recent events that have led to a person's current medical condition.

HIV Human immunodeficiency virus, transmitted via contaminated blood, injection with non-sterile needles, or sexual intercourse. It is the cause of AIDS (acquired immune deficiency syndrome).

Hives Urticaria, an itchy rash often caused by an allergic reaction.

Holistic Term used to describe treatments that consider the whole person rather than simply the diseased part or symptoms.

Hormone Chemical substance produced by one part of the body to create a specific effect elsewhere. For example, insulin is produced by the pancreas and regulates the level of glucose in the blood.

HRT Hormone replacement therapy, in which oestrogen and progesterone are used to alleviate symptoms of the menopause.

Hyperglycaemia Abnormally high level of blood sugar in those suffering from untreated diabetes.

Hypertension High blood pressure.

Hyperventilation Rapid breathing, usually caused by anxiety or panic, that leads to dizziness and cramps.

Hypoglycaemia Abnormally low level of blood sugar, usually in diabetics.

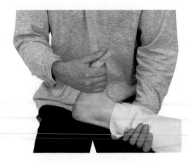

Hypotension Low blood pressure.

Hypothermia Fall in core body temperature to below 35°C (95°F).

Immobilization Supporting an injured person in a stable position to prevent further damage from body movement.

Immune Protected against contracting an infectious disease. People may become immune after an initial infection, as occurs with chickenpox, or after being vaccinated against a specific disease such as rubella.

Immunization Administering antibodies or altered forms of disease-causing micro-organisms in order to stimulate the body's immune system to resist disease.

Immunosuppressant Substance that suppresses the body's immune responses.

Incision Clean-edged cut. An incision resulting from an accident or attack may be deep and involve damage to underlying tissues and organs.

Insulin Hormone produced by the pancreas that regulates blood sugar. Too little or no insulin is produced by diabetics.

Labyrinthitis Inflammation of the chambers of the inner ear, causing vertigo.

Laceration Wound with jagged edges, which may bleed heavily.

Laparoscopy Inspection of the abdominal cavity using a fibre-optic viewing tube.

Laxative Substance that encourages the bowels to pass faeces or increases fluid in the bowel, relieving constipation.

Ligaments Strong bands of fibrous tissue that connect bone ends in joints and support various organs, such as the uterus.

Lithotripsy Technique used to break up kidney stones using ultrasonic shockwaves.

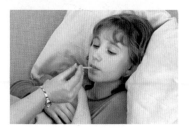

Log roll Method of turning an injured person (if essential) without changing the relative positions of the head and spine.

Meningitis Inflammation of the membranes covering the brain and spinal cord caused by bacterial or viral infection.

Metabolism General term for all the chemical processes in the body.

Metastasis The spread of cancer from one area of the body to another, resulting in metastases, or secondary tumours.

MRI Magnetic resonance imaging: radiation-free scanning technique that produces detailed images of "slices" of the body to examine the content of tissues. The images are created by a computer, using magnets and radio waves.

Neurology Branch of medicine dealing with the nervous system.

Nonsteroidal anti-inflammatory drugs (NSAIDs) Drugs used to reduce both pain and inflammation, for example in the treatment of arthritis.

Obstetrics Branch of medicine dealing with pregnancy and labour.

Occupational therapy Treatment, using both therapy and physical exercises, that helps people return to everyday life following a period of ill health.

Oncology Branch of medicine dealing with the treatment of cancer.

Ophthalmology Branch of medicine dealing with the eyes and sight.

Opioids Painkilling drugs that are powerful but potentially addictive.

Orthopaedics Branch of medicine dealing with the bones and joints.

Paediatrics Branch of medicine dealing with children's health.

Palliative medicine Medical care that focuses on relief of symptoms rather than curing disease, as in the final stages of terminal illness.

Palpitation Irregular heart rate experienced as a "thump" or missed beat.

Paramedic Any healthcare worker who is not a doctor, nurse or dentist.

Parasites Organisms that live on or within a host, causing it harm. Worms, fungi, bacteria and viruses are all forms of parasite.

Partial-thickness burn Burn limited to the epidermis that causes blisters and fluid loss.

Pathogen Disease-producing substance or micro-organism.

Pathology Branch of medicine dealing with the causes of disease and the changes it effects in the body.

Peritonitis Inflammation of the membrane lining the abdominal cavity, almost always caused by another abdominal disorder.

Physiotherapy Hands-on physical therapy and exercise techniques used to help people recover from injuries or to relieve pain resulting from chronic illness.

Placebo Inactive substance administered as if it were therapy, used as a control to test the efficacy of drugs in clinical trials.

Placebo effect Remedial effect of treatment stemming from the belief or expectation of the receiver, regardless of the efficacy of the drugs or techniques used.

Psychiatry Branch of medicine dealing with mental health.

Psychology Scientific study of the mind and behaviour. Psychologists are not usually medical doctors.

Pulled elbow Dislocation of a forearm bone from the elbow joint.

Puncture wound Wound inflicted by long, needle-like object, whose depth is difficult to assess.

Radiography Photography of the inside of the body by means of X-rays (radiation).

Radiotherapy Cancer treatment involving the use of large doses of X-rays.

Recovery position Secure pose for someone who is unconscious but breathing, which ensures that their airway stays open.

Rehydration salts Commercial preparations containing sodium chloride, glucose and other substances, to be added to water for the treatment of dehydration.

Rescue breathing Artificial respiration.

RICE guidelines Procedure (Rest, Ice, Compression, Elevation) to be followed in the treatment of sprains.

Sedatives Drugs that reduce the activity of the brain, and are used to treat anxiety, insomnia or psychiatric disturbance.

Sepsis Bacterial infection of a wound,

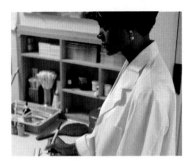

leading to the formation of pus or the multiplication of bacteria in the blood.

Septicaemia Blood poisoning due to the escape of bacteria from a site of infection and their rapid multiplication in the blood.

Shock Serious physiological condition caused by a sudden drop in blood pressure, which deprives the body of oxygen.

Slipped disc Rupture of an intervertebral disc, causing the inner pulp to protrude and press on a nerve.

Soft-tissue injury Damage to tissues – including ligaments, tendons and muscles – surrounding bones and joints.

Solvent abuse Inhalation of intoxicating fumes from volatile liquids such as glue, paint or lighter fuel.

Spacer Device used in conjunction with an asthma inhaler to improve drug take-up.

Speech therapy Treatment to help people to speak more clearly. It is often used to help people who have suffered a stroke.

Splint Rigid support bound to a fractured limb to prevent movement.

Sprain Either the tearing or the overstretching of a ligament.

Steroids Powerful substances that can be used to reduce inflammation and immune responses. They are used in the treatment of many conditions including asthma.

Stoma Surgically created opening, such as at the front of the neck to act as an airway if the windpipe is severed, or in the abdomen to act as an artificial anus if part of the intestine is removed.

Strain Either the tearing or the overstretching of a muscle.

Swab Specimen (of bodily fluids, for

example) taken for examination. The term also describes a piece of material, such as cotton or gauze, used to clean wounds or take specimens.

Systemic Term used to describe a disease that affects the body as a whole rather than a particular area or organ.

Tetanus Serious disease caused by the contamination of a wound by a bacterium found in soil and animal faeces. Painful muscular spasms can lead to respiratory failure. Contraction of tetanus is prevented by regular immunization.

Thrombosis Abnormal formation of a blood clot inside an undamaged blood vessel, which may cause blockage.

Tourniquet Emergency device to stem bleeding, such as a tight bandage. It should not normally be used in first aid.

Transient ischaemic attack (TIA) Brief interruption of blood supply to the brain, causing temporary sensory impairment. It may be a warning sign of full-scale stroke.

Ulcer Open sore on skin or mucous membrane resulting from surface damage.

Ultrasound scan Technique using sound waves to produce images of internal organs.

Urology Branch of medicine dealing with the urinary system in men and women, and with the male genital organs.

Vaccination Administering killed or weakened forms of a disease-causing micro-organism, usually by injection, to help the body fight that disease.

Vein Blood vessel carrying deoxygenated blood back to the lungs. Veinous blood is dark red; bleeding is steady and slower than from an artery.

Vital signs Breathing, coughing, movement, pulse, skin colour, warmth and other signs of life.

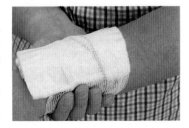

Useful addresses

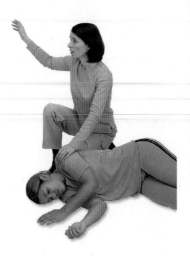

IMPORTANT NOTES:
This is simply a contact listing of relevant bodies that may be helpful to the reader – inclusion here does not indicate endorsement of the book by the bodies listed. Note also that certain first-aid and medical practices differ from one country to another.

Websites: many relevant organizations have websites that are constantly updated with the very latest guidelines. Such sites can be a good source of information, but only if they originate with an authoritative medical organization. Health information from a website or helpline must be considered alongside your doctor's advice.

All address listings are correct at time of going to press.

UNITED KINGDOM

Action for Sick Children (NAWCH;
    National Association for the Welfare of
    Children in Hospital)
c/o National Children's Bureau
8 Wakley Street, London EC1V 7QE
Tel: 020 7843 6444
www.actionforsickchildren.org

Alcoholics Anonymous (AA)
Helpline Tel: 0845 769 7555
www.alcoholics-anonymous.org.uk

Allergy UK
3 White Oak Square
London Road, Swanley
Kent
BR8 7AG
Helpline Tel: 01322 619864
www.allergyfoundation.com

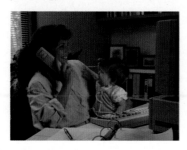

Ambulance Service Association
Friars House
157–168 Blackfriars Road
London SE1 8EU
Tel: 020 7928 9620
www.asa.uk.net

Arthritis Research Campaign
Copeman House, St Mary's Gate
Chesterfield, Derbyshire S41 7TD
Tel: 0870 850 5000
www.arc.org.uk; info@arc.org.uk

Asthma UK
Providence House
Providence Place
London N1 0NT
Tel: 020 7226 2260
www.asthma.org.uk

The British Epilepsy Association, known
    as Epilepsy Action
New Anstey House
Gateway Drive
Yeadon
Leeds LS19 7XY
Tel: 0113 210 8800
www.epilepsy.org.uk

British Heart Foundation
14 Fitzhardinge Street
London W1H 6DH
Tel: 020 7935 0185
www.bhf.org.uk

British Red Cross
9 Grosvenor Crescent
London SW1X 7EJ
Tel: 020 7235 5454
www.redcross.org.uk

British Safety Council
70 Chancellors Road
Hammersmith
London W6 9RS
Tel: 020 8741 1231
www.britishsafetycouncil.org

CancerBACUP
3 Bath Place, Rivington Street
London EC2A 3DR
Tel: 0808 800 1234
www.cancerbacup.org.uk
info@cancerbacup.org.uk

The Child Accident Prevention
    Trust
18–20 Farringdon Lane
London EC1R 3HA
Tel: 020 7608 3828
www.capt.org.uk

ChildLine
Freepost 1111
London N1 0BR (no stamp
    needed)
Tel: 0800 1111 (Freefone)
www.childline.org.uk

Cry-sis
BM Cry-sis
London WC1N 3XX
Tel: 020 7404 5011
www.cry-sis.com

Dept of Health
Tel: 020 7210 4850
www.doh.gov.uk

Diabetes UK
10 Parkway
London NW1 7AA
Tel: 020 7424 1000
www.diabetes.org.uk

Eating Disorders Association
Wensum House
103 Prince of Wales Road
Norwich NR1 1DW
Tel: 0845 634 1414 (helpline)
www.edauk.com; info@edauk.com

Family Planning Association
2–12 Pentonville Road
London N1 9FP
Tel: 0845 310 1334 (helpline)
www.fpa.org.uk

Foundation for the Study of
 Infant Deaths
Artillery House
11–19 Artillery Row
London SW1P 1RH
Helpline Tel: 0870 7870554
www.sids.org.uk/fsid/

Headway – the Brain Injury Association
4 King Edward Court
King Edward St
Nottingham NG1 1EW
Tel: 0115 924 0800
www.headway.org.uk

Help the Aged
207–221 Pentonville Road
London N1 9UZ
Tel: 020 7278 1114
www.helptheaged.org.uk
info@helptheaged.org.uk

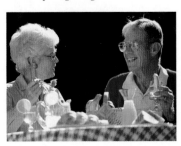

Institute of Complementary Medicine
Send SAE for information about your
 local practitioners to:
PO Box 194, London SE16 7QZ
Tel: 020 7237 5165
www.icmedicine.co.uk

MedicAlert
1 Bridge Wharf, 156 Caledonian Road
London N1 9UU
Tel: 020 7833 3034
www.medicalert.org.uk

The Meningitis Trust
Fern House, Bath Road, Stroud
Glos GL5 3TJ
Tel: 01453 768000
24-hour helpline: 0845 6000 800
www.meningitis-trust.org.uk

Narcotics Anonymous (NA)
Helpline Tel: 020 7730 0009
www.na.org

National Childbirth Trust (NCT)
Alexandra House, Oldham Terrace
London W3 6NH
Tel: 0870 7703236
www.pregnancyandbabycare.com

National Eczema Society
Hill House, Highgate Hill
London N19 5NA
Tel: 0870 241 3604 (helpline)
www.eczema.org

NHS Direct
Tel: 0845 4647
www.nhsdirect.nhs.uk

Parentline Plus
Tel: 0808 800 2222
www.parentlineplus.org.uk

Resuscitation Council (UK)
5th Floor, Tavistock House North
Tavistock Square
London WC1H 9HR
Tel: 020 7388 4678
www.resus.org.uk (gives latest guidelines)

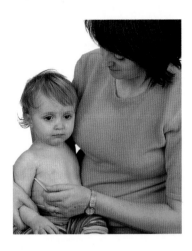

Royal College of General Practitioners
14 Princess Gate, Hyde Park
London SW7 1PU
www.rcgp.org.uk

Royal Society for the Prevention of
 Accidents (RoSPA)
Edgbaston Park, 353 Bristol Rd
Birmingham B5 7ST
Tel: 0121 248 2046
www.rospa.co.uk

St John Ambulance
27 St John's Lane
London EC1M 4BU
Tel: 08700 10 49 50
www.sja.org.uk

Samaritans
Tel: 0845 790 9090

Spinal Injuries Association
Suite J, 3rd Floor
Acorn House
387–391 Midsummer Boulevard
Milton Keynes MK9 3HP
Helpline Tel: 0800 980 0501
www.spinal.co.uk

The Stroke Association
240 City Road
London EC1V 2PR
Tel: 020 7566 0300
www.stroke.org.uk

USA

American Academy of Family Physicians
11400 Tomahawk Creek Parkway
Leawood, Kansas 66211-2672
Tel: (800) 274-2237
www.aafp.org; fp@aafp.org

American Heart Association
7272 Greenville Avenue
Dallas, Texas 75231
Tel: (800) 242-8721
www.americanheart.org

American Lung Association
61 Broadway, 6th Floor
New York 10006
Tel: (212) 315-8700
www.lungusa.org; info@lungusa.org

American Red Cross National HQ
2025E Street NW
Washington DC 20006
Tel: (202) 303-4498
www.redcross.org

Child Family Health International
953 Mission Street, Suite 220
San Francisco, California 94103
Tel: (415) 957-9000
www.cfhi.org; cfhi@cfhi.org

National Safety Council
1121 Spring Lake Drive, Itasca
Illinois 60143-3201
Tel: (630) 285 1121
www.nsc.org

Occupational Safety and Health
    Administration, US Dept of Labor
200 Constitution Avenue NW
Washington DC 20210
Tel: (800) 321 6742
www.osha.gov

CANADA

Asthma Society of Canada
130 Bridgeland Avenue, Suite 425
Toronto, Ontario M6A 1Z4
Tel: (866) 787-4050
www.asthma.ca; info@asthma.ca

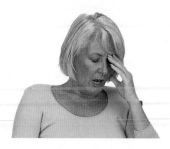

Canada Safety Council
1020 Thomas Spratt Place
Ottawa ON K1G 5L5
Tel: (613) 739-1535
www.safety-council.org

Canadian Cancer Society
Suite 200, 10 Alcorn Avenue
Toronto, Ontario M4V 3B1
Tel: (416) 961-7223
www.cancer.ca; ccs@cancer.ca

Canadian Red Cross National Office
170 Metcalfe Street, Suite 300
Ottawa, Ontario K2P 2P2
Tel: (613) 740-1900
www.redcross.ca

College of Family Physicians of Canada
2630 Skymark Avenue
Mississauga
Ontario L4W 5A4
Tel: (905) 629-0900
www.cfpc.ca

Heart and Stroke Foundation
    of Canada
222 Queen Street
Suite 1402
Ottawa, Ontario K1P 5V9
Tel: (613) 569-4361
ww1.heartandstroke.ca

National Safe Kids Campaign
1301 Pennsylvania Avenue NW
Suite 1000
Washington DC 20004
Tel: (202) 662-0600
www.safekids.org

St John Ambulance Canada
1900 City Park Drive, Suite 400
Ottawa, Ontario K1A 1A3
Tel: (613) 236-7461
www.sja.ca

Safe Kids Canada
180 Dundas Street West
Toronto ON M5G 1Z8
Tel: (888) SAFE TIPS (723-3847)
www.safekidscanada.ca

AUSTRALIA

Australian Red Cross
155 Pelham Street
Carlton, Victoria 3053
Tel: 03 9345 1800
www.redcross.org.au

Cancer Council Australia
Level 5, Medical Foundation Building
92–94 Parramatta Road
Camperdown, New South Wales 2050
Tel: 02 9036 3100
www.cancer.org.au; info@cancer.org.au

Children's Health Development Foundation
8th Floor, Samuel Way Building
Women's and Children's Hospital
72 King William Road
North Adelaide, South Australia, 5006
Tel: 08 8161 7777
www.chdf.org.au; chdf@wch.sa.gov.au

Kidsafe Australia
Safety Centre, Royal Children's Hospital
Flemington Road, Parkville
Victoria 3052
Tel: 03 9345 6471
www.kidsafevic.com.au

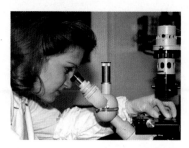

National Asthma Council Australia
1 Palmerston Crescent
South Melbourne, Victoria 3205
Tel: 03 8699 0476
www.nationalasthma.org.au
nac@nationalasthma.org.au

National Heart Foundation of Australia
15 Denison Street, Deakin ACT 2600
Tel: 1300 36 27 87
www.heartfoundation.com.au
heartlinesa@heartfoundation.com.au

National Safety Council of Australia
322 Glenferrie Road
Malvern
Victoria 3144
Tel: 03 9832 1555
www.safetynews.com

St John Ambulance Australia
PO Box 3895
Manuka ACT 2603
Tel: 02 6295 3777
www.stjohn.org.au

NEW ZEALAND
Asthma and Respiratory Foundation NZ
Level 9, Clayton Ford House
132 The Terrace
PO Box 1459, Wellington
Tel: 04 499 4592
www.asthmanz.co.nz; arf@asthma.co.nz

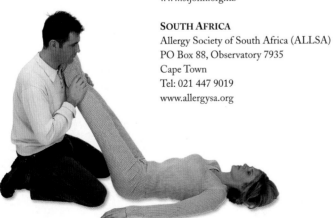

Cancer Society of New Zealand
PO Box 10847, Wellington
Tel: 04 494 7270
www.cancernz.org.nz
admin@cancernz.org.nz

National Heart Foundation NZ
9 Kalmia Street, Ellerslie, PO Box 17160,
Greenlane, Auckland 1130
Tel: 09 571 9191
www.nhf.org.nz; info@nhf.org.nz

New Zealand Red Cross
PO Box 12–140
Thorndon
Wellington 6038
Tel: 04 472 3750
www.redcross.org.nz

Safekids New Zealand
162 Blockhouse Bay Rd
PO Box 19544
Avondale
Auckland 7
Tel: 64-9-820 1190
www.safekids.org.nz

St John Ambulance National Office
St John House
114 The Terrace
PO Box 10043
Wellington
Tel: 04 472 3600
www.stjohn.org.nz

SOUTH AFRICA
Allergy Society of South Africa (ALLSA)
PO Box 88, Observatory 7935
Cape Town
Tel: 021 447 9019
www.allergysa.org

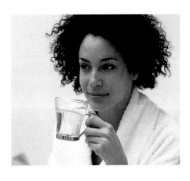

Cancer Association of South Africa
  (CANSA)
26 Concorde Road West
Bedfordview, 2007
PO Box 2121, Bedfordview 2008
Tel: 021 689 5381
Helpline: 0800 226622
www.cansa.org.za; cansainfo@cansa.org.uk

Heart Foundation South Africa
PO Box 15139
Vlaeberg 8018
Tel: 021 447 4222
www.heartfoundation.co.za
heart@heartfoundation.co.za

St John Ambulance
The Order of St John
PO Box 7137
2000 Johannesburg
Tel: 011 646 5520
www.stjohn.org.za

South African Red Cross Society
PO Box 50696, Waterfront
Cape Town 8002
Tel: 021 4186640
www.redcross.org.za
info@redcross.org.za

The KidSafe Project
c/o PASASA
Suite 10, 10 Pepper St.
PO Box 16225
Vlaeberg 8018
Cape Town
Tel: 021 424 3473
www.pasasa.org

Index

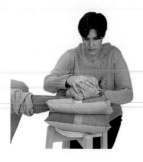

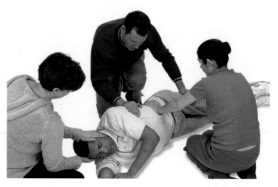

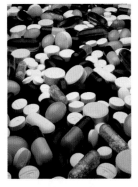

locations 457
myeloma 456
transplant 454
bones 152, 354
cancer 358
effect of gravity 357
fractures 368–369
function 354
healing 369
metastases 358
needs 152
osteomalacia and rickets 357
osteoporosis 356–357
skeleton 152
structure 354
see also fractures
bowel
Crohn's disease 308
habit 294, 295
irritable bowel syndrome
(IBS) 305
ulcerative colitis 309
brain 82–83, 322
epilepsy 86–87, 330–331
head injury 327
Huntington's disease 341
injury 84–85
meningitis 332–333
Parkinson's disease 340–341
stroke 88–89, 328–329
structure 322
tumours 331
viral encephalitis 333
breast
cancer 273, 401
cysts 401
fibroadenoma 400
lumpiness 400

pain 400
structure 400
breathing 58–59, 374–375
child 122–123
difficulties 59, 60–61
mouth-to-mouth rescue
34–35
bronchiolitis in children 475
bronchitis 381
bruises 130, 131
complementary therapies 220
bulimia 352
bunions 366
Burkitt's lymphoma 458
burns 178–181
chemical 184–185
complementary therapies 220
electrical 185
facial 186
inhalation 185
kitchen safety 230–231
sunburn 187, 221, 245
treatment of 182–183
types 178
bursitis 371

C
caffeine 263
calcium 356, 357
calluses 446
calories 265
cancer
bone 358
bone-marrow 456
brain tumours 331
breast 273, 401
cervix 406
colorectal 306–307
larynx 424
leukaemias 454–455
lung 384
lymphomas 458
oesophagus 297
ovarian 405
pancreas 301
prostate 273, 409
skin 442–443
stomach 300
testicular 410
thyroid 317
uterine 403
car accidents 226–227

carbon monoxide poisoning 63
cardiac arrest 78–79
cardiac compressions 36–37
cardiopulmonary resuscitation
(CPR) 30–31
baby and child 48–49
cardiovascular system 70–71,
276–277
carpal tunnel syndrome 337
cartilage, torn or damaged 370
cataracts 432
cellulitis 444
central nervous system 322, 323
cervical spondylosis 360
cervix
cancer 406
dysplasia 406
smear test 273
cheekbone fractures 157
chemicals
burns 184–185
garden safety 234
poisoning, first aid for
child 199
chest wound 139, 165
chicken pox 466
childbirth, emergency 98–99
childhood problems 114–127
abdominal pain 120
alcohol poisoning 198
appendicitis 121
asthma 123
breathing difficulty 122–123
chemical poisoning 199
choking 54, 55
constipation 121
coughing 122
diarrhoea 119
drug poisoning 199
earache 126
fever 118
headaches 124–125
intussusception 121
meningitis 125
plant poisoning 199, 235
poisoning in 198–199
pulled elbow 171
rashes 125
recognizing 114
resuscitation 48–49, 51–53
seriously ill child 115
solvent abuse 195

sore throat 127
swallowed objects 148
toothache 127
urinary tract infections 127
vomiting 119
children
balanitis 479
bronchiolitis 475
Burkitt's lymphoma 458
colds 474
constipation 477
croup 475
diarrhoea 476
earache 474
eczema 480
febrile convulsions 479
gastroenteritis 477
gigantism 320
healthy lifestyle 259
heart problems 482
migraine 478
Perthes' disease 483
phimosis 479
pneumonia 475
protection against infection
472–473
rickets 357
sore throats 474
urinary tract infection 481
vomiting 476
chiropractic 494
chlamydia 411
choking 42–45
baby 54
child 55
cholesterol test 272, 281
chondromalacia 370–371
chronic obstructive pulmonary
disease (COPD) 380–381

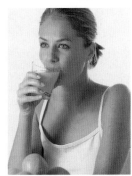

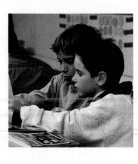
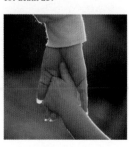

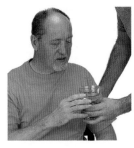

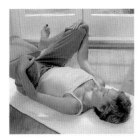

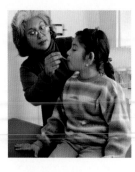

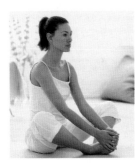

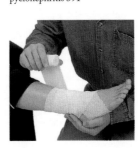

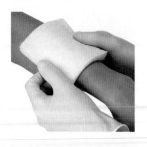

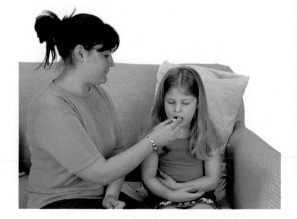

trigeminal neuralgia 337
tuberculosis 465
tumours, brain 331

U

ulcerative colitis 309
ulcers
   corneal 428
   Helicobacter pylori 298,
    299
   leg 446
   peptic 298–299
   rodent 442
urinary system 386–387
   incontinence 392
   tract infections (UTIs)
    390–391, in children 127,
    481
urticaria 440
uterus
   cancer 403
   endometriosis 403
   fibroids 402

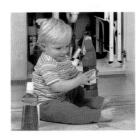

V

vaccination 472–473
   MMR 473
vaginal bleeding 146
vaginal infections 407
varicocele 410
varicose veins 290
veins 277
   clots 288
   deep vein thrombosis (DVT)
    288
   varicose veins 290

verrucas 445
vertebral column, see spine
vertigo 92, 418
Viagra 412
viruses
   encephalitis 333
   infectious disease 462,
    466–467
   skin infections 445
voice, hoarseness of 424
vomiting 102
   blood 146
   child 119, 476
   complementary therapies
    218
   terminally ill 488

W

walking hazards 245
warts 445
wasp stings 108
water sports safety 246–247
weight control 264–265

whiplash injury 335
whooping cough 464
wounds
   abdominal 139
   amputation 130, 140
   bleeding, control 142–143
   chest 139, 165
   cleaning and dressing 133
   embedded objects 134–135
   healing process 132
   infected 136–137
   major 138–139
   types 130–131
wrist fracture 163

Acknowledgements – Step-by-step First Aid

The publishers would like to thank the following people for their assistance in creating the first aid section of this book:

The models:
Peter Akinola, Neil Barnes, Sue Barraclough, Heather Batchelor and Angus (18 months), Aaron Beha-Parks, Lesley Betts, Neil Bradbury, Jim Britton, Natasha Brown, Iva Buckova, Matthew Charlton, Rachel Chilcott and Tabitha (18 months), Valerie Ferguson, Jack France (18 months), John France, Tom France (6 years), Irene Halton, Jane Harris, Hannah Higgins, Lydia Hitchings, Simona Hill, Oliver Hitchings, Louise

Hughes, Brian Jackson, Emma Jackson, Sam Jones, Pippa Keech and William (aged 7), Dallas Kidman, Ralph Leming, Helen Lowe, Debra Mayhew and Jamie Austin (18 months), Emily MacQueen, Denise Olive, Alan Powell, Joanne Rippin, David Spicer, Helen Sudell, Vivien Tobies, Melanie Ward, Evie Wyld. Thanks to Dammers Model and Promotion Agency, Bristol, for providing some of the models listed above.

Others:
Two Wheels Service, Bath, for the loan of a crash helmet. Pat Coward, for compiling the index.

Photographic acknowledgements

All photographs other than those listed below are copyrighted to Anness Publishing Ltd.
   The publishers would like to thank the agencies listed below for their kind permission to reproduce the following images in the first aid section of this book:

l=left; r=right; t=top; b=bottom; c=centre

pp12/13 Tom Stewart/Corbis; p71bc Medical-On-Line/Mediscan; p75t Garry Watson/Science Photo Library; p125t image courtesy of Meningitis

Trust © 2003; p137b Jim Selby/Science Photo Library; p141b Marcelo Brodsky/Latin Stock/Science Photo Library; p246br Robert Harding Picture Library Ltd; p247bl Sinclair Stammers/Science Photo Library; p248b Robert Harding Picture Library Ltd.

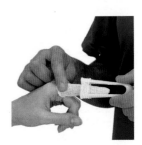

Acknowledgements – Family Health Guide

The publishers would like to thank the following people for their assistance in creating the family health section of this book:

Everyone at the Royal College of General Practitioners, London, for their patient and scholarly help, from the Chairman of Council, Professor David Haslam FRCGP and Helen Farrelly, Publications Manager, to the team of painstaking verifiers: Dr Rodger Charlton FRCGP, Dr Helen Liley, and Krysia Saul. Additional verifying and advice: Dr Tim Wallington, consultant immunologist at the National Blood Service, Bristol, and his colleague, haematologist Dr Edwin Massey; Margaret Hallendorff, Chief Executive, The Royal College of Ophthalmologists, London.

Thanks also to Luci Gosling and Arran Frood at the Science Photo Library for all their cheerful, highly efficient help, and to Pat Coward for compiling the family health index.

Dr Peter Fermie would like to thank his wife Ellen and daughter Anna for putting up with his long periods spent in front of the computer while working on his text!

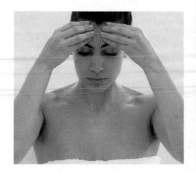

Photographic acknowledgements

All photographs other than those listed below are copyrighted to Anness Publishing Ltd.

The publishers would like to thank the agencies listed below for their kind permission to reproduce the following images in the family health guide:

l=left; r=right; t=top; b=bottom

Corbis: pp254/5; p270bl; p274tl
John Birdsall Photo Library: p267t; p268bl; p281b.
Robert Harding Picture Library Ltd: p286t; p300bl.
The Hutchison Library: p308t.
The Meningitis Trust: p333t.

Science Photo Library: p258t: Ruth Jenkinson/Midirs; p265bl: BSIP, JPL/Anne; p268br: Dr Clive Kocher; p269tr: Francoise Sauze; p269b: Andrew McClenaghan; p271t: Astrid & Hanns-Frieder Michler; p271b: Hank Morgan; p272t: Claire Paxton & Jacqui Farrow; p272b: Sean O'Brien/Custom Medical Stock Photo; p273t: Samuel Ashfield; p273b: Antonia Reeve; p274bl: Mauro Fermariello; p278b: Antonia Reeve; p279b: Science Photo Library; p281t: BSIP/VEM; p282t: Mike Agliolo; p282b: BSIP/Ducloux; p283t: David Campione; p283b: BSIP/VEM; p284: BSIP/Laurent B./Hop Ame; p285: Tim Beddow; p286b: Mike Devlin; p287: BSIP/Beranger; p288b: Dr P. Marazzi; p289t: James King-Holmes; p289b: John Radcliffe Hospital;

p292: Eye of Science; p294t: CC Studio; p294b: Ron Sutherland; p295: Innerspace Imaging; p296t: Dr P. Marazzi; p296b: Science Photo Library; p297: Mehau Kulyk; p298: Juergen Berger/Max Planck; p299t: Pascal Geotgheluck; p300br: Science Photo Library; p303tl: Jim Varney; p303tr: Dr P. Marazzi; p303b: John Radcliffe Hospital; p306: Andrew Syred; p307b: Mehau Kulyk; p308b: G JLP; p309: Alfred Pasieka; p314: Science Photo Library; p315t: Saturn Stills; p316: SNRI; p317l: Quest; p317r: Science Photo Library; p319l: Science Photo Library; p319r: Ovellette & Theroux/Publiphoto diffusion; p323: Astrid & Hanns-Frieder Michler; p324t: Zephyr; p324b: Oscar Burriel; p325t: Custom Medical Stock; p327t: Scott Camazine; p328: Scotte Camazine; p329t: Colin Cuthbert; p330t: BSIP VEM; p330b: Science Photo Library; p331bl: MIT AI LAB/Surgical Planning Lab, Brigham & Women's Hospital; p331br: Sam Ogden; p332l: Dr Kari Lounatmaa; p332r: CDC; p336: Dept. of Clinical Radiology, Salisbury District Hospital; p337: Szuson Jwong/Peter Arnold Inc.; p338t: Alfred Pasieka; p339t: Catherine Povedras; p339b: Simon Fraser/Royal Victoria Infirmary, Newcastle-upon-Tyne; p340: Catherine Povedras; p341l: Prof. K. Seddon & Dr T. Evans/Queen's University, Belfast; p341r: Simon Fraser/Royal Victoria Infirmary, Newcastle-upon-Tyne; p343t: John Greim; p347br: Pascal Goetgheluck; p348b: John Greim; p349t: BSIP/Laurent; p349b: Hattie Young; p350l: Ed Young; p350r: Alain Dex/Publiphoto Diffusion; p351: BSIP/Laurent/Carlo; p352b: Science Photo Library; p354r: Andrew Syred; p354b: Prof. P. Motta/Dept of Anatomy, University 'La Sapienza', Rome; p356l: Dr Tony Brain; p356r: Dr P. Marazzi; p357r: Biophotos Associates; p358t: St Bartholomew's Hospital; p358b: Martin Dohr; p359t: CNRI; p359bl: Chris Priest; p359br: Biophoto Associates; p361r: Tek Image; p362: David M. Campione; p363t: CC Studio; p363bl: Dr P. Marazzi; p363br: Alfred Pasieka; p364t: Jerrican Faure Felix; p364b: St Bartholomew's Hospital; p365: Antonia Reeve; p366: Francoise Sauze; p367: Will & Deni McIntyre; p368: Mark Clarke; p370: Brad Nelson/Custom Medical Stock Photo; p374: Science Photo Library; p376tl: Alfred Pasieka; p376b: Science Photo Library; p379tl: Eye of Science; p379tr, 379b: Damien Lovegrove; p380bl: CC Studio; p380br: Josh Sher; p381t: Science Photo Library; p382t: Eye of Science; p382b: Mehau Kulyk; p384tl: Peter Menzel; p384tr:

Philippe Plailly; p384b: Scott Camazine; p388t: CNRI; p389: Geoff Tompkinson; p390bl: Juergen Berger/Max-Planck Institute; p391tr: Science Photo Library; p396t: Josh Sher; p396b: Faye Norman; p398: Dr Yorgos Nikas; p400: Bates/Custom Medical Stock Photo; p402: Science Photo Library; p403: Science Photo Library; p404r: Z. Binor/Custom Medical Stock Photo; p404b: Dr P. Marazzi; p405: BSIP/Edwige; p406: Hattie Young; p409b: BSIP/Chassenet; p415: Dave Roberts; p416: Brian Yarvin; p419bl: Mark Clarke; p419br: Dr P. Marrazi; p421t: Andrew Syred; p421bl: Science Photo Library; p423bl: Dr P. Marazzi; p426t: Wellcome Department of Cognitive Neurology; p427: Ralph Eagle; p428bl, p428br: Dr P. Marazzi; p429t: Western Opthalmic Hospital; p429b: Dr P. Marazzi; p430: Custom Medical Stock Photo; p432t: Dr P. Marazzi; p434t: Adam Hart-Davis; p434b: Omikran; p436t: Martin Dohrn; p438t: Dr P. Marazzi; p438b: John Radcliffe Hospital; p439t: St Bartholomew's Hospital; p439b: Scott Camazine; p440t, p440b, p441bl, p441br: Dr P. Marazzi; p442tl: Dr Chris Hale; p442tr: Dr P. Marazzi; p443t: James Stevenson; p443b: Dr P. Marazzi; p444: Science Photo Library; p445bl: Jane Shemilt/Cosine Graphics; p445br, p446: Dr P. Marazzi; p450: Susumu Nishinga; p452: Alex Bartel; p454bl: Geoff Tompkinson; p454br: Simon Fraser; p455t: Science Photo Library; p456t: Maximilian Stock Ltd; p457: CNRI; p458t: Dr P. Marazzi; p458b: John Greim; p459t, p459b: Dr P. Marazzi; p460r: James Stevenson; p462t: Dr P. Marazzi; p462bl: Dr Kari Lounatmaa; p463t: Saturn Stills; p464r: Alfred Pasieka; p465r: Biophotos Associates; p466l: Science Photo Library; p466r: Dr P. Marazzi; p467tr: Georgia Lowell; p467b: Science Photo Library; p468: John Greim; p469r: NIBSC; p469b: Department of Medical Photography, St Stephen's Hospital, London; p470bl: CNRI; p470br: Andy Crump/Tdr/WHO; p473b: Saturn Stills; p474: Ruth Jenkinson/MIDIRS; p477t: Mark Clarke; p481t: Alexander Tsiaras; p481b: Hattie Young; p483t: BSIP/Astier; p483b: Dr P. Marazzi; p484tl: Chris Priest; p484tr: BSIP/Astier; p484b: Larry Mulvehill; p486bl: Colin Cuthbert; p486b: James King-Holmes; p487tl: Stevie Grand; 487tr: Mark Thomas; p487b: Antonia Reeve; p488t: Deep Light Production; p488bl: Will & Reni McIntyre; p488br: Chris Priest; p493tr: Matt Meadows/Peter Arnold Inc; p494tl: Mark de Fraeye.

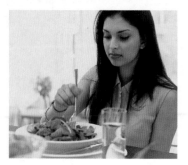